Kowalski. ("9 ments to

THE BESTSELLING CHOLESTEROL COUNTER—ADVICE YOU CAN TRUST FROM HEALTH EXPERTS!

The National Cholesterol Education Program of the National Institutes of Health recently celebrated its twelfth anniversary of teaching Americans about cholesterol. Thanks to the NCEP, we know the importance of having our cholesterol level checked, and of monitoring cholesterol intake through our food choices. This is the cholesterol counter that takes the guesswork out of healthy eating.

Revised and updated for this expansive fifth edition, *THE CHOLESTEROL COUNTER* supplies the most up-to-date information on cholesterol—how much you should eat, where to cut down, and how to choose foods for optimal health benefits. Packed with listings for thousands of supermarket foods as well as popular menu items from dozens of chain restaurants, this accessible guide makes controlling your cholesterol a reachable goal, and the best thing you can do for yourself and your family.

Don't miss
THE EATING OUT FOOD COUNTER

**A guide for healthy dining at your favorite restaurants
Annette B. Natow, Ph.D., R.D. and
Jo-Ann Heslin, M.A., R.D.**

Coming soon from Pocket Books

Books by Annette B. Natow and Jo-Ann Heslin

The
CHOLESTEROL
COUNTER

FIFTH EDITION
REVISED AND UPDATED

ANNETTE B. NATOW, Ph.D., R.D.
and JO-ANN HESLIN, M.A., R.D.

POCKET BOOKS
New York   London   Toronto   Sydney   Singapore

POCKET BOOKS, a division of Simon & Schuster Inc.
1230 Avenue of the Americas, New York, NY 10020

Copyright © 1993, 1996, 1998 by Annette Natow and Jo-Ann Heslin

All rights reserved, including the right to reproduce
this book or portions thereof in any form whatsoever.
For information address Pocket Books, 1230 Avenue
of the Americas, New York, NY 10020

ISBN: 0-671-00451-4

First Pocket Books printing of this revised edition August 1998

10 9 8 7 6 5 4 3

POCKET and colophon are registered trademarks of
Simon & Schuster Inc.

Front cover photo © FoodPix

Printed in the U.S.A.

To our families, who support us through every project: Harry, Allen, Irene, Sarah, Meryl, Marty, Laura, George, Emily, Steven, Joseph, Kristen and Karen.

ACKNOWLEDGMENTS

Without the tireless cooperation of Steven and Stephen, *The Cholesterol Counter* would never have been completed. A special thanks to our agent, Nancy Trichter, and Jane Cavolina, our editor, and her assistant, Brett Freese.

Our thanks also to all the food manufacturers who graciously shared their data.

"If only half a dozen foods were available, the matter would be quickly settled."

MARY SWARTZ ROSE, PH.D.
Feeding the Family
The Macmillan Company, 1919

SOURCES OF DATA

Values in this counter have been obtained from the Composition of Foods, United States Department of Agriculture, Agricultural Handbooks: No. 8-1, Dairy and Egg Products; No. 8-2, Spices and Herbs; No. 8-3, Baby Foods; No. 8-4, Fats and Oils; No. 8-5, Poultry Products; No. 8-6, Soups, Sauces and Gravies; No. 8-7, Sausages and Luncheon Meats; No. 8-8, Breakfast Cereals; No. 8-9, Fruit and Fruit Juices; No. 8-10, Pork Products, Revised; No. 8-11, Vegetables and Vegetable Products; No. 8-12, Nut and Seed Products; No. 8-13, Beef Products; No. 8-14, Beverages; No. 8-15, Finfish and Shellfish Products; No. 8-16, Legumes and Legume Products; No. 8-17, Lamb, Veal and Game Products; No. 8-19, Snacks and Sweets; No. 8-20, Cereal Grains and Pasta; No. 8-21, Fast Foods; Supplements 1989, 1990, 1991, 1992.

"Nutritive Value of Foods," United States Department of Agriculture, Home and Garden Bulletin No. 72.

J. Davies and J. Dickerson, *Nutrient Content of Food Portions.* Cambridge, UK: The Royal Society of Chemistry, 1991.

G. A. Leveille, M. E. Zabik, K. J. Morgan, *Nutrients in Foods.* Cambridge, MA: The Nutrition Guild, 1983.

A. Moller, E. Saxholt, B. E. Mikkelsen, *Food Composition*

Tables: Amino Acids, Carbohydrates and Fatty Acids in Danish Foods, 1991.

Souci, Fachman, Kraut, *Food Composition and Nutrition Tables.* Stuttgart: Wissenschaftliche Verlagsgesellschaft MbH, 1989.

Information from food labels, manufacturers and processors. The values are based on research conducted through 1997. Manufacturers' ingredients are subject to change, so current values may vary from those listed in the book.

INTRODUCTION

High Cholesterol is a major risk factor for heart
  disease.
High Cholesterol is a major risk factor for stroke.
High Cholesterol increases your risk of colon and
  rectal cancer.
High Cholesterol plus high blood pressure may
  cause hearing loss.
High Cholesterol, fat-rich diets may cause gallstones.

Cardiovascular disease (CVD) is the leading cause of death
in the United States. Over 900,000 Americans died from CVD
in 1993—mainly heart attack and stroke. That's one person
every thirty-three seconds! Heart attack and stroke disable
even more people than they kill, more than the number of
people who die from all forms of cancer! CVD is not only a
disease of older people; 45 percent of all heart attacks occur
in people under age 65. Often, a heart attack or stroke that
causes death or disability is the first sign that something is
wrong. In 48 percent of the men and 63 percent of the
women who died suddenly of CVD, there had been no previous signs of this disease, making prevention very important.
   Research in the United States and many other countries

shows that high cholesterol levels in the blood are one of the most important risk factors for heart disease. The higher the cholesterol, the greater the risk. Lowering your cholesterol lowers your risk.

Note: Blood cholesterol is measured in milligrams. A milligram is one thousandth of a gram. The number of milligrams of cholesterol in a deciliter (dL), which is a little less than one-half cup, is the ratio used to measure the cholesterol level in the blood. When describing the cholesterol level of the blood, usually just the number is given, such as 180 rather than the more complete 180 milligrams per dL. For simplicity, all cholesterol measurements in the following pages are given as numbers without the mg/dL abbreviation.

For Women Only

Heart disease is often thought of as a disease of men. Unfortunately that's not true.

- Heart attack is the single largest killer of American women. It kills ten times more women than breast cancer.
- Cardiovascular disease has killed more women than men every year since 1984.
- In 1995, 455,000 men and 505,000 women died from cardiovascular disease.
- 20,000 women under age 65 die of heart attacks each year; more than 31 percent of them are under age 55.
- The death rate from heart attack for black women is two to three times that of all other women.
- In 63 percent of the women who die suddenly of cardio-

vascular disease, there were no previous signs of this disease.

- Women's cholesterol levels are higher than men's beginning at age 55.
- Before age 45 women's cholesterol level averages 185–207. Between ages 45 and 65 it increases to 217–237.
- In 1994, over 50 million women had cholesterol levels of 200 or higher and over 22 percent had levels above 240.
- When total cholesterol is between 200 and 239, the risk for heart attack doubles compared to a person with a cholesterol level of 200 or less. As cholesterol rises above 240, the risk is greater.

A Word About Men

- Almost two times as many men die of cardiovascular disease as die from cancer.
- In 1994, 1,219,000 men were diagnosed with heart disease.
- In 48 percent of men who die suddenly of heart disease, there was no previous sign of this disease.
- Over 53 percent of men age 20 and older have cholesterol levels over 200 and almost 20 percent have levels at or over 240.

WHAT IS CHOLESTEROL?

Cholesterol is a white, waxy, fatlike substance that is part of every cell in your body. Cholesterol is important to body function. Hormones, nerve coverings, vitamin D, bile (used for digestion), and the fat that keeps your skin soft (sebum) are all made from cholesterol. Cholesterol makes up a major part of your brain. Cholesterol is needed by the body but when the level of cholesterol in your blood gets too high, it's not healthy. Some of that extra cholesterol can be deposited on the artery wall, narrowing it and interfering with normal blood flow.

Where does cholesterol come from?

We get some cholesterol every time we eat any animal foods. Meat, poultry, fish, eggs, milk, yogurt, cheese and butter are all animal foods and contain cholesterol. Egg yolk is a major source of cholesterol. An average yolk contains about 213 milligrams. The egg white does not have any cholesterol. Caviar and organ meats like liver, heart and brains are very high in cholesterol.

There is no cholesterol in any food that grows in the ground. Vegetable oils, peanut butter, vegetables, fruits, cereals and grains contain no cholesterol.

Cholesterol is also made in the body. In fact, most people make three times as much cholesterol as they get in the food they eat.

How do I know if my blood cholesterol is too high?

Surveys show that the percentage of Americans who have had their cholesterol level checked rose from 35 percent in 1983 to 65 percent in 1990. The National Cholesterol Education Program recommends that all adults over age twenty have their total and high-density lipoprotein (HDL) cholesterol levels measured at least once every five years so they know their numbers. In 1995 only 49 percent of Americans knew their cholesterol level.

For adults, a range from 150 to 200 is best. A cholesterol

level over 200 is considered too high. If your cholesterol is above 200, your risk for heart disease and other problems is increased. The Center for Disease Control of the National Center for Health Statistics reports that average blood cholesterol levels have declined from 1960 to 1994, with the average falling from 220 to 203. Over time, the average low-density lipoprotein (LDL), "bad" cholesterol, levels fell from 136 to 128. Even with this decline, 20 percent of Americans have very high cholesterol levels over 240. And as many as one third need diet changes to lower their cholesterol.

National Institutes of Health, National Heart, Lung and Blood Institute, Detection, Evaluation, and Treatment of High Blood Cholesterol in Adults, 1993 Executive Summary.

What is the difference between "good" cholesterol and "bad" cholesterol?

Cholesterol is coated with protein so it can travel in the blood. These packages of protein, cholesterol and other fats are called "lipoproteins." Two kinds of lipoproteins are low-density lipoproteins (LDL) and high-density lipoproteins (HDL).

LDL cholesterol is called "bad" cholesterol. LDLs contain large amounts of cholesterol that may be deposited in the artery walls. Levels of LDL cholesterol above 130 are considered unhealthy.

HDL cholesterol is called "good" cholesterol. HDLs contain small amounts of cholesterol. They take the cholesterol away from the cells in the artery walls and carry it to the liver where it is processed and removed from the body. People with higher levels of HDL cholesterol (over 60) have less heart disease. Levels of HDL cholesterol under 35 are considered too low. Every 1% increase in HDLs reduces the risk of heart disease by 3 percent.

We are often asked, "What foods contain 'good' cholesterol?" Cholesterol in foods is simply cholesterol and is converted to LDL cholesterol (bad cholesterol) and HDL cholesterol (good cholesterol) after it is eaten. LDL cholesterol and HDL cholesterol refer to forms of cholesterol in your body, not the form of cholesterol in the food you eat.

CLASSIFICATIONS OF CHOLESTEROL VALUES IN ADULTS*

Total Cholesterol

less than 200 mg/dl	Desirable Blood Cholesterol
200 to 239 mg/dl	Borderline High Blood Cholesterol
240 mg/dl and over	High Blood Cholesterol

*National Institutes of Health, National Heart, Lung and Blood Institute, Detection, Evaluation, and Treatment of High Blood Cholesterol in Adults, 1993 Publication No. 93-3095.

If my cholesterol is higher than 200, what should I do?

In late 1987 the federal government, along with over twenty health organizations, issued guidelines, which were updated in 1993, to help identify and treat people whose blood cholesterol levels are too high. This affected one in four Americans.

People with desirable cholesterol levels of under 200 were advised to recheck the level every 5 years.

People with levels above 200 are advised to go on a cholesterol lowering diet that is low in cholesterol, fats and saturated fats.

Many foods are high in all three—cholesterol, fats and saturated fats. By lowering your intake of high cholesterol foods, you reduce your intake of other fats as well and lower your risk for heart disease.

For each 1 percent decrease in blood cholesterol level, you reduce your risk of heart disease by 2 percent. Even the smallest change is to your benefit.

The ratio of total cholesterol to HDL cholesterol has been found to be a good predictor of increased coronary risk especially in those under age sixty. You can figure your own risk level by dividing your total cholesterol (TC) value by your HDL cholesterol. For example, if your TC is 250 and HDL is 50, the average ratio of TC/HDL is 5. This is considered average risk but is actually not very healthy. A ratio of 9.6 indicates twice the average risk of coronary heart disease, while a ratio of 3.5 signals half the risk.

How much cholesterol should I eat each day?

The National Cholesterol Education Program recommends less than 300 milligrams of cholesterol a day for everyone over the age of two. In the government guidelines for lowering cholesterol, the Step 1 diet for those whose cholesterol levels are 200 to 239 milligrams recommends eating less than 300 milligrams of cholesterol a day. Those people whose cholesterol levels are 240 and over are advised to restrict their cholesterol intake to less than 200 milligrams per day.

The cholesterol intake for men averages 360 milligrams a day. For women it ranges from 220 to 260 milligrams. For children, the average intake is less than 300 milligrams a day.

GUIDELINES FOR CHOLESTEROL INTAKE*

Cholesterol Level In the Blood	MG of Cholesterol You Can Eat Each Day
less than 200 mg/dl	300 mg or less a day
200 to 239 mg/dl	less than 300 mg a day
240 mg and over/dl	less than 200 mg a day

*Adapted from material provided by the National Cholesterol Education Program, Second Report, National Heart, Lung and Blood Institute, National Institutes of Health 1993.

What about taking drugs to lower my cholesterol?

Some people who have a high cholesterol level may not be able to lower it enough by diet changes alone. They may need to use a drug in addition to making changes in the way they eat. Drugs used most often are the "statins," cholestyramine, colestipol, and niacin. The following are some blood cholesterol lowering drugs.

Statins, a family of drugs, are considered effective and safe. Mevacor (*lovastatin*), Zocor (*simvastatin*), Pravachol (*pravastatin*) and Lipitor (*atorvastatin*) are well tolerated by most people. The most common side effects are mild gastrointestinal disturbances, which subside as therapy continues; infrequently, "statins" can cause liver problems.

Questran (*cholestyramine*) and Colestid (*colestipol*) are resins that increase the excretion of cholesterol from the body. Major side effects are constipation, bloating and gas. They are unpleasant to take.

Niacin (nicotinic acid, a B vitamin) causes intense flushing and itching of the skin right after you take it. Major side effects are rashes and upset stomach. It can worsen diabetes and gout.

Lorelco (*probucol*) and Lopid (*gemfibrozil*) are reserved for use when diet and other medications are not effective.

What about cholesterol levels in children?

It is recommended that children and adolescents be screened for blood cholesterol levels if there is a family history of heart disease. If parents have high blood cholesterol levels or if grandparents had heart disease before age fifty-five, children should be checked.

According to the 1987–88 Nationwide Food Consumption Survey children and adolescents eat 193 to 296 milligrams of cholesterol daily. This is in line with the recommendation of less than 300 milligrams daily. Even so one third of children have cholesterol levels of over 170 milligrams.

CLASSIFICATIONS OF VALUES FOR CHOLESTEROL IN CHILDREN
AGES 2–19*

	Total Cholesterol	LDL Cholesterol
Acceptable	less than 170	less than 110
Borderline	170 to 199	110–129
High	equal to or greater than 200	equal to or greater than 130

*Report of the Expert Panel on Blood Cholesterol Levels in Children and Adolescents, US Department of Health and Human Services, Public Health Service, National Institutes of Health, Sept. 1991, Publication No. 91-2732.

FACTS ON FIBER

While you are eating less cholesterol to lower its level in your blood, try eating more fiber, too. Besides helping to fill you up with fewer calories, fiber itself helps cholesterol levels go down. And that's not all. Fiber is believed to help prevent breast and colon cancer, normalize blood sugar levels and help your digestive tract function by preventing constipation.

Animal foods like meat, chicken, milk and cheese do not contain any fiber. Fiber is found in plant foods like whole grains, beans, brown rice, dried fruit, vegetables and fruits. Because fiber is not digested and absorbed, it combines with fat preventing its absorption. The result is that there is less fat available to raise blood cholesterol levels. There is also less fat available to make you fat! This helps to lower cholesterol too.

There are actually two types of fiber: soluble and insoluble. The first dissolves in water and the second doesn't. Both types fill you up, but each one has special health benefits. Soluble fiber helps lower cholesterol. The best food sources of soluble fiber are apples, barley, beans, carrots, grapefruit, oats, oranges, peas, rice bran and berries.

Insoluble fiber comes from the outer hard shell of grains. It bulks up your stools helping to prevent or relieve constipation and also is believed to help prevent breast and colon cancer. Bran, celery, green beans, green leafy vegetables, potato skins, flaxseed and whole grains are all good sources of insoluble fiber.

The American Dietetic Association, National Cancer Institute and other experts recommend fiber intake of 20 to 30 or even 35 grams a day. To reach this level you would need to eat 3 to 5 servings of whole grain bread and cereals, 3 servings of fruit, and 3 servings of vegetables a day. Most Americans are not eating that much; fiber intake averages only 10 to 20 grams a day.

Start adding more fiber to your diet slowly so that your body can adjust to it. And don't go overboard. Excess intake of fiber—over 50 grams a day—can displace other foods that contain needed nutrients and may block the absorption of vital minerals like iron, zinc, calcium and magnesium.

Children, too, benefit from fiber in their diet and studies show they do not eat enough for good health. Experts recommend that children age two and older eat grams of fiber each day equal to their age + five. Following this rule, a five-year-old should eat 10 grams a day ($5 + 5 = 10$) while for a fifteen-year-old, 20 grams is right ($15 + 5 = 20$). After age twenty, fiber levels of 25 to 35 grams a day are advised.

Note: Throughout the counter, fiber listings refer to dietary fiber. This is the residue of plant foods that remains after digestion.

Add some fiber to your life:

1. It's healthier to get fiber in your food. Fiber pills or supplements are usually not necessary.
2. Eat whole fruits and vegetables instead of drinking their juices.
3. Enjoy the fiber-rich skins of apples, pears and potatoes.
4. Choose whole grains like brown rice, oats, cracked wheat and whole wheat spaghetti, cereal and bread whenever you can.
5. Enjoy beans, lentils and dried split peas. They are often on restaurant menus and in salad bars.
6. Try soybeans or one of its forms—soynuts, tofu, tempeh—for an interesting food or snack.
7. Dried fruits and raisins are favorites. Try some of the more unusual kinds like pineapple, mango and persimmon.

Along with fiber, studies suggest that some foods and drinks can affect cholesterol levels. Drinking five or six cups of "French-pressed" coffee a day can increase cholesterol by as much as 14 percent. Boiled coffee, as it is made in Europe, increases cholesterol levels much more than the filtered coffee used in the U.S. Garlic, small amounts of nuts, especially walnuts and almonds, green tea, olive and canola oils may lower LDL cholesterol. Try to include some of these in your diet. One or two alcoholic drinks a day, especially red wine, may raise HDL "good" cholesterol levels.

COUNT UP YOUR CHOLESTEROL

Most of us eat too much cholesterol. We eat on the run and pick foods high in fat. By the end of the day we've often eaten too much cholesterol.

You know that you shouldn't be eating a lot of cholesterol.

You want to cut back. But it's not easy since you are not really sure which foods are high in cholesterol and which foods are not. With *The Cholesterol Counter* it's easy to find out which foods have cholesterol and to reduce the amount you are eating.

Let's look at a typical day. Are the food choices familiar? Let's see just how much cholesterol this sample day contains and how we can reduce the amount with better food choices.

CHOLESTEROL COUNTING

A SAMPLE DAY OF FOOD CHOICES

Breakfast	CHOLESTEROL (MG)
Orange juice (½ cup)	0
Scrambled egg (w/ milk & margarine)	215
Bacon (2 slices)	27
Toast (1 slice)	0
Butter (1 pat)	11
Coffee &	0
Half & half (1 tbsp)	6
Lunch	
Double burger with cheese & bun	110
Ketchup	0
French fries	0
Vanilla shake (10 oz)	32
Snack	
Pound cake (1 slice)	66
Coffee &	0
Half & half (1 tbsp)	6
Dinner	
Batter dipped fried chicken w/ skin (½ breast)	119
Baked potato &	0
Sour cream (2 tbsp)	10
Tossed salad &	0
Reduced calorie French dressing (2 tbsp)	2
Chocolate pudding cup	5
Tea &	0
Sugar	0
TV Snack	
Rich vanilla ice cream (1 cup)	90
TOTAL CHOLESTEROL	699

This is too much cholesterol for one day—more than double the recommended level of 300 milligrams a day. Now you can see how easy it is to take in more cholesterol than you need.

CHOLESTEROL COUNTING

A SAMPLE DAY OF BETTER FOOD CHOICES

	CHOLESTEROL (MG)
Breakfast	
Orange juice (½ cup)	0
All Bran &	0
Lowfat milk, 1% (½ cup)	5
Toast (1 slice) &	0
Jelly	0
Coffee &	0
Lowfat milk (2 tbsp)	1
Lunch	
Hamburger with bun	71
Ketchup	0
French fries	0
Cola	0
Snack	
Fat-free pound cake (1 slice)	0
Coffee &	
Lowfat milk (1 tbsp)	tr
Dinner	
Roasted chicken breast, no skin	
(½ breast)	73
Baked potato &	0
Plain lowfat yogurt (2 tbsp or 1 oz)	2
Tossed salad &	0
Oil & vinegar dressing (2 tbsp)	0
Lemon pudding cup	0
Tea &	0
Sugar	0
TV Snack	
Vanilla light ice cream (1 cup)	18
TOTAL CHOLESTEROL	170

Better food choices! A much healthier intake of cholesterol for the day.

Check your fiber values regularly. Aim for 20 to 30 grams a day.

TEN STEPS TO LOWER CHOLESTEROL

1. Use liquid vegetable oils. Choose olive, canola, corn, soybean, sunflower, safflower and cottonseed oils.
2. Limit amount of meat eaten to 3–4 ounce portions. Poultry, shellfish and other fish also should be eaten in small portions. Eat liver, brains, or other organ meats infrequently.
3. Use lean cuts of meat; trim off all visible fat. Cook without added fat. Bake, broil or roast to further reduce fat. Remove skin from poultry and fish.
4. Use more beans, grains, pasta, rice and vegetables to make up for the smaller portions of meat, fish and poultry.
5. Avoid nondairy creamers (coffee whiteners) and whipped toppings.
6. Limit eggs to four a week including those used in cooking and desserts. Egg substitutes and egg whites can be eaten as desired. Two egg whites can be substituted for one egg.
7. Use lowfat or nonfat milk and cheese, yogurt, ice cream and fat free sour cream. Avoid butter, cream, regular ice cream, regular sour cream and whole milk.
8. When using margarine, salad dressing or gravy, use a teaspoon or tablespoon to measure out a portion.
9. Eat fiber-rich foods—beans, whole grains, bran, brown rice, dried fruits, fruits and vegetables.
10. Substitute soy foods—soynuts, tofu, soymilk, soy ice cream, soy yogurt—often. Soy protein lowers cholesterol.

Now it's your turn to *count your cholesterol*. Note everything you eat today, then look up the cholesterol in each food you have eaten and see how much cholesterol you had. While you're at it, jot down the calories too! Don't forget to count up your fiber at least once a week.

CHOLESTEROL COUNTING

A SAMPLE WORKSHEET

FOOD	AMOUNT	CHOLESTEROL (Mg)	CALORIES	FIBER
Breakfast				
Snack				
Lunch				
Snack				
Dinner				
Snack				
Total		Cholesterol: ___	Calories: ___	Fiber: ___

Did your cholesterol total more than 300 milligrams for the day? If it did, you need to start counting cholesterol and making better food choices. What about fiber? Did you reach the target of 20 to 30 grams a day?

USING YOUR CHOLESTEROL COUNTER

This book lists the cholesterol, fiber and calorie content of over 20,000 foods. Now you can compare the cholesterol values in your favorite foods and choose substitutes for them before you go out to grocery shop or eat. This will help you save time when you are deciding what to buy or eat.

The Cholesterol Counter has foods listed alphabetically. For each category, you will find nonbranded (generic) foods listed first in alphabetical order, followed by an alphabetical listing of brand name foods. The nonbranded listing will help you determine cholesterol values for foods when you do not find your favorite brand listed. They also help you to evaluate generic and store brands. Large categories are divided into subcategories such as canned, fresh, frozen, and ready-to-eat to make it easier to find what you are looking for. Many categories have a take-out subcategory. Look there for foods you take out or order in a store or restaurant because these foods are not nutrition labeled.

If you want to know how much cholesterol is in the hamburger you are having for lunch, look under HAMBURGER where you will find all kinds of hamburgers listed, or if you are making a homemade hamburger, look under ROLL where you will find the hamburger roll listed alphabetically, and under BEEF where you will find a cooked chopped beef patty. For foods like FRENCH TOAST, HONEY or SALAD DRESSING, simply look for the specific food alphabetically in the complete listing. For example, FRENCH TOAST is found on page 211, listed alphabetically between FRENCH BEANS and FROG'S LEGS. One slice has about 48 milligrams of cholesterol.

If you are having dinner from your favorite take-out place or eating out, many food categories will have a take-out subcategory. Items found in the take-out subcategory will help you estimate the cholesterol, fiber and calories in similar restaurant or take-out menu items. Simply look up the individual foods you are eating under the take-out subcategory and total the cholesterol for the meal. For example, on a typical take-out night you may have:

	CHOLESTEROL MILLIGRAMS
Wonton soup, 1 cup	89
Vegetable egg roll	0
Chicken teriyaki w/rice, 1 serv.	25
Fortune cookie	0
Orange sherbet	5
Green tea	0
TOTAL CHOLESTEROL FOR THE MEAL =	119

Most foods are listed alphabetically. But, in some cases, foods are grouped by category. For example, all pasta dishes, like spaghetti and meatballs, lasagna and fettucine, are found under the category PASTA DINNERS.

Other group categories include:

DELI MEATS/COLD CUTS   page 182
   includes all sandwich meats except
      chicken, ham and turkey
DINNER   page 187
   includes all frozen dinners by brand name
ICE CREAM AND FROZEN DESSERTS   page 252
   includes all dairy and nondairy ice cream
LIQUOR/LIQUEUR   page 286
   includes all alcoholic beverages except
      wine or beer
NUTRITIONAL SUPPLEMENTS   page 313
   includes all meal replacers, energy bars
     and drinks

Part Two, Restaurant Chains, contains an alphabetical listing of over 75 popular chains. Fast foods like BURGER KING, DOMINO'S PIZZA, TACO BELL and WENDY'S are listed alphabetically under the chain's name. For example MCDONALD'S is listed on page 587 under M.

We have tried to include all foods for which cholesterol values are known. There will be some foods, however, that are not listed in *The Cholesterol Counter* because the cholesterol values are not available for that particular food.

When you can't locate your favorite brand, look at other similar foods. You will probably find a brand name food, a generic product or a take-out item that is like your favorite food.

With *The Cholesterol Counter* as your guide, you will never again wonder how much cholesterol is in food. You will always be able to tell if a food is high in cholesterol, moderate in cholesterol or low in cholesterol. *Your goal is to pick low cholesterol foods most times.*

Finding cholesterol in the foods you eat

When you know the ingredients in a food, you can tell if that food contains cholesterol. Read the ingredient list on the label or, if you are making a homemade recipe, read through the recipe ingredients. To find cholesterol-containing ingredients you need only remember these two simple rules:

If it grows in the ground, the food does not contain cholesterol.

If it has a face, the food contains cholesterol.

Try out the rules. Which of the following foods have cholesterol?

	YES	NO
Hamburger		
Sardines		
Lobster		
Chicken leg		
Cheddar cheese		
Milk		
Egg		
Peanut butter		
Apple		
Olive oil		

The first seven foods all contain cholesterol. Hamburger comes from a steer. Sardines and lobster are seafood. Chicken leg comes from a chicken. All of these have faces, therefore, they all contain cholesterol. Cheddar cheese, milk and egg have cholesterol because they all come from an animal that has a face.

Peanut butter, apples and olive oil are all from plants that grow in the ground. Therefore, they do not have cholesterol.

Now you know why all of the ingredients on the following list have cholesterol. These are the ingredients to limit.

INGREDIENTS THAT CONTAIN CHOLESTEROL

whole eggs	butter
egg yolks	lard
whole milk	chicken fat
lowfat milk	beef suet or tallow
cream	liver

ice cream   kidney
sour cream   brains
yogurt   meat
cheese   fish
bacon or bacon fat   poultry

Some packaged foods that do not contain any cholesterol suggest adding ingredients that do contain cholesterol when you prepare the food. For example, instant mashed potatoes made with potato flakes do not contain any cholesterol. The package directions, however, tell you to add butter and milk. *Both are sources of cholesterol.* By adding butter and milk, you add cholesterol to the mashed potatoes so that each one-half-cup serving contains 15 mg of cholesterol. To cut down on the cholesterol in the instant mashed potatoes, use margarine and nonfat milk.

DEFINITIONS

as prep (as prepared): refers to food that has been prepared according to package directions.

home recipe: describes homemade dishes; those included can be used as a guide to the cholesterol and calorie values of similar products you may prepare or take-out food you buy ready-to-eat.

lean and fat: describes meat with some fat on its edges that is not cut away before cooking or poultry prepared with skin and fat as purchased.

lean only: lean portion, trimmed of all visible fat.

shelf stable: refers to prepared products found on the supermarket shelf that are ready to eat or be heated and do not require refrigeration.

take-out: describes prepared dishes that you purchase ready-to-eat; those included serve as a guide to the cholesterol and calorie values of similar products you may purchase.

tr (trace): value used when a food contains less than 1 calorie, less than 1 milligram of cholesterol, or less than 1 gram of fiber.

ABBREVIATIONS

avg	=	average
diam	=	diameter
fl	=	fluid
frzn	=	frozen
g	=	gram
in	=	inch
lb	=	pound
lg	=	large
med	=	medium
mg	=	milligram
oz	=	ounce
pkg	=	package
prep	=	prepared
pt	=	pint
qt	=	quart
reg	=	regular
serv	=	serving
sm	=	small
sq	=	square
tbsp	=	tablespoon
tr	=	trace
tsp	=	teaspoon
w/	=	with
w/o	=	without
<	=	less than

EQUIVALENT MEASURES

3 teaspoons	=	1 tablespoon
4 tablespoons	=	¼ cup
8 tablespoons	=	½ cup
12 tablespoons	=	¾ cup
16 tablespoons	=	1 cup
1000 milligrams	=	1 gram
28 grams	=	1 ounce

Liquid Measurements

2 tablespoons	=	1 ounce
¼ cup	=	2 ounces
½ cup	=	4 ounces
¾ cup	=	6 ounces
1 cup	=	8 ounces
2 cups	=	1 pint
4 cups	=	1 quart

Dry Measurements

4 ounces	=	¼ pound
8 ounces	=	½ pound
12 ounces	=	¾ pound
16 ounces	=	1 pound

NOTES

Discrepancies in figures are due to rounding, product reformulation and reevaluation. Labeling law allows rounding of values. Because most of the data in this book is analysis data, obtained directly from manufacturers, not from labels, in some cases our values may not be exactly the same as label information because they have not been rounded.

The fiber values listed are for dietary fiber.

Throughout the Counter portion of this book, CALS. indicates calories, CHOL. indicates cholesterol and FIB. indicates fiber.

All cholesterol values are given in milligrams (mg), and all fiber values are given in grams (g).

A dash (—) indicates data is not available.

BRAND NAME,

NONBRANDED

(GENERIC)

AND

TAKE-OUT FOODS

FOOD	PORTION	CALS.	FIB.	CHOL.
ABALONE				
fresh fried	3 oz	161	—	80
raw	3 oz	89	—	72
ACEROLA				
fresh	1	2	—	0
ACEROLA JUICE				
juice	1 cup	51	—	0
ADZUKI BEANS				
CANNED				
sweetened	1 cup	702	—	0
Eden				
Organic	½ cup (4.1 oz)	100	5	0
DRIED				
cooked	1 cup	294	—	0
READY-TO-EAT				
yokan sliced	3¼ in slices	112	—	0
AKEE				
fresh	3½ oz	223	—	0
ALE				
(*see* BEER AND ALE, MALT)				
ALFALFA				
sprouts	1 tbsp	1	—	0
sprouts	1 cup	40	—	0
ALLIGATOR				
tail cooked	3½ oz	143	—	65
ALLSPICE				
ground	1 tsp	5	—	0
ALMONDS				
almond butter honey & cinnamon	1 tbsp	96	—	0
almond butter w/ salt	1 tbsp	101	—	0
almond butter w/o salt	1 tbsp	101	—	0
almond meal	1 oz	116	—	0
almond paste	1 oz	127	—	0
dried blanched	1 oz	166	—	0
dried unblanched	1 oz	167	—	0
dry roasted unblanched	1 oz	167	—	0
dry roasted unblanched salted	1 oz	167	—	0
oil roasted blanched	1 oz	174	3	0
oil roasted blanched salted	1 oz	174	—	0

FOOD	PORTION	CALS.	FIB.	CHOL.
oil roasted unblanched	1 oz	176	—	0
toasted unblanched	1 oz	167	3	0
Beer Nuts				
Almonds	1 pkg (1 oz)	180	—	0
Dole				
Blanched Slivered	1 oz	170	—	0
Blanched Whole	1 oz	170	—	0
Chopped Natural	1 oz	170	—	0
Sliced Natural	1 oz	170	—	0
Whole Natural	1 oz	170	—	0
Erewhon				
Almond Butter	1 tbsp (16 g)	90	—	0
Hain				
Almond Butter Natural Raw	2 tbsp	190	—	0
Almond Butter Toasted	2 tbsp	220	—	0
Lance				
Smoked	1 pkg (0.7 oz)	120	—	0
Nutella				
Spread	1 tbsp (0.5 oz)	85	—	0
Planters				
Almonds	1 oz	170	3	0
Gold Measure Slivered	1 pkg (2 oz)	340	4	0
Honey Roasted	1 oz	160	2	0

AMARANTH
(*see also* CEREAL, COOKIES)

FOOD	PORTION	CALS.	FIB.	CHOL.
cooked	½ cup	59	—	0
uncooked	½ cup	366	—	0
Arrowhead				
Seeds	¼ cup (1.6 oz)	170	3	0
Health Valley				
Amaranth Cereal With Bananas	½ cup (1 oz)	110	4	0
Amaranth Crunch With Raisins	¼ cup (1 oz)	110	3	0
Amaranth Flakes 100% Organic	½ cup (1 oz)	90	3	0
Fast Menu Amaranth With Garden Vegetables	7½ oz	140	8	0

ANASAZI BEANS
Arrowhead

FOOD	PORTION	CALS.	FIB.	CHOL.
Dried	¼ cup (1.5 oz)	150	9	0
Bean Cuisine				
Dried	½ cup	115	5	0

ANISE

FOOD	PORTION	CALS.	FIB.	CHOL.
seed	sp	7	—	0

FOOD	PORTION	CALS.	FIB.	CHOL.
ANTELOPE				
roasted	3 oz	127	—	107
APPLE				
CANNED				
sliced sweetened	1 cup	136	—	0
White House				
Escalloped Apples	4 oz	120	1	0
Sliced	4 oz	55	1	0
Spiced Apple Rings	1 ring	25	tr	0
DRIED				
cooked w/ sugar	½ cup	116	—	0
cooked w/o sugar	½ cup	172	—	0
rings	10	155	—	0
Del Monte				
Sliced	⅓ cup (1.4 oz)	80	5	0
Mariani				
Apples	¼ cup	150	—	0
Sonoma				
Pieces	10-12 pieces (1.4 oz)	110	4	0
FRESH				
apple	1	81	3	0
w/o skin sliced	1 cup	62	2	0
w/o skin sliced & cooked	1 cup	91	—	0
w/o skin sliced & microwaved	1 cup	96	—	0
Dole				
Apple	1	80	5	0
Tastee				
Candy Apple	1 (3 oz)	160	4	0
Caramel Apple	1 (3 oz)	160	4	0
FROZEN				
sliced w/o sugar	½ cup	41	—	0
Mrs. Paul's				
Apple Fritters	2	270	—	5
APPLE JUICE				
frzn as prep	1 cup	111	—	0
frzn not prep	6 oz	349	—	0
juice	1 cup	116	tr	0
After The Fall				
Organic	1 bottle (10 oz)	110	—	0
Vermont Apple	1 bottle (8 oz)	90	—	0
Vermont Apple	1 bottle (10 oz)	110	—	0
Vermont Harvest Moon Sparkling Apple Cider	8 fl oz	110	—	0

FOOD	PORTION	CALS.	FIB.	CHOL.
Apple & Eve				
Cider	6 fl oz	80	—	0
Juice	6 fl oz	80	—	0
Nothin' But Juice	6 fl oz	78	—	0
Bruce				
Lite	½ cup	88	—	0
Hi-C				
Jammin' Apple	8 fl oz	130	—	0
Hood				
Select Cider	1 cup (8 oz)	120	—	0
Juice Works	6 oz	100	—	0
Minute Maid				
Box	8.45 fl oz	120	—	0
Juices To Go	1 can (11.5 fl oz)	160	—	0
Juices To Go	1 bottle (10 fl oz)	140	—	0
Juices To Go	1 bottle (16 fl oz)	110	—	0
Naturals	8 fl oz	110	—	0
Mott's				
From Concentrate as prep	8 fl oz	120	0	0
Fruit Basket Cocktail as prep	8 fl oz	120	0	0
Natural	8 fl oz	120	0	0
Ocean Spray				
Juice	8 fl oz	110	0	0
Odwalla				
Live Apple	8 fl oz	140	0	0
Red Cheek				
From Concentrate	8 fl oz	120	0	0
Natural	8 fl oz	120	0	0
S&W				
100% Unsweetened	6 oz	85	—	0
Seneca				
Clarified frzn, as prep	8 fl oz	120	0	0
Granny Smith frzn as prep	8 fl oz	120	0	0
Natural frzn as prep	8 fl oz	120	0	0
Sippin' Pak				
100% Pure	8.45 fl oz	110	—	0
Sipps				
Juice	8.45 oz	130	—	0
Snapple				
Apple Crisp	10 fl oz	140	—	0
Tree Of Life				
East Coast Apple	8 fl oz	120	—	0

FOOD	PORTION	CALS.	FIB.	CHOL.
Tree Top				
Cider	6 oz	90	—	0
Cider frzn as prep	6 oz	90	—	0
Frzn, as prep	6 oz	90	—	0
Juice	6 oz	90	—	0
Sparkling Juice	6 oz	90	—	0
Unfiltered	6 oz	90	—	0
Unfiltered frzn as prep	6 oz	90	—	0
w/ Vitamin C	6 oz	90	—	0
Tropicana				
Season's Best	1 bottle (10 fl oz)	140	—	0
Season's Best	1 can (11.5 fl oz)	160	—	0
Season's Best	1 bottle (7 fl oz)	100	—	0
Season's Best	8 fl oz	110	—	0
Season's Best	1 container (10 fl oz)	140	—	0
Season's Best	1 container (8 fl oz)	110	—	0
Season's Best	1 container (6 fl oz)	80	—	0
Veryfine				
100%	8 oz	107	—	0
White House				
Juice	6 oz	90	0	0
APPLESAUCE				
sweetened	½ cup	97	2	0
unsweetened	½ cup	53	2	0
Eden				
Applesauce	½ cup (4.3 oz)	50	2	0
Mott's				
Chunky	5 oz	110	2	0
Cinnamon	5 oz	120	1	0
Fruit Snacks Apple Spice	4 oz	70	1	0
Fruit Snacks Cinnamon	4 oz	90	1	0
Fruit Snacks Strawberry	4 oz	80	1	0
Fruit Snacks Sweetened	4 oz	90	1	0
Sweetened	5 oz	110	1	0
S&W				
Diet	½ cup	55	—	0
Gravenstein Sweetened	½ cup	90	—	0
Gravenstein Unsweetened	½ cup	55	—	0
Sweetened	½ cup	55	—	0
Seneca				
Cinnamon	½ cup	100	3	0
Golden Delicious	½ cup	100	3	0

FOOD	PORTION	CALS.	FIB.	CHOL.
Seneca (CONT.)				
McIntosh	½ cup	100	3	0
Natural	½ cup	60	3	0
Regular	½ cup	100	3	0
Tree Of Life				
Applesauce	½ cup (4.3 oz)	50	2	0
Tree Top				
Cinnamon	½ cup	80	—	0
Natural	½ cup	60	—	0
Original	½ cup	80	—	0
White House				
Chunky	4 oz	80	1	0
Cinnamon	4 oz	100	1	0
Natural Packed w/ Apple Juice	4 oz	60	1	0
Regular	4 oz	80	1	0
Unsweetened	4 oz	50	2	0

APRICOT JUICE

FOOD	PORTION	CALS.	FIB.	CHOL.
nectar	1 cup	141	2	0
Del Monte				
Nectar	8 fl oz	140	1	0
Kern's				
Nectar	6 fl oz	110	—	0
Libby				
Nectar	1 can (11.5 fl oz)	220	—	0
S&W				
Nectar	6 oz	35	—	0

APRICOTS
CANNED

FOOD	PORTION	CALS.	FIB.	CHOL.
halves heavy syrup pack w/ skin	1 cup (9.1 oz)	214	—	0
halves water pack w/ skin	1 cup (8.5 oz)	65	—	0
halves water pack w/o skin	1 cup (8 oz)	51	—	0
heavy syrup w/ skin	3 halves	70	—	0
juice pack w/ skin	3 halves	40	—	0
light syrup w/ skin	3 halves	54	—	0
puree from heavy syrup pack w/ skin	¾ cup (9.1 oz)	214	—	0
puree from light pack w/ skin	¾ cup (8.9 oz)	160	—	0
puree from water pack w/ skin	¾ cup (8.5 oz)	65	—	0
puree juice pack w/ skin	1 cup (8.7 oz)	119	—	0
water pack w/ skin	3 halves	22	—	0
water pack w/o skin	4 halves	20	—	0
Del Monte				
Halves Unpeeled In Heavy Syrup	½ cup (4.5 oz)	100	1	0

FOOD	PORTION	CALS.	FIB.	CHOL.
Del Monte (CONT.)				
Halves Unpeeled Lite	½ cup (4.3 oz)	60	1	0
Libby				
Halves Unpeeled Lite	½ cup (4.4 oz)	60	1	0
S&W				
Halves Diet	½ cup	35	—	0
Halves Unpeeled In Heavy Syrup	½ cup	110	—	0
Halves Unsweetened	½ cup	35	—	0
Whole Peeled Diet	½ cup	28	—	0
Whole Peeled In Heavy Syrup	½ cup	100	—	0
DRIED				
halves	10	83	3	0
halves cooked w/o sugar	½ cup	106	—	0
Del Monte				
Sun Dried	⅓ cup (1.4 oz)	80	6	0
Mariani				
Apricots	¼ cup	140	—	0
Sonoma				
Dried	10 pieces (1.4 oz)	120	1	0
FRESH				
apricots	3	51	—	0
FROZEN				
sweetened	½ cup	119	—	0
ARROWHEAD				
fresh boiled	1 med (⅓ oz)	9	—	0
ARROWROOT				
flour	1 cup	457	4	0
ARTICHOKE				
CANNED				
Progresso				
Hearts	2 pieces (2.9 oz)	35	1	0
Hearts Marinated	⅓ cup (3 oz)	160	1	0
S&W				
Hearts Marinated	½ cup	225	—	0
FRESH				
boiled	1 med (4 oz)	60	—	0
hearts cooked	½ cup	42	—	0
Dole				
Large	1	23	3	0
FROZEN				
cooked	1 pkg (9 oz)	108	—	0

FOOD	PORTION	CALS.	FIB.	CHOL.
Birds Eye				
Hearts Deluxe	½ cup	30	3	0
ARUGULA				
raw	½ cup	2	—	0
ASPARAGUS				
CANNED				
spears	½ cup	24	—	0
Del Monte				
Salad Tips Tender Green	½ cup (4.4 oz)	20	1	0
Spears Cut Tender Green	½ cup (4.4 oz)	20	1	0
Spears Extra Long Tender Green	½ cup (4.4 oz)	20	1	0
Spears Tender Green	½ cup (4.4 oz)	20	1	0
Tips Tender Green	½ cup (4.4 oz)	20	1	0
Owatonna				
Spears Cut	½ cup	20	—	0
S&W				
Points Water Pack	½ cup	17	—	0
Spears Colossal Fancy	½ cup	20	—	0
Spears Fancy	½ cup	18	—	0
Seneca				
Asparagus	½ cup	20	2	0
FRESH				
cooked	4 spears	14	—	0
cooked	½ cup	22	—	0
raw	½ cup	16	—	0
raw	4 spears	14	—	0
Dole				
Spears	5	18	2	0
FROZEN				
cooked	4 spears	17	—	0
cooked	1 pkg (10 oz)	82	—	0
Big Valley				
Spears	5–6 (3 oz)	20	1	0
Birds Eye				
Cut	½ cup	23	—	0
Spears	½ cup	25	—	0
Green Giant				
Harvest Fresh Cuts	½ cup	25	2	0
AVOCADO				
FRESH				
avocado	1	324	—	0
mashed	1 cup	370	—	0

FOOD	PORTION	CALS.	FIB.	CHOL.

BABY FOOD

Nutritional guidelines for infants are different from those recommended for older children and adults. Check with a pediatrician for advice on feeding children under the age of 2.

CEREAL

Earth's Best

FOOD	PORTION	CALS.	FIB.	CHOL.
Brown Rice	5 tbsp (0.5 oz)	60	—	0
Mixed Grain	5 tbsp (0.5 oz)	60	—	0
Peach Oatmeal Banana	1 jar (4.5 fl oz)	60	—	0
Prunes & Oatmeal	1 jar (4.5 fl oz)	100	—	0

Gerber

FOOD	PORTION	CALS.	FIB.	CHOL.
2nd Foods Rice With Applesauce & Bananas	1 jar (4 oz)	90	—	0

Health Valley

FOOD	PORTION	CALS.	FIB.	CHOL.
Brown Rice 100% Organic	1 tbsp (0.5 oz)	60	1	0
Sprouted Baby Cereal 100% Organic	1 tbsp (0.5 oz)	60	—	0

DESSERT

Gerber

FOOD	PORTION	CALS.	FIB.	CHOL.
2nd Foods Banana Apple Dessert	1 jar (4 oz)	80	—	0
2nd Foods Cherry Vanilla Pudding	1 jar (4 oz)	80	—	0
2nd Foods Fruit Dessert	1 jar (4 oz)	100	—	0

DINNER

Earth's Best

FOOD	PORTION	CALS.	FIB.	CHOL.
Corn Rice & Cheese Dinner	1 jar (4.5 fl oz)	120	—	10
Macaroni & Cheese	1 jar (4.5 oz)	100	—	13
Pasta Dinner	1 jar (4.5 fl oz)	90	—	0
Potato & Green Bean Dinner	1 jar (4.5 fl oz)	100	—	10
Rice & Lentil Dinner	1 jar (4.5 fl oz)	80	—	7
Summer Vegetable Dinner	1 jar (4.5 oz)	90	—	0

FRUIT

Beech-Nut

FOOD	PORTION	CALS.	FIB.	CHOL.
Stage 1 Bananas Chiquita	1 jar (2.5 oz)	70	1	0
Stage 1 Peaches Yellow Cling	1 jar (2.5 oz)	45	2	0
Stage 1 Pears Bartlett	1 jar (2.5 oz)	50	2	0

Earth's Best

FOOD	PORTION	CALS.	FIB.	CHOL.
Apples	1 jar (4.5 oz)	70	—	0
Apples & Apricots	1 jar (4.5 fl oz)	70	—	0
Apples & Blueberries	1 jar (4.5 fl oz)	70	—	0
Apples & Plums	1 jar (4.5 fl oz)	70	—	0
Bananas	1 jar (4.5 oz)	90	—	0

FOOD	PORTION	CALS.	FIB.	CHOL.
Earth's Best (CONT.)				
Pear	1 jar (4.5 fl oz)	60	—	0
Plums Bananas & Rice	1 jar (4.5 fl oz)	90	—	0
Gerber				
1st Foods Applesauce	1 jar (2.5 oz)	25	—	0
1st Foods Bananas	1 jar (2.5 oz)	70	—	0
1st Foods Peaches	1 jar (2.5 oz)	30	—	0
1st Foods Pears	1 jar (2.5 oz)	40	—	0
1st Foods Prunes	1 jar (2.5 oz)	70	—	0
2nd Foods Apple Blueberry	1 jar (4 oz)	50	—	0
2nd Foods Applesauce	1 jar (4 oz)	60	—	0
2nd Foods Applesauce Apricot	1 jar (4 oz)	60	—	0
JUICE				
Beech-Nut				
Stage 2 Apple Banana	4 fl oz	70	0	0
Stage 2 Apple Cherry	4 fl oz	70	0	0
Stage 2 Apple Cranberry	4 fl oz	60	0	0
Stage 2 Apple Grape	4 fl oz	70	0	0
Stage 2 Juice Plus Grape	4 fl oz	100	0	0
Stage 2 Mango Nectar (Spanish Label)	4 fl oz	80	0	0
Stage 2 Mixed Fruit	4 fl oz	70	0	0
Stage 2 Papaya Nectar (Spanish Label)	4 fl oz	80	0	0
Stage 2 Tropical Blend	4 fl oz	90	0	0
Stage 2 Tropical Blend Nectar (Spanish Label)	4 fl oz	90	0	0
Stage 3 Orange	4 fl oz	60	0	0
Earth's Best				
Apple	1 bottle (4.2 fl oz)	60	—	0
Apple Banana	1 bottle (4.2 fl oz)	60	—	0
Apple Grape	1 bottle (4.2 fl oz)	60	—	0
Apples & Bananas	1 jar (4.5 fl oz)	80	—	0
Pear	1 bottle (4.2 fl oz)	60	—	0
Gerber				
1st Foods Apple	4 fl oz	60	—	0
1st Foods Pear	4 fl oz	60	—	0
1st Foods Red Grape	4 fl oz	80	—	0
1st Foods White Grape	4 fl oz	80	—	0
2nd Foods Apple Banana	4 fl oz	60	—	0
2nd Foods Apple Cherry	4 fl oz	60	—	0
2nd Foods Apple Grape	4 fl oz	60	—	0
2nd Foods Apple Peach	4 fl oz	60	—	0
2nd Foods Apple Plum	4 fl oz	60	—	0

FOOD	PORTION	CALS.	FIB.	CHOL.
Gerber (CONT.)				
2nd Foods Apple Prune	4 fl oz	60	—	0
3rd Foods Apple Carrot	4 fl oz	50	—	0
3rd Foods Apple Sweet Potato	4 fl oz	60	—	0
3rd Foods Orange Carrot	4 fl oz	50	—	0
3rd Foods Pineapple Carrot	4 fl oz	60	—	0
Tropical Foods Guava With Mixed Fruit	4 fl oz	70	—	0
Tropical Foods Mango With Mixed Fruit	4 fl oz	70	—	0
Tropical Foods Papaya With Mixed Fruit	4 fl oz	70	—	0
VEGETABLE				
Beech-Nut				
Stage 1 Carrots Tender Sweet	1 jar (2.5 oz)	30	2	0
Stage 1 Green Beans (Spanish Label)	1 jar (2.5 oz)	20	2	0
Earth's Best				
Carrots	1 jar (4.5 fl oz)	40	—	0
Carrots & Parsnips	1 jar (4.5 fl oz)	60	—	0
Corn & Butternut Squash	1 jar (4.5 fl oz)	90	—	0
Garden Vegetables	1 jar (4.5 fl oz)	70	—	0
Green Beans & Rice	1 jar (4.5 fl oz)	40	—	0
Peas & Brown Rice	1 jar (4.5 fl oz)	80	—	0
Spinach & Potatoes	1 jar (4.5 fl oz)	60	—	0
Sweet Potatoes	1 jar (4.5 fl oz)	60	—	0
Winter Squash	1 jar (4.5 fl oz)	50	—	0
Gerber				
1st Foods Carrots	1 jar (2.5 oz)	25	—	0
1st Foods Green Beans	1 jar (2.5 oz)	25	—	0
1st Foods Peas	1 jar (2.5 oz)	30	—	0
1st Foods Squash	1 jar (2.5 oz)	25	—	0
1st Foods Sweet Potatoes	1 jar (2.5 oz)	45	—	0
3rd Foods Carrots	1 jar (6 oz)	50	—	0
3rd Foods Mixed Vegetables	1 jar (6 oz)	70	—	0
3rd Foods Sweet Potatoes	1 jar (6 oz)	100	—	0
BACON				
(*see also* BACON SUBSTITUTES)				
breakfast strips cooked	3 strips (34 g)	156	—	36
breakfast strips beef cooked	3 strips (34 g)	153	—	40
cooked	3 strips	109	—	16
grilled	2 slices (1.7 oz)	86	—	27
Armour				
Lower Salt cooked	1 strip	38	—	6

FOOD	PORTION	CALS.	FIB.	CHOL.
Armour (CONT.)				
Star cooked	1 strip	38	—	6
Black Label				
Center Cut cooked	3 slices (0.5 oz)	70	0	15
Cooked	2 slices (0.5 oz)	80	0	15
Low Salt cooked	2 slices (0.5 oz)	80	0	15
Hormel				
Bacon Bits	1 tsp (7 g)	30	0	5
Bacon Pieces	1 tsp (7 g)	25	0	10
Microwave cooked	2 slices (0.5 oz)	70	0	15
Jones				
Sliced	1 slice	130	—	25
Nathan's				
Beef cooked	3 slices	100	—	20
Old Smokehouse				
Cooked	2 slices (0.5 oz)	80	0	15
Oscar Mayer				
Bacon Bits	1 tbsp (7 g)	25	0	5
Center Cut cooked	3 slices (0.5 oz)	70	0	15
Cooked	2 slices (0.4 oz)	60	0	10
Lower Sodium cooked	2 slices (0.5 oz)	60	0	15
Thick Cut cooked	1 slice (0.4 oz)	50	0	10
Range Brand				
Cooked	2 slices (0.7 oz)	100	0	20
Red Label				
Cooked	2 slices (0.5 oz)	80	0	15

BACON SUBSTITUTES

bacon substitute	1 strip	25	—	0
Bac-Os				
Pieces	2 tsp (5 g)	25	—	0
Harvest Direct				
Bacon Bits	3.5 oz	320	17	0
Lightlife				
Fakin' Bacon	3 strips (2 oz)	79	—	0
Louis Rich				
Turkey Bacon	1 slice (0.5 oz)	30	0	10
McCormick				
Bac'n Pieces	2 tsp	20	—	0
Mr. Turkey				
Slice	1	25	—	10

BAGEL

FRESH

cinnamon raisin	1 (3½ in)	194	—	0

FOOD	PORTION	CALS.	FIB.	CHOL.
cinnamon raisin toasted	1 (3½ in)	194	—	0
egg	1 (3½ in)	197	—	17
egg toasted	1 (3½ in)	197	—	17
oat bran	1 (3½ in)	181	—	0
oat bran toasted	1 (3½ in)	181	—	0
onion	1 (3½ in)	195	2	0
plain	1 (3½ in)	195	2	0
plain toasted	1 (3½ in)	195	2	0
poppy seed	1 (3½ in)	195	2	0
Alvarado St. Bakery				
Sprouted Wheat	1 (3.3 oz)	260	2	0
Sprouted Wheat Cinnamon/ Raisin	1 (3.3 oz)	280	3	0
Sprouted Wheat Onion/ Poppyseed	1 (3.3 oz)	320	2	0
Sprouted Wheat Sesame	1 (3.3 oz)	320	2	0
FROZEN				
Lender's				
Cinnamon'N Raisin	1 (2.5 oz)	200	1	0
Egg	1 (2 oz)	150	—	5
Onion	1 (2 oz)	160	1	0
Plain	1 (2 oz)	150	—	0
Sara Lee				
Cinnamon & Raisin	1 (3 oz)	240	—	0
Cinnamon Raisin	1 (2.5 oz)	200	—	0
Egg	1 (2.5 oz)	200	—	15
Egg	1 (3 oz)	250	—	20
Oat Bran	1 (3 oz)	220	—	0
Oat Bran	1 (2.5 oz)	180	—	0
Onion	1 (3 oz)	230	—	0
Onion	1 (2.5 oz)	190	—	0
Plain	1 (3 oz)	230	—	0
Plain	1 (2.5 oz)	190	—	0
Poppy Seed	1 (3 oz)	230	—	0
Poppy Seed	1 (2.5 oz)	190	—	0
Sesame Seed	1 (3 oz)	240	—	0
Sesame Seed	1 (2.5 oz)	190	—	0
Tree Of Life				
Onion	1 (3 oz)	210	0	0
Plain	1 (3 oz)	210	0	0
Poppy	1 (3 oz)	210	0	0
Raisin	1 (3 oz)	210	tr	0
Sesame	1 (3 oz)	210	0	0

FOOD	PORTION	CALS.	FIB.	CHOL.
Weight Watchers				
Sandwich Ham And Cheese	1 (3 oz)	200	1	15
BAKING POWDER				
baking powder	1 tsp	2	—	0
low sodium	1 tsp	5	—	0
Calumet				
Baking Powder	1 tsp	3	—	0
Clabber Girl				
Baking Powder	1 tsp	0	—	0
Davis				
Baking Powder	1 tsp	6	—	0
Watkins				
Baking Powder	¼ tsp (1 g)	0	0	0
BAKING SODA				
baking soda	1 tsp	0	—	0
Arm & Hammer				
Baking Soda	1 tsp	0	—	0
BALSAM PEAR				
leafy tips cooked	½ cup	10	—	0
leafy tips raw	½ cup	7	—	0
pods cooked	½ cup	12	—	0
BAMBOO SHOOTS				
CANNED				
sliced	1 cup	25	—	0
Empress				
Sliced	2 oz	14	—	0
Ka-Me				
Sliced	½ cup (4.5 oz)	15	1	0
La Choy				
Sliced	¼ cup	6	tr	0
FRESH				
cooked	½ cup	15	—	0
raw	½ cup	21	—	0
BANANA				
banana chips	1 oz	147	2	0
DRIED				
powder	1 tbsp	21	—	0
FRESH				
banana	1	105	2	0
mashed	1 cup	207	4	0
Chiquita				
Fresh	1 (3½ oz)	110	—	0

FOOD	PORTION	CALS.	FIB.	CHOL.
Dole				
Banana	1	120	3	0
BANANA JUICE				
Libby				
Nectar	1 can (11.5 fl oz)	190	—	0
BARBECUE SAUCE				
(see also SAUCE*)*				
barbecue	1 cup	188	—	0
Bull's Eye				
Original	2 tbsp	50	—	0
Hain				
Honey	1 tbsp	14	—	0
Healthy Choice				
Hickory	2 tbsp (1.1 oz)	26	tr	0
Hot & Spicy	2 tbsp (1.1 oz)	25	tr	0
Original	2 tbsp (1.1 oz)	25	tr	0
Heinz				
Select	1 oz	40	—	0
Select Hickory	1 oz	35	—	0
Thick & Rich Cajun Style	1 oz	35	—	0
Thick & Rich Chunky	1 oz	30	—	0
Thick & Rich Hawaiian Style	1 oz	40	—	0
Thick & Rich Hickory Smoke	1 oz	35	—	0
Thick & Rich Mesquite Smoke	1 oz	30	—	0
Thick & Rich Mushroom	1 oz	30	—	0
Thick & Rich Old Fashioned	1 oz	35	—	0
Thick & Rich Onion	1 oz	30	—	0
Thick & Rich Original	1 oz	35	—	0
Thick & Rich Texas Hot	1 oz	30	—	0
House Of Tsang				
Hong Kong	1 tbsp (0.6 oz)	10	0	0
Hunt's				
Bold Hickory	2 tbsp (1.2 oz)	47	1	0
Bold Original	2 tbsp (1.2 oz)	46	1	0
Hickory	2 tbsp (1.2 oz)	38	1	0
Hickory & Brown Sugar	2 tbsp (1.3 oz)	75	1	0
Honey Hickory	2 tbsp (1.2 oz)	38	1	0
Honey Mustard	2 tbsp (1.2 oz)	48	1	0
Hot & Spicy	2 tbsp (1.2 oz)	48	1	0
Light	2 tbsp (1.2 oz)	23	1	0
Mesquite Barbecue	2 tbsp (1.2 oz)	40	1	0
Mild	2 tbsp (1.2 oz)	41	1	0
Mild Dijon	2 tbsp (1.2 oz)	39	tr	0

FOOD	PORTION	CALS.	FIB.	CHOL.
Hunt's (CONT.)				
Original	2 tbsp (1.2 oz)	39	1	0
Teriyaki	2 tbsp (1.2 oz)	46	1	0
Kraft				
Char-Grill	2 tbsp (1.2 oz)	60	0	0
Extra Rich Original	2 tbsp (1.2 oz)	50	0	0
Garlic	2 tbsp (1.2 oz)	40	0	0
Hickory Smoke	2 tbsp (1.2 oz)	40	0	0
Hickory Smoke Onion Bits	2 tbsp (1.2 oz)	50	tr	0
Honey	2 tbsp (1.2 oz)	50	0	0
Hot	2 tbsp (1.2 oz)	40	0	0
Hot Hickory Smoke	2 tbsp (1.2 oz)	40	0	0
Italian Seasonings	2 tbsp (1.2 oz)	45	0	0
Kansas City Style	2 tbsp (1.2 oz)	45	tr	0
Mesquite Smoke	2 tbsp (1.2 oz)	40	0	0
Onion Bits	2 tbsp (1.2 oz)	50	0	0
Original	2 tbsp (1.2 oz)	40	0	0
Teriyaki	2 tbsp (1.2 oz)	60	0	0
Thick'N Spicy Hickory Smoke	2 tbsp (1.2 oz)	50	0	0
Thick'N Spicy Honey	2 tbsp (1.2 oz)	60	0	0
Thick'N Spicy Kansas City Style	2 tbsp (1.2 oz)	60	tr	0
Thick'N Spicy Mesquite Smoke	2 tbsp (1.2 oz)	50	0	0
Thick'N Spicy Original	2 tbsp (1.2 oz)	50	0	0
Lawry's				
Dijon Honey	¼ cup	203	tr	0
Maull's				
Beer Non-Alcoholic	3.5 oz	128	—	1
Regular	3.5 oz	123	—	1
Smoky	3.5 oz	124	—	1
Sweet-N-Mild	3.5 oz	167	—	1
Sweet-N-Smoky	3.5 oz	160	—	1
With Onion Bits	3.5 oz	126	—	1
Red Wing				
"K" Sauce	2 tbsp (1.2 oz)	45	0	0
Watkins				
Bold	2 tsp (0.4 oz)	25	0	0
Honey	2 tsp (0.4 oz)	25	0	0
Mesquite	2 tsp (0.4 oz)	25	0	0
Original	2 tsp (0.4 oz)	25	0	0
Smokehouse	2 tsp (0.4 oz)	25	0	0
BARLEY				
pearled cooked	½ cup	97	—	0
pearled uncooked	½ cup	352	16	0

FOOD	PORTION	CALS.	FIB.	CHOL.
Arrowhead				
Barley	¼ cup (1.7 oz)	170	6	0
Hulless	¼ cup (1.6 oz)	140	6	0
Quaker				
Medium Pearled	¼ cup	172	5	0
Quick Pearled	¼ cup	172	5	0
Scotch				
Medium Pearled	¼ cup	172	5	0
Quick Pearled	¼ cup	172	5	0
BASIL				
fresh chopped	2 tbsp	1	—	0
ground	1 tsp	4	—	0
leaves fresh	5	1	—	0
Watkins				
Liquid Spice	1 tbsp (0.5 oz)	120	0	0
BASS				
freshwater raw	3 oz	97	—	58
sea cooked	3 oz	105	—	45
sea raw	3 oz	82	—	35
striped baked	3 oz	105	—	87
BAY LEAF				
crumbled	1 tsp	2	—	0
Watkins				
Bay Leaves	¼ tsp (0.5 g)	0	0	0
BEAN SPROUTS				
(see also individual bean names)				
CANNED				
La Choy	⅔ cup	8	tr	0
BEANS				
(see also individual names)				
CANNED				
baked beans plain	½ cup	118	10	0
baked beans vegetarian	½ cup	118	10	0
baked beans w/ beef	½ cup	161	—	29
baked beans w/ franks	½ cup	182	9	8
baked beans w/ pork	½ cup	133	7	9
baked beans w/ pork & sweet sauce	½ cup	140	7	9
baked beans w/ pork & tomato sauce	½ cup	123	7	9
Allen				
Baked	½ cup (4.5 oz)	150	8	0

FOOD	PORTION	CALS.	FIB.	CHOL.
B&M				
99% Fat Free Baked Beans	½ cup (4.6 oz)	160	7	0
Baked With Honey	½ cup (4.7 oz)	170	8	0
Barbeque Baked Beans	½ cup (4.7 oz)	170	6	<5
Brick Oven Baked	½ cup (4.6 oz)	180	7	5
Extra Hearty Baked	½ cup (4.6 oz)	190	8	<5
Brown Beauty				
Mexican Beans With Jalapeno	½ cup (4.5 oz)	120	7	0
Bush's				
Baked	½ cup (4.6 oz)	150	7	<5
Baked With Onions	½ cup (4.6 oz)	150	6	5
Homestyle Baked	½ cup (4.6 oz)	160	8	5
Vegetarian	½ cup (4.6 oz)	140	6	0
Chi-Chi's				
Ranchero Beans	½ cup (4.3 oz)	100	1	0
Refried	½ cup (4.2 oz)	130	4	0
Crest Top				
Pork And Beans	½ cup (4.5 oz)	130	6	0
Friend's				
Maple Baked	8 oz	240	11	<5
Original Baked	½ cup (4.6 oz)	170	7	<5
Gebhardt				
Chili	4 oz	115	5	0
Refried	4 oz	100	7	2
Refried Jalapeno	4 oz	115	7	2
Green Giant				
Pork And Beans In Tomato Sauce	½ cup	90	6	0
Three Bean Salad	½ cup	70	3	0
Hanover				
Four Bean Salad	½ cup	80	—	0
Health Valley				
Boston Baked	7½ oz	190	5	0
Boston Baked No Salt Added	7.5 oz	190	5	0
Fast Menu Honey Baked Organic Beans With Tofu Weiner	7½ oz	150	16	0
Vegetarian With Miso	7½ oz	180	5	0
Heartland				
Iron Kettle Baked	½ cup (4.6 oz)	150	5	<5
Hormel				
Beans & Wieners	1 can (7.5 oz)	290	6	45
Hunt's				
Big John's Beans & Fixin's	½ cup (4.7 oz)	127	6	3

FOOD	PORTION	CALS.	FIB.	CHOL.
Hunt's (CONT.)				
Pork & Beans	½ cup (4.5 oz)	130	4	tr
Kid's Kitchen				
Beans & Weiners	1 cup (7.5 oz)	310	8	45
Little Pancho				
Refried & Green Chili	½ cup	80	—	0
McIlhenny				
Spicy	1 oz	7	1	0
Old El Paso				
Mexe-Beans	½ cup (4.6 oz)	110	7	0
Refried	½ cup (4.2 oz)	110	5	<5
Refried Fat Free	½ cup (4.4 oz)	110	6	0
Refried Spicy	½ cup (4.3 oz)	140	6	<5
Refried Vegetarian	½ cup (4.1 oz)	100	6	0
Refried With Cheese	½ cup (4.2 oz)	130	6	5
Refried With Green Chilies	½ cup (4.3 oz)	110	6	<5
Refried With Sausage	½ cup (4.1 oz)	200	8	10
Rosarita				
Refried	4 oz	100	6	0
Refried Spicy	4 oz	100	6	0
Refried Vegetarian	4 oz	100	6	0
Refried With Bacon	4 oz	110	6	14
Refried With Green Chilies	4 oz	90	6	0
Refried With Nacho Cheese	4 oz	110	6	2
Refried With Onions	4 oz	110	6	0
S&W				
Maple Sugar Beans	½ cup	150	—	0
Mixed Bean Salad Marinated	½ cup	90	—	0
Smokey Ranch	½ cup	130	—	0
Trappey				
Mexi-Beans With Jalapeno	½ cup (4.5 oz)	130	8	0
Pork And Beans	½ cup (4.5 oz)	110	7	0
Pork And Beans With Jalapeno	½ cup (4.5 oz)	130	6	0
Van Camp's				
Baked Beans Fat Free	½ cup (4.6 oz)	130	5	0
Baked Beans Premium	½ cup (4.6 oz)	140	5	0
Beanee Weenee	1 cup (9 oz)	320	8	40
Beanee Weenee Baked Flavor	1 cup (9 oz)	410	10	40
Beanee Weenee Barbeque	1 cup (9 oz)	340	8	40
Brown Sugar Beans	½ cup (4.6 oz)	170	6	5
Mexican Style Chili Beans	½ cup (4.6 oz)	110	8	0
Pork And Beans	½ cup (4.6 oz)	110	6	0
Vegetarian In Tomato Sauce	½ cup (4.6 oz)	110	5	0

FOOD	PORTION	CALS.	FIB.	CHOL.
Wagon Master				
Pork And Beans	½ cup (4.5 oz)	110	7	0
FROZEN				
Hanover				
Romano Bean Medley	½ cup	25	—	0
MIX				
Bean Cuisine				
Florentine Beans With Bow Ties	½ cup	199	—	6
Pasta & Beans Country French With Gemelli	½ cup	214	—	tr
TAKE-OUT				
baked beans	½ cup	190	—	6
barbecue beans	3.5 oz	120	—	0
four bean salad	3.5 oz	100	—	0
refried beans	½ cup	43	—	2
three bean salad	¾ cup	230	1	0

BEECHNUTS

dried	1 oz	164	—	0

BEEF

(*see also* BEEF DISHES, VEAL)

Beef is graded according to its marbling, the little flecks of fat in the muscle. Beef graded "Prime" has the highest percentage of fat, followed by "Choice" with less fat and "Select" with the least fat. Note that the values for cooked beef may differ slightly from values for raw beef. When meat is cooked some moisture and fat is lost changing the nutrition value slightly. As a rule of thumb it can be assumed that a 4 oz raw portion will equal a 3 oz cooked portion of meat.

CANNED				
corned beef	1 oz	71	—	24
Armour				
Chopped Beef	2 oz	170	—	49
Corned Beef	2 oz	120	—	45
Potted Meat	¼ cup (2.2 oz)	90	—	60
Potted Meat	1 can (3 oz)	120	—	80
Tripe	3 oz	90	—	125
Hormel				
Corned Beef	2 oz	120	0	50
Potted Meat	4 tbsp (2 oz)	60	0	50
Treet				
50% Less Fat	2 oz	120	—	45
Beef	2 oz	150	—	50

FOOD	PORTION	CALS.	FIB.	CHOL.
Underwood				
Roast Beef	2.08 oz	140	—	45
Roast Beef Mesquite Smoked	2.08 oz	126	—	45
Roast Beef Light	2.08 oz	90	—	30
DRIED				
Hormel				
Pillow Pack	10 slices (1 oz)	45	0	20
Sliced	10 slices (1 oz)	50	0	25
FRESH				
bottom round lean & fat trim 0 in Choice roasted	3 oz	172	—	66
bottom round lean & fat trim 0 in Select braised	3 oz	171	—	82
bottom round lean & fat trim 0 in Select roasted	3 oz	150	—	66
bottom round lean & fat trim 0 in braised	3 oz	193	—	82
bottom round lean & fat trim ¼ in Choice braised	3 oz	241	—	81
bottom round lean & fat trim ¼ in Choice roasted	3 oz	221	—	68
bottom round lean & fat trim ¼ in Select braised	3 oz	220	—	81
bottom round lean & fat trim ¼ in Select roasted	3 oz	199	—	68
brisket flat half lean & fat trim 0 in braised	3 oz	183	—	81
brisket flat half lean & fat trim ¼ in braised	3 oz	309	—	81
brisket point half lean & fat trim 0 in braised	3 oz	304	—	78
brisket point half lean & fat trim ¼ in braised	3 oz	343	—	79
brisket whole lean & fat trim 0 in braised	3 oz	247	—	79
brisket whole lean & fat trim ¼ in braised	3 oz	327	—	80
chuck arm pot roast lean & fat trim 0 in braised	3 oz	238	—	85
chuck arm pot roast lean & fat trim ¼ in braised	3 oz	282	—	85
chuck blade roast lean & fat trim 0 in braised	3 oz	284	—	88
chuck blade roast lean & fat trim ¼ in braised	3 oz	293	—	88

FOOD	PORTION	CALS.	FIB.	CHOL.
corned beef brisket cooked	3 oz	213	—	83
eye of round lean & fat trim 0 in Choice roasted	3 oz	153	—	59
eye of round lean & fat trim 0 in Select roasted	3 oz	137	—	59
eye of round lean & fat trim ¼ in Choice roasted	3 oz	205	—	62
eye of round lean & fat trim ¼ in Select roasted	3 oz	184	—	61
flank lean & fat trim 0 in braised	3 oz	224	—	62
flank lean & fat trim 0 in broiled	3 oz	192	—	58
ground extra lean broiled medium	3 oz	217	—	71
ground extra lean broiled well done	3 oz	225	—	84
ground extra lean fried medium	3 oz	216	—	69
ground extra lean fried well done	3 oz	224	—	79
ground extra lean raw	4 oz	265	—	78
ground lean broiled medium	3 oz	231	—	74
ground lean broiled well done	3 oz	238	—	86
ground regular broiled medium	3 oz	246	—	76
ground regular broiled well done	3 oz	248	—	86
ground low-fat w/ carrageenan raw	4 oz	160	—	53
porterhouse steak lean & fat trim ¼ in Choice broiled	3 oz	260	—	70
porterhouse steak lean only trim ¼ in Prime broiled	3 oz	185	—	68
rib eye small end lean & fat trim 0 in Choice broiled	3 oz	261	—	70
rib large end lean & fat trim 0 in roasted	3 oz	300	—	72
rib large end lean & fat trim ¼ in broiled	3 oz	295	—	69
rib large end lean & fat trim ¼ in roasted	3 oz	310	—	72
rib small end lean & fat trim 0 in broiled	3 oz	252	—	70
rib small end lean & fat trim ¼ in broiled	3 oz	285	—	71
rib small end lean & fat trim ¼ in roasted	3 oz	295	—	71
rib whole lean & fat trim ¼ in Choice broiled	3 oz	306	—	70
rib whole lean & fat trim ¼ in Choice roasted	3 oz	320	—	72

FOOD	PORTION	CALS.	FIB.	CHOL.
rib whole lean & fat trim ¼ in Prime roasted	3 oz	348	—	72
rib whole lean & fat trim ¼ in Select broiled	3 oz	274	—	69
rib whole lean & fat trim ¼ in Select roasted	3 oz	286	—	71
shank crosscut lean & fat trim ¼ in Choice simmered	3 oz	224	—	68
short loin top loin lean & fat trim 0 in Choice broiled	1 steak (5.4 oz)	353	—	119
short loin top loin lean & fat trim 0 in Choice broiled	3 oz	193	—	65
short loin top loin lean & fat trim 0 in Select broiled	1 steak (5.4 oz)	309	—	119
short loin top loin lean & fat trim ¼ in Choice braised	3 oz	253	—	68
short loin top loin lean & fat trim ¼ in Choice broiled	1 steak (6.3 oz)	536	—	143
short loin top loin lean & fat trim ¼ in Prime broiled	1 steak (6.3 oz)	582	—	143
short loin top loin lean & fat trim ¼ in Select broiled	1 steak (6.3 oz)	473	—	140
short loin top loin lean only trim 0 in Choice broiled	1 steak (5.2 oz)	311	—	113
short loin top loin lean only trim ¼ in Choice broiled	1 steak (5.2 oz)	314	—	112
shortribs lean & fat Choice braised	3 oz	400	—	80
t-bone steak lean & fat trim ¼ in Choice broiled	3 oz	253	—	70
t-bone steak lean only trim ¼ in Choice broiled	3 oz	182	—	68
tenderloin lean & fat trim 0 in Select broiled	3 oz	194	—	72
tenderloin lean & fat trim ¼ in Choice broiled	3 oz	259	—	73
tenderloin lean & fat trim ¼ in Choice roasted	3 oz	288	—	73
tenderloin lean & fat trim ¼ in Choice broiled	3 oz	208	—	72
tenderloin lean & fat trim ¼ in Prime broiled	3 oz	270	—	73
tenderloin lean & fat trim ¼ in Select roasted	3 oz	275	—	73

FOOD	PORTION	CALS.	FIB.	CHOL.
tenderloin lean only trim 0 in Select broiled	3 oz	170	—	71
tenderloin lean only trim ¼ in Choice broiled	3 oz	188	—	71
tenderloin lean only trim ¼ in Select broiled	3 oz	169	—	71
tip round lean & fat trim 0 in Choice roasted	3 oz	170	—	69
tip round lean & fat trim 0 in Select roasted	3 oz	158	—	69
tip round lean & fat trim ¼ in Choice roasted	3 oz	210	—	70
tip round lean & fat trim ¼ in Prime roasted	3 oz	233	—	70
tip round lean & fat trim ¼ in Select roasted	3 oz	191	—	70
top round lean & fat trim 0 in Choice braised	3 oz	184	—	77
top round lean & fat trim 0 in Select braised	3 oz	170	—	77
top round lean & fat trim ¼ in Choice braised	3 oz	221	—	77
top round lean & fat trim ¼ in Choice broiled	3 oz	190	—	72
top round lean & fat trim ¼ in Choice fried	3 oz	235	—	82
top round lean & fat trim ¼ in Prime broiled	3 oz	195	—	72
top round lean & fat trim ¼ in Select braised	3 oz	199	—	77
top sirloin lean & fat trim 0 in Choice broiled	3 oz	194	—	76
top sirloin lean & fat trim 0 in Select broiled	3 oz	166	—	76
top sirloin lean & fat trim ¼ in Choice broiled	3 oz	228	—	76
top sirloin lean & fat trim ¼ in Choice fried	3 oz	277	—	83
top sirloin lean & fat trim ¼ in Select broiled	3 oz	208	—	76
tripe raw	4 oz	111	—	107
Dakota Lean				
Chuck Roast raw	3 oz	80	—	48
Eye Round raw	3 oz	80	—	40

FOOD	PORTION	CALS.	FIB.	CHOL.
Dakota Lean (CONT.)				
Flank Steak raw	3 oz	80	—	40
Ground raw	3 oz	88	—	50
Outside Round raw	3 oz	80	—	40
Ribeye raw	3 oz	90	—	45
Sirloin Tip raw	3 oz	90	—	40
Strip Loin raw	3 oz	90	—	45
Tenderloin raw	3 oz	70	—	45
Top Round raw	3 oz	80	—	40
Double J				
Filet	3.5 oz	130	—	51
NY Strip	3.5 oz	133	—	52
Rib Eye	3.5 oz	134	—	54
Top Butt	3.5 oz	136	—	50
Healthy Choice				
Ground Extra Lean	4 oz	130	0	55
Laura's Lean				
Eye Of Round	4 oz	150	—	60
Flank Steak	4 oz	160	—	65
Ground	4 oz	180	—	60
Ground Round	4 oz	160	—	65
Ribeye Steak	4 oz	150	—	65
Sirloin Tip Round	4 oz	140	—	65
Sirloin Top Butt	4 oz	140	—	60
Strip Steak	4 oz	150	—	50
Tenderloins	4 oz	150	—	75
Top Round	4 oz	140	—	65
Maverick Ranch				
Ground Round Extra Lean	4 oz	130	—	60
FROZEN				
patties broiled medium	3 oz	240	—	80
READY-TO-EAT				
Healthy Choice				
Deli-Thin Roast Beef	6 slices (2 oz)	60	0	25
Fresh-Trak Roast Beef	1 slice (1 oz)	30	0	10
Jordan's				
Healthy Trim 97% Fat Free Roast Beef Medium	1 slice (1 oz)	30	0	20
Healthy Trim 97% Fat Free Roast Beef Rare	1 slice (1 oz)	30	0	20
Oscar Mayer				
Deli-Thin Roast Beef	4 slices (1.8 oz)	60	0	25
Weight Watchers				
Deli Thin Oven Roasted Cured	5 slices (⅓ oz)	10	—	5

FOOD	PORTION	CALS.	FIB.	CHOL.
TAKE-OUT				
roast beef medium	2 oz	70	—	30
roast beef rare	2 oz	70	—	30
BEEF DISHES				
CANNED				
Armour				
Corned Beef Hash	1 cup (8.3 oz)	440	—	100
Roast Beef Hash	1 cup (8.4 oz)	400	—	95
Roast Beef In Gravy	½ cup (4.6 oz)	150	—	75
Stew	1 cup (8.6 oz)	220	—	30
Dinty Moore				
Meatball Stew	1 cup (8.4 oz)	250	2	40
Stew	1 cup (8.2 oz)	230	2	40
Hormel				
Beef Goulash	1 can (7.5 oz)	230	3	50
Corned Beef Hash	1 cup (8.3 oz)	390	2	70
Roast Beef Hash	1 cup (8.3 oz)	390	2	70
Roast Beef With Gravy	2 oz	60	0	30
Mary Kitchen				
Corned Beef Hash	1 can (7.5 oz)	350	2	60
Roast Beef Hash	1 can (7.5 oz)	348	2	58
FROZEN				
Chefwich				
Beef w/ Barbecue Sauce	1	340	—	29
Hot Pocket				
Stuffed Sandwich Barbecue	1 (4.5 oz)	340	1	25
Stuffed Sandwich Beef & Cheddar	1 (4.5 oz)	360	tr	50
Stuffed Sandwich Beef Fajita	1 (4.5 oz)	360	5	40
Lean Pockets				
Stuffed Sandwich Beef & Broccoli	1 (4.5 oz)	250	7	50
Luigino's				
Creamed Sauce Shaved Cured Beef With Croutons	1 pkg (8 oz)	360	3	60
Egg Noodles Rich Gravy Swedish Meatballs	1 pkg (9 oz)	340	3	80
Egg Noodles Rich Gravy Swedish Meatballs	1 cup (7.5 oz)	280	3	70
Tyson				
Microwave BBQ Sandwich	1 sandwich	200	—	30

FOOD	PORTION	CALS.	FIB.	CHOL.
Weight Watchers				
Reuben Pocket Sandwich	1 (5 oz)	250	5	20
MIX				
Casbah				
Gyro as prep	1 patty (2 oz)	145	tr	63
SHELF-STABLE				
Dinty Moore				
Microwave Cup Corned Beef Hash	1 cup (7.5 oz)	350	1	60
Microwave Cup Hearty Burger Stew	1 cup (7.5 oz)	240	3	40
Microwave Cup Stew	1 cup (7.5 oz)	190	2	40
Lunch Bucket				
Beef Stew	1 pkg (7.5 oz)	180	—	40
Micro Cup Meals				
Beef Stew	1 cup (7.5 oz)	180	2	30
TAKE-OUT				
roast beef sandwich plain	1	346	—	52
roast beef sandwich w/ cheese	1	402	—	77
roast beef submarine sandwich w/ tomato lettuce & mayonnaise	1	411	—	73
steak sandwich w/ tomato lettuce salt & mayonnaise	1	459	—	73
stew w/ vegetables	1 cup	220	—	71
stroganoff	¾ cup	260	—	69
swiss steak	4.6 oz	214	2	61
BEEFALO				
roasted	3 oz	160	—	49
BEER AND ALE				
alcohol free beer	7 fl oz	50	—	0
ale brown	10 oz	77	0	0
ale pale	10 oz	88	0	0
beer light	12 oz can	100	—	0
beer regular	12 oz can	146	—	0
lager	10 oz	80	0	0
pilsener lager beer	7 fl oz	85	—	0
stout	10 oz	102	0	0
Amstel				
Light	12 oz	95	—	0
Anheuser Busch				
Natural Light	12 oz	110	—	0

FOOD	PORTION	CALS.	FIB.	CHOL.
Bud				
Light	12 oz	108	—	0
Coors				
Beer	12 oz	132	—	0
Extra Gold	12 oz	147	—	0
Light	12 oz	101	—	0
Guinness				
Kaliber	12 oz	43	—	0
Hamm's				
Beer	12 oz	137	—	0
Nonalcoholic	12 oz	55	—	0
Killian's				
Beer	12 oz	212	—	0
Kingsbury				
Nonalcoholic	12 fl oz	60	—	0
Michelob				
Light	12 oz	134	—	0
Miller				
Lite	12 oz	96	—	0
Molson				
Light	12 oz	109	—	0
Old Milwaukee				
Beer	12 oz	145	—	0
Light	12 oz	122	—	0
Olympia				
Beer	12 oz	143	—	0
Pabst				
Beer	12 oz	143	—	0
Nonalcoholic	12 oz	55	—	0
Piels				
Light	12 oz	136	—	0
Schaefer				
Beer	12 oz	138	—	0
Light	12 oz	111	—	0
Schlitz				
Beer	12 oz	145	—	0
Light	12 oz	99	—	0
Schmidts				
Light	12 oz	96	—	0
Signature				
Beer	12 oz	150	—	0
Spirit				
Nonalcoholic	12 oz	80	—	0

FOOD	PORTION	CALS.	FIB.	CHOL.
Stroh				
Beer	12 oz	142	—	0
Light	12 oz	115	—	0
Winterfest				
Beer	12 oz	167	—	0
BEET JUICE				
juice	3½ oz	36	—	0
BEETS				
CANNED				
harvard	½ cup	89	—	0
pickled	½ cup	75	—	0
sliced	½ cup	27	—	0
Del Monte				
Pickled Crinkle Style Sliced	½ cup (4.5 oz)	80	2	0
Sliced	½ cup (4.3 oz)	35	2	0
Whole	½ cup (4.3 oz)	35	2	0
Whole Tiny	½ cup (4.3 oz)	35	2	0
S&W				
Diced Tender	½ cup	40	—	0
Julienne French Style	½ cup	40	—	0
Pickled Whole Extra Small	½ cup	70	—	0
Pickled w/ Red Wine Vinegar Sliced	½ cup	70	—	0
Sliced Small Premium	½ cup	40	—	0
Sliced Water Pack	½ cup	35	—	0
Whole Small	½ cup	40	—	0
Seneca				
Cut	½ cup	35	2	0
Diced	½ cup	35	2	0
Harvard	½ cup	90	1	0
Pickled	2 tbsp	20	0	0
Pickled With Onions	2 tbsp	20	0	0
Sliced	½ cup	35	2	0
Whole	½ cup	35	2	0
FRESH				
greens cooked	½ cup	20	—	0
greens raw	½ cup	4	—	0
greens raw chopped	½ cup	4	—	0
raw sliced	½ cup (2.4 oz)	29	—	0
sliced cooked	½ cup (3 oz)	38	—	0
whole cooked	2 (3.5 oz)	44	—	0
whole raw	2 (5.7 oz)	70	—	0

FOOD	PORTION	CALS.	FIB.	CHOL.

BEVERAGES

(*see* BEER AND ALE, CHAMPAGNE, COFFEE, DRINK MIXERS, FRUIT DRINKS, ICED TEA, LIQUOR/LIQUEUR, MALT, MILKSHAKE, MINERAL/BOTTLED WATER, SODA, SPORTS DRINKS, TEA/HERBAL TEA, WINE, WINE COOLERS)

BISCUIT

FROZEN

Jimmy Dean

FOOD	PORTION	CALS.	FIB.	CHOL.
Chicken Twin	2 (3.2 oz)	280	2	25
Sausage Twin	2 (3.4 oz)	330	2	30
Steak Twin	2 (3.2 oz)	270	2	25

Rudy's Farm

Ham Twin	2 (3 oz)	160	1	20
Sausage & Cheese Twin	2 (3 oz)	290	1	30
Sausage Twin	2 (2.7 oz)	296	1	30

Weight Watchers

Sausage Biscuit	1 (3 oz)	230	4	25

HOME RECIPE

buttermilk	1 (2 oz)	212	—	2
plain	1 (2 oz)	212	—	2

MIX

Arrowhead

Biscuit Mix	¼ cup (1.2 oz)	120	3	0

Bisquick

Mix	½ cup (2 oz)	240	—	0
Reduced Fat	½ cup (2 oz)	210	—	0

Health Valley

Buttermilk Biscuit Mix not prep	1 oz	100	3	0

Jiffy

As prep	1	150	2	3
Biscuit	¼ cup (1.1 oz)	130	1	0
Buttermilk as prep	1	170	tr	5

REFRIGERATED

buttermilk	1 (1 oz)	98	—	0

1869 Brand

Baking Powder	1	100	—	0
Butter Tastin'	1	100	—	0
Buttermilk	1	100	—	0

Ballard

Ovenready	1	50	—	0
Ovenready Buttermilk	1	50	—	0

Big Country

Southern Style	1	100	—	0

Hungry Jack

Butter Tastin' Flaky	1	90	—	0

FOOD	PORTION	CALS.	FIB.	CHOL.
Hungry Jack (CONT.)				
Buttermilk Flaky	1	90	—	0
Buttermilk Fluffy	1	90	—	0
Extra Rich Buttermilk	1	50	—	0
Flaky	1	80	—	0
Honey Tastin' Flaky	1	90	—	0
Pillsbury				
Big Country Butter Tastin'	1	100	—	0
Big Country Buttermilk	1	100	—	0
Butter	1	50	—	0
Buttermilk	1	50	—	0
Country	1	50	—	0
Deluxe Heat N' Eat Buttermilk	2	170	—	0
Good'N Buttery Fluffy	1	90	—	0
Hearty Grains Multi-Grain	1	80	—	0
Hearty Grains Oatmeal Raisin	1	90	—	0
Heat N' Eat Big Premium	2	280	—	0
Tender Layer Buttermilk	1	50	—	0
Roman Meal				
Biscuit	2 (2.4 oz)	180	1	0
Honey Nut Oat Bran	1 (1.5 oz)	131	1	0
TAKE-OUT				
plain	1 (35 g)	276	—	5
w/ egg	1	315	—	232
w/ egg & bacon	1	457	—	353
w/ egg & sausage	1	582	—	302
w/ egg & steak	1	474	—	272
w/ egg cheese & bacon	1	477	—	261
w/ ham	1	387	—	25
w/ sausage	1	485	—	34
w/ steak	1	456	—	26

BISON
roasted	3 oz	122	—	70

BLACK BEANS
CANNED

FOOD	PORTION	CALS.	FIB.	CHOL.
Allen				
Seasoned	½ cup (4.5 oz)	120	7	0
Eden				
Organic	½ cup (4.3 oz)	100	6	0
Health Valley				
Fast Menu Organic Black Beans With Tofu Weiners	7½ oz	150	15	0

FOOD	PORTION	CALS.	FIB.	CHOL.
Health Valley (CONT.)				
Fast Menu Western Black Beans With Garden Vegetable	7½ oz	160	14	0
Old El Paso				
Black Beans	½ cup (4.6 oz)	100	7	0
Refried	½ cup (4.2 oz)	120	6	0
Progresso				
Black Beans	½ cup (4.6 oz)	100	7	0
Trappey				
Seasoned	½ cup (4.5 oz)	120	7	0
DRIED				
cooked	1 cup	227	—	0
MIX				
Bean Cuisine				
Black Turtle	½ cup	115	5	0
Pasta & Beans Black Beans With Fusilli	½ cup	174	—	tr
Mahatma				
Black Beans & Rice	1 cup	200	6	0

BLACKBERRIES

FOOD	PORTION	CALS.	FIB.	CHOL.
CANNED				
in heavy syrup	½ cup	118	—	0
Allen-Wolco				
Blackberries	½ cup (5.3 oz)	60	9	0
FRESH				
blackberries	½ cup	37	3	0
FROZEN				
unsweetened	1 cup	97	—	0
Big Valley				
Blackberries	⅔ cup (4.9 oz)	70	4	0

BLACKEYE PEAS

FOOD	PORTION	CALS.	FIB.	CHOL.
CANNED				
w/pork	½ cup	199	—	17
Allen				
Blackeye Peas	½ cup (4.5 oz)	110	4	0
Fresh Shell	½ cup (4.4 oz)	120	6	0
With Bacon	½ cup (4.5 oz)	105	5	0
With Snaps	½ cup (4.4 oz)	120	5	0
Dorman				
Fresh Shell	½ cup (4.4 oz)	120	6	0
East Texas Fair				
Blackeye Peas	½ cup (4.5 oz)	110	4	0

FOOD	PORTION	CALS.	FIB.	CHOL.
East Texas Fair (CONT.)				
Fresh Shell	½ cup (4.4 oz)	120	6	0
With Snaps	½ cup (4.4 oz)	120	5	0
Homefolks				
Fresh Shell	½ cup (4.4 oz)	120	6	0
With Jalapeno	½ cup (4.4 oz)	120	5	0
With Snaps	½ cup (4.4 oz)	120	5	0
Sunshine				
With Bacon	½ cup (4.5 oz)	105	5	0
Trappey				
With Bacon	½ cup (4.5 oz)	120	5	0
With Bacon & Jalapeno	½ cup (4.4 oz)	110	5	0
DRIED				
cooked	1 cup	198	16	0
BLINTZE				
Empire				
Apple	2 (4.4 oz)	220	5	<5
Blueberry	2 (4.4 oz)	190	2	10
Cheese	2 (4.4 oz)	200	3	20
Cherry	2 (4.4 oz)	200	3	10
Potato	2 (4.4 oz)	190	3	10
Golden				
Apple Raisin	1 (2.25 oz)	80	—	10
Blueberry	1 (2.25 oz)	90	—	10
Cheese	1 (2.25 oz)	80	—	13
Cherry	1 (2.25 oz)	95	—	5
Potato	1 (2.25 oz)	90	—	5
TAKE-OUT				
cheese	2	186	tr	149
BLUEBERRIES				
CANNED				
in heavy syrup	1 cup	225	—	0
S&W				
In Heavy Syrup	½ cup	111	—	0
DRIED				
Sonoma				
Dried	¼ cup (1.3 oz)	140	5	0
FRESH				
blueberries	1 cup	82	—	0
FROZEN				
unsweetened	1 cup	78	—	0

FOOD	PORTION	CALS.	FIB.	CHOL.
Big Valley				
Blueberries	¾ cup (4.9 oz)	70	4	0
BLUEBERRY JUICE				
After The Fall				
Maine Coast	1 cup (8 oz)	90	0	0
BLUEFIN				
fillet baked	4.1 oz	186	—	88
BLUEFISH				
fresh baked	3 oz	135	—	64
BOK CHOY				
Dole				
Shredded	½ cup	5	—	0
BORAGE				
fresh chopped cooked	3½ oz	25	—	0
raw chopped	½ cup	9	—	0
BOYSENBERRIES				
in heavy syrup	1 cup	226	—	0
unsweetened frzn	1 cup	66	—	0
BOYSENBERRY JUICE				
Smucker's				
Juice	8 oz	120	—	0
BRAINS				
beef pan-fried	3 oz	167	—	1696
beef simmered	3 oz	136	—	1746
lamb braised	3 oz	124	—	1737
lamb fried	3 oz	232	—	2128
pork braised	3 oz	117	—	2169
veal braised	3 oz	115	—	2635
veal fried	3 oz	181	—	1802
Armour				
Pork Brains In Milk Gravy	⅔ cup (5.5 oz)	150	—	3500
BRAN				
corn	⅓ cup	56	21	0
oat cooked	½ cup	44	—	0
oat dry	½ cup	116	7	0
rice dry	⅓ cup	88	6	0
wheat dry	½ cup	65	13	0
Arrowhead				
Oat Bran	⅓ cup (1.4 oz)	150	7	0
Wheat Bran	¼ cup (0.6 oz)	30	6	0

FOOD	PORTION	CALS.	FIB.	CHOL.
Good Shepherd				
Wheat Bran	1 oz	80	3	0
H-O				
Super Bran	⅓ cup	110	3	0
Health Valley				
Fast Menu Oat Bran Pilaf With Garden Vegetables	7½ oz	210	15	0
Hodgson Mill				
Oat	¼ cup (1.3 oz)	120	6	0
Wheat	¼ cup (0.5 oz)	30	7	0
Kretschmer				
Toasted Wheat Bran	⅓ cup	57	3	0
Mother's				
Oat Bran	½ cup	150	6	0
Quaker				
Oat Bran	½ cup	150	6	0
Unprocessed	2 tbsp	8	3	0
Roman Meal				
Oat	1 oz	94	5	0
Stone-Buhr				
Oat	⅓ cup (1 oz)	90	4	0
BRAZIL NUTS				
dried unblanched	1 oz	186	—	0
BREAD				

(*see also* BAGEL, BISCUIT, BREADSTICKS, CROISSANT, ENGLISH MUFFIN, MUFFIN, ROLL, SCONE)

FOOD	PORTION	CALS.	FIB.	CHOL.
CANNED				
B&M				
Brown Bread	½ in slice (2 oz)	130	2	0
Brown Bread Raisins	½ in slice (2 oz)	130	2	0
S&W				
Brown Bread New England Recipe	2 slices	76	—	0
FROZEN				
Kineret				
Challah	⅛ loaf (2 oz)	150	1	15
HOME RECIPE				
banana	1 slice (2 oz)	195	—	26
cornbread as prep w/ 2% milk	1 piece (2.3 oz)	173	—	26
cornbread as prep w/ whole milk	1 piece (2.3 oz)	176	—	28
datenut	½ in slice	92	—	15
irish soda bread	1 slice (2 oz)	174	—	11
pita whole wheat	1 (6 in diam)	247	—	0

FOOD	PORTION	CALS.	FIB.	CHOL.
pumpkin	1 slice (1 oz)	94	—	13
white as prep w/ nonfat dry milk	1 slice	78	—	0
white as prep w/ 2% milk	1 slice	81	—	1
white as prep w/ whole milk	1 slice	82	—	1
whole wheat	1 slice	79	—	0
MIX				
cornbread	1 piece (2 oz)	189	1	37
Aunt Jemima				
Corn Bread Easy Mix	⅓ cup (1.3 oz)	150	1	0
Natural Ovens				
Cracked Wheat	2 slices (2.4 oz)	140	4	0
English Muffin Bread	2 slices (2.4 oz)	140	2	0
Executive Fitness Sunny Millet	2 slices (2.6 oz)	160	4	0
Garden Bread	1 oz	50	1	0
Glorious Cinnamon & Raisin Fat Free	2 slices (2.1 oz)	110	3	0
Honey 'N Flax	2 slices (2.5 oz)	140	4	0
Hunger Filler Bread	2 slices (2.1 oz)	110	5	0
Light Wheat	2 slices (2.2 oz)	84	5	0
Nutty Natural Wheat Bread	2 slices (2.5 oz)	140	6	0
Seven Grain Herb	2 slices (2.5 oz)	140	4	0
Soft Hearth Whole Wheat	2 slices (2 oz)	100	4	0
Soft Sandwich Very Low Fat	2 slices (2.3 oz)	110	2	0
Stay Slim	2 slices (2 oz)	100	4	0
Zia Foods				
Cornbread Blue Cornmeal	1 piece (1.2 oz)	110	—	41
READY-TO-EAT				
egg	1 slice (1.4 oz)	115	—	20
french	1 loaf (1 lb)	1270	—	0
french	1 slice (1 oz)	78	1	0
gluten	1 slice	47	—	0
italian	1 loaf (1 lb)	1255	—	0
italian	1 slice (1 oz)	81	1	0
navajo fry	1 (5 in diam)	296	—	0
navajo fry	1 (10.5 in diam)	527	—	0
oat bran	1 slice	71	1	0
oat bran reduced calorie	1 slice	46	—	0
oatmeal reduced calorie	1 slice	48	—	0
pita	1 reg (2 oz)	165	1	0
pita	1 sm (1 oz)	78	1	0
pita whole wheat	1 reg (2 oz)	170	5	0
pita whole wheat	1 sm (1 oz)	76	2	0
protein	1 slice	47	—	0
pumpernickel	1 slice	80	2	0

FOOD	PORTION	CALS.	FIB.	CHOL.
raisin	1 slice	71	—	0
rice bran	1 slice	66	—	0
rye	1 slice	83	2	0
rye reduced calorie	1 slice	47	—	0
seven grain	1 slice	65	2	0
sourdough	1 slice (1 oz)	78	1	0
vienna	1 slice (1 oz)	78	1	0
wheat berry	1 slice	65	1	0
wheat bran	1 slice	89	3	0
white	1 slice	67	1	0
white reduced calorie	1 slice	48	2	0
white toasted	1 slice	67	—	0
white cubed	1 cup	80	—	0
Alvarado St. Bakery				
Barley	1 slice (1.2 oz)	70	2	0
California Style	1 slice (1.2 oz)	60	2	0
French	1 slice (1.2 oz)	80	2	0
Multi-Grain	1 slice (1.2 oz)	60	2	0
Multi-Grain No-Salt	1 slice (1.2 oz)	60	2	0
Oat Berry	1 slice (1.2 oz)	70	2	0
Raisin	1 slice (1.1 oz)	80	2	0
Rye Seed	1 slice (1.2 oz)	60	2	0
Sourdough	1 slice (1.2 oz)	80	2	0
Wheat	1 slice (1.3 oz)	90	3	0
America's Own				
Wheat Cottage	1 slice	70	—	0
White Cottage	1 slice	70	—	0
Arnold				
12 Grain Natural	1 slice (0.8 oz)	60	1	0
Augusto Pan De Aqua	1 oz	80	1	0
Bran'nola Country Oat	1 slice (1.3 oz)	90	3	0
Bran'nola Dark Wheat	1 slice (1.3 oz)	90	3	0
Bran'nola Hearty Wheat	1 slice (1.3 oz)	100	3	0
Bran'nola Nutty Grains	1 slice (1.3 oz)	90	3	0
Bran'nola Original	1 slice (1.3 oz)	90	3	0
Cinnamon Chip	1 slice	80	tr	0
Cinnamon Raisin	1 slice (0.9 oz)	70	1	0
Country Bran Bakery Light	1 slice (0.8 oz)	40	3	0
Cranberry	1 slice (0.9 oz)	70	1	0
French Stick Savoni	1 oz	80	1	0
Italian Bakery Light	1 slice (0.7 oz)	40	1	0
Oatmeal Bakery	1 slice	60	2	0
Oatmeal Bakery Light	1 slice	40	2	0
Oatmeal Raisin	1 slice (0.9 oz)	60	2	0

FOOD	PORTION	CALS.	FIB.	CHOL.
Arnold (CONT.)				
Pumpernickel	1 slice (1.1 oz)	70	1	0
Rye Bakery Soft Light	1 slice (1.1 oz)	40	2	0
Rye Bakery Soft Seeded	1 slice (1.1 oz)	70	1	0
Rye Bakery Soft Unseeded	1 slice (1.1 oz)	70	1	0
Rye Dill	1 slice (1.1 oz)	60	1	0
Rye Real Jewish Dijon	1 slice	70	1	0
Rye Real Jewish Melba Thin	1 slice (0.7 oz)	40	1	0
Rye Real Jewish Unseeded	1 slice	80	1	0
Rye Real Jewish With Caraway	1 slice	70	1	0
Rye Real Jewish Without Seeds	1 slice (1.1 oz)	70	1	0
Sourdough Francisco	1 slice	90	1	0
Wheat Brick Oven	1 slice (0.8 oz)	60	2	0
Wheat Golden Light	1 slice (0.8 oz)	40	2	0
Wheat Natural	1 slice (1.3 oz)	80	2	0
Wheat Berry Honey	1 slice (1.1 oz)	80	2	0
White Brick Oven	1 slice (0.8 oz)	60	1	0
White Country	1 slice (1.3 oz)	100	1	0
White Extra Fiber Brick Oven	1 slice (0.9 oz)	50	2	0
White Light Brick Oven	1 slice (0.8 oz)	40	2	0
White Premium Light	1 slice	40	2	0
White Thin Sliced Brick Oven	1 slice	40	tr	0
Whole Wheat 100% Light Brick Oven	1 slice (0.8 oz)	40	3	0
Whole Wheat 100% Stoneground	1 slice (0.8 oz)	50	2	<5
August Bros.				
Pumpernickel	1 slice	80	1	0
Rye Onion	1 slice	80	1	0
Rye Thin Unseeded	1 slice	40	1	0
Rye With Seeds	1 slice (1 lb loaf)	80	1	0
Rye Without Seeds	1 slice	80	1	0
Rye N' Pump	1 slice	90	1	0
Beefsteak				
Pumpernickel	1 slice (1 oz)	70	1	0
Rye Hearty	1 slice (1 oz)	70	1	0
Rye Light	2 slices (1.6 oz)	70	5	0
Rye Mild	2 slices (1.4 oz)	90	2	0
Rye Soft	1 slice (1 oz)	70	1	0
Wheat Hearty	1 slice (1 oz)	70	1	0
Wheat Soft	1 slice (1 oz)	70	tr	0
White Robust	1 slice (1 oz)	70	tr	0
Bread Du Jour				
Austrian Wheat	3 in slice (1 oz)	130	2	0

FOOD	PORTION	CALS.	FIB.	CHOL.
Bread Du Jour (CONT.)				
French	3 in slice (1 oz)	130	1	0
Brownberry				
Bran'nola Country Oat	1 slice	90	3	0
Bran'nola Hearty Wheat	1 slice	88	3	0
Bran'nola Nutty Grains	1 slice	85	3	0
Bran'nola Original	1 slice	85	3	0
Health Nut	1 slice	71	3	0
Oatmeal Natural	1 slice	63	1	0
Oatmeal Soft	1 slice	48	2	0
Raisin Bran	1 slice	61	2	0
Raisin Cinnamon	1 slice	66	1	0
Raisin Walnut	1 slice	68	2	0
Wheat Apple Honey	1 slice	69	2	0
Wheat Soft	1 slice	74	1	0
Cedar's				
Mountain Bread Six Grain	1 piece (2.4 oz)	200	4	0
Damascus Bakeries				
Mountain Shepard Lahvash	⅓ loaf (2 oz)	135	2	0
Dicarlo's				
Foccaccia	⅛ bread (2 oz)	130	1	0
French Parisian	2 slices (1 oz)	70	tr	0
Freihofer's				
Country Potato	1 slice (1.3 oz)	100	1	0
Country White	1 slice (1.3 oz)	100	tr	0
Wheat	1½ slices	70	—	0
Wheat Light	1 slice (1.6 oz)	80	4	0
White Light	2 slices (1.6 oz)	80	4	0
Whole Wheat 100%	1 slice (1.3 oz)	90	2	0
Home Pride				
Hearty Buttermilk & Biscuit White	1 slice (1.3 oz)	100	tr	0
Hearty Deli Rye	1 slice (2 oz)	140	3	0
Hearty Golden Honey Wheat	1 slice (1.3 oz)	90	2	0
Hearty Honey Oats & Cracked Wheat	1 slice (1.4 oz)	100	2	0
Hearty Seven Grain Multi Grain	1 slice (1.3 oz)	100	2	0
Honey Wheat	1 slice (1 oz)	70	1	0
Seven Grain	1 slice (0.9 oz)	60	1	0
Wheat	1 slice (0.9 oz)	70	1	0
Wheat Light	3 slices (2.1 oz)	110	6	0
White	1 slice (0.9 oz)	70	0	0
White Grain	1 slice (1 oz)	60	1	0
White Light	3 slices (0.9 oz)	110	6	0

FOOD	PORTION	CALS.	FIB.	CHOL.
Home Pride (CONT.)				
Whole Wheat Hearty 100% Stoneground	1 slice (1.4 oz)	90	3	0
Malsovit				
Bread	1 slice	66	4	0
Raisin	1 slice	77	3	0
Matthew's				
9 Grain & Nut	1 slice	80	2	0
Cinnamon	1 slice	70	2	0
Golden	1 slice	70	1	0
Oat Bran	1 slice	65	2	0
Pita Whole Wheat	1	210	7	0
Sodium Free	1 slice	70	2	0
Whole Wheat	1 slice	70	2	0
Mediterranean Magic				
Focaccia	1/5 loaf (1.8 oz)	140	tr	0
Monks' Bread				
Hi-Fibre	1 slice	50	—	0
Raisin	1 slice	70	—	0
Sunflower & Bran	1 slice	70	2	0
White	1 slice	60	—	0
Whole Wheat 100% Stoneground	1 slice	70	—	0
Pepperidge Farm				
7 Grain Hearty Slice	2 slices	180	2	0
Cinnamon	1 slice	90	2	0
Cracked Wheat	1 slice	70	1	0
Crunchy Oat 1½ lb Loaf	2 slices	190	3	0
Date Walnut	1 slice	90	2	0
French Fully Baked	2 oz	150	1	0
French Twin	1 oz	80	0	0
Honey Bran	1 slice	90	1	0
Italian Brown & Serve	1 oz	80	0	0
Italian Sliced	1 slice	70	—	0
Oatmeal	1 slice	70	1	0
Oatmeal 1½ lb Loaf	1 slice	90	1	0
Oatmeal Light	1 slice	45	1	0
Oatmeal Very Thin Sliced	1 slice	40	—	0
Pumpernickel Family	1 slice	80	2	0
Pumpernickel Party	4 slices	60	1	0
Raisin With Cinnamon	1 slice	90	1	0
Rye Dijon	1 slice	50	1	0
Rye Dijon Thick Sliced	1 slice	70	2	0
Rye Family	1 slice (32 g)	80	2	0

FOOD	PORTION	CALS.	FIB.	CHOL.
Pepperidge Farm (CONT.)				
Rye Party	4 slices	60	1	0
Rye Seedless Family	1 slice	80	2	0
Rye Soft	1 slice	70	—	0
Sesame Wheat	2 slices	190	3	0
Sprouted Wheat	1 slice	70	2	0
Vienna Light	1 slice	45	1	0
Vienna Thick Sliced	1 slice	70	0	0
Wheat 1½ lb Loaf	1 slice	90	2	0
Wheat Family	1 slice	70	2	0
Wheat Light	1 slice	45	1	0
Wheat Very Thin Sliced	1 slice	35	0	0
White Country	2 slices	190	2	0
White Large Family Thin Slice	1 slice	70	0	0
White Sandwich	2 slices	130	0	0
White Thin Slice	1 slice	80	0	0
White Toasting	1 slice	90	1	0
White Very Thin Sliced	1 slice	40	0	0
Whole Wheat Thin Slice	1 slice	60	2	0
Roman Meal				
Brown & Serve Mini Loaf	½ loaf (2 oz)	136	1	0
Cracked Wheat	1 slice (1.4 oz)	92	2	0
Hearty Wheat Light	1 slice (0.8 oz)	42	2	0
Honey Nut Oat Bran	1 slice (1 oz)	72	1	0
Honey Oat Bran	1 slice (1 oz)	70	1	0
Oat	1 slice (1 oz)	69	1	0
Oat Bran	1 slice (1 oz)	68	1	0
Oat Bran Light	1 slice (0.8 oz)	42	2	0
Round Top	1 slice (1 oz)	67	1	0
Sandwich	1 slice (0.8 oz)	55	1	0
Seven Grain	1 slice (1 oz)	67	1	0
Seven Grain Light	1 slice (0.8 oz)	42	3	0
Sourdough Light	1 slice (0.8 oz)	41	3	0
Sourdough Whole Grain Light	1 slice (0.8 oz)	40	3	0
Sun Grain	1 slice (1 oz)	70	1	0
Twelve Grain	1 slice (1 oz)	70	1	0
Twelve Grain Light	1 slice (0.8 oz)	42	3	0
Wheat Light	1 slice (0.8 oz)	41	3	0
Wheatberry Honey	1 slice (1 oz)	67	1	0
Wheatberry Light	1 slice (0.8 oz)	42	2	0
White Light	1 slice (0.8 oz)	41	3	0
Whole Grain 100%	1 slice (1.4 oz)	91	2	0
Whole Grain Sourdough	1 slice (1 oz)	66	1	0
Whole Wheat 100%	1 slice (1 oz)	64	2	0

FOOD	PORTION	CALS.	FIB.	CHOL.
Roman Meal (CONT.)				
Whole Wheat 100% Light	1 slice (0.8 oz)	42	2	0
Sahara				
Pita Oat Bran	½ pocket (1 oz)	66	2	0
Stroehmann				
White Whole Special Recipe	1 slice	70	—	0
White Whole Special Recipe Kids	1 slice	60	—	0
Sunmaid				
Raisin	1 slice	70	1	0
Tree Of Life				
100% Spelt	1 slice (1.8 oz)	130	3	10
Millet	1 slice (1.8 oz)	130	2	0
Rye Sour Dough	1 slice (1.8 oz)	110	5	0
Sprouted Seven Grain	1 slice (1.8 oz)	110	2	0
Wonder				
Calcium Enriched	1 slice (1 oz)	70	tr	0
Cinnamon Raisin	1 slice (1 oz)	70	tr	0
Cracked Wheat	1 slice (1 oz)	70	1	0
French	1 slice (1 oz)	80	tr	0
French Light	2 slices (1.6 oz)	80	5	0
Granola	1 slice (1.5 oz)	100	2	0
Honey Bran Light	2 slices (1.6 oz)	80	6	0
Italian	1 slice (1.1 oz)	80	tr	0
Italian Family	1 slice (1 oz)	70	tr	0
Italian Light	2 slices (1.6 oz)	80	5	0
Kid	1 slice (0.9 oz)	70	tr	0
Light Calcium Enriched	2 slices (1.6 oz)	80	5	<5
Nine Grain Light	2 slices (1.6 oz)	80	6	0
Oatmeal Light	2 slices (1.6 oz)	90	4	0
Rye	1 slice (1 oz)	70	1	0
Rye Light	2 slices (1.6 oz)	70	5	0
Sourdough	1 slice (1.2 oz)	90	tr	0
Sourdough Light	2 slices (1.6 oz)	80	5	0
Texas Toast	1 slice (1.4 oz)	100	1	0
Vienna	1 slice (1 oz)	70	tr	0
Wheat Calcium Light	2 slices (1.6 oz)	80	6	0
Wheat Family	1 slice (0.9 oz)	70	tr	0
Wheat Golden Country Style	2 slices (1.4 oz)	100	1	0
Wheat Light	2 slices (1.6 oz)	80	6	0
White	1 slice (0.9 oz)	70	tr	0
White Calcium	2 slices (1.6 oz)	100	1	0
White Calcium Light	2 slices (1.6 oz)	80	5	0
White Light	2 slices (1.6 oz)	80	5	0

FOOD	PORTION	CALS.	FIB.	CHOL.
Wonder (CONT.)				
White With Buttermilk	1 slice (1 oz)	80	tr	0
Whole Wheat 100%	1 slice (1 oz)	70	2	0
Whole Wheat 100% Soft	2 slices (1.6 oz)	110	1	0
Whole Wheat 100% Stoneground	1 slice (1.2 oz)	80	2	0
ZA				
Pit-Za Hearty Multi-Grain	⅛ bread (2 oz)	130	2	0
Pit-Za Salt-Free Garlic Whole Wheat	⅛ bread (2 oz)	150	3	0
REFRIGERATED				
Pillsbury				
Crusty French Loaf	1 in slice	60	—	0
Hearty Grains Country Oatmeal Twists	1	80	—	0
Hearty Grains Cracked Wheat Twists	1	80	—	0
Pipin'Hot Wheat Loaf	1 in slice	70	—	0
Pipin'Hot White Loaf	1 in slice	70	—	0
Roman Meal				
Loaf	1 slice (1 oz)	85	1	0
Stefano's				
Stuffed Bread Broccoli & Cheese	½ bread (6 oz)	450	7	25
TAKE-OUT				
cornbread	2 in x 2 in (1.4 oz)	107	—	28
cornstick	1 (1.3 oz)	101	tr	30
focaccia onion	1 piece (4.6 oz)	282	2	0
focaccia rosemary	1 piece (3.5 oz)	251	2	0
focaccia tomato olive	1 piece (4.7 oz)	270	2	0
BREAD COATING				
Don's Chuck Wagon				
All Purpose Mix	¼ cup (1 oz)	100	1	0
Fish & Chips Mix	¼ cup (1 oz)	100	1	0
Fish Mix	¼ cup (1 oz)	95	1	0
Frying Mix Chicken	¼ cup (1 oz)	95	1	0
Frying Mix Seafood Seasoned	¼ cup (1 oz)	95	1	0
Mushroom Mix	¼ cup (1 oz)	95	1	0
Onion Ring Mix	¼ cup (1 oz)	100	1	0
Golden Dipt				
Breading Frying Mix	1 oz	90	—	0
Chicken Frying Mix	1 oz	90	—	0
Onion Ring Mix	1 oz	100	—	0

FOOD	PORTION	CALS.	FIB.	CHOL.
Ka-Me				
Tempura Batter Mix	1 oz	100	0	0
Little Crow				
Fryin' Magic	0.5 oz	43	—	0
Mrs. Dash				
Crispy Coating	2 tbsp (0.6 oz)	65	—	0
Shake 'N Bake				
Extra Crispy Oven Fry For Pork	¼ pkg (1 oz)	120	—	0
Italian Herb Recipe	¼ pkg (½ oz)	77	—	1
Original Barbecue For Chicken	¼ pkg (½ oz)	93	—	0
Original Barbecue For Pork	¼ pkg (½ oz)	38	—	0
Original Country Mild	¼ pkg (½ oz)	76	—	0
Original For Chicken	¼ pkg (½ oz)	75	—	0
Original For Fish	¼ pkg (½ oz)	73	—	0
Original For Pork	¼ pkg (½ oz)	41	—	0

BREAD MACHINE MIX

FOOD	PORTION	CALS.	FIB.	CHOL.
Dromedary				
Country White	½ in slice (2 oz)	140	1	0
Italian Herb	½ in slice (1.8 oz)	140	1	0
Stoneground Wheat	½ in slice (1.8 oz)	140	2	0
Pillsbury				
Cracked Wheat	¹⁄₁₂ pkg (1.3 oz)	130	2	0
Sassafras				
Apricot Oatmeal	1 slice (1.4 oz)	140	2	0
Wanda's				
Dried Tomato Cheddar	¼ cup mix per serv (1.2 oz)	140	3	0
European White	¼ cup mix per serv (1.2 oz)	130	1	0
Oatmeal	¼ cup mix per serv (1.2 oz)	120	1	0
Oatmeal Cinnamon	¼ cup mix per serv (1.2 oz)	120	1	0
Old World Rye	¼ cup mix per serv (1.9 oz)	90	3	0
Onion	¼ cup mix per serv (1.2 oz)	120	1	0
Orange Cinnamon	¼ cup mix per serv (1.3 oz)	130	1	0
Oregano Garlic	¼ cup mix per serv (1.2 oz)	130	2	0
Rosemary Basil	¼ cup mix per serv (1.2 oz)	130	1	0

FOOD	PORTION	CALS.	FIB.	CHOL.
Wanda's (CONT.)				
Rye	¼ cup mix per serv (1.2 oz)	120	1	0
Rye Caraway	¼ cup mix per serv (1.2 oz)	120	1	0
Sourdough	¼ cup mix per serv (1.2 oz)	120	1	0
Sunflower Sesame Poppyseed	¼ cup mix per serv (1.2 oz)	120	2	0
Ten Grain	¼ cup mix per serv (1.4 oz)	140	3	0
Wheat	¼ cup mix per serv (1.2 oz)	130	2	0
White	¼ cup mix per serv (1.2 oz)	130	1	0
Whole Wheat	¼ cup mix per serv (1.3 oz)	130	4	0

BREADCRUMBS

FOOD	PORTION	CALS.	FIB.	CHOL.
fresh	⅔ cup	76	1	0
Arnold				
Italian	½ oz	50	tr	0
Plain	½ oz	50	tr	0
Devonsheer				
Italian Style	1 oz	104	1	0
Plain	1 oz	108	1	0
Friday's				
Seasoned	1 oz	56	—	0
Jaclyn's				
Organic Whole Wheat Italian Style	½ oz	28	—	0
Organic Whole Wheat Plain	½ oz	28	—	0
Progresso				
Italian Style	¼ cup (1 oz)	110	1	0
Lemon Herb	¼ cup (0.9 oz)	100	2	0
Plain	¼ cup (1 oz)	100	1	0
Tomato Basil	¼ cup (1.1 oz)	120	2	0

BREADFRUIT

FOOD	PORTION	CALS.	FIB.	CHOL.
breadfruit	3.5 oz	109	—	0
fresh	¼ small	99	—	0
seeds cooked	1 oz	48	—	0
seeds raw	1 oz	54	—	0
seeds roasted	1 oz	59	—	0

FOOD	PORTION	CALS.	FIB.	CHOL.
BREADNUTTREE SEEDS				
dried	1 oz	104	—	0
BREADSTICKS				
onion poppyseed home recipe	1	64	—	10
plain	1	41	—	0
plain	1 sm	25	—	0
Angonoa				
Cheese	5 (1 oz)	120	1	0
Cheese Mini	16 (1 oz)	120	1	0
Garlic	6 (1 oz)	120	1	0
Italian Style Plain	5 (1 oz)	120	1	0
Low Sodium With Sesame Seed	6 (1 oz)	130	2	0
Onion	6 (1 oz)	120	2	0
Pizza Mini	26 (1 oz)	120	1	0
Sesame Mini	16 (1 oz)	130	2	0
Sesame Royale	6 (1 oz)	130	2	0
Whole Wheat Mini	14 (1 oz)	130	3	0
Bread Du Jour				
Italian	1 (1.9 oz)	130	1	0
Sourdough	1 (1.9 oz)	130	1	0
J.J. Cassone				
Garlic	1 (1.6 oz)	150	2	0
Keebler				
Garlic	2	30	—	0
Onion	2	30	—	0
Plain	2	30	—	0
Sesame	2	30	—	0
Lance				
Cheese	2	20	—	0
Garlic	2	30	—	0
Plain	2	30	—	0
Sesame	2	30	—	0
Pillsbury				
Soft Bread Sticks	1	100	—	0
Roman Meal				
Brown & Serve Soft	1 (2.7 oz)	181	3	0
Refrigerated	1 (1.4 oz)	117	1	0
Stella D'Oro				
Deli Garlic Fat Free	5	60	—	0
Deli Original Fat Free	5	60	—	0
Garlic	1	35	—	0
Grissini Garlic Fat Free	3	60	—	0

FOOD	PORTION	CALS.	FIB.	CHOL.
Stella D'Oro (CONT.)				
Grissini Original Fat Free	3	60	—	0
Onion	1	40	—	0
Regular	1	40	—	0
Regular Sodium Free	2	80	—	0
Sesame Low Fat	2	70	—	0
Sesame Sodium Free	1	50	—	0
Traditional Garlic Fat Free	2	70	—	0
Traditional Original Fat Free	2	70	—	0
Wheat	1	40	—	0

BREAKFAST BAR

(see also BREAKFAST DRINKS, NUTRITIONAL SUPPLEMENTS)

Carnation				
Chewy Chocolate Chip	1 (1.26 oz)	150	tr	0
Chewy Peanut Butter Chocolate Chip	1 (1.26 oz)	140	tr	0
Nutri-Grain				
Apple Cinnamon	1 (1.3 oz)	140	1	0
Blueberry	1 (1.3 oz)	140	1	0
Peach	1 (1.3 oz)	140	1	0
Raspberry	1 (1.3 oz)	140	1	0
Strawberry	1 (1.3 oz)	140	1	0

BREAKFAST DRINKS

(see also BREAKFAST BAR, NUTRITIONAL SUPPLEMENTS)

orange drink powder	3 rounded tsp	93	—	0
orange drink powder as prep w/ water	6 oz	86	—	0
Carnation				
Instant Breakfast Cafe Mocha	1 pkg + skim milk (9 fl oz)	220	1	6
Instant Breakfast Cafe Mocha	1 pkg	130	1	<5
Instant Breakfast Cafe Mocha	1 can (10 fl oz)	220	0	5
Instant Breakfast Classic Chocolate Malt	1 pkg + skim milk (9 fl oz)	220	1	6
Instant Breakfast Classic Chocolate Malt	1 pkg	130	1	<5
Instant Breakfast Creamy Milk Chocolate	1 pkg + skim milk (9 fl oz)	220	1	8
Instant Breakfast Creamy Milk Chocolate	1 pkg	130	1	<5
Instant Breakfast Creamy Milk Chocolate	8 fl oz	220	1	10
Instant Breakfast Creamy Milk Chocolate	1 can (10 fl oz)	220	1	5

FOOD	PORTION	CALS.	FIB.	CHOL.
Carnation (CONT.)				
Instant Breakfast French Vanilla	1 pkg	130	0	<5
Instant Breakfast French Vanilla	1 pkg + skim milk	220	0	6
Instant Breakfast No Sugar Added Classic Chocolate	1 pkg	70	1	<5
Instant Breakfast No Sugar Added Classic Chocolate	1 pkg + skim milk (9 fl oz)	160	1	6
Instant Breakfast No Sugar Added Creamy Milk Chocolate	1 pkg	70	1	<5
Instant Breakfast No Sugar Added Creamy Milk Chocolate	1 pkg + skim milk (9 fl oz)	160	1	6
Instant Breakfast No Sugar Added French Vanilla	1 pkg + skim milk (9 fl oz)	150	0	6
Instant Breakfast No Sugar Added French Vanilla	1 pkg	70	0	<5
Instant Breakfast No Sugar Added Strawberry Creme	1 pkg + skim milk (9 fl oz)	150	0	6
Instant Breakfast No Sugar Added Strawberry Creme	1 pkg	70	0	<5
Instant Breakfast Strawberry Creme	1 pkg + skim milk	220	0	6
Instant Breakfast Strawberry Creme	1 pkg	130	0	<5
BROAD BEANS				
canned	1 cup	183	—	0
dried cooked	1 cup	186	—	0
fresh cooked	3½ oz	56	—	0
BROCCOFLOWER				
fresh raw	½ cup (1.8 oz)	16	—	0
Dole				
Fresh	⅕ head	35	—	0
BROCCOLI				
FRESH				
chopped cooked	½ cup	22	2	0
raw chopped	½ cup	12	1	0
Dole				
Spear	1 med	40	5	0
FROZEN				
chopped cooked	½ cup	25	—	0
spears cooked	½ cup	25	3	0
spears cooked	10 oz pkg	69	4	0

FOOD	PORTION	CALS.	FIB.	CHOL.
Big Valley				
Chopped	¾ cup (3 oz)	25	2	0
Cuts	¾ cup (3 oz)	25	2	0
Birds Eye				
Baby Spears Deluxe	⅔ cup	30	3	0
Chopped	⅔ cup	25	3	0
Farm Fresh Spears	¾ cup	30	2	0
Florets Deluxe	½ cup	25	3	0
Polybag Cuts	½ cup	25	3	0
Polybag Deluxe Florets	⅔ cup	25	3	0
Spears	⅔ cup	25	3	0
With Cheese Sauce	½ pkg	110	1	15
Green Giant				
Cut	½ cup	16	2	0
Cuts	½ cup	12	2	0
Harvest Fresh Spears	½ cup	20	2	0
In Butter Sauce	½ cup	40	—	5
In Cheese Sauce	½ cup	60	2	2
Mini Spears Select	4-5 spears	18	3	0
One Serve Cuts In Butter Sauce	1 pkg	45	3	5
Valley Combinations Broccoli Fanfare	½ cup	80	—	0
Hanover				
Cut	½ cup	25	—	0
Florets	½ cup	30	—	0
Tree Of Life				
Broccoli	1 cup (3.1 oz)	25	2	0

BROWNIE
FROZEN
Pepperidge Farm

Monterey Hot Fudge Chocolate Chunk Brownie	1	480	—	65
Newport Hot Fudge Brownie	1	400	—	80
Weight Watchers				
Brownie A La Mode	1 (6.42 oz)	190	4	5
Chocolate Frosted Brownie	1 (1.25 oz)	100	3	0
Deluxe Fudge Brownie Parfait	1 (5.3 oz)	190	2	5
Peanut Butter Double Fudge	1 (1.23 oz)	110	3	0
HOME RECIPE				
plain	1 (0.8 oz)	112	1	17
w/nuts	1 (0.8 oz)	95	—	18
MIX				
plain	1 (1.2 oz)	139	1	9
plain low calorie	1 (0.8 oz)	84	1	0

FOOD	PORTION	CALS.	FIB.	CHOL.
Betty Crocker				
Brownie With Hot Fudge MicroRave Single	1	350	—	0
Frosted MicroRave	1	180	—	0
Fudge Family Size	1	150	—	10
Fudge Light	1	100	—	0
Fudge MicroRave	1	150	—	0
Fudge Regular Size	1	150	—	15
Supreme Caramel	1	120	—	10
Supreme Frosted	1	160	—	10
Supreme German Chocolate	1	160	—	10
Supreme Original	1	140	—	10
Supreme Party	1	160	—	10
Supreme Walnut	1	140	—	10
Walnut MicroRave	1	160	—	0
Estee				
Lite	2	100	1	0
Jiffy				
Fudge as prep	1	160	tr	7
READY-TO-EAT				
plain	1 lg (2 oz)	227	1	10
plain	1 sm (1 oz)	115	1	5
w/ nuts	1 (1 oz)	100	—	14
w/o nuts	1 (2 oz)	243	—	9
Frito Lay				
Fudge Nut	3 oz	360	—	8
Greenfield				
Brownie HomeStyle	1 (1.4 oz)	120	1	0
Hostess				
Brownie Bites	5 (2 oz)	260	2	50
Brownie Bites Walnut	5 (2 oz)	270	2	50
Lance				
Brownie	1 pkg (78 g)	320	—	5
Little Debbie				
Fudge	1 pkg (2.1 oz)	270	1	15
Fudge	1 pkg (3.6 oz)	450	2	20
Fudge	1 pkg (2.5 oz)	310	1	15
Fudge	1 pkg (2.9 oz)	360	1	15
Pepperidge Farm				
Charlotte Fudgey Brownie	1	220	2	25
Tahoe Milk Chocolate Pecan	1	210	1	25
Westport Fudgey Brownies w/ Walnuts	1	220	2	25

FOOD	PORTION	CALS.	FIB.	CHOL.
Sweet Rewards				
Double Fudge	1 (1.1 oz)	110	tr	0
Fat Free Brownie	1 bar (1 oz)	90	<1	0
Tastykake				
Brownie	1 (85 g)	340	5	20

BRUSSELS SPROUTS
FRESH

FOOD	PORTION	CALS.	FIB.	CHOL.
cooked	½ cup	30	3	0
cooked	1 sprout	8	—	0
raw	½ cup	19	—	0
raw	1 sprout	8	1	0
Dole				
Sprouts	½ cup	19	2	0
FROZEN				
cooked	½ cup	33	—	0
Big Valley				
Whole	5-8 pieces (3 oz)	35	1	0
Birds Eye				
Brussels Sprouts	½ cup	35	3	0
Green Giant				
In Butter Sauce	½ cup	40	—	5
Sprouts	½ cup	25	2	0
Hanover				
Brussels Sprouts	½ cup	40	—	0

BUCKWHEAT

FOOD	PORTION	CALS.	FIB.	CHOL.
flour whole groat	1 cup	402	—	0
groats roasted cooked	½ cup	91	—	0
groats roasted uncooked	½ cup	283	—	0
Wolff's				
Kasha Coarse cooked	¼ cup (1.6 oz)	170	2	0
Kasha Fine cooked	¼ cup (1.6 oz)	170	2	0
Kasha Medium cooked	¼ cup (1.6 oz)	170	2	0
Kasha Whole cooked	¼ cup (1.6 oz)	170	2	0

BUFFALO

FOOD	PORTION	CALS.	FIB.	CHOL.
water buffalo roasted	3 oz	111	—	52

BULGUR

FOOD	PORTION	CALS.	FIB.	CHOL.
cooked	½ cup	76	—	0
uncooked	½ cup	239	—	0
Casbah				
Pilaf Mix as prep	1 cup	200	4	0
Salad Mix as prep	⅔ cup	90	1	0

FOOD	PORTION	CALS.	FIB.	CHOL.
Good Shepherd				
Bulgur	¼ cup (43 g)	150	1	0
Hodgson Mill				
Bulgur	¼ cup (1.4 oz)	120	1	0

BURBOT (FISH)
fresh baked	3 oz	98	—	65

BURDOCK ROOT
cooked	1 cup	110	—	0
raw	1 cup	85	—	0

BUTTER
(*see also* BUTTER BLENDS, BUTTER SUBSTITUTES, MARGARINE)

FOOD	PORTION	CALS.	FIB.	CHOL.
clarified butter	3½ oz	876	—	256
stick	1 pat (5 g)	36	—	11
stick	1 stick (4 oz)	813	—	248
whipped	1 pat (4 g)	27	—	8
whipped	4 oz	542	—	165
Cabot				
Stick	1 tsp	35	—	11
Unsalted Stick	1 tsp	35	—	11
Crystal				
Salted Stick	1 tbsp (0.5 oz)	102	0	43
Unsalted Stick	1 tbsp (0.5 oz)	102	0	43
Land O'Lakes				
Light Stick	1 tbsp	50	—	20
Light Unsalted Stick	1 tbsp	50	—	15
Stick	1 tbsp (0.5 oz)	100	—	30
Unsalted Stick	1 tbsp (0.5 oz)	100	—	30
Unsalted Tub	1 tbsp	60	—	20
Whipped	1 tbsp (0.3 oz)	70	—	20

BUTTER BEANS
CANNED
FOOD	PORTION	CALS.	FIB.	CHOL.
Allen				
Baby	½ cup (4.5 oz)	120	6	0
Large	½ cup (4.5 oz)	120	7	0
Hanover				
Butter Beans	½ cup	80	—	0
In Sauce	½ cup	100	—	0
S&W				
Tender Cooked	½ cup	100	—	0
Sunshine				
Butter Beans	½ cup (4.5 oz)	120	8	0

FOOD	PORTION	CALS.	FIB.	CHOL.
Trappey				
Baby White With Bacon	½ cup (4.5 oz)	130	6	0
Large White With Bacon	½ cup (4.5 oz)	110	6	0
Van Camp's				
Butter Beans	½ cup	110	7	0

BUTTER BLENDS

(*see also* BUTTER, BUTTER SUBSTITUTES, MARGARINE)

stick	1 stick	811	—	99
Blue Bonnet				
Better Blend Tub	1 tbsp	90	—	0
Better Blend Unsalted Stick	1 tbsp	90	—	5
Country Morning				
Blend Light Stick	1 tbsp (0.5 oz)	50	—	10
Blend Light Tub	1 tbsp (0.5 oz)	50	—	5
Blend Stick	1 tbsp	100	—	0
Blend Tub	1 tbsp	100	—	0
Blend Unsalted Stick	1 tbsp	100	—	0
Downey's				
Cinnamon Honey-Butter Tub	1 tbsp	52	—	tr
Original Honey-Butter Tub	1 tbsp	52	—	tr
Le Slim Cow				
Tub	1 tbsp	40	—	7
Touch Of Butter				
Tub	1 tbsp (0.5 oz)	60	0	0

BUTTER SUBSTITUTES

(*see also* BUTTER BLENDS, MARGARINE)

Butter Buds				
Mix	1 tsp (2 g)	5	—	0
Sprinkles	1 tsp (2 g)	5	—	0
Molly McButter				
Cheese	1 tsp	5	—	0
Light Sodium	1 tsp	5	—	0
Natural Butter	1 tsp	5	—	0
Roasted Garlic	1 tsp	5	—	0
Mrs. Bateman's				
Butterlike Baking Butter	1 tbsp (0.5 oz)	36	0	<5
Butterlike Saute Butter	1 tbsp (0.5 oz)	40	0	5
Watkins				
Butter Sprinkles	1 tsp (2 g)	5	0	0
Imitation Butter Flavored Mist	1 tbsp (0.5 oz)	120	0	0

BUTTERBUR

canned fuki chopped	1 cup	3	—	0
fresh fuki raw	1 cup	13	—	0

FOOD	PORTION	CALS.	FIB.	CHOL.
BUTTERFISH				
baked	3 oz	159	—	71
fillet baked	1 oz	47	—	21
BUTTERNUTS				
dried	1 oz	174	—	0
BUTTERSCOTCH				
(see CANDY)				
CABBAGE				
FRESH				
chinese pak-choi raw shredded	½ cup	5	—	0
chinese pak-choi shredded cooked	½ cup	10	—	0
chinese pe-tsai raw shredded	1 cup	12	—	0
chinese pe-tsai shredded cooked	1 cup	16	—	0
danish raw	1 head (2 lbs)	228	18	0
danish raw shredded	½ cup (1.2 oz)	9	tr	0
danish shredded cooked	½ cup (2.6 oz)	17	1	0
green raw	1 head (2 lbs)	228	18	0
green raw shredded	½ cup (1.2 oz)	9	tr	0
green shredded cooked	½ cup (2.6 oz)	17	1	0
red raw shredded	½ cup	10	1	0
red shredded cooked	½ cup	16	—	0
savoy raw shredded	½ cup	10	—	0
savoy shredded cooked	½ cup	18	—	0
Dole				
Cabbage	1/12 med head	18	2	0
Napa shredded	½ cup	6	tr	0
Fresh Express				
Cole Slaw	1½ cups (3 oz)	25	2	0
HOME RECIPE				
coleslaw w/ dressing	¾ cup	147	—	5
TAKE-OUT				
coleslaw w/ dressing	½ cup	42	—	5
stuffed cabbage	1 (6 oz)	373	—	95
vinegar & oil coleslaw	3.5 oz	150	—	0
CAKE				
(see also BROWNIE, COOKIES, DANISH PASTRY, DOUGHNUTS, PIE)				
FROSTING/ICING				
chocolate as prep w/ butter	1 box (13.7 oz)	1908	—	121
chocolate as prep w/ butter	1/12 box (1.5 oz)	161	—	10
chocolate as prep w/ butter home recipe	1/12 recipe (1.8 oz)	200	—	15

FOOD	PORTION	CALS.	FIB.	CHOL.
chocolate as prep w/ butter home recipe	1 recipe (21.1 oz)	2409	—	176
chocolate as prep w/ margarine	1/12 box (1.5 oz)	161	—	0
chocolate as prep w/ margarine	1 box (13.7 oz)	1909	—	0
chocolate as prep w/ margarine home recipe	1 recipe (21.1 oz)	2411	—	5
chocolate as prep w/ margarine home recipe	1/12 recipe (1.8 oz)	200	—	0
chocolate ready-to-use	1/12 pkg (1.3 oz)	151	—	0
chocolate ready-to-use	1 pkg (16 oz)	1834	—	0
coconut ready-to-use	1/12 pkg (1.3 oz)	157	—	0
coconut ready-to-use	1 pkg (16 oz)	1903	—	0
cream cheese ready-to-use	1/12 pkg (1.3 oz)	157	—	0
cream cheese ready-to-use	1 pkg (16 oz)	1906	—	0
glaze home recipe	1 recipe (11.5 oz)	1173	—	7
glaze home recipe	1/12 recipe (1 oz)	97	—	1
seven minute home recipe	1/12 recipe (1.1 oz)	102	—	0
seven minute home recipe	1 recipe (13.6 oz)	1231	—	0
vanilla as prep w/ butter	1 pkg (14.5 oz)	2188	—	126
vanilla as prep w/ butter	1/12 pkg (1.5 oz)	182	—	10
vanilla as prep w/ butter home recipe	1 recipe (20.1 oz)	1972	—	67
vanilla as prep w/ butter home recipe	1/12 recipe (1.7 oz)	165	—	6
vanilla as prep w/ margarine	1 pkg (14.5 oz)	2190	—	0
vanilla as prep w/ margarine	1/12 pkg (1.5 oz)	182	—	0
vanilla as prep w/ margarine home recipe	1/12 recipe (1.7 oz)	195	—	0
vanilla as prep w/ margarine home recipe	1 recipe (20.1 oz)	2326	—	5
vanilla ready-to-use	1/12 pkg (1.3 oz)	159	—	0
vanilla ready-to-use	1 pkg (16 oz)	1936	—	0
Betty Crocker				
Butter Pecan Ready-to-Spread	1/12 tub	170	—	0
Cherry Ready-to-Spread	1/12 tub	160	—	0
Chocolate Ready-to-Spread	1/12 tub	160	—	0
Chocolate Chip Ready-to-Spread	1/12 tub	170	—	0
Chocolate Fudge as prep	1/12 mix	180	—	0
Chocolate Light Ready-to-Spread	1/12 tub	130	—	0
Chocolate With Candy Coated Chocolate Chips Ready-to-Spread	1/12 tub	160	—	0

FOOD	PORTION	CALS.	FIB.	CHOL.
Betty Crocker (CONT.)				
Chocolate With Dinosaurs Ready-to-Spread	1/12 tub	160	—	0
Chocolate With Turbo Racers Ready-to-Spread	1/12 tub	160	—	0
Coconut Pecan Ready-to-Spread	1/12 tub	160	—	0
Coconut Pecan as prep	1/12 mix	180	—	0
Cream Cheese Ready-to-Spread	1/12 tub	170	—	0
Creamy Milk Chocolate as prep	1/12 mix	170	—	0
Creamy Vanilla as prep	1/12 mix	170	—	0
Dark Dutch Fudge Ready-to-Spread	1/12 tub	160	—	0
Lemon Ready-to-Spread	1/12 tub	170	—	0
Milk Chocolate Light Ready-to-Spread	1/12 tub	140	—	0
Milk Chocolate Ready-to-Spread	1/12 tub	160	—	0
Rainbow Chip Ready-to-Spread	1/12 tub	170	—	0
Sour Cream Chocolate Ready-to-Spread	1/12 tub	160	—	0
Sour Cream White Ready-to-Spread	1/12 tub	160	—	0
Vanilla Ready-to-Spread	1/12 tub	160	—	0
Vanilla Light Ready-to-Spread	1/12 tub	140	—	0
Vanilla With Teddy Bears Ready-to-Spread	1/12 tub	160	—	0
White Fluffy as prep	1/12 mix	70	—	0
Duncan Hines				
Chocolate Creamy Homestyle	1 oz	130	2	0
Milk Chocolate Creamy Homestyle	1 oz	130	1	0
Vanilla Creamy Homestyle	1 oz	140	1	0
Estee				
Lite Frosting as prep	3 tbsp (0.7 oz)	100	0	0
Jiffy				
Fudge	1/4 cup (1.2 oz)	150	tr	0
White	1/4 cup (1.2 oz)	150	0	0
Pillsbury				
Fluffy White Frosting Mix	for 1/12 cake	60	—	0
Frost It Hot Chocolate	for 1/8 cake	50	—	0
Frost It Hot Fluffy White	for 1/8 cake	50	—	0
FROZEN				
boston cream pie	1/8 cake (3.2 oz)	232	1	34

FOOD	PORTION	CALS.	FIB.	CHOL.
eclair w/ chocolate icing & custard filling	1	205	—	35
Pepperidge Farm				
Amhurst Apple Crumb Coffee Cake	1	220	—	20
Apple 'N Spice Bake Dessert Lights	1 piece (4¼ oz)	170	—	10
Berkshire Apple Crisp	1	250	1	40
Boston Cream Supreme	1 piece (2⅞ oz)	290	—	50
Butter Pound	1 slice (1 oz)	130	—	60
Carrot Classic	1 cake	260	—	50
Carrot w/ Cream Cheese Icing	1 slice (1½ oz)	150	—	15
Charleston Peach Melba Shortcake	1	220	—	135
Cherries Supreme Dessert Lights	1 piece (3¼ oz)	170	—	80
Chocolate Supreme	1 piece (2⅞ oz)	300	—	25
Chocolate Fudge Large Layer	1 slice (1⅝ oz)	180	—	20
Chocolate Fudge Strip Large Layer	1 piece (1⅝ oz)	170	—	20
Chocolate Mousse Cake Dessert Lights	1 piece (2½ oz)	190	—	5
Cholesterol Free Pound	1 slice (1 oz)	110	—	0
Coconut Classic	1 cake	230	—	20
Coconut Large Layer	1 slice (1⅝ oz)	180	—	20
Devil's Food Large Layer	1 slice (1⅝ oz)	180	—	20
Double Chocolate Classic	1 cake	250	—	35
Fudge Golden Classic	1 cake	260	—	40
German Chocolate Classic	1 cake	250	—	45
German Chocolate Large Layer	1 slice (1⅝ oz)	180	—	20
Golden Large Layer	1 slice (1⅝ oz)	180	—	20
Lemon Cake Supreme Dessert Lights	1 piece (2¾ oz)	170	—	50
Lemon Coconut Supreme	1 piece (3 oz)	280	—	30
Lemon Cream Supreme	1 piece (1⅝ oz)	170	—	20
Manhattan Strawberry Cheesecake	1	300	—	150
Peach Melba Supreme	1 (3⅛ oz)	270	—	35
Peach Parfait Dessert Lights	1 piece (4¼ oz)	150	—	10
Pineapple Cream Supreme	1 piece (2 oz)	190	—	20
Raspberry Vanilla Swirl Dessert Lights	1 piece (3¼ oz)	160	—	15
Strawberry Shortcake Dessert Lights	1 piece (3 oz)	170	1	70

FOOD	PORTION	CALS.	FIB.	CHOL.
Pepperidge Farm (CONT.)				
Strawberry Cream Supreme	1 piece (2 oz)	190	—	20
Strawberry Strip Large Layer	1 piece (1½ oz)	160	—	20
Vanilla Fudge Swirl Classic	1 cake	250	—	35
Vanilla Large Layer	1 slice (1⅝ oz)	190	—	20
Sara Lee				
Apple Crisp Light	1 (3 oz)	150	—	5
Black Forest Light	1 (3.6 oz)	170	—	10
Carrot Light	1 (2.5 oz)	170	—	5
Carrot Single Layer Iced	1 slice (2.4 oz)	250	—	25
Chocolate Free & Light	1 slice (1.7 oz)	110	—	0
Double Chocolate Light	1 (2.5 oz)	150	—	10
Double Chocolate Three Layer	1 slice (2.2 oz)	220	—	20
French Cheesecake Light	1 (3.2 oz)	150	—	15
French Cheese	1 slice (2.9 oz)	250	—	20
Lemon Cream Light	1 (3.2 oz)	180	—	10
Pound Free & Light	1 slice (1 oz)	70	—	0
Strawberry French Cheesecake Light	1 (3.5 oz)	150	—	5
Strawberry Yogurt Dessert Free & Light	1 slice (2.2 oz)	120	—	0
Weight Watchers				
Brownie Cheesecake	1 cake (3.5 oz)	200	4	5
Caramel Fudge A La Mode	1 cake (6.07 oz)	180	0	0
Chocolate Eclair	1 (2.1 oz)	150	2	0
Coffee Cake Cinnamon Streusel	1 (2.25 oz)	190	2	0
Double Fudge	1 piece (2.75 oz)	190	2	0
Strawberry Cheesecake	1 (3.9 oz)	190	5	15
Strawberry Shortcake A La Mode	1 (6.49 oz)	180	1	5
Toasted Almond Amaretto Cheesecake	1 (3 oz)	170	3	5
Triple Chocolate Cheesecake	1 (3.15 oz)	200	1	10
HOME RECIPE				
angelfood	1/12 cake (1.9 oz)	142	1	0
apple crisp	1 recipe 6 serv (29.6 oz)	1377	—	1
apple crisp	½ cup (5 oz)	230	—	0
boston cream pie	1/6 cake (3.3 oz)	293	1	43
carrot w/ cream cheese icing	1/12 cake (3.9 oz)	484	—	60
carrot w/ cream cheese icing	1 cake 10 in diam	6175	—	1183
cheesecake	1/12 cake (4.5 oz)	456	—	155
cheesecake w/ cherry topping	1/12 cake (5 oz)	359	—	106
chocolate cupcake creme filled w/ frosting	1 (1.8 oz)	188	—	9

FOOD	PORTION	CALS.	FIB.	CHOL.
chocolate w/o frosting	1/12 cake (3.3 oz)	340	—	55
chocolate w/o frosting	2 layers (39.9 oz)	4067	—	661
coffeecake crumb topped cinnamon	1/12 cake (2.1 oz)	240	2	36
cream puff shell	1 (2.3 oz)	239	—	129
cream puff w/ custard filling	1 (4.6 oz)	336	—	174
eclair	1 (3 oz)	262	—	127
fruitcake	1/36 cake (2.9 oz)	302	3	24
fruitcake dark	1 cake 7½ in x 2¼ in	5185	—	640
gingerbread	1/9 cake (2.6 oz)	264	2	24
pineapple upside down	1/9 cake (4 oz)	367	—	25
pound	1 loaf 8½ in x 3½ in	1935	—	1100
pound cake	1 slice (1 oz)	120	—	32
sheet cake w/ white frosting	1 cake 9 in sq	4020	—	636
sheet cake w/ white frosting	1/9 cake	445	—	70
sheet cake w/o frosting	1 cake 9 in sq	2830	—	552
sheet cake w/o frosting	1/9 cake	315	—	61
shortcake	1 (2.3 oz)	225	—	2
sponge	1/12 cake (2.2 oz)	140	—	80
white w/ coconut frosting	1/12 cake (3.9 oz)	399	—	2
white w/o frosting	1/12 cake (2.6 oz)	264	—	2
yellow w/o frosting	1/12 cake (2.4 oz)	245	—	37
yellow w/o frosting	2 layers (28.7 oz)	2947	—	443
MIX				
angelfood	10 in cake (20.9 oz)	1535	9	0
angelfood	1/12 cake (1.8 oz)	129	1	0
chocolate w/o frosting	1/12 cake (2.3 oz)	198	—	35
chocolate w/o frosting	2 layers (26.8 oz)	2393	—	425
chocolate w/o frosting low sodium	1/10 cake (1.3 oz)	116	—	0
coffeecake crumb topped cinnamon	1/8 cake (2 oz)	178	2	28
devil's food w/o frosting	1/12 cake (2.3 oz)	198	—	35
devil's food w/ chocolate frosting	1 cake 9 in diam	3755	—	598
devil's food w/ chocolate frosting	1/16 cake	235	—	37
fudge w/o frosting	1/12 cake (2.3 oz)	198	—	35
german chocolate pudding type w/ coconut nut frosting	1/12 cake (3.9 oz)	404	—	53
gingerbread	1 cake 8 in sq	1575	—	6
gingerbread	1/9 cake (2.4 oz)	207	2	24
lemon w/o frosting no sugar low sodium	1/10 cake (1.3 oz)	118	—	0
marble pudding type w/o frosting	2 layers (30.6 oz)	3021	—	638

FOOD	PORTION	CALS.	FIB.	CHOL.
marble pudding type w/o frosting	1/12 cake (2.6 oz)	253	—	53
white w/o frosting no sugar low sodium	1/10 cake (1.3 oz)	118	—	0
yellow w/ chocolate frosting	1/16 cake	235	—	36
yellow w/o frosting	2 layers (26.5 oz)	2415	—	437
yellow w/o frosting	1/12 cake (2.2 oz)	202	—	37
yellow w/ chocolate frosting	1 cake 9 in diam	3895	—	609
Aunt Jemima				
Coffee Cake Easy Mix	1/3 cup (1.4 oz)	170	1	0
Betty Crocker				
Angel Food Confetti	1/12 cake	150	—	0
Angel Food Traditional	1/12 cake	130	—	0
Angel Food White	1/12 cake	150	—	0
Angel Food Lemon Custard	1/12 cake	150	—	0
Apple Streusel MicroRave	1/6 cake	240	—	45
Apple Streusel MicroRave No Cholesterol Recipe	1/6 cake	210	—	0
Butter Chocolate	1/12 cake	280	—	75
Butter Pecan No Cholesterol Recipe	1/12 cake	220	—	0
Butter Pecan SuperMoist	1/12 cake	250	—	55
Butter Yellow	1/12 cake	260	—	75
Carrot	1/12 cake	250	—	55
Carrot No Cholesterol Recipe	1/12 cake	210	—	0
Cherry Chip	1/12 cake	190	—	0
Chocolate Chocolate Chip	1/12 cake	260	—	55
Chocolate Chip	1/12 cake	290	—	55
Chocolate Chip No Cholesterol Recipe	1/12 cake	220	—	0
Chocolate Fudge	1/12 cake	260	—	55
Cinnamon Pecan Streusel Microwave	1/6 cake	280	—	35
Cinnamon Pecan Streusel Microwave No Cholesterol	1/6 cake	230	—	0
Devil's Food	1/12 cake	260	—	55
Devil's Food Chocolate Frosting MicroRave	1/6 cake	310	—	35
Devil's Food No Cholesterol Recipe	1/12 cake	220	—	0
Devil's Food SuperMoist Light	1/12 cake	200	—	55
Devil's Food SuperMoist Light No Cholesterol Recipe	1/12 cake	180	—	0
Devils Food With Chocolate Frosting MicroRave Single	1	440	—	50

FOOD	PORTION	CALS.	FIB.	CHOL.
Betty Crocker (CONT.)				
German Chocolate	1/12 cake	260	—	55
German Chocolate Chocolate Frosting MicroRave	1/6 cake	320	—	35
German Chocolate No Cholesterol Recipe	1/12 cake	220	—	0
Gingerbread Classic Dessert	1/9 cake	22	—	30
Gingerbread Classic Dessert No Cholesterol Recipe	1/9 cake	210	—	0
Golden Pound Classic Dessert	1/12 cake	200	—	35
Golden Vanilla	1/12 cake	280	—	55
Golden Vanilla No Cholesterol Recipe	1/12 cake	220	—	0
Golden Vanilla Rainbow Chip Frosting MicroRave	1/6 cake	320	—	35
Lemon	1/12 cake	260	—	55
Lemon No Cholesterol Recipe	1/12 cake	220	—	0
Marble	1/12 cake	260	—	55
Marble No Cholesterol Recipe	1/12 cake	220	—	0
Milk Chocolate	1/12 cake	260	—	55
Milk Chocolate No Cholesterol Recipe	1/12 cake	210	—	0
Pineapple Upsidedown Classic Dessert	1/9 cake	250	—	40
Rainbow Chip	1/12 cake	250	—	55
Sour Cream Chocolate	1/12 cake	260	—	55
Sour Cream Chocolate No Cholesterol Recipe	1/12 cake	220	—	0
Sour Cream White	1/12 cake	180	—	0
Spice	1/12 cake	260	—	55
Spice No Cholesterol Recipe	1/12 cake	220	—	0
White	1/12 cake	240	—	0
White No Cholesterol Recipe	1/12 cake	220	—	0
White SuperMoist Light	1/12 cake	180	—	0
Yellow	1/12 cake	260	—	55
Yellow Chocolate Frosting MicroRave	1/6 cake	300	—	35
Yellow No Cholesterol Recipe	1/12 cake	220	—	0
Yellow SuperMoist Light	1/12 cake	200	—	55
Yellow SuperMoist Light No Cholesterol Recipe	1/12 cake	190	—	0
Yellow With Chocolate Frosting MicroRave Single	1	440	—	50
Bisquick				
Mix	1/2 cup (2 oz)	240	—	0

FOOD	PORTION	CALS.	FIB.	CHOL.
Bisquick (CONT.)				
Reduced Fat	½ cup (2 oz)	210	—	0
Duncan Hines				
Angel Food	1/12 pkg (1.3 oz)	140	1	0
Cupcake Yellow With Chocolate Frosting	1	180	—	6
Devil's Food Moist Deluxe	1/12 cake (1.5 oz)	290	1	45
French Vanilla Moist Deluxe	1/12 cake (1.5 oz)	250	0	45
Fudge Marble Moist Deluxe	1/12 cake (1.5 oz)	250	0	45
Lemon Supreme Moist Deluxe	1/12 cake (1.5 oz)	250	0	45
Yellow Moist Deluxe	1/12 cake (1.5 oz)	250	—	45
Estee				
Lite White as prep	1/5 cake (1.7 oz)	200	tr	0
Lite Chocolate	1/5 cake (1.7 oz)	190	1	0
Lite Pound as prep	1/5 cake (1.7 oz)	200	tr	0
Jell-O				
Cheesecake	1/8 cake	277	—	28
Cheesecake New York Style	1/8 cake	283	—	28
Jiffy				
Devil's Food as prep	1/5 cake	220	1	42
Golden Yellow as prep	1/5 cake	220	1	36
White as prep	1/5 cake	210	tr	0
Royal				
Cheese Cake Lite No-Bake	1/8 pie	130	—	5
Wanda's				
Double Chocolate	¼ cup mix per serv (1.4 oz)	170	2	0
READY-TO-EAT				
angelfood	1 cake (11.9 oz)	876	5	0
angelfood	1/12 cake (1 oz)	73	1	0
cheesecake	1/6 cake (2.8 oz)	256	2	44
cheesecake	1 cake 9 in diam	3350	—	2053
coffeecake crumb topped cinnamon	1/8 cake (2.2 oz)	263	2	20
fruitcake	1 piece (1.5 oz)	139	—	2
panettone dal forno	1/8 cake (1.9 oz)	212	0	25
pound	1 cake (8½ x 3½ x 3 in)	1935	—	1100
pound	1/10 cake (1 oz)	117	—	66
pound fat free	1 oz	80	—	0
pound fat free	1 cake (12 oz)	961	—	0
sour cream pound	1/10 cake (1 oz)	117	tr	17
sponge	1/12 cake (1.3 oz)	110	—	39
tiramisu	1 piece (5.1 oz)	409	tr	171

FOOD	PORTION	CALS.	FIB.	CHOL.
tiramisu	1 cake (4.4 lbs)	5732	3	2395
white w/ white frosting	1 cake 9 in diam	4170	—	46
white w/ white frosting	1/16 cake	260	—	3
yellow w/ chocolate frosting	1 cake 9 in diam	3895	—	609
yellow w/ chocolate frosting	1/8 cake (2.2 oz)	242	1	35
Baker Maid				
Creole Royal Pineapple Apricot	1 slice (1.7 oz)	90	1	5
Creole Royal Pineapple Apricot	3 slices (5 oz)	270	4	20
Dutch Mill				
Dessert Shells Chocolate Covered	1 (0.5 oz)	80	0	0
Freihofer's				
Angel Food	1/5 cake (2 oz)	150	0	0
Cinnamon Swirl Buns	1 (2.8 oz)	290	1	30
Coffee Cake Cinnamon Pecan	1/8 cake (2 oz)	220	1	25
Crumb	1/8 cake (2 oz)	240	1	15
Homestyle Golden Loaf	1/8 cake (1.8 oz)	200	0	50
Pound	1/5 cake (2.8 oz)	330	0	65
Hostess				
Angel Food Ring	1/6 cake (1.6 oz)	150	0	<5
Fruit Cake Holiday	1/6 cake (5.3 oz)	490	3	10
Pound Cake	1/5 cake (3.2 oz)	350	1	55
Perugina				
Pannettone Au Beurre	1/6 cake (2.9 oz)	310	2	110
Sinbad				
Baklava	1 piece (2 oz)	337	2	10
Thomas'				
Date Nut Loaf	1 oz	90	1	<5
REFRIGERATED				
Baby Watson				
Cheesecake	1 slice (3.8 oz)	390	2	142
Cheesecake Light	1/16 cake (3.9 oz)	280	3	33
Pillsbury				
Apple Turnovers	1	170	—	0
Cherry Turnovers	1	170	—	0
Coffee Cake Cinnamon Swirl	1/8 of cake	180	—	0
Coffee Cake Pecan Streusel	1/8 of cake	180	—	0
Pastry Pockets	1	240	—	0
SNACK				
devil's food cupcake w/ chocolate frosting	1	120	—	19
devil's food w/ creme filling	1 (1 oz)	105	—	15
sponge w/ creme filling	1 (1.5 oz)	155	—	7

FOOD	PORTION	CALS.	FIB.	CHOL.
Drake's				
Coffee Cake	1 (1.1 oz)	140	—	10
Coffee Cake Chocolate Crumb	1 (2.5 oz)	245	—	18
Coffee Cake Cinnamon Crumb	¹⁄₁₂ cake (1.3 oz)	150	—	10
Coffee Cake Small	1 (2 oz)	220	—	15
Devil Dog	1 (1.5 oz)	160	—	0
Funny Bones	1 (1.25 oz)	150	—	0
Light & Fruity Apple	1 (1.2 oz)	90	—	0
Light & Fruity Blueberry	1 (1.2 oz)	90	—	0
Light & Fruity Cinnamon Raisin	1 (1.2 oz)	90	—	0
Pound Cake	1	110	—	25
Ring Ding	1 (1.5 oz)	180	—	0
Ring Ding Mint	1 (1.5 oz)	190	—	0
Sunny Doodle	1 (1 oz)	100	—	10
Yankee Doodle	1 (1 oz)	100	—	0
Yodel's	1 (1 oz)	150	—	5
Greenfield				
Blondie Apple Spice	1 (1.4 oz)	120	0	0
Blondie Chocolate Chip	1 (1.4 oz)	120	0	0
Hostess				
Apple Twist	1 (2.5 oz)	220	tr	15
Baseball Yellow Cakes	1 (1.6 oz)	160	0	<5
Choco Licious	1 (1.5 oz)	170	1	10
Choco-Diles	1 (1.8 oz)	210	1	20
Cinnaminis Original	5 (2.4 oz)	300	2	20
Cinnamon Roll	1 (2.3 oz)	220	1	25
Crumb Cake	1 (1.9 oz)	210	1	15
Crumb Cake Light	1 (1.8 oz)	150	tr	0
Cup Cakes Chocolate	1 (1.6 oz)	170	tr	<5
Cup Cakes Chocolate Light	1 (1.4 oz)	120	tr	0
Cup Cakes Orange	1 (1.5 oz)	160	0	10
Dessert Cups	1 (1 oz)	90	0	10
Ding Dongs	1 (1.3 oz)	160	tr	5
Fruit Loaf	1 (3.8 oz)	350	2	5
Ho Ho's	1 (1 oz)	130	tr	10
Holiday Cakes	1 (1.6 oz)	160	0	<5
Honey Bun Glazed	1 (2.7 oz)	320	2	15
Honey Bun Iced	1 (3.4 oz)	390	2	15
Hopper Cakes	1 (1.6 oz)	160	0	<5
Lil Angels	1 (1 oz)	90	0	<5
Pecan Spinners	1 (1 oz)	110	tr	0
Sno Balls	1 (1.6 oz)	160	1	0
Suzy Q's	1 (2 oz)	220	2	10
Suzy Q's Banana	1 (2 oz)	220	tr	25

FOOD	PORTION	CALS.	FIB.	CHOL.
Hostess (CONT.)				
Swirls Caramel Pecan	1 (2 oz)	140	1	15
Tiger Tails	1 (1.5 oz)	160	tr	15
Twinkies	1 (1.4 oz)	140	0	15
Twinkies Banana	2 (2.7 oz)	300	tr	35
Twinkies Devil Food	2 (2.7 oz)	300	2	15
Twinkies Lights	1 (1.4 oz)	120	0	0
Twinkies Strawberry Fruit 'n Creme	1 (1.6 oz)	150	tr	20
Kellogg's				
Pop-Tarts Apple Cinnamon	1 (1.8 oz)	210	1	0
Pop-Tarts Blueberry	1 (1.8 oz)	210	1	0
Pop-Tarts Brown Sugar Cinnamon	1 (1.8 oz)	220	1	0
Pop-Tarts Cherry	1 (1.8 oz)	200	1	0
Pop-Tarts Chocolate Graham	1 (1.8 oz)	210	1	0
Pop-Tarts Frosted Blueberry	1 (1.8 oz)	200	1	0
Pop-Tarts Frosted Brown Sugar Cinnamon	1 (1.8 oz)	210	1	0
Pop-Tarts Frosted Cherry	1 (1.8 oz)	200	1	0
Pop-Tarts Frosted Chocolate Vanilla Creme	1 (1.8 oz)	200	1	0
Pop-Tarts Frosted Chocolate Fudge	1 (1.8 oz)	200	1	0
Pop-Tarts Frosted Grape	1 (1.8 oz)	200	1	0
Pop-Tarts Frosted Raspberry	1 (1.8 oz)	210	1	0
Pop-Tarts Frosted S'mores	1 (1.8 oz)	200	1	0
Pop-Tarts Frosted Strawberry	1 (1.8 oz)	200	1	0
Pop-Tarts Strawberry	1 (1.8 oz)	200	1	0
Pop-Tarts Minis Frosted Chocolate	1 pkg (1.5 oz)	170	1	0
Pop-Tarts Minis Frosted Grape	1 pkg (1.5 oz)	170	0	0
Pop-Tarts Minis Frosted Strawberry	1 pkg (1.5 oz)	170	0	0
Rice Krispies Treats	1 (0.8 oz)	90	0	0
Lance				
Apple Oatmeal	1 pkg (51 g)	200	—	10
Dunking Sticks	1 (39 g)	190	—	5
Fig Cake	1 pkg (60 g)	210	—	0
Honey Buns	1 (85 g)	330	—	0
Oatmeal Cake	1 (57 g)	240	—	0
Pecan Twirls	1 pkg (57 g)	220	—	0
Raisin Cake	1 (57 g)	230	—	0

FOOD	PORTION	CALS.	FIB.	CHOL.
Little Debbie				
Apple Delights	1 pkg (1.2 oz)	140	1	5
Apple-Roos	1 pkg (1.5 oz)	150	1	0
Banana Nut Muffin Loaves	1 pkg (1.9 oz)	210	1	10
Banana Twins	1 pkg (2.2 oz)	250	0	10
Be My Valentine	1 pkg (2.2 oz)	280	1	0
Cherry Cordials	1 pkg (1.3 oz)	160	1	0
Choc-o-Jel	1 pkg (1.2 oz)	150	1	0
Choco-Cakes	1 pkg (2.2 oz)	240	1	0
Choco-Cakes	1 pkg (2.1 oz)	250	1	0
Chocolate	1 pkg (3 oz)	360	1	0
Chocolate Chip	1 pkg (2.4 oz)	290	1	0
Chocolate Twins	1 pkg (2.4 oz)	240	1	20
Christmas Tree Cakes	1 pkg (1.5 oz)	190	0	0
Coconut	1 pkg (2.1 oz)	270	1	5
Coconut	1 pkg (2.4 oz)	300	0	5
Coconut Rounds	1 pkg (1.2 oz)	140	1	0
Coffee Cake Apple	1 pkg (1.9 oz)	220	1	10
Coffee Cake Apple Streusel	1 pkg (2 oz)	220	1	10
Devil Cremes	1 pkg (1.6 oz)	190	0	0
Devil Cremes	1 pkg (3.2 oz)	380	1	5
Devil Squares	1 pkg (2.2 oz)	260	1	0
Easter Basket Cakes	1 pkg (2.5 oz)	310	1	0
Fancy Cakes	1 pkg (2.4 oz)	300	0	0
Fudge Crispy	1 pkg (1.1 oz)	170	1	0
Fudge Rounds	1 pkg (2.5 oz)	290	2	5
Fudge Rounds	1 pkg (3 oz)	350	2	5
Fudge Rounds	1 pkg (1.2 oz)	140	1	5
Golden Cremes	1 pkg (1.5 oz)	170	0	0
Golden Cremes	1 pkg (3 oz)	330	0	10
Holiday Cake Chocolate	1 pkg (2.4 oz)	290	1	0
Holiday Cake Vanilla	1 pkg (2.5 oz)	310	1	0
Honey Bun	1 pkg (3 oz)	380	4	0
Honey Bun	1 pkg (4 oz)	510	5	0
Jelly Rolls	1 pkg (2.1 oz)	230	0	15
Lemon Stix	1 pkg (1.5 oz)	210	1	0
Marshmallow Supremes	1 pkg (1.1 oz)	130	1	0
Mint Sprints	1 pkg (1.5 oz)	230	1	0
Nutty Bar	1 pkg (2 oz)	290	1	0
Pecan Twins	1 pkg (2 oz)	220	1	0
Pumpkin Delights	1 pkg (1.1 oz)	130	1	5
Smiley Faces Cherry	1 pkg (1.2 oz)	140	1	5
Smiley Faces Pumpkin	1 pkg (1 oz)	130	1	0
Snack Cake Chocolate	1 pkg (2.5 oz)	300	1	0

FOOD	PORTION	CALS.	FIB.	CHOL.
Little Debbie (CONT.)				
Snack Cake Vanilla	1 pkg (2.6 oz)	320	1	0
Spice	1 pkg (2.5 oz)	300	1	10
Star Crunch	1 pkg (1.1 oz)	140	1	0
Star Crunch	1 pkg (2.6 oz)	330	1	0
Swiss Rolls	1 pkg (2.1 oz)	250	1	15
Swiss Rolls	1 pkg (3.2 oz)	380	1	20
Swiss Rolls	1 pkg (2.7 oz)	320	1	15
Teddy Berries	1 pkg (1.2 oz)	130	1	5
Vanilla	1 pkg (3 oz)	370	0	0
Vanilla Cremes	1 pkg (1.4 oz)	170	0	0
Zebra Cakes	1 pkg (2.6 oz)	150	1	0
Nabisco				
Frosted Strawberry	1 (1.7 oz)	190	1	0
Pepperidge Farm				
Toaster Tart Apple Cinnamon	1	170	—	0
Toaster Tart Cheese	1	190	—	14
Toaster Tart Strawberry	1	190	—	0
Tastykake				
Butter Cream Cream Filled Cupcake	1 (32 g)	120	1	5
Chocolate Cream Filled Cupcake	1 (34 g)	130	1	5
Chocolate Cupcake	1 (30 g)	100	1	5
Honeybun Glazed	1 pkg (92 g)	360	4	0
Honeybun Iced	1 pkg (92 g)	350	1	50
Junior Chocolate	1 pkg (94 g)	340	4	60
Junior Coconut	1 pkg (94 g)	300	3	50
Junior Lemon	1 pkg (94 g)	310	1	75
Junior Orange	1 pkg (94 g)	340	1	50
Kandy Kake Chocolate	1 (19 g)	80	1	0
Kandy Kake Coconut	1 (19 g)	80	1	0
Kandy Kake Peanut Butter	1 (19 g)	90	1	5
Koffee Kake Cream Filled	1 (29 g)	110	0	15
Koffee Kake Junior	1 pkg (71 g)	260	1	40
Kreme Kup	1 (25 g)	90	1	5
Krimpet Butterscotch	1 (28 g)	100	0	19
Krimpet Jelly	1 (28 g)	90	1	20
Krimpet Strawberry	1 (28 g)	100	0	20
Pastry Pocket Apple	1 (85 g)	320	—	10
Pastry Pocket Cheese	1 (85 g)	330	1	10
Pastry Pocket Cherry	1 (85 g)	330	1	10
Royale Chocolate Cupcake	1 (46 g)	170	2	5
Tasty Too Chocolate Cream Filled Cupcake	1 (32 g)	100	1	0

FOOD	PORTION	CALS.	FIB.	CHOL.
Tastykake (CONT.)				
Tasty Too Vanilla Cream Filled Cupcake	1 (32 g)	100	1	0
Toastettes				
Frosted Blueberry	1 (1.7 oz)	190	1	0
Frosted Brown Sugar Cinnamon	1 (1.7 oz)	190	1	0
Frosted Cherry	1 (1.7 oz)	190	1	0
Frosted Fudge	1 (1.7 oz)	190	3	0
Strawberry	1 (1.7 oz)	190	1	0
Well-Bred Loaf				
Banana Bread	1 slice (3.5 oz)	330	tr	60
Banana Nut	1 slice (4.3 oz)	440	2	85
Blueberry	1 slice (4.3 oz)	440	1	110
Carrot	1 slice (4.3 oz)	480	2	125
Carrot Traditional	1 slice (4.3 oz)	440	2	40
Chocolate Chip	1 slice (4.3 oz)	490	2	105
Cinnamon Walnut	1 slice (4.3 oz)	480	1	110
Coconut Rum	1 slice (4.3 oz)	490	tr	95
Cranberry	1 slice (4.3 oz)	460	1	100
Marble	1 slice (4.3 oz)	530	1	115
Pound All Butter	1 slice (4.3 oz)	470	tr	115
Pound Mandarin Orange	1 slice (4 oz)	460	tr	70
Raisin	1 slice (4.3 oz)	460	2	105
TAKE-OUT				
baklava	1 oz	126	1	23
strudel	1 piece (4.1 oz)	272	3	39

CALZONE
TAKE-OUT

cheese	1 (12 oz)	1020	8	100

CANADIAN BACON

unheated	2 slices (1.9 oz)	89	—	28
Hormel				
Canadian Bacon	2 oz	70	0	30
Jones				
Slices	1	30	—	7
Oscar Mayer				
Canadian Bacon	2 slices (1.6 oz)	50	0	25

CANDY
(*see also* MARSHMALLOW)

butterscotch	1 oz	112	—	3
butterscotch	1 piece (6 g)	24	—	1

FOOD	PORTION	CALS.	FIB.	CHOL.
candied cherries	1 (4 g)	12	—	0
candied citron	1 oz	89	—	0
candied lemon peel	1 oz	90	—	0
candied orange peel	1 oz	90	—	0
candied pineapple slice	1 slice (2 oz)	179	—	0
candy corn	1 oz	105	—	0
caramels	1 pkg (2.5 oz)	271	—	5
caramels	1 piece (8 g)	31	—	1
caramels chocolate	1 bar (2.3 oz)	231	—	0
caramels chocolate	1 piece (6 g)	22	—	0
crisped rice bar almond	1 bar (1 oz)	130	1	0
crisped rice bar chocolate chip	1 bar (1 oz)	115	1	0
dark chocolate	1 oz	150	—	0
fondant chocolate coated	1 lg (1.2 oz)	128	—	0
fondant chocolate coated	1 sm (0.4 oz)	40	—	0
fondant mint	1 oz	105	—	0
gumdrops	10 sm (0.4 oz)	135	—	0
gumdrops	10 lg (3.8 oz)	420	—	0
hard candy	1 oz	106	—	0
jelly beans	10 sm (0.4 oz)	40	—	0
jelly beans	10 lg (1 oz)	104	—	0
lollipop	1 (6 g)	22	—	0
milk chocolate	1 bar (1.55 oz)	226	—	10
milk chocolate crisp	1 bar (1.45 oz)	203	—	8
milk chocolate w/ almonds	1 bar (1.45 oz)	215	—	8
peanuts chocolate covered	1 cup (5.2 oz)	773	—	13
peanuts chocolate covered	10 (1.4 oz)	208	—	4
sesame crunch	1 oz	146	—	0
sesame crunch	20 pieces (1.2 oz)	181	—	0
sweet chocolate	1 bar (1.45 oz)	201	—	0
sweet chocolate	1 oz	143	—	0
100 Grand				
Bar	1 bar (1.5 oz)	200	tr	10
3 Musketeers				
Bar	2 fun size (1.2 oz)	140	0	5
Bar	1 (2.1 oz)	260	1	5
5th Avenue				
Bar	1 (2.1 oz)	290	—	5
Almond Joy				
Bar	1 (1.76 oz)	250	—	0
Bar None				
Candy	1 (1.5 oz)	240	—	10
Bits O Brickle				
Candy	1 tbsp (0.5 oz)	80	0	5

FOOD	PORTION	CALS.	FIB.	CHOL.
Bonus				
Bar	1 bar (2.1 oz)	290	2	0
Brock				
Butterscotch Discs	3 pieces (0.6 oz)	70	—	0
Candy Corn	21 pieces (1.4 oz)	150	—	0
Candy Rolls	2 rolls (0.5 oz)	50	—	0
Cinnamon Discs	3 pieces (0.6 oz)	70	—	0
Circus Peanuts	11 pieces (2.5 oz)	260	—	0
Fruit Basket	3 pieces (0.6 oz)	60	—	0
Fruit Kisses	3 pieces (0.6 oz)	70	—	0
Glitters	2 pieces (0.5 oz)	50	—	0
Gummy Bears	5 pieces (1.4 oz)	130	—	0
Gummy Squirms	5 pieces (1.3 oz)	120	—	0
Jelly Beans	12 pieces (1.4 oz)	140	—	0
Lemon Drops	3 pieces (0.5 oz)	60	—	0
Orange Slices	4 pieces (1.5 oz)	140	—	0
Party Mints	9 pieces (0.5 oz)	60	—	0
Pops Assorted	2 (0.5 oz)	60	—	0
Sour Balls	3 pieces (0.6 oz)	70	—	0
Spearmint Starlights	3 pieces (0.6 oz)	60	—	0
Spice Drops	12 pieces (1.4 oz)	130	—	0
Starlight Mints	3 pieces (0.6 oz)	60	—	0
Butterfinger				
BB's	1 pkg (1.7 oz)	230	1	0
Bar	1 (2.1 oz)	280	1	0
Caramello				
Candy	1 (1.6 oz)	220	—	10
Cellas				
Chocolate Covered Cherries Milk Chocolate	2 pieces (1 oz)	110	2	0
Certs				
Breath Mints	1 piece (1.67 g)	6	—	0
Mini Sugar Free	1 piece (0.365 g)	1	—	0
Sugar Free	1 piece (1.67 g)	7	—	0
Charms				
Blow Pop	1 (0.7 oz)	80	—	0
Pop	1 (0.6 oz)	70	—	0
Chuckles				
Candy	4 pieces (1.4 oz)	140	—	0
Chunky				
Bar	1 (1.4 oz)	200	2	<5
Clorets				
Mints	1 piece (1.67 g)	6	—	0

FOOD	PORTION	CALS.	FIB.	CHOL.
Crunch				
Fun Size	4 bars (1.5 oz)	200	1	5
Dove				
Dark Chocolate	¼ bar (1.5 oz)	230	3	5
Dark Chocolate	1 bar (1.3 oz)	200	2	5
Dark Chocolate Miniatures	7 (1.5 oz)	220	2	5
Milk Chocolate	¼ bar (1.5 oz)	230	1	10
Milk Chocolate	1 bar (1.3 oz)	200	1	5
Milk Chocolate Miniatures	7 (1.5 oz)	230	1	10
Truffles	3 (1.2 oz)	200	1	5
Dream				
Caramel & Nougat In Milk Chocolate	1 bar (1 oz)	90	1	<5
Estee				
Caramels Chocolate & Vanilla No Sugar Added	5 (1.3 oz)	150	0	0
Dark Chocolate	½ bar (1.4 oz)	200	0	10
Gum Drops Assorted Fruit Sugar Free	23 (1.4 oz)	140	0	0
Gum Drops Licorice	23 (1.4 oz)	140	—	0
Gummy Bears Sugar Free	16 (1.4 oz)	140	—	0
Hard Candies Assorted Fruit Sugar Free	5 (0.5 oz)	60	0	0
Hard Candies Assorted Mint Sugar Free	5 (0.5 oz)	60	0	0
Hard Candies Butterscotch Sugar Free	2 (0.4 oz)	50	—	0
Hard Candies Peppermint Swirls Sugar Free	3 (0.5 oz)	60	—	0
Hard Candies Tropical Fruit Sugar Free	5 (0.5 oz)	60	0	0
Lollipops Assorted Fruit Sugar Free	2 (0.5 oz)	60	—	0
Milk Chocolate	½ bar (1.4 oz)	230	0	20
Milk Chocolate With Almonds	½ bar (1.4 oz)	230	0	20
Milk Chocolate With Crisp Rice	1 bar (2.3 oz)	370	0	30
Milk Chocolate With Fruit & Nuts	½ bar (1.4 oz)	220	0	20
Mint Chocolate	½ bar (1.4 oz)	200	0	10
Peanut Brittle No Sugar Added	⅓ box (1.5 oz)	210	1	10
Peanut Butter Cups	1 (0.3 oz)	40	0	0
Peanut Butter Cups	5 (1.3 oz)	200	1	5
Toffee Sugar Free	5 (0.5 oz)	60	—	0

FOOD	PORTION	CALS.	FIB.	CHOL.
Ferrero Rocher				
Candy	2 pieces (0.9 oz)	150	0	0
Franklin				
Crunch 'N Munch Candied	1.25 oz	170	1	0
Crunch 'N Munch Caramel	1.25 oz	160	1	13
Crunch 'N Munch Maple Walnut	1.25 oz	160	1	6
Crunch 'N Munch Toffee	1.25 oz	160	1	6
Glenny's				
Brown Rice Treats Toasted Almond With Oat Bran	1 bar (1.75 oz)	200	2	34
Godiva				
Bouchee Au Chocolat	1 piece (1.5 oz)	210	0	5
Bouchee Ivory Raspberry	1 piece (1 oz)	160	0	5
Gold Ballotin	3 pieces (1.5 oz)	210	0	5
Truffle Amaretto Di Saronno	2 pieces (1.5 oz)	210	0	5
Truffle Deluxe Liqueur	2 pieces (1.5 oz)	210	0	5
Golden Almond				
Bar	½ bar	260	—	5
Golden III				
Bar	½ bar	250	—	10
Goldenberg's				
Peanut Chews	3 pieces (1.3 oz)	180	1	0
Goo Goo Supreme				
With Pecans	1 pkg (1.5 oz)	188	4	0
Goobers				
Peanuts	1 pkg (1.38 oz)	210	3	<5
Good & Plenty				
Snacksize	3 boxes (1.5 oz)	140	—	0
Heath				
Bar	1 (1.4 oz)	210	0	20
Hershey				
Amazin'Fruit Gummy Candy	2 snack pkg (1.4 oz)	130	—	0
Bar	1 (1.55 oz)	240	—	10
Bar With Almonds	1 (1.45 oz)	230	—	15
Kisses	9 pieces (1.46 oz)	220	—	10
Special Dark Sweet Chocolate Bar	1 (1.45 oz)	220	—	0
Jolly Rancher				
Candies	3 pieces (0.6 oz)	60	—	0
Joyva				
Halvah	1.5 oz	240	2	0
Halvah Chocolate Covered	1 bar (2 oz)	380	3	0
Jells Raspberry	3 pieces (1.6 oz)	200	tr	0

FOOD	PORTION	CALS.	FIB.	CHOL.
Joyva (CONT.)				
Joys Raspberry	1 (1.6 oz)	200	1	0
Marshmallow Twists Chocolate Covered	2 (1.5 oz)	190	0	0
Rings Orange & Raspberry	3 pieces (1.5 oz)	190	tr	0
Sesame Crunch	3 pieces (0.5 oz)	80	0	0
Sticks Orange	3 pieces (1.6 oz)	200	tr	0
Twists Vanilla & Cherry	2 pieces (1.5 oz)	190	0	0
Juicefuls				
Candy	3 pieces (0.5 oz)	60	—	0
Kit Kat				
Bar	1 (1.625 oz)	250	—	10
Krackel				
Bar	1 (1.55 oz)	230	—	10
Kraft				
Butter Mints	7 (0.5 oz)	60	0	0
Caramels	5 (1.4 oz)	170	0	<5
Fudgies	5 (1.4 oz)	180	0	<5
Party Mints	7 (0.5 oz)	60	0	0
Peanut Brittle	5 pieces (1.3 oz)	170	1	0
Lance				
Chocolaty Peanut Bar	1 (57 g)	320	—	0
Peanut Bar	1 pkg (50 g)	260	—	0
Popscotch	1 pkg (35 g)	160	—	0
Lifesavers				
Fruit Juicers Lollipops	1	40	0	0
Holes Tangerine	1 candy	2	0	0
Holes Wild Fruits	20 pieces (5 g)	20	—	<5
Lollipops Fruit Flavors	1 (0.4 oz)	45	0	0
M&M's				
Almond	1 pkg (1.3 oz)	200	2	5
Almond	1.5 oz	220	2	5
Mint	1.5 oz	200	1	5
Mint	1 pkg (1.7 oz)	230	1	10
Peanut	½ bag king size (1.6 oz)	240	2	5
Peanut	1 pkg (1.7 oz)	250	2	5
Peanut	1 fun size (0.7 oz)	110	1	5
Peanut	1.5 oz	220	2	5
Peanut Butter	1 pkg (1.6 oz)	240	2	5
Peanut Butter	1 fun size (0.7 oz)	110	1	0
Peanut Butter	1.5 oz	220	2	5
Plain	1 pkg fun size (0.7 oz)	100	0	5

FOOD	PORTION	CALS.	FIB.	CHOL.
M&M's (CONT.)				
Plain	1.5 oz	200	1	5
Plain	1 pkg (1.7 oz)	230	1	6
Plain	½ pkg king size (1.6 oz)	220	1	5
Mars				
Almond Bar	2 fun size (1.3 oz)	190	1	5
Almond Bar	1 bar (1.8 oz)	240	1	5
Mayfair				
Mints	5 pieces (1.3 oz)	180	tr	0
Milk Duds				
Pieces	1 box (1.8 oz)	230	0	0
Snack Size	4 boxes (1.3 oz)	160	0	0
Milkshake				
Bar	1 bar (1.8 oz)	220	0	0
Milky Way				
Bar	2 fun size (1.4 oz)	180	0	5
Bar	⅓ king size (1.2 oz)	160	0	5
Bar	1 (2.1 oz)	280	1	5
Dark	1 bar (1.8 oz)	220	1	5
Dark	1 fun size (0.7 oz)	90	0	0
Miniature	5 (1.5 oz)	190	0	5
Mounds				
Bar	1 (1.9 oz)	260	—	0
Mr. Goodbar				
Candy	1 (1.75 oz)	290	—	15
NECCO				
Mint	1 piece	12	—	0
Nestle				
Areo Bar	1 bar (1.45 oz)	210	2	10
Buncha Crunch	1 pkg (1.4 oz)	90	tr	5
Crunch	1 bar (1.55 oz)	230	1	5
Milk Chocolate	1 bar (1.45 oz)	220	2	10
Turtles Pecan Caramel Candy	2 pieces (1.2 oz)	160	1	<5
Newman's Own				
Organics Espresso Sweet Dark Chocolate	1 bar (1.2 oz)	190	0	0
Ocean Spray				
Fruit Waves Assorted	3 pieces (0.3 oz)	35	—	0
Oh Henry!				
Bar	1 (1.8 oz)	230	2	<5
PayDay				
Bar	1 (1.85 oz)	240	2	0

FOOD	PORTION	CALS.	FIB.	CHOL.
Pez				
Candy	1 roll (0.3 oz)	30	—	0
Planters				
Original Peanut Bar	1 pkg (1.6 oz)	230	2	0
Raisinets				
Raisins	1 pkg (1.58 oz)	200	2	<5
Reese's				
Peanut Butter Cups	1 (1.8 oz)	280	—	10
Pieces	1.85 oz	260	—	5
Riesen				
Candy	5 pieces (1.4 oz)	180	3	<5
Rolo				
Carmels In Milk Chocolate	8 pieces (1.93 oz)	270	—	15
Russell Stover				
Assorted Creams	3 pieces (1.4 oz)	180	0	<5
Pecan Roll	1 (2 oz)	300	3	5
Skittles				
Original	2 pkg fun size (1.6 oz)	180	0	0
Original	1.5 oz	170	0	0
Original	1 pkg (2.8 oz)	250	0	0
Original	½ king size (1.3 oz)	150	0	0
Tropical	1.5 oz	170	0	0
Tropical	2 bags fun size (1.4 oz)	160	0	0
Tropical	1 bag (2.2 oz)	250	0	0
Wild Berry	1 bag (2.2 oz)	250	0	0
Wild Berry	1.5 oz	170	0	0
Wild Berry	2 bags fun size (1.4 oz)	160	0	0
Skor				
Toffee Bar	1 (1.4 oz)	220	—	25
Smucker's				
Jelly Beans	1 pkg (0.7 oz)	70	0	0
Snickers				
Bar	1 bar (2.1 oz)	280	1	10
Bar	2 bars fun size (1.4 oz)	190	1	5
Bar	⅓ king size (1.2 oz)	170	1	5
Miniatures	4 (1.3 oz)	170	1	5
Munch Bar	1 (1.4 oz)	230	2	10
Peanut Butter	1 bar (2 oz)	310	1	5
Solitaires				
Candies	½ bag	260	—	5

FOOD	PORTION	CALS.	FIB.	CHOL.
Sour Punch				
Candy Straws Sour Apple	6 pieces (1.4 oz)	130	—	0
Spice Stix				
And Drops	14 pieces (1.6 oz)	140	—	0
Starburst				
California Fruits	8 pieces (1.4 oz)	160	0	0
California Fruits	1 stick (2.1 oz)	240	0	2
Original Fruits	⅓ king size (1.2 oz)	140	0	0
Original Fruits	8 pieces (1.4 oz)	160	0	0
Orignal Fruits	1 stick (2.1 oz)	240	0	0
Strawberry Fruits	8 pieces (1.4 oz)	160	0	0
Strawberry Fruits	1 stick (2.1 oz)	240	0	0
Tropical Fruits	8 pieces (1.4 oz)	160	0	0
Tropical Fruits	1 stick (2.1 oz)	240	0	0
Swedish Red Fish				
Candy	19 pieces (1.4 oz)	150	—	0
Sweet Escapes				
Triple Chocolate Wafer Bars	1 (0.7 oz)	80	—	0
Switzer				
Cherry Bites	12 pieces (1.6 oz)	50	—	0
Licorice Bites	12 pieces (1.6 oz)	46	—	0
Symphony				
Milk Chocolate	1 (1.4 oz)	220	—	10
Terry's				
Orange Milk Chocolate	5 pieces (1.5 oz)	240	1	10
Tootsie Roll				
Dots	12 (1.5 oz)	160	—	0
Pop	1 (0.6 oz)	60	—	0
Twix				
Caramel	1 fun size (0.5 oz)	80	0	0
Caramel	1 (1 oz)	140	0	0
Caramel	1 pkg (2 oz)	280	0	5
Caramel	1 king size (0.8 oz)	120	1	0
Peanut Butter	1 (0.9 oz)	130	1	0
Twizzlers				
Pull-N-Peel Cherry	1 piece (1.1 oz)	110	—	0
Velamints				
Cocoamint	1 piece (1.7 g)	5	—	0
Peppermint	1 piece (1.7 g)	5	—	0
Spearmint	1 piece (1.7 g)	5	—	0
Wintergreen	1 piece (1.7 g)	5	—	0
Very Special				
Chocolate Bottles Liquor Filled	3 pieces (1 oz)	150	2	0

FOOD	PORTION	CALS.	FIB.	CHOL.
Whatchamacallit				
Bar	1 (1.8 oz)	260	—	10
Whitman's				
Assorted	3 pieces (1.4 oz)	190	0	5
Dark Chocolate	3 pieces (1.4 oz)	200	1	<5
Little Ambassadors	7 pieces (1.4 oz)	190	1	5
Pecan Delight	1 bar (2 oz)	310	2	10
Pecan Roll	1 bar (2 oz)	300	1	5
Sampler	3 pieces (1.4 oz)	200	1	5
Whoppers				
Candy	1 pkg (1.8 oz)	230	1	0
Y&S				
Bites Cherry	1 oz	100	—	0
York				
Peppermint Patty	1 snack size (0.5 oz)	57	—	0
Peppermint Patty	1 (1.5 oz)	180	—	0
Zero				
Bar	2 pieces (1.4 oz)	170	0	0
HOME RECIPE				
divinity	1 recipe 48 pieces (19 oz)	1891	—	0
divinity	1 (11 g)	38	—	0
fondant	1 piece (0.6 oz)	57	—	0
fondant	1 recipe 60 pieces (32.6 oz)	3327	—	0
fudge brown sugar w/ nuts	1 piece (0.5 oz)	56	—	1
fudge brown sugar w/ nuts	1 recipe 60 pieces (30.7 oz)	3453	—	49
fudge chocolate	1 piece (0.6 oz)	65	—	2
fudge chocolate	1 recipe 48 pieces (29 oz)	3161	—	120
fudge chocolate marshmallow	1 piece (0.7 oz)	84	—	5
fudge chocolate marshmallow	1 recipe (43.1 oz)	5182	—	304
fudge chocolate marshmallow w/ nuts	1 piece (0.8 oz)	96	—	5
fudge chocolate marshmallow w/ nuts	1 recipe 60 pieces (46.1 oz)	5742	—	291
fudge chocolate marshmallow w/ nuts	1 recipe 60 pieces (43.1 oz)	5182	—	304
fudge chocolate w/ nuts	1 recipe 48 pieces (32.7 oz)	3967	—	130
fudge chocolate w/ nuts	1 piece (0.7 oz)	81	—	3
fudge peanut butter	1 recipe 36 pieces (20.4 oz)	2161	—	25

FOOD	PORTION	CALS.	FIB.	CHOL.
fudge peanut butter	1 piece (0.6 oz)	59	—	1
fudge vanilla	1 piece (0.6 oz)	59	—	3
fudge vanilla	1 recipe 48 pieces (27.5 oz)	2893	—	125
fudge vanilla w/ nuts	1 recipe 60 pieces (31 oz)	3666	—	125
fudge vanilla w/ nuts	1 piece (0.5 oz)	62	—	2
peanut brittle	1 recipe (17.6 oz)	2288	—	66
peanut brittle	1 oz	128	—	4
praline	1 recipe 23 pieces (31.8 oz)	4116	—	0
praline	1 piece (1.4 oz)	177	—	0
taffy	1 piece (0.5 oz)	56	—	1
taffy	1 recipe 48 pieces (25 oz)	2677	—	63
toffee	1 piece (0.4 oz)	65	—	13
toffee	1 recipe 48 pieces (19.4 oz)	2997	—	580
truffles	1 recipe 49 pieces (21.5 oz)	2985	—	318
truffles	1 piece (0.4 oz)	59	—	6

CANTALOUPE

fresh cubed	1 cup	57	1	0
fresh half	½	94	2	0
Big Valley				
Balls frzn	¾ cup (4.9 oz)	40	0	0
Chiquita				
Fresh	1 cup	70	—	0
Dole				
Fresh	¼	50	0	0

CAPERS

Progresso				
Capers	1 tsp (5 g)	0	0	0
Reese				
Capers	1 tsp (5 g)	0	—	0

CARAWAY

seed	1 tsp	7	—	0

CARDAMOM

ground	1 tsp	6	—	0

CARDOON

fresh cooked	3½ oz	22	—	0
raw shredded	½ cup	36	—	0

FOOD	PORTION	CALS.	FIB.	CHOL.
CARIBOU				
roasted	3 oz	142	—	93
CARISSA				
fresh	1	12	—	0
CAROB				
carob mix	3 tsp	45	—	0
carob mix as prep w/ whole milk	9 oz	195	—	33
flour	1 tbsp	14	—	0
flour	1 cup	185	—	0
CARP				
fresh cooked	3 oz	138	—	72
fresh cooked	1 fillet (6 oz)	276	—	143
raw	3 oz	108	—	56
roe raw	3½ oz	130	—	360
CARROT JUICE				
canned	6 oz	73	—	0
Hain				
Juice	6 fl oz	80	—	0
Hollywood				
Juice	6 fl oz	80	2	0
Odwalla				
Juice	8 fl oz	70	2	0
CARROTS				
CANNED				
slices	½ cup	17	1	0
slices low sodium	½ cup	17	1	0
Allen				
Sliced	½ cup (4.5 oz)	35	3	0
Crest Top				
Sliced	½ cup (4.5 oz)	35	3	0
Del Monte				
Cut	½ cup (4.3 oz)	35	3	0
Sliced	½ cup (4.3 oz)	35	3	0
S&W				
Diced Fancy	½ cup	30	—	0
Julienne French Style Fancy	½ cup	30	—	0
Sliced Fancy	½ cup	30	—	0
Sliced Water Pack	½ cup	30	—	0
Whole Tiny Fancy	½ cup	30	—	0
Seneca				
Diced	½ cup	30	2	0

FOOD	PORTION	CALS.	FIB.	CHOL.
Seneca (CONT.)				
Sliced	½ cup	30	2	0
FRESH				
baby raw	1 (½ oz)	6	—	0
raw	1 (2.5 oz)	31	2	0
raw shredded	½ cup	24	2	0
slices cooked	½ cup	35	—	0
Dole				
Medium	1	40	1	0
FROZEN				
slices cooked	½ cup	26	—	0
Big Valley				
Carrots	½ cup (3 oz)	35	2	0
Birds Eye				
Baby Whole Deluxe	½ cup	40	2	0
Polybag Sliced	¾ cup	35	1	0
Green Giant				
Harvest Fresh Baby	½ cup	18	2	0
Hanover				
Crinkle Sliced	½ cup	35	—	0
CASABA				
cubed	1 cup	45	—	0
fresh	⅒	43	—	0
CASHEWS				
cashew butter w/o salt	1 tbsp	94	—	0
dry roasted	1 oz	163	—	0
dry roasted salted	1 oz	163	—	0
oil roasted	1 oz	163	—	0
oil roasted salted	1 oz	163	—	0
Beer Nuts				
Cashews	1 pkg (1 oz)	170	—	0
Fisher				
Honey Roasted Halves	1 oz	150	—	0
Honey Roasted Whole	1 oz	150	—	0
Oil Roasted Halves	1 oz	170	—	0
Oil Roasted Whole	1 oz	170	—	0
Frito Lay				
Cashews	1 oz	170	—	0
Guy's				
Whole Salted	1 oz	170	—	0
Hain				
Cashew Butter Raw	2 tbsp	190	—	0
Cashew Butter Toasted	2 tbsp	210	—	0

FOOD	PORTION	CALS.	FIB.	CHOL.
Lance				
Cashews	1 pkg (32 g)	190	—	0
Planters				
Fancy Oil Roasted	1 oz	170	1	0
Fancy Oil Roasted	1 pkg (2 oz)	340	3	0
Halves Lightly Salted Oil Roasted	1 oz	160	2	0
Halves Oil Roasted	1 oz	170	2	0
Honey Roasted	1 oz	150	1	0
Honey Roasted	1 pkg (2 oz)	310	3	0
Munch'N Go Honey Roasted	1 pkg (2 oz)	310	3	0
Munch'N Go Singles Oil Roasted	1 pkg (2 oz)	330	3	0
Oil Roasted	1 pkg (1 oz)	160	1	0
Oil Roasted	1 pkg (1.5 oz)	250	2	0

CASSAVA

FOOD	PORTION	CALS.	FIB.	CHOL.
raw	3½ oz	120	—	0

CATFISH

FOOD	PORTION	CALS.	FIB.	CHOL.
channel breaded & fried	3 oz	194	—	69
channel raw	3 oz	99	—	49

CATSUP
(*see* KETCHUP)

CAULIFLOWER
FRESH

FOOD	PORTION	CALS.	FIB.	CHOL.
cooked	½ cup (2.2 oz)	14	1	0
flowerets cooked	3 (2 oz)	12	1	0
flowerets raw	3 (2 oz)	14	1	0
green cooked	½ cup (2.2 oz)	20	—	0
raw	½ cup (1.8 oz)	13	1	0
Dole				
Cauliflower	⅙ med head	18	2	0
FROZEN				
cooked	½ cup	17	—	0
Big Valley				
Florets	¾ cup (3 oz)	25	1	0
Birds Eye				
Frzn	⅔ cup	25	2	0
Polybag	½ cup	20	—	0
With Cheese Sauce	½ pkg	90	1	15
Green Giant				
Cuts	½ cup	12	1	0
In Cheese Sauce	½ cup	60	2	2

FOOD	PORTION	CALS.	FIB.	CHOL.
Green Giant (CONT.)				
One Serve In Cheese Sauce	1 pkg	80	2	5
Hanover				
Cauliflower	½ cup	20	—	0
Florets	½ cup	20	—	0
JARRED				
Vlasic				
Hot & Spicy	1 oz	4	—	0
Sweet	1 oz	35	—	0

CAVIAR

FOOD	PORTION	CALS.	FIB.	CHOL.
black	1 oz	71	—	165
black	1 tbsp	40	—	94
red	1 oz	71	—	165
red	1 tbsp	40	—	94

CELERIAC

FOOD	PORTION	CALS.	FIB.	CHOL.
fresh cooked	3½ oz	25	—	0
raw	½ cup	31	—	0

CELERY
DRIED

FOOD	PORTION	CALS.	FIB.	CHOL.
seed	1 tsp	8	—	0
FRESH				
diced cooked	½ cup	13	—	0
raw	1 stalk (1.3 oz)	6	1	0
raw diced	½ cup	10	1	0
Dole				
Stalks	2 med	20	4	0

CELTUCE

FOOD	PORTION	CALS.	FIB.	CHOL.
raw	3½ oz	22	—	0

CEREAL

FOOD	PORTION	CALS.	FIB.	CHOL.
all bran	½ cup (1 oz)	76	—	0
bran flakes	¾ cup (1 oz)	90	—	0
corn flakes	1¼ cup (1 oz)	110	—	0
corn flakes low sodium	1 cup	100	—	0
corn grits instant	1 pkg (0.8 oz)	82	—	0
corn grits quick	1 cup	146	—	0
corn grits quick not prep	1 cup	579	—	0
corn grits quick not prep	1 tbsp	36	—	0
corn grits regular	1 cup	146	—	0
corn grits regular not prep	1 cup	579	—	0
crispy rice	1 cup	111	—	0
farina	¾ cup	87	3	0

FOOD	PORTION	CALS.	FIB.	CHOL.
farina not prep	1 tbsp	40	tr	0
oatmeal	1 cup	145	—	0
oatmeal instant cooked w/o salt	1 cup	145	—	0
oatmeal not prep	1 cup	311	9	0
oatmeal quick cooked w/o salt	1 cup	145	—	0
oatmeal regular cooked w/o salt	1 cup	145	—	0
puffed rice	1 cup	57	—	0
puffed wheat	1 cup	44	—	0
shredded wheat	1 biscuit	83	—	0
sugar-coated corn flakes	¾ cup (1 oz)	110	—	0
Albers				
Hominy Quick Grits uncooked	¼ cup	140	1	0
Arrowhead				
4 Grain + Flax	¼ cup (1.6 oz)	150	6	0
7 Grain	⅓ cup (1.4 oz)	140	5	0
Amaranth Flakes	1 cup (1.2 oz)	130	3	0
Apple Corns	1 cup (1.5 oz)	150	4	0
Bear Mush	¼ cup (1.6 oz)	160	2	0
Bran Flakes	1 cup (1 oz)	100	4	0
Kamut Flakes	1 cup (1.1 oz)	120	3	0
Maple Corns	1 cup (1.9 oz)	190	6	0
Multi Grain Flakes	1 cup (1.2 oz)	140	3	0
Nature O's	1 cup (1.1 oz)	130	3	0
Oat Bran Flakes	1 cup (1.2 oz)	110	4	0
Oat Flakes Rolled	⅓ cup (1.2 oz)	130	4	0
Oat Groats	¼ cup (1.5 oz)	160	4	0
Puffed Corn	1 cup (0.8 oz)	80	1	0
Puffed Kamut	1 cup (0.6 oz)	50	2	0
Puffed Millet	1 cup (0.9 oz)	90	1	0
Puffed Rice	1 cup (0.8 oz)	90	1	0
Puffed Wheat	1 cup (0.9 oz)	90	2	0
Rice & Shine	¼ cup (1.5 oz)	150	2	0
Spelt Flakes	1 cup (1.1 oz)	100	3	0
Wheat Flakes Rolled	⅓ cup (1.2 oz)	110	5	0
Aunt Jemima				
Enriched White Hominy Grits Regular	3 tbsp	101	1	0
Chex				
Corn	1¼ cup (1 oz)	110	1	0
Double	1¼ cup (1 oz)	120	0	0
Graham	1 cup (1.8 oz)	210	1	0
Rice	1 cup (1.1 oz)	120	0	0
Wheat	¾ cup (1.8 oz)	190	5	0

FOOD	PORTION	CALS.	FIB.	CHOL.
Erewhon				
Aztec	1 oz	100	1	0
Barley Plus	1 oz	110	1	0
Crispy Brown Rice	1 oz	110	4	0
Fruit 'n Wheat	1 oz	100	3	0
Oat Bran With Toasted Wheat Germ	1 oz	115	3	0
Oatmeal Instant Apple Cinnamon	1.25 oz	145	—	0
Raisin Bran	1 oz	100	3	0
Super-O's	1 oz	110	4	0
Wheat Flakes	1 oz	100	4	0
Estee				
Corn Flakes	1 pkg (1 oz)	90	4	0
Raisin Bran	1 pkg (1 oz)	90	3	0
General Mills				
Basic 4	¾ cup	130	2	0
Body Buddies Natural Fruit	1 cup (1 oz)	110	—	0
Booberry	1 cup (1 oz)	110	—	0
Cheerios	1¼ cup (1 oz)	110	2	0
Cheerios Apple Cinnamon	¾ cup (1 oz)	110	2	0
Cheerios Honey Nut	¾ cup (1 oz)	110	2	0
Cheerios-to-Go	1 pkg (0.75 oz)	80	2	0
Cheerios-to-Go Apple Cinnamon	1 pkg (1 oz)	110	2	0
Cheerios-to-Go Honey Nut	1 pkg (1 oz)	110	2	0
Cinnamon Toast Crunch	¾ cup (1 oz)	120	1	0
Clusters	½ cup (1 oz)	110	2	0
Cocoa Puffs	1 cup (1 oz)	110	—	0
Count Chocula	1 cup (1 oz)	110	—	0
Country Corn Flakes	1 cup (1 oz)	110	—	0
Crispy Wheats 'N Raisins	¾ cup (1 oz)	100	2	0
Fiber One	½ cup (1 oz)	60	13	0
Frankenberry	1 cup (1 oz)	110	—	0
Fruity Yummy Mummy	1 cup (1 oz)	110	—	0
Golden Grahams	¾ cup (1 oz)	110	—	0
Kaboom	1 cup (1 oz)	110	—	0
Kix	1½ cup (1 oz)	110	—	0
Lucky Charms	1 cup (1 oz)	110	—	0
Oatmeal Crisp	½ cup (1 oz)	110	1	0
Oatmeal Raisin Crisp	½ cup (1.2 oz)	130	2	0
Raisin Nut Bran	½ cup (1 oz)	110	3	0
S'Mores Grahams	¾ cup (1 oz)	120	—	0
Sun Crunchers	1 cup (1.9 oz)	210	3	0

FOOD	PORTION	CALS.	FIB.	CHOL.
General Mills (CONT.)				
Total	1 cup (1 oz)	100	3	0
Total Corn Flakes	1 cup (1 oz)	110	—	0
Total Raisin Bran	1 cup (1.5 oz)	140	4	0
Triples	¾ cup (1 oz)	110	—	0
Trix	1 cup (1 oz)	110	—	0
Wheaties	1 cup (1 oz)	100	3	0
Good Shepherd				
Millet Rice Flakes Wheat Free	1 oz	95	1	0
Spelt	1 oz	90	3	0
Spelt Flakes	1 oz	100	2	0
Grist Mill				
Apple Cinnamon Natural	½ cup (1.9 oz)	260	3	0
Bran	½ cup (1.9 oz)	250	11	0
Oat & Honey Natural	½ cup (1.9 oz)	270	4	0
Oat Honey & Raisin Natural	½ cup (1.9 oz)	260	4	0
H-O				
Farina Instant	1 pkg	110	3	0
Farina not prep	3 tbsp	120	3	0
Oatmeal Instant	1 pkg	110	3	0
Oatmeal Instant	½ cup	130	3	0
Oatmeal Instant Apple Cinnamon	1 pkg	130	3	0
Oatmeal Instant Maple Brown Sugar	1 pkg	160	3	0
Oatmeal Instant Raisin & Spice	1 pkg	150	3	0
Oatmeal Instant Sweet 'n Mellow	1 pkg	150	3	0
Oats 'n Fiber	1 pkg	110	3	0
Oats 'n Fiber	⅓ cup	100	3	0
Oats 'n Fiber Apple & Bran	1 pkg	130	3	0
Oats 'n Fiber Raisin & Bran	1 pkg	150	3	0
Oats Gourmet	⅓ cup	100	3	0
Oats Quick	½ cup	130	3	0
Health Valley				
100% Natural Bran With Apples & Cinnamon	¼ cup (1 oz)	100	5	0
Blue Corn Flakes 100% Organic	½ cup (1 oz)	90	3	0
Bran Cereal With Dates 100% Organic	¼ cup (1 oz)	100	5	0
Bran Cereal With Raisins 100% Organic	¼ cup (1 oz)	100	5	0
Fiber 7 Flakes 100% Organic	½ cup (1 oz)	90	5	0
Fiber 7 Flakes With Raisins 100% Organic	½ cup (1 oz)	90	5	0

FOOD	PORTION	CALS.	FIB.	CHOL.
Health Valley (CONT.)				
Fruit & Fitness	1 cup (2 oz)	220	11	0
Fruit Lites Corn	½ cup (0.5 oz)	45	tr	0
Fruit Lites Rice	½ cup (0.5 oz)	45	tr	0
Fruit Lites Wheat	½ cup (0.5 oz)	45	2	0
Healthy Crunch Almond Date	¼ cup (1 oz)	110	4	0
Healthy Crunch Apple Cinnamon	¼ cup (1 oz)	110	4	0
Healthy O's 100% Organic	¾ cup (1 oz)	90	3	0
Lites Puffed Corn	½ cup (1 oz)	50	tr	0
Lites Puffed Rice	½ cup (1 oz)	50	tr	0
Lites Puffed Wheat	½ cup (1 oz)	50	1	0
Oat Bran Flakes 100% Organic	½ cup (1 oz)	100	4	0
Oat Bran Flakes Almonds/Dates 100% Organic	½ cup (1 oz)	100	4	0
Oat Bran Flakes With Raisins 100% Organic	½ cup (1 oz)	100	4	0
Oat Bran Natural Apples & Cinnamon	¼ cup (1 oz)	100	4	0
Oat Bran Natural Raisins & Spice	¼ cup	100	4	0
Oat Bran O's 100% Organic	½ cup (1 oz)	110	3	0
Oat Bran O's Fruit & Nuts	½ cup (1 oz)	110	3	0
Orangeola Almonds & Dates	¼ cup	110	4	0
Orangeola Bananas & Hawaiian Fruit	¼ cup (1 oz)	120	4	0
Raisin Bran Flakes 100% Organic	½ cup (1 oz)	100	6	0
Real Oat Bran Almond Crunch	¼ cup (1 oz)	110	4	0
Real Oat Bran Hawaiian Fruit	¼ cup (1 oz)	130	5	0
Real Oat Bran Raisin Nut	¼ cup (1 oz)	130	5	0
Rice Bran O's	½ cup	110	2	0
Rice Bran With Almonds & Dates	½ cup (1 oz)	110	2	0
Sprouts 7 Bananas & Hawaiian Fruit	¼ cup (1 oz)	90	4	0
Sprouts 7 Raisin	¼ cup	90	5	0
Swiss Breakfast Raisin Nut	¼ cup (1 oz)	100	3	0
Swiss Breakfast Tropical Fruit	¼ cup (1 oz)	100	3	0
Healthy Choice				
Multi-Grain Flakes	1 cup (1.1 oz)	100	3	0
Multi-Grain Raisins & Almonds	1¼ cup (2 oz)	200	4	0
Multi-Grain Squares	1¼ cup (2 oz)	190	6	0

FOOD	PORTION	CALS.	FIB.	CHOL.
Heartland				
Coconut	1 oz	130	2	0
Plain	1 oz	130	2	0
Raisin	1 oz	130	2	0
Kellogg's				
All-Bran	½ cup (1 oz)	80	10	0
All-Bran With Extra Fiber	½ cup (1 oz)	50	15	0
Apple Cinnamon Rice Krispies	¾ cup (1 oz)	110	1	0
Apple Cinnamon Squares	¾ cup (1.9 oz)	180	0	0
Apple Jacks	1 cup (1 oz)	110	1	0
Apple Raisin Crisp	1 cup (1.9 oz)	180	4	0
Blueberry Squares	¾ cup (1.9 oz)	180	5	0
Bran Buds	⅓ cup (1 oz)	70	11	0
Cinnamon Mini Buns	¾ cup (1 oz)	120	1	0
Cocoa Krispies	¾ cup (1 oz)	120	0	0
Common Sense Oat Bran	¾ cup (1 oz)	110	4	0
Complete Bran Flakes	¾ cup (1 oz)	100	5	0
Corn Flakes	1 cup (1 oz)	110	1	0
Corn Pops	1 cup (1 oz)	110	1	0
Cracklin' Oat Bran	¾ cup (1.9 oz)	230	6	0
Crispix	1 cup (1 oz)	110	1	0
Double Dip Crunch	¾ cup (1 oz)	110	0	0
Froot Loops	1 cup (1 oz)	120	1	0
Frosted Bran	¾ cup (1 oz)	100	3	0
Frosted Flakes	¾ cup (1 oz)	120	0	0
Frosted Krispies	¾ cup (1 oz)	110	0	0
Frosted Mini-Wheats	1 cup (1.9 oz)	190	6	0
Frosted Mini-Wheats Bite Size	1 cup (1.9 oz)	190	6	0
Fruitful Bran	1¼ cup (1.9 oz)	170	6	0
Fruity Marshmallow Krispies	¾ cup (1 oz)	110	0	0
Just Right Crunchy Nuggets	1 cup (1.9 oz)	200	3	0
Just Right Fruit & Nut	1 cup (1.9 oz)	210	3	0
Mueslix Golden Crunch	¾ cup (1.9 oz)	210	6	0
Nut & Honey Crunch	1¼ cup (1.9 oz)	220	1	0
Oatbake Raisin Nut	⅓ cup (1 oz)	110	3	0
Pop-Tart Crunch Frosted Brown Sugar Cinnamon	¾ cup (1 oz)	120	0	0
Pop-Tart Crunch Frosted Strawberry	¾ cup (1 oz)	120	0	0
Product 19	1 cup (1 oz)	110	1	0
Raisin Bran	1 cup (1.9 oz)	170	7	0
Raisin Squares	¾ cup (1.9 oz)	180	5	0
Rice Krispies	1¼ cup (1 oz)	110	1	0
Special K	1 cup (1 oz)	110	1	0

FOOD	PORTION	CALS.	FIB.	CHOL.
Kellogg's (CONT.)				
Strawberry Squares	¾ cup (1.9 oz)	180	5	0
Temptations French Vanilla Almond	¾ cup (1 oz)	120	1	0
Temptations Honey Roasted Pecan	1 cup (1 oz)	120	0	0
Kolln				
Crispy Oats	1 cup (1.8 oz)	190	2	0
Oat Bran Crunch	⅔ cup (2.1 oz)	220	9	0
Oat Muesli Fruit	¾ cup (2 oz)	200	4	0
LaLoma				
Ruskets Biscuits	2 biscuits (30 g)	110	—	0
Little Crow				
Coco Wheat	3 tbsp (36 g)	130	4	0
Maltex				
Cereal	1 oz	105	3	0
Maypo				
30 Second	1 oz	100	2	0
Vermont Style	1 oz	105	2	0
With Oat Bran	1 oz	130	4	0
McCann's				
Irish Oatmeal	1 oz	110	3	0
Mother's				
Oatmeal Instant	½ cup (1.4 oz)	150	4	0
Whole Wheat Natural	½ cup (1.4 oz)	130	4	0
Mueslix				
Crispy Blend	⅔ cup (1.9 oz)	200	4	0
Nabisco				
100% Bran	⅓ cup (1 oz)	70	10	1
Cream Of Rice	1 oz	100	—	0
Fruit Wheats Apple	1 oz	90	3	0
Mix'n Eat Cream Of Wheat Apple & Cinnamon	1 pkg (1¼ oz)	130	1	0
Mix'n Eat Cream Of Wheat Brown Sugar Cinnamon	1 pkg (1¼ oz)	130	1	0
Mix'n Eat Cream Of Wheat Maple Brown Sugar	1 pkg (1¼ oz)	130	1	0
Mix'n Eat Cream Of Wheat Our Original	1 pkg (1¼ oz)	100	1	0
Shredded Wheat 'n Bran	⅔ cup (1 oz)	90	4	0
Shredded Wheat Spoon Size	⅔ cup (1 oz)	90	3	0
Shredded Wheat With Oat Bran	⅔ cup (1 oz)	100	4	0
Nut & Honey				
Crunch O's	¾ cup (1 oz)	120	2	0

FOOD	PORTION	CALS.	FIB.	CHOL.
Nutri-Grain				
Almond Raisin	1¼ cup (2 oz)	200	4	0
Golden Wheat	¾ cup (1.1 oz)	100	4	0
Golden Wheat & Raisin	1¼ cup (2 oz)	180	6	0
Post				
Crispy Critters	1 cup (1 oz)	110	1	0
Grape-Nuts	¼ cup (1 oz)	105	3	0
Grape-Nuts Raisin	¼ cup (1 oz)	102	2	0
Honey Bunches Of Oats Honey Roasted	⅔ cup (1 oz)	111	2	0
Honey Bunches Of Oats With Almonds	⅔ cup (1 oz)	115	2	0
Honeycomb	1⅓ cups (1 oz)	110	1	0
Natural Bran Flakes	⅔ cup (1 oz)	88	6	0
Post Toasties Corn Flakes	1¼ cup (1 oz)	111	1	0
Super Golden Crisp	⅞ cup (1 oz)	104	tr	0
Waffle Crisp	1 cup (1 oz)	130	0	0
Pritikin				
Apple Raisin Spice	1 pkg (1.6 oz)	170	—	0
Multigrain	1 pkg	160	—	0
Quaker				
Enriched White Hominy Grits Quick	3 tbsp	101	1	0
Enriched Yellow Hominy Quick Grits	3 tbsp	101	1	0
Instant Grits White Hominy	1 pkg	79	1	0
Instant Grits With Imitation Ham Bits	1 pkg	99	2	0
Instant Grits With Real Cheddar Cheese	1 pkg	104	1	0
Multigrain	½ cup	130	5	0
Oatmeal Instant	1 pkg (1.2 oz)	130	3	0
Oatmeal Instant Apples & Cinnamon	1 pkg (1.2 oz)	130	3	0
Oatmeal Instant Cinnamon Graham Cookie	1 pkg (1.4 oz)	150	3	0
Oatmeal Instant Cinnamon Spice	1 pkg (1.6 oz)	170	3	0
Oatmeal Instant Cinnamon Toast	1 pkg (1.2 oz)	130	2	0
Oatmeal Instant Fruit & Cream Blueberry	1 pkg (1.2 oz)	130	2	0
Oatmeal Instant Honey Nut	1 pkg (1.2 oz)	130	2	0
Oatmeal Instant Kids Choice Radical Raspberry	1 pkg (1.4 oz)	150	3	0

FOOD	PORTION	CALS.	FIB.	CHOL.
Quaker (CONT.)				
Oatmeal Instant Maple Brown Sugar	1 pkg (1.5 oz)	160	3	0
Oatmeal Instant Peaches & Cream	1 pkg (1.2 oz)	130	2	0
Oatmeal Instant Raisin & Walnut	1 pkg (1.3 oz)	140	3	0
Oatmeal Instant Raisin Date Walnut	1 pkg (1.3 oz)	130	3	0
Oatmeal Instant Raisin Spice	1 pkg (1.5 oz)	160	3	0
Oatmeal Instant Strawberries & Cream	1 pkg (1.2 oz)	130	2	0
Oatmeal Instant Strawberries 'N Stuff	1 pkg (1.4 oz)	150	3	0
Oats Old Fashion	½ cup	150	4	0
Oats Quick	½ cup	150	4	0
Puffed Rice	1 cup	54	tr	0
Puffed Wheat	1 cup	50	1	0
Ralston				
Almond Delight	1 cup (1.8 oz)	210	4	0
Bran Flakes	¾ cup (1.1 oz)	110	5	0
Chex Multi-Bran	1¼ cup (2 oz)	220	7	0
Cocoa Crispy Rice	1 cup (1.8 oz)	200	tr	0
Cocoa Crunchies	¾ cup (1.1 oz)	120	0	0
Cookie Crisp	1 cup (1 oz)	120	0	0
Corn Flakes	1¼ cup (1.1 oz)	120	1	0
Crisp Crunch	¾ cup (1.1 oz)	120	tr	0
Crisp Rice	1¼ cup (1.2 oz)	130	0	0
Frosted Flakes	¾ cup (1.1 oz)	120	1	0
Fruit Rings	¾ cup (0.9 oz)	100	0	0
Magic Stair	¾ cup (1.1 oz)	120	tr	0
Muesli Blueberry	1 cup (1.9 oz)	200	4	0
Muesli Cranberry	¾ cup (1.9 oz)	200	4	0
Muesli Peach	¾ cup (1.9 oz)	200	4	0
Muesli Raspberry	¾ cup (2 oz)	220	4	0
Muesli Strawberry	1 cup (1.9 oz)	210	4	0
Multi Vitamin Whole Grain Flakes	1 cup (1.1 oz)	120	3	0
Nutty Nuggets	½ cup (1.7 oz)	180	5	0
Raisin Bran	¾ cup (1.9 oz)	190	6	0
Tasteeos	1¼ cup (1.1 oz)	130	3	0
Tasteeos Apple Cinnamon	1 cup (1.2 oz)	130	1	0
Tasteeos Honey Nut	1 cup (1.2 oz)	130	1	0

FOOD	PORTION	CALS.	FIB.	CHOL.
Rice Krispies				
Treats	¾ cup (1 oz)	120	0	0
Roman Meal				
Apple Cinnamon	1.2 oz	105	6	0
Cream Of Rye	1.3 oz	111	5	0
Oats Wheat Dates Raisins Almonds	1.3 oz	129	3	0
Oats Wheat Honey Coconut Almonds	1.3 oz	155	3	0
Original	1 oz	83	5	0
Original With Oats	1.2 oz	108	5	0
Smacks				
Cereal	¾ cup (1 oz)	110	1	0
Stone-Buhr				
4 Grain	⅓ cup (1.6 oz)	140	5	0
7 Grain	⅓ cup (1.6 oz)	140	7	0
Bran Flakes	¼ cup (0.6 oz)	64	2	0
Cracked Wheat	¼ cup (2.4 oz)	210	6	0
Manna Golden	6 tsp (1.6 oz)	160	1	0
Rolled Oats Old Fashion	6 tsp (1.6 oz)	150	5	0
Scotch Oats	¼ cup (1.6 oz)	150	4	0
Sunbelt				
Muesli	1.9 oz	210	3	1
Team				
Cereal	1 cup	110	—	0
US Mills				
Uncle Sam	1 oz	110	7	0
Uncle Roy's				
Muesli Swiss Style	½ cup (1.6 oz)	170	3	0
Wheatena				
Cereal	⅓ cup (1.4 oz)	150	5	0

CEREAL BARS

(*see also* NUTRITIONAL SUPPLEMENTS)

Cap'n Crunch				
Bar	1 (0.8 oz)	90	—	0
Berries Bar	1 (0.8 oz)	90	—	0
Rice Krispies				
Treats	1 bar (0.8 oz)	90	0	0
Treats Chocolate Chip	1 (1 oz)	120	1	0

CHAMPAGNE

sekt german champagne	3.5 fl oz	84	—	0
Andre				
Blush	1 fl oz	22	—	0

FOOD	PORTION	CALS.	FIB.	CHOL.
Andre (CONT.)				
Brut	1 fl oz	21	—	0
Cold Duck	1 fl oz	25	—	0
Extra Dry	1 fl oz	23	—	0
Ballatore				
Spumante	1 fl oz	23	—	0
Eden Roc				
Brut	1 fl oz	21	—	0
Brut Rose	1 fl oz	22	—	0
Extra Dry	1 fl oz	21	—	0
Tott's				
Blanc de Noir	1 fl oz	22	—	0
Brut	1 fl oz	20	—	0
Extra Dry	1 fl oz	21	—	0

CHAYOTE

fresh cooked	1 cup	38	—	0
raw	1 (7 oz)	49	—	0
raw cut up	1 cup	32	—	0

CHEESE

(*see also* CHEESE DISHES, CHEESE SUBSTITUTES, COTTAGE CHEESE, CREAM CHEESE)

american	1 oz	93	—	18
american cheese food	1 pkg (8 oz)	745	—	145
american cheese spread	1 jar (5 oz)	412	—	78
american cold pack	1 pkg (8 oz)	752	—	144
american cheese spread	1 oz	82	—	16
blue	1 oz	100	—	21
blue crumbled	1 cup (4.7 oz)	477	—	102
brick	1 oz	105	—	27
brie	1 oz	95	—	28
cacio di roma sheep's milk cheese	1 oz	130	—	30
camembert	1 oz	85	—	20
camembert	1 wedge (1⅓ oz)	114	—	27
cheddar	1 oz	114	—	30
cheddar low fat	1 oz	49	—	6
cheddar low sodium	1 oz	113	—	28
cheddar shredded	1 cup	455	—	119
cheshire	1 oz	110	—	29
colby	1 oz	112	—	27
colby low fat	1 oz	49	—	6
colby low sodium	1 oz	113	—	28
edam	1 oz	101	—	25
emmentaler	3½ oz	403	—	92

FOOD	PORTION	CALS.	FIB.	CHOL.
feta	1 oz	75	—	25
fontina	1 oz	110	—	33
goat hard	1 oz	128	—	30
goat semi-soft	1 oz	103	—	22
goat soft	1 oz	76	—	13
gouda	1 oz	101	—	32
gruyere	1 oz	117	—	31
limburger	1 oz	93	—	26
mozzarella	1 lb	1276	—	356
mozzarella	1 oz	80	—	22
mozzarella low moisture	1 oz	90	—	25
mozzarella low moisture part skim	1 oz	79	—	15
mozzarella part skim	1 oz	72	—	16
muenster	1 oz	104	—	27
parmesan grated	1 tbsp (5 g)	23	—	4
parmesan grated	1 oz	129	—	22
parmesan hard	1 oz	111	—	19
pimento	1 oz	106	—	27
port du salut	1 oz	100	—	35
provolone	1 oz	100	—	20
quark 20% fat	3½ oz	116	—	17
quark 40% fat	3½ oz	167	—	37
quark made w/ skim milk	3½ oz	78	—	1
queso anego	1 oz	106	—	30
queso asadero	1 oz	101	—	30
queso chihuahua	1 oz	106	—	30
ricotta part skim	1 cup (8.6 oz)	340	—	76
ricotta part skim	½ cup (4.4 oz)	171	—	38
ricotta whole milk	1 cup (8.6 oz)	428	—	124
ricotta whole milk	½ cup (4.4 oz)	216	—	63
romano	1 oz	110	—	29
roquefort	1 oz	105	—	26
swiss	1 oz	107	—	26
swiss cheese food	1 pkg (8 oz)	734	—	186
swiss processed	1 oz	95	—	24
tilsit	1 oz	96	—	29
yogurt cheese	1 oz	20	—	7
Alouette				
Brie Baby	1 oz	110	0	30
Brie Baby With Herbs	1 oz	110	0	30
French Onion	2 tbsp (0.8 oz)	70	0	30
Garlic	2 tbsp (0.8 oz)	70	0	30
Light Dill	2 tbsp (0.8 oz)	50	0	20
Light Garlic	2 tbsp (0.8 oz)	50	1	20

FOOD	PORTION	CALS.	FIB.	CHOL.
Alouette (CONT.)				
Light Herb	2 tbsp (0.8 oz)	50	0	20
Light Herbs & Garlic	2 tbsp (0.8 oz)	50	0	20
Light Spring Vegetable	2 tbsp (0.8 oz)	50	0	20
Salmon	2 tbsp (0.8 oz)	60	0	15
Scallions	2 tbsp (0.8 oz)	70	0	30
Spinach	2 tbsp (0.8 oz)	60	0	25
Alpine Lace				
American	1 slice (0.66 oz)	50	0	10
American Fat Free	1 piece (1 oz)	45	0	<5
American Hot Pepper Less Fat Less Sodium	1 piece (1 oz)	80	0	6
American Less Fat Less Sodium	1 piece (1 oz)	80	0	20
Cheddar Fat Free	1 piece (1 oz)	45	0	<5
Cheddar Reduced Fat	1 piece (1 oz)	80	0	15
Colby Reduced Fat	1 piece (1 oz)	80	0	15
Fat Free For Parmesan Lovers	2 tsp (5 g)	10	0	0
Fat Free Mexican Macho	2 tbsp (1 oz)	30	0	3
Fat Free Singles	1 slice (0.66 oz)	25	0	<5
Feta Reduced Fat	1 piece (1 oz)	60	0	10
Goat	1 oz	40	—	5
Mozzarella Fat Free	1 piece (1 oz)	45	0	<5
Mozzarella Reduced Sodium Part Skim	1 piece (1 oz)	70	0	15
Muenster Reduced Sodium	1 piece (1 oz)	100	0	25
Provolone Smoked Reduced Fat	1 piece (1 oz)	70	0	15
Swiss Reduced Fat	1 piece (1 oz)	90	0	20
Armour				
Cheddar	1 oz	110	—	30
Cheddar Lower Salt	1 oz	110	—	30
Monterey Jack	1 oz	110	—	30
Monterey Jack Lower Salt	1 oz	110	—	30
Babybel				
Mini Light	1 (0.7 oz)	45	0	5
Bongrain				
Chevre	2 tbsp (0.8 oz)	40	0	15
Montrachet	1 oz	70	0	30
Montrachet Chive	1 oz	70	0	30
Montrachet Classic	1 oz	70	0	30
Montrachet Classic Herb	1 oz	70	0	30
Montrachet Herbs & Garlic	1 oz	70	0	30
Montrachet In Oil drained	1 oz	70	0	30

FOOD	PORTION	CALS.	FIB.	CHOL.
Bongrain (CONT.)				
Montrachet With Ash	1 oz	70	0	30
Borden				
American Slices	1 oz	110	—	25
American Very Sharp	1 oz	110	—	25
Swiss Slices	1 oz	100	—	20
Breakstone				
Ricotta	¼ cup (2.2 oz)	110	0	25
Bresse				
Brie	1 oz	110	0	30
Brie Light	1 oz	70	tr	20
Brie With Herbs	1 oz	110	0	30
Creme De Brie	2 tbsp (1 oz)	90	0	25
Creme De Brie Herb	2 tbsp (1 oz)	90	0	25
Brier Run				
Chevre	1 oz	61	—	18
Quark	1 oz	34	—	10
Bristol Gold				
Cheddar Light	1 oz	70	—	15
French Onion Light	1 oz	70	—	15
Garlic & Herb Light	1 oz	70	—	15
Horseradish Light	1 oz	70	—	15
Smoke Light	1 oz	70	—	15
Wine Light	1 oz	70	—	15
Cabot				
Cheddar	1 oz	110	—	30
Mediterranean Cheddar	1 oz	110	0	30
Monterey Jack	1 oz	80	—	15
Vermont Cheddar 50% Light	1 oz	70	0	15
Vitalait	1 oz	70	—	15
Vitalait Jalapeno	1 oz	70	—	15
Cheez Whiz				
Light	2 tbsp (1.2 oz)	80	0	15
Spread	2 tbsp (1.2 oz)	90	0	20
Spread Hot Salsa	2 tbsp (1.2 oz)	90	0	25
Spread Jalapeno Peppers	2 tbsp (1.2 oz)	90	0	25
Spread Mild Salsa	2 tbsp (1.2 oz)	90	0	25
Squeezable	2 tbsp (1.2 oz)	100	0	15
Zap-A-Pack Cheese Sauce	2 tbsp (1.2 oz)	90	0	20
Zap-A-Pack Cheese Sauce With Mild Salsa	2 tbsp (1.2 oz)	90	0	20
Churney				
Diet Snack Cheddar Flavored	1 oz	70	—	10
Diet Snack Port Wine Flavored	1 oz	70	—	10

FOOD	PORTION	CALS.	FIB.	CHOL.
Churney (CONT.)				
Feta	1 oz	80	0	20
Cracker Barrel				
Cheddar Extra Sharp	2 tbsp (1.1 oz)	100	0	25
Cheddar Sharp	2 tbsp (1.1 oz)	100	0	25
Cheddar Sharp Reduced Fat	1 oz	80	0	20
Cheddar Sharp Reduced Fat Shredded	¼ cup (0.9 oz)	80	0	20
Delice De France				
Cheese	1 oz	110	0	30
With Herbs	1 oz	110	0	30
Delico				
Alouette Cajun	2 tbsp (0.8 oz)	70	0	30
Alouette French Onion	2 tbsp (0.8 oz)	70	0	30
Alouette Garden Vegetable	2 tbsp (0.8 oz)	60	0	30
Alouette Garlic	2 tbsp (0.8 oz)	70	0	30
Alouette Horseradish & Chive	2 tbsp (0.8 oz)	60	0	30
Alouette Spinach	2 tbsp (0.8 oz)	60	0	25
Di Giorno				
Parmesan	2 tsp (5 g)	20	0	5
Parmesan Grated	2 tsp (5 g)	20	0	5
Parmesan Shredded	2 tsp (5 g)	20	0	<5
Romano	2 tsp (5 g)	20	0	5
Romano Grated	2 tsp (5 g)	25	0	5
Romano Shredded	2 tsp (5 g)	20	0	5
Dorman				
Cheda-Jack Reduced Fat Low Sodium	1 oz	80	—	19
Cheddar Reduced Fat Low Sodium	1 oz	80	—	20
Monterey Reduced Fat Low Sodium	1 oz	80	—	20
Mozzarella Reduced Fat Low Sodium	1 oz	80	—	17
Muenster Reduced Fat Low Sodium	1 oz	80	—	20
Provolone Reduced Fat Low Sodium	1 oz	80	—	17
Swiss Reduced Fat Low Sodium	1 oz	90	—	15
Easy Cheese				
Spread American	2 tbsp (1.2 oz)	100	0	25
Spread Cheddar	2 tbsp (1.2 oz)	100	0	25
Spread Cheddar'n Bacon	2 tbsp (1.2 oz)	100	0	25

FOOD	PORTION	CALS.	FIB.	CHOL.
Easy Cheese (CONT.)				
Spread Nacho	2 tbsp (1.2 oz)	100	0	25
Spread Sharp Cheddar	2 tbsp (1.2 oz)	100	0	25
Father Time				
Cheddar Extra-Sharp Premium	1 oz	110	0	30
Formagg				
Formaggio D'Oro	1 oz	70	0	15
Friendship				
Farmer	2 tbsp (1 oz)	50	0	10
Farmer No Salt Added	2 tbsp (1 oz)	50	0	10
Hoop	2 tbsp (1 oz)	20	0	0
Frigo				
Cheddar	1 oz	110	—	30
Cheddar Lite	1 oz	80	—	17
Impastata	1 oz	60	—	15
Mozzarella Part Skim Low Moisture	1 oz	80	—	10
Mozzarella Whole Milk Low Moisture	1 oz	90	—	15
Mozzarella Lite Whole Milk Low Moisture	1 oz	60	—	8
Pizza Shredded	1 oz	65	—	10
Provolone	1 oz	100	—	20
Provolone Lite	1 oz	70	—	10
Ricotta Low Fat Low Salt	1 oz	30	—	5
Ricotta Part Skim	1 oz	40	—	10
Ricotta Whole Milk	1 oz	60	—	15
Romano Dry Grated	1 oz	130	—	35
Romano Grated	1 oz	110	—	30
Romano Whole	1 oz	110	—	30
String	1 oz	80	—	10
String Lite	1 oz	60	—	8
Gerard				
Brie	1 oz	90	0	25
Handi-Snacks				
Cheez'n Breadsticks	1 pkg (1.1 oz)	130	0	14
Cheez'n Crackers	1 pkg (1.1 oz)	130	0	15
Cheez'n Pretzels	1 pkg (1 oz)	110	tr	15
Mozzarella String Cheese	1 stick (1 oz)	80	0	20
Harvest Moon				
American	1 slice (0.7 oz)	70	0	20
American	0.7 oz	50	0	10
Spread American	0.7 oz	60	0	15

FOOD	PORTION	CALS.	FIB.	CHOL.
Healthy Choice				
American Singles White	1 slice (0.7 oz)	30	—	<5
American Singles Yellow	1 slice (0.7 oz)	30	—	<5
Cheddar Fancy Shreds	¼ cup (1 oz)	45	—	<5
Cheddar Shreds	¼ cup (1 oz)	45	—	<5
Loaf	1 in cube (1 oz)	35	—	<5
Mexican Shreds	¼ cup (1 oz)	45	—	<5
Mozzarella	1 oz	45	—	<5
Mozzarella Fancy Shreds	¼ cup (1 oz)	45	—	<5
Mozzarella Shreds	¼ cup (1 oz)	45	—	<5
Mozzarella String Cheese	1 stick (1 oz)	45	—	<5
Pizza Fancy Shreds	¼ cup (1 oz)	45	—	<5
Pizza String	1 stick (1 oz)	45	—	<5
Heluva Good Cheese				
American	1 slice (0.7 oz)	45	0	15
Cheddar Curds Snack	1 oz	113	0	28
Cheddar Extra-Sharp	1 oz	110	0	30
Cheddar Mild	1 oz	110	0	30
Cheddar Mild Reduced Fat	1 oz	80	0	15
Cheddar Mild White	1 oz	110	0	30
Cheddar Sharp	1 oz	110	0	30
Cheddar Sharp White	1 oz	110	0	30
Cheddar Shredded	¼ cup (1 oz)	110	0	30
Cheddar Very Low Sodium	1 oz	110	0	25
Cheddar White Extra-Sharp	1 oz	110	0	30
Cheddar White Very Low Sodium	1 oz	110	0	25
Cheddar White Shredded	¼ cup (1 oz)	110	0	30
Colby	1 oz	117	0	30
Colby-Jack	1 oz	110	0	30
Cold Pack Cheddar Sharp	2 tbsp (1 oz)	90	0	20
Cold Pack Cheddar Sharp With Bacon	2 tbsp (1 oz)	90	0	20
Cold Pack Cheddar Sharp With Horseradish	2 tbsp (1 oz)	90	0	20
Cold Pack Cheddar Sharp With Jalapenos	2 tbsp (1 oz)	90	0	20
Cold Pack Cheddar Sharp With Port Wine	2 tbsp (1 oz)	90	0	20
Monterey Jack	1 oz	100	0	25
Monterey Jack Shredded	¼ cup (1 oz)	100	0	30
Monterey Jack With Jalapenos	1 oz	100	0	25
Mozzarella Part Skim Low Moisture Shredded	¼ cup (1 oz)	80	0	15

FOOD	PORTION	CALS.	FIB.	CHOL.
Heluva Good Cheese (CONT.)				
Mozzarella Whole Milk	1 oz	80	0	20
Muenster	1 oz	100	0	25
Swiss	1 oz	112	0	28
Washed Curd Cheese	1 oz	110	0	30
Hoffman				
American Yellow	1 oz	110	0	25
Hot Pepper	1 oz	90	0	20
Super Sharp	1 oz	110	0	25
Holland Farm				
Edam	1 oz	97	—	25
Farmer	1 oz	102	—	26
Gouda	1 oz	103	—	27
Monterey Jack	1 oz	102	—	27
Muenster	1 oz	102	—	27
Hollow Road Farms				
Sheep's Milk	1 oz	45	—	15
Keller's				
Chub	2 tbsp (1 oz)	100	0	35
Kraft				
American Grated	1 tbsp (0.2 oz)	25	0	<5
American Shredded	¼ cup (0.9 oz)	110	0	30
Baby Swiss	1 oz	110	0	25
Blue	1 oz	100	0	30
Blue Crumbles	1 oz	100	0	30
Brick	1 oz	110	0	30
Cheddar	1 oz	110	0	30
Cheddar Fat Free Shredded	¼ cup (1 oz)	45	0	<5
Cheddar Mild Reduced Fat	1 oz	80	0	20
Cheddar Mild Reduced Fat Shredded	¼ cup (1.1 oz)	90	0	20
Cheddar Nacho Blend With Peppers	1 oz	110	0	30
Cheddar Sharp Reduced Fat	1 oz	80	0	20
Cheddar Shredded Finely	¼ cup (0.8 oz)	90	0	25
Cheese With Garlic	1 oz	90	0	20
Cheese With Jalapeno Peppers	1 oz	60	0	20
Colby	1 oz	110	0	30
Colby Reduced Fat	1 oz	80	0	20
Colby And Monterey Jack	1 oz	110	0	30
Colby And Monterey Jack Shredded	¼ cup (1 oz)	120	0	30
Colby And Monterey Jack Shredded Reduced Fat Light	1 oz	80	—	20

FOOD	PORTION	CALS.	FIB.	CHOL.
Kraft (CONT.)				
Deluxe 25% Less Fat American	0.7 oz	70	0	15
Deluxe American	1 oz	100	0	25
Deluxe American	1 slice (1 oz)	110	0	25
Deluxe American	1 slice (0.7 oz)	70	0	15
Deluxe American White	1 slice (1 oz)	110	0	25
Deluxe American White	1 slice (0.7 oz)	70	0	15
Deluxe American White	1 oz	100	0	25
Deluxe Pimento	1 slice (1 oz)	100	0	25
Deluxe Swiss	1 slice (0.7 oz)	70	0	20
Deluxe Swiss	1 slice (1 oz)	90	0	25
Farmers	1 oz	100	0	25
Free Singles	1 slice (0.7 oz)	30	0	<5
Free Singles Sharp Cheddar	1 slice (0.7 oz)	30	0	<5
Free Singles Swiss	1 slice (0.7 oz)	30	0	<5
Free Singles White	1 slice (0.7 oz)	30	0	<5
Gouda	1 oz	110	0	25
Havarti	1 oz	120	0	35
House Italian ⅓ Less Fat Grated	2 tsp (0.2 oz)	25	0	<5
Italian Blend Grated	2 tsp (0.2 oz)	25	0	<5
Limburger	1 oz	90	0	25
Monterey Jack	1 oz	110	0	30
Monterey Jack Reduced Fat	1 oz	80	0	20
Monterey Jack Shredded	¼ cup (1 oz)	110	0	30
Monterey Jack With Jalapeno Peppers	1 oz	110	0	30
Monterey Jack With Peppers Reduced Fat	1 oz	80	0	20
Mozzarella Fat Free Shredded	¼ cup (1 oz)	50	tr	<5
Mozzarella Low Moisture Part Skim Reduced Fat Shredded	¼ cup (1.1 oz)	80	0	15
Mozzarella Low Moisture Part Skim Shredded	¼ cup (1 oz)	90	0	20
Mozzarella Low Moisture Part Skim Shredded Finely	¼ cup (0.8 oz)	70	0	15
Mozzarella Low Moisture Whole Milk Shredded	¼ cup (1 oz)	90	0	25
Mozzarella Part Skim Low Moisture	1 oz	80	0	15
Mozzarella String Cheese Low Moisture Part Skim	1 stick (1 oz)	80	0	20
Muenster	1 oz	110	0	30
Parmesan Grated	2 tsp (0.2 oz)	20	0	5
Parmesan Shredded	2 tsp (0.2 oz)	20	0	<5

FOOD	PORTION	CALS.	FIB.	CHOL.
Kraft (CONT.)				
Pizza Four Cheeses Shredded	¼ cup (0.9 oz)	90	0	20
Pizza Mild Cheddar & Mozzarella Shredded	¼ cup (0.9 oz)	90	0	20
Pizza Mozzarella & Cheddar	¼ cup (0.9 oz)	100	0	25
Pizza Mozzarella & Provolone	¼ cup (0.9 oz)	90	0	20
Provolone Smoke Flavor	1 oz	100	0	25
Romano Grated	2 tsp (0.2 oz)	25	0	5
Shredded	¼ cup (1 oz)	120	0	30
Singles ⅓ Less Fat American	0.7 oz	40	0	10
Singles ⅓ Less Fat American White	0.7 oz	50	0	10
Singles ⅓ Less Fat Sharp Cheddar	0.7 oz	50	0	10
Singles ⅓ Less Fat Swiss	0.7 oz	50	0	10
Singles American	1 slice (1.2 oz)	110	0	30
Singles American	1 slice (0.7 oz)	70	0	15
Singles American White	1 slice (0.7 oz)	70	0	15
Singles Mild Mexican Jalapeno Peppers	1 slice (0.7 oz)	70	0	15
Singles Monterey	1 slice (0.7 oz)	70	0	15
Singles Pimento	1 slice (0.7 oz)	60	0	15
Singles Sharp	1 slice (0.7 oz)	70	0	15
Singles Swiss	1 slice (0.7 oz)	70	0	15
Spread Jalapeno Pepper	1 oz	80	0	20
Spread Olive & Pimento	2 tbsp (1.1 oz)	70	0	20
Spread Pimento	2 tbsp (1.1 oz)	80	0	20
Spread Pineapple	2 tbsp (1.1 oz)	70	0	15
String With Jalapeno Peppers	1 oz	80	—	20
Swiss	1 oz	110	0	30
Swiss Shredded	¼ cup (1 oz)	80	0	30
Taco Cheddar & Monterey Jack Shredded	¼ cup (0.9 oz)	100	0	25
Lactaid				
American	3.5 oz	328	0	64
Land O'Lakes				
American	2 slices (1 oz)	100	0	25
American	1 slice (0.75 oz)	80	0	20
American	1 oz	110	0	30
American Less Salt	1 oz	110	0	30
American Light	1 oz	70	0	20
American Sharp	1 oz	110	0	30
American & Swiss	1 oz	100	0	35
Baby Swiss	1 oz	110	0	25

FOOD	PORTION	CALS.	FIB.	CHOL.
Land O'Lakes (CONT.)				
Brick	1 oz	100	0	30
Chedarella	1 oz	100	0	25
Cheddar Light	1 oz	70	0	10
Gouda	1 oz	110	—	30
Jalapeno Light	1 oz	70	0	15
Monterey Jack	1 oz	110	0	30
Mozzarella	1 oz	80	0	15
Muenster	1 oz	100	0	25
Provolone	1 oz	100	0	20
Swiss	1 oz	110	0	25
Swiss Light	1 oz	80	0	15
Laughing Cow				
Assorted Wedge	1 (1 oz)	70	0	20
Babybel	1 oz	90	0	10
Babybel Mini	1 (0.7 oz)	70	0	15
Bonbel	1 oz	100	0	25
Bonbel Mini	1 (0.7 oz)	70	0	15
Cheesebits	6 pieces (1 oz)	70	0	20
Gouda Mini	1 (0.7 oz)	80	0	20
Original Wedge	1 (1 oz)	70	0	20
Wedge Light	1 (1 oz)	50	0	10
Lifetime				
Cheddar Fat Free	1 oz	40	0	<5
Cheddar Fat Free Lactose Free	1 oz	40	0	<5
Garden Vegetable Fat Free	1 oz	40	0	<5
Jalapeno Jack Fat Free	1 oz	40	0	<5
Jalapeno Jack Fat Free Lactose Free	1 oz	40	0	<5
Mild Mexican Fat Free	1 oz	40	0	<5
Monterey Jack Fat Free	1 oz	40	0	<5
Mozzarella Fat Free	1 oz	40	0	<5
Mozzarella Fat Free Lactose Free	1 oz	40	0	<5
Onions & Chives Fat Free	1 oz	40	0	<5
Sharp Cheddar Fat Free	1 oz	40	0	<5
Smoked Cheddar Fat Free	1 oz	40	0	<5
Swiss Fat Free	1 oz	40	0	<5
Light N'Lively				
Singles 50% Less Fat American	0.7 oz	50	0	10
Singles 50% Less Fat American White	0.7 oz	50	0	10
MayBud				
Edam	1 oz	100	0	25

FOOD	PORTION	CALS.	FIB.	CHOL.
MayBud (cont.)				
Gouda	1 oz	100	0	25
Gouda Round	1 oz	100	0	25
Mohawk Valley				
Spread Limburger	2 tbsp (1.1 oz)	80	0	20
New Holland				
Cheese	1 oz	90	0	30
Garlic	1 oz	90	0	30
Havarti Lower Fat Garden Vegetable	1 oz	80	0	25
Jalapeno	1 oz	80	0	25
Natural Vegetable	1 oz	80	0	25
Northfield				
Naturally Slender	1 oz	90	—	10
Old English				
American Sharp	1 oz	100	0	25
Spread Sharp	2 tbsp (1.1 oz)	70	0	25
Polly-O				
Mozzarella Free	1 oz	35	—	<5
Mozzarella Lite	1 oz	60	—	10
Mozzarella Part Skim	1 oz	70	—	15
Mozzarella Part Skim Shredded	1/4 cup	80	—	15
Mozzarella Shredded Free	1/4 cup	45	—	<5
Mozzarella Shredded Lite	1/4 cup	60	—	15
Mozzarella Whole Milk	1 oz	80	—	20
Mozzarella Whole Milk Shredded	1/4 cup	90	—	20
Ricotta Free	1/4 cup	50	—	<5
Ricotta Lite	1/4 cup	70	—	10
Ricotta Part Skim	1/4 cup	90	—	20
Ricotta Whole Milk	1/4 cup	110	—	25
String	1 oz	80	—	15
String Lite	1 piece (1 oz)	60	0	10
Price's				
Cheese & Bacon Spread	2 tbsp (1.1 oz)	90	0	15
Jalapeno Nacho Dip Hot	2 tbsp (1.1 oz)	80	0	15
Jalapeno Nacho Dip Mild	2 tbsp (1.1 oz)	80	0	15
Pimento Cheese Spread	2 tbsp (1.1 oz)	80	0	15
Pimento Cheese Spread Light	2 tbsp (1.1 oz)	60	0	10
Vegetable Garden	2 tbsp (1.1 oz)	70	0	15
Quaker				
Chub	2 tbsp (1 oz)	100	0	35
Roka				
Spread Blue	2 tbsp (1.1 oz)	80	0	20

FOOD	PORTION	CALS.	FIB.	CHOL.
Rondele				
Light Soft Spreadable Garlic & Herb	2 tbsp (0.9 oz)	60	0	10
Soft Spreadable Garlic & Herbs	2 tbsp (1 oz)	100	0	25
Sargento				
4 Cheese Mexican Recipe Blend Shredded	¼ cup (1 oz)	110	0	25
6 Cheese Italian Recipe Blend Shredded	¼ cup (1 oz)	90	0	20
Blue Crumbled	¼ cup (1 oz)	100	0	20
Cheddar	1 slice (1 oz)	110	0	30
Cheddar Mild Shredded Classic Supreme	¼ cup (1 oz)	110	0	30
Cheddar Mild Shredded Fancy Supreme	¼ cup (1 oz)	110	0	30
Cheddar Mild Shredded Preferred Light	¼ cup (1 oz)	70	0	10
Cheddar Mild White Shredded Classic Supreme	¼ cup (1 oz)	110	0	30
Cheddar New York Sharp Shredded Classic Supreme	¼ cup (1 oz)	110	0	30
Cheddar Sharp Shredded Classic Supreme	¼ cup (1 oz)	110	0	30
Cheddar Sharp Shredded Fancy Supreme	¼ cup (1 oz)	110	0	30
Cheese For Nachos & Tacos Shredded	¼ cup (1 oz)	110	0	25
Cheese For Pizza Shredded	¼ cup (1 oz)	90	0	20
Cheese For Tacos Shredded	¼ cup (1 oz)	110	0	25
Cheese For Tacos Shredded Preferred Light	¼ cup (1 oz)	70	0	15
Colby	1 slice (1 oz)	110	0	30
Colby-Jack Shredded Fancy Supreme	¼ cup (1 oz)	110	0	25
Gourmet Parm	1 tbsp	20	—	5
Jarlsberg	1 slice (1.2 oz)	120	0	20
Monterey Jack	1 slice (1 oz)	100	0	30
MooTown Snackers Cheddar	1 piece (0.8 oz)	100	0	25
MooTown Snackers Cheddar Mild Light	1 piece (0.8 oz)	60	0	10
MooTown Snackers Cheese & Pretzels	1 pkg (1 oz)	90	0	10
MooTown Snackers Cheese & Sticks	1 pkg (1 oz)	100	0	10

FOOD	PORTION	CALS.	FIB.	CHOL.
Sargento (CONT.)				
MooTown Snackers Colby-Jack	1 piece (0.8 oz)	90	0	20
MooTown Snackers Pizza Cheese & Sticks	1 pkg (1 oz)	100	0	10
MooTown Snackers String	1 piece (0.8 oz)	70	0	15
MooTown Snackers String Light	1 piece (0.8 oz)	60	0	10
Mozzarella	1 slice (1.5 oz)	130	0	25
Mozzarella Preferred Light	1 slice (1.5 oz)	100	0	15
Mozzarella Shredded Classic Supreme	¼ cup (1 oz)	80	0	15
Mozzarella Shredded Fancy Supreme	¼ cup (1 oz)	80	0	15
Mozzarella Shredded Preferred Light	¼ cup (1 oz)	70	0	10
Muenster	1 slice (1 oz)	100	0	25
Parmesan Fresh	1 oz	111	—	19
Parmesan Shredded	¼ cup (1 oz)	110	0	25
Parmesan & Romano Shredded	¼ cup (1 oz)	110	0	25
Pizza Double Cheese Shredded	¼ cup (1 oz)	90	0	20
Provolone	1 slice (1 oz)	100	0	25
Ricotta Light	¼ cup (2.2 oz)	60	0	15
Ricotta Old Fashioned	¼ cup (2.2 oz)	90	0	25
Ricotta Part Skim	¼ cup (2.2 oz)	80	0	20
Swiss	1 slice (0.7 oz)	80	0	20
Swiss Preferred Light	1 slice (1 oz)	80	0	15
Swiss Shredded Fancy Supreme	¼ cup (1 oz)	110	0	30
Swiss Wafer Thin	2 slices (1 oz)	110	0	25
Smart Beat				
American Fat Free	1 slice (0.6 oz)	25	—	0
Lactose Free Fat Free	1 slice (0.6 oz)	25	—	0
Mellow Cheddar Fat Free	1 slice (0.6 oz)	25	—	0
Sharp Cheddar Fat Free	1 slice (0.6 oz)	25	—	0
Spreadery				
Medium Cheddar	2 tbsp (1.1 oz)	80	0	15
Pimento Spread	2 tbsp (1.1 oz)	100	0	20
Sharp Cheddar	2 tbsp (1.1 oz)	80	0	15
Vermont Sharp White Cheddar	2 tbsp (1.1 oz)	80	0	15
Squeez-A-Snak				
Spread Sharp	2 tbsp (1.1 oz)	90	0	25
Treasure Cave				
Blue Crumbled	1 oz	110	0	25
Feta Crumbled	1 oz	80	0	20

FOOD	PORTION	CALS.	FIB.	CHOL.
Tree Of Life				
Cheddar 33% Reduced Fat Organic Milk	1 oz	90	—	15
Cheddar Low Sodium Raw Milk	1 oz	110	—	24
Cheddar Mild Organic Milk	1 oz	110	—	25
Cheddar Mild Raw Milk	1 oz	110	—	25
Cheddar Razor Sharp Raw Milk	1 oz	110	—	25
Cheddar Sharp Organic Milk	1 oz	110	—	25
Cheddar Sharp Raw Milk	1 oz	110	—	25
Colby Organic Milk	1 oz	120	—	30
Colby Raw Milk	1 oz	110	—	30
Farmer Part-Skim Organic Milk	1 oz	90	—	15
Jalapeno Jack Organic Milk	1 oz	110	—	20
Jalapeno Jack Semi-Soft Organic Milk	1 oz	110	—	25
Monterey Jack 35% Reduced Fat Organic Milk	1 oz	80	—	15
Monterey Jack Organic Milk	1 oz	100	—	20
Monterey Jack Semi-Soft Raw Milk	1 oz	110	—	25
Mozzarella Low Moisture Part Skim	1 oz	80	—	15
Mozzarella Low Moisture Part Skim Organic Milk	1 oz	80	—	16
Muenster Organic Milk	1 oz	100	—	25
Muenster Semi-Soft Raw Milk	1 oz	100	—	30
Provolone	1 oz	100	—	20
Swiss Raw Milk	1 oz	110	—	25
Velveeta				
Cheese	1 slice (0.7 oz)	60	0	15
Cheese	1 slice (1.2 oz)	100	0	25
Cheese	1 slice (0.8 oz)	70	0	15
Hot Mexican With Jalapeno Peppers Shredded	¼ cup (1.3 oz)	130	0	30
Light	1 oz	60	0	10
Mild Mexican With Jalapeno Peppers Shredded	¼ cup (1.3 oz)	130	0	30
Shredded	¼ cup (1.3 oz)	130	0	30
Spread	1 oz	80	0	20
Spread Hot Mexican Jalapeno Pepper	1 oz	80	0	20
Spread Italiana	1 oz	60	0	20
Spread Mild Mexican With Jalapeno Pepper	1 oz	80	0	20

FOOD	PORTION	CALS.	FIB.	CHOL.
Weight Watchers				
Cheddar Mild Yellow	1 oz	80	0	15
Cheddar Sharp Yellow	1 oz	80	0	15
Fat Free Grated Parmesan	1 tbsp	15	0	0
Fat Free Sharp Cheddar	2 slices (0.75 oz)	30	0	0
Fat Free Swiss	2 slices (0.75 oz)	30	0	0
Fat Free White	2 slices (0.75 oz)	30	0	0
Fat Free Yellow	2 slices (0.75 oz)	30	0	0
Low Sodium Cheddar Mild	1 oz	80	0	15
Monterey Jack	1 oz	80	0	15
Reduced Sodium American White	2 slices (0.75 oz)	30	0	0
Reduced Sodium American Yellow	2 slices (0.75 oz)	30	0	0
White Clover				
Cheddar Light With Simplesse	1 oz	80	—	15
Colby Light With Simplesse	1 oz	80	—	15
Monterey Jack Light With Simplesse	1 oz	70	—	15
Muenster Light With Simplesse	1 oz	70	—	15
WisPride				
Chunk	1 oz	110	0	20
Garlic & Herb Cup	2 tbsp (1.1 oz)	100	0	20
Hickory Smoked Cup	2 tbsp (1.1 oz)	100	0	20
Port Wine Ball	2 tbsp (1.1 oz)	100	0	20
Port Wine Cup	2 tbsp (1.1 oz)	100	0	20
Port Wine Light Cup	2 tbsp (1.1 oz)	80	0	10
Sharp Ball	2 tbsp (1.1 oz)	100	0	20
Sharp Cheddar Ball	2 tbsp (1.1 oz)	100	0	20
Sharp Cup	2 tbsp (1.1 oz)	100	0	20
Sharp Light Cup	2 tbsp (1.1 oz)	80	0	10
Swiss Ball	2 tbsp (1.1 oz)	110	0	20

CHEESE DISHES
FROZEN
Stouffer's

FOOD	PORTION	CALS.	FIB.	CHOL.
Welsh Rarebit	¼ cup (1.1 oz)	120	—	20

TAKE-OUT

FOOD	PORTION	CALS.	FIB.	CHOL.
fondue	1 cup (7.5 oz)	492	—	97
fondue	½ cup (3.8 oz)	247	—	49

CHEESE SUBSTITUTES

FOOD	PORTION	CALS.	FIB.	CHOL.
mozzarella	1 oz	70	—	0
Borden				
Cheese Two	1 oz	90	—	<5

FOOD	PORTION	CALS.	FIB.	CHOL.
Borden (CONT.)				
Taco-Mate	1 oz	100	—	10
Formagg				
American White	1 slice (0.66 oz)	60	0	0
American Yellow	1 slice (0.66 oz)	60	0	0
Caesar's Italian Garden American	1 oz	60	0	0
Cheddar	1 slice (0.66 oz)	60	0	0
Cheddar Shredded	1 oz	60	0	0
Classic American	1 oz	60	0	0
Macaroni And Cheese Sauce	⅔ cup (5 oz)	190	0	0
Mozzarella Shredded	1 oz	60	0	0
Old World Mozzarella	1 oz	60	0	0
Parmesan Grated	2 tsp (5 g)	15	tr	0
Swiss	1 oz	60	0	0
Swiss White	1 slice (0.66 oz)	60	0	0
Vintage Provolone	1 oz	60	0	0
Zesty Jalapeno American	1 oz	60	0	0
Georgio's				
Imitation Cheddar Shredded	¼ cup (1 oz)	90	0	0
Imitation Mozzarella Shredded	¼ cup (1 oz)	90	0	0
Golden Image				
American	0.7 oz	70	0	5
Harvest Moon				
American Shredded	¼ cup (1.3 oz)	120	0	0
Cheddar Shredded	¼ cup (1.3 oz)	120	0	0
Mozzarella Shredded	¼ cup (1.3 oz)	110	1	0
Lunchwagon				
American	1 slice (0.7 oz)	70	0	0
Sargento				
Classic Supreme Cheddar Shredded	¼ cup (1 oz)	90	0	0
Classic Supreme Mozzarella Shredded	¼ cup (1 oz)	80	0	0
Fancy Supreme Cheddar Shredded	¼ cup (1 oz)	90	0	0
White Wave				
Soy A Melt Cheddar	1 oz	80	—	0
Soy A Melt Fat Free Cheddar	1 oz	40	—	0
Soy A Melt Fat Free Mozzarella	1 oz	40	—	0
Soy A Melt Garlic Herb	1 oz	80	—	0
Soy A Melt Jalapeno Jack	1 oz	80	—	0
Soy A Melt Monterey Jack	1 oz	80	—	0
Soy A Melt Mozzarella	1 oz	80	—	0

FOOD	PORTION	CALS.	FIB.	CHOL.
White Wave (CONT.)				
Soy A Melt Singles American	1 slice (¾ oz)	60	—	0
Soy A Melt Singles Mozzarella	1 slice (¾ oz)	60	—	0
CHERIMOYA				
fresh	1	515	—	0
CHERRIES				
CANNED				
sour in heavy syrup	½ cup	232	—	0
sour in light syrup	½ cup	189	—	0
sour water packed	1 cup	87	—	0
sweet in heavy syrup	½ cup	107	—	0
sweet in light syrup	½ cup	85	—	0
sweet juice pack	½ cup	68	—	0
sweet water pack	½ cup	57	—	0
Del Monte				
Dark Pitted In Heavy Syrup	½ cup (4.2 oz)	120	tr	0
Sweet Dark Whole Unpitted In Heavy Syrup	½ cup (4.2 oz)	120	tr	0
DRIED				
Chukar				
Bing	2 oz	160	—	0
Rainer	2 oz	160	—	0
Tart	2 oz	170	—	0
Tart 'n Sweet	2 oz	180	—	0
Sonoma				
Pitted	¼ cup (1.4 oz)	140	2	0
FRESH				
sour	1 cup	51	—	0
sweet	10	49	—	0
Dole				
Cherries	1 cup	90	3	0
FROZEN				
sour unsweetened	1 cup	72	—	0
sweet sweetened	1 cup	232	—	0
Big Valley				
Dark Sweet	¾ cup (4.9 oz)	90	3	0
CHERRY JUICE				
After The Fall				
Black Cherry	1 can (12 oz)	170	0	0
Hi-C				
Box	8.45 fl oz	140	—	0
Drink	8 fl oz	130	—	0

FOOD	PORTION	CALS.	FIB.	CHOL.
Juice Works				
Drink	6 oz	100	—	0
Juicy Juice				
Drink	1 box (8.45 fl oz)	130	—	0
Drink	1 bottle (6 fl oz)	90	—	0
Kool-Aid				
Black Cherry	8 oz	98	—	0
Drink	8 oz	98	—	0
Sugar Free	8 oz	3	—	0
Sipps				
Wild Cherry	8.45 oz	130	—	0
Smucker's				
Black Cherry	8 oz	130	—	0
Tang				
Fruit Box	8.45 oz	121	—	0
Tree Of Life				
Concentrate	8 tsp (1.4 oz)	110	—	0
CHERVIL				
seed	1 tsp	1	—	0
CHESTNUTS				
chinese cooked	1 oz	44	—	0
chinese dried	1 oz	103	—	0
chinese raw	1 oz	64	—	0
chinese roasted	1 oz	68	—	0
cooked	1 oz	37	—	0
dried peeled	1 oz	105	—	0
japanese cooked	1 oz	16	—	0
japanese dried	1 oz	102	—	0
japanese raw	1 oz	44	—	0
japanese roasted	1 oz	57	—	0
raw peeled	1 oz	56	—	0
roasted	1 cup	350	—	0
roasted	2 to 3 (1 oz)	70	—	0
CHEWING GUM				
bubble gum	1 block (8 g)	27	—	0
stick	1 (3 g)	10	—	0
Bazooka				
Fruit Chunk	1 piece (6 g)	25	—	0
Fruit Soft	1 piece (6 g)	25	—	0
Gum	1 piece (4 g)	15	—	0
Gum	1 piece (6 g)	25	—	0
Beech-Nut				
Peppermint	1 stick (3 g)	10	0	0

FOOD	PORTION	CALS.	FIB.	CHOL.
Beech-Nut (CONT.)				
Spearmint	1 stick (3 g)	10	0	0
Big Red				
Stick	1	10	—	0
Brock				
Bubble Gum	1 piece (0.2 oz)	20	—	0
Bubble Yum				
Bananaberry Split	1 piece (0.3 oz)	25	—	0
Cotton Candy	1 piece (0.3 oz)	25	—	0
Grape	1 piece (0.3 oz)	25	—	0
Luscious Lime	1 piece (0.3 oz)	25	—	0
Regular	1 piece (0.3 oz)	25	0	0
Sour Apple	1 piece (0.3 oz)	25	1	0
Sour Cherry	1 piece (0.3 oz)	25	0	0
Variety Pack	1 piece (0.3 oz)	25	0	0
Watermelon	1 piece (0.3 oz)	25	0	0
Wild Strawberry	1 piece (0.3 oz)	25	0	0
Bubblicious				
Gum	1 piece (7.9 g)	25	—	0
Chiclets				
Original	1 piece (1.59 g)	6	—	0
Tiny Size	8 pieces (0.13 g)	tr	—	0
Clorets	1 piece (1.59 g)	6	—	0
Dentyne				
Cinn-A-Burst	1 piece (3.2 g)	9	—	0
Gum	1 piece (1.88 g)	6	—	0
Sugar Free	1 piece (1.88 g)	5	—	0
Doublemint				
Chewing Gum	1 piece	10	—	0
Extra Sugar Free				
Cinnamon	1 piece	8	—	0
Spearmint & Peppermint	1 stick	8	—	0
Winter Fresh	1 piece	8	—	0
Freedent				
Spearmint Peppermint & Cinnamon	1 stick	10	—	0
Freshen-Up				
Gum	1 piece (4.2 g)	13	—	0
Fruit Stripe				
Bubble Gum Jumbo Pack	1 stick (3 g)	10	0	0
Variety Pack Chewing & Bubble Gum	1 stick (3 g)	10	0	0
Hubba Bubba				
Bubble Gum Cola	1 piece	23	—	0

FOOD	PORTION	CALS.	FIB.	CHOL.
Hubba Bubba (CONT.)				
Bubble Gum Sugarfree Grape	1 piece	13	—	0
Bubble Gum Sugarfree Original	1 piece	14	—	0
Original	1 piece	23	—	0
Strawberry Grape Raspberry	1 piece	23	—	0
Juicy Fruit				
Stick	1	10	—	0
Rain-Blo				
Bubble Gum Balls	1 piece (2 g)	5	—	0
Swell				
Bubble Gum	1 piece (3 g)	10	—	0
Trident				
Gum	1 piece (1.88 g)	5	—	0
Soft Bubble Gum	1 piece (3.3 g)	9	—	0
Wrigley's				
Spearmint	1 stick	10	—	0

CHIA SEEDS

dried	1 oz	134	—	0

CHICKEN

(*see also* CHICKEN DISHES, CHICKEN SUBSTITUTES, DINNER, HOT DOG)

CANNED

Hormel				
Chunk	2 oz	70	0	35
Chunk Breast	2 oz	60	0	25
No Salt Chunk Breast	2 oz	60	0	30
Underwood				
Chunky	2.08 oz	150	—	40
Chunky Light	2.08 oz	80	—	30
Smoky	2.08 oz	150	—	40
FRESH				
broiler/fryer back w/ skin batter dipped & fried	½ back (2.5 oz)	238	—	63
broiler/fryer back w/ skin floured & fried	1.5 oz	146	—	39
broiler/fryer back w/ skin roasted	1 oz	96	—	28
broiler/fryer back w/ skin stewed	½ back (2.1 oz)	158	—	48
broiler/fryer back w/o skin fried	½ back (2 oz)	167	—	54
broiler/fryer breast w/ skin batter dipped & fried	2.9 oz	218	—	72
broiler/fryer breast w/ skin batter dipped & fried	½ breast (4.9 oz)	364	—	119
broiler/fryer breast w/ skin roasted	2 oz	115	—	49

FOOD	PORTION	CALS.	FIB.	CHOL.
broiler/fryer breast w/ skin roasted	½ breast (3.4 oz)	193	—	83
broiler/fryer breast w/ skin stewed	½ breast (3.9 oz)	202	—	83
broiler/fryer breast w/o skin fried	½ breast (3 oz)	161	—	78
broiler/fryer breast w/o skin roasted	½ breast (3 oz)	142	—	73
broiler/fryer breast w/o skin stewed	2 oz	86	—	44
broiler/fryer dark meat w/ skin batter dipped & fried	5.9 oz	497	—	149
broiler/fryer dark meat w/ skin floured & fried	3.9 oz	313	—	101
broiler/fryer dark meat w/ skin roasted	3.5 oz	256	—	92
broiler/fryer dark meat w/ skin stewed	3.9 oz	256	—	90
broiler/fryer dark meat w/o skin fried	1 cup (5 oz)	334	—	135
broiler/fryer dark meat w/o skin roasted	1 cup (5 oz)	286	—	130
broiler/fryer dark meat w/o skin stewed	3 oz	165	—	76
broiler/fryer dark meat w/o skin stewed	1 cup (5 oz)	269	—	123
broiler/fryer drumstick w/ skin batter dipped & fried	1 (2.6 oz)	193	—	62
broiler/fryer drumstick w/ skin floured & fried	1 (1.7 oz)	120	—	44
broiler/fryer drumstick w/ skin roasted	1 (1.8 oz)	112	—	48
broiler/fryer drumstick w/ skin stewed	1 (2 oz)	116	—	48
broiler/fryer drumstick w/o skin fried	1 (1.5 oz)	82	—	40
broiler/fryer drumstick w/o skin roasted	1 (1.5 oz)	76	—	41
broiler/fryer drumstick w/o skin stewed	1 (1.6 oz)	78	—	40
broiler/fryer leg w/ skin batter dipped & fried	1 (5.5 oz)	431	—	142
broiler/fryer leg w/ skin floured & fried	1 (3.9 oz)	285	—	105
broiler/fryer leg w/ skin roasted	1 (4 oz)	265	—	105
broiler/fryer leg w/ skin stewed	1 (4.4 oz)	275	—	105

FOOD	PORTION	CALS.	FIB.	CHOL.
broiler/fryer leg w/o skin fried	1 (3.3 oz)	195	—	93
broiler/fryer leg w/o skin roasted	1 (3.3 oz)	182	—	89
broiler/fryer leg w/o skin stewed	1 (3.5 oz)	187	—	90
broiler/fryer light meat w/ skin batter dipped & fried	4 oz	312	—	94
broiler/fryer light meat w/ skin floured & fried	2.7 oz	192	—	68
broiler/fryer light meat w/ skin roasted	2.8 oz	175	—	67
broiler/fryer light meat w/ skin stewed	3.2 oz	181	—	66
broiler/fryer light meat w/o skin fried	1 cup (5 oz)	268	—	125
broiler/fryer light meat w/o skin roasted	1 cup (5 oz)	242	—	118
broiler/fryer light meat w/o skin stewed	1 cup (5 oz)	223	—	107
broiler/fryer neck w/ skin stewed	1 (1.3 oz)	94	—	27
broiler/fryer neck w/o skin stewed	1 (0.6 oz)	32	—	14
broiler/fryer skin batter dipped & fried	from ½ chicken (6.7 oz)	748	—	140
broiler/fryer skin batter dipped & fried	4 oz	449	—	84
broiler/fryer skin floured & fried	1 oz	166	—	24
broiler/fryer skin floured & fried	from ½ chicken (2 oz)	281	—	41
broiler/fryer skin roasted	from ½ chicken (2 oz)	254	—	46
broiler/fryer skin stewed	from ½ chicken (2.5 oz)	261	—	45
broiler/fryer thigh w/ skin batter dipped & fried	1 (3 oz)	238	—	80
broiler/fryer thigh w/ skin floured & fried	1 (2.2 oz)	162	—	60
broiler/fryer thigh w/ skin roasted	1 (2.2 oz)	153	—	58
broiler/fryer thigh w/ skin stewed	1 (2.4 oz)	158	—	57
broiler/fryer thigh w/o skin fried	1 (1.8 oz)	113	—	53
broiler/fryer thigh w/o skin roasted	1 (1.8 oz)	109	—	49
broiler/fryer thigh w/o skin stewed	1 (1.9 oz)	107	—	49
broiler/fryer w/ skin floured & fried	½ chicken (11 oz)	844	—	283
broiler/fryer w/ skin floured & fried	½ breast (3.4 oz)	218	—	88

FOOD	PORTION	CALS.	FIB.	CHOL.
broiler/fryer w/ skin fried	½ chicken (16.4 oz)	1347	—	404
broiler/fryer w/ skin roasted	½ chicken (10.5 oz)	715	—	263
broiler/fryer w/ skin stewed	½ chicken (11.7 oz)	730	—	262
broiler/fryer w/ skin neck & giblets batter dipped & fried	1 chicken (2.3 lbs)	2987	—	1054
broiler/fryer w/ skin neck & giblets roasted	1 chicken (1.5 lbs)	1598	—	730
broiler/fryer w/ skin neck & giblets stewed	1 chicken (1.6 lbs)	1625	—	726
broiler/fryer w/o skin fried	1 cup	307	—	131
broiler/fryer w/o skin roasted	1 cup (5 oz)	266	—	125
broiler/fryer w/o skin stewed	1 cup (5 oz)	248	—	116
broiler/fryer w/o skin stewed	1 oz	54	—	22
broiler/fryer wing w/ skin batter dipped & fried	1 (1.7 oz)	159	—	39
broiler/fryer wing w/ skin floured & fried	1 (1.1 oz)	103	—	26
broiler/fryer wing w/ skin roasted	1 (1.2 oz)	99	—	29
broiler/fryer wing w/ skin stewed	1 (1.4 oz)	100	—	28
capon w/ skin neck & giblets roasted	1 chicken (3.1 lbs)	3211	—	1458
cornish hen w/o skin & bone roasted	½ hen (2 oz)	72	—	57
cornish hen w/o skin & bone roasted	1 hen (3.8 oz)	144	—	113
cornish hen w/skin roasted	1 hen (8 oz)	595	—	299
cornish hen w/skin roasted	½ hen (4 oz)	296	—	149
roaster dark meat w/o skin roasted	1 cup (5 oz)	250	—	104
roaster light meat w/o skin roasted	1 cup (5 oz)	214	—	105
roaster w/ skin neck & giblets roasted	1 chicken (2.4 lbs)	2363	—	1003
roaster w/ skin roasted	½ chicken (1.1 lbs)	1071	—	365
roaster w/o skin roasted	1 cup (5 oz)	469	—	160
stewing dark meat w/o skin stewed	1 cup (5 oz)	361	—	132
stewing w/ skin neck & giblets stewed	1 chicken (1.3 lbs)	1636	—	603
stewing w/ skin stewed	6.2 oz	507	—	140
stewing w/ skin stewed	½ chicken (9.2 oz)	744	—	205
Perdue				
Boneless Breasts Cooked	3 oz	120	—	70
Boneless Breast Tenderloins Cooked	3 oz	100	—	55

FOOD	PORTION	CALS.	FIB.	CHOL.
Perdue (CONT.)				
Boneless Thighs Roasted	2 (3.5 oz)	200	—	130
Breast Quarters Cooked	3 oz	180	—	90
Burger Cooked	1 (3 oz)	170	—	120
Chicken Breast Seasoned Barbecue Cooked	3 oz	110	—	60
Chicken Breast Seasoned Italian Cooked	3 oz	100	—	55
Chicken Breast Seasoned Lemon Pepper Cooked	3 oz	90	—	55
Chicken Breast Seasoned Oriental Cooked	3 oz	100	—	55
Cornish Hen Split Dark Meat Roasted	1 half (6.5 oz)	210	0	130
Cornish Hen White Meat Cooked	3 oz	170	—	100
Drumsticks Roasted	1 (2 oz)	110	—	85
Drumsticks Skinless Roasted	2 (3.5 oz)	150	—	135
Ground Cooked	3 oz	180	—	145
Jumbo Drumsticks Roasted	1 (2 oz)	110	—	85
Jumbo Split Breast Roasted	1 (7 oz)	370	—	175
Jumbo Thighs Roasted	1 (3 oz)	240	—	125
Jumbo Whole Leg Roasted	2 (5.5 oz)	360	—	205
Jumbo Wings Roasted	2 (3 oz)	210	—	125
Leg Quarters Cooked	3 oz	210	—	115
Oven Stuffer Boneless Breast Cooked	3 oz	120	—	70
Oven Stuffer Boneless Breast Thin Sliced Cooked	1 slice (2 oz)	80	—	50
Oven Stuffer Boneless Thighs Roasted	1 (3.5 oz)	170	—	125
Oven Stuffer Dark Meat Roasted	3 oz	200	—	105
Oven Stuffer Drumstick Roasted	1 (3.5 oz)	190	—	135
Oven Stuffer White Meat Roasted	3 oz	160	—	80
Oven Stuffer Whole Breast Cooked	3 oz	150	—	75
Oven Stuffer Wing Drummettes Roasted	2 (2.5 oz)	170	—	90
Split Breast Skinless Roasted	1 (6 oz)	250	—	140
Split Breasts Roasted	1 (7 oz)	370	—	175
Thighs Roasted	1 (3 oz)	240	—	125

FOOD	PORTION	CALS.	FIB.	CHOL.
Perdue (CONT.)				
Thighs Skinless Roasted	1 (2.5 oz)	160	—	100
Whole White Meat Cooked	3 oz	160	0	85
Whole Leg Roasted	1 (5.5 oz)	360	—	200
Wingettes Roasted	3 (3 oz)	200	0	120
Wings Roasted	2 (3 oz)	210	—	125
Tyson				
Breast	3 oz	116	—	72
Cornish Hen	3.5 oz	250	—	155
Drumstick	3 oz	131	—	79
Thigh	3 oz	152	—	81
Whole	3 oz	134	—	76
Wing	3 oz	147	—	72
Wampler Longacre				
Ground raw	1 oz	50	—	30
FROZEN				
Banquet				
Country Fried	1 serv (3 oz)	270	1	65
Drum Snackers	2.25 oz	190	1	25
Fried Breast	1 piece (4.45 oz)	240	4	85
Fried Hot & Spicy	1 serv (3 oz)	260	1	65
Fried Original	1 serv (3 oz)	270	1	65
Fried Thigh & Drumsticks	1 serv (3 oz)	260	2	65
Hot & Spicy Nuggets	2.5 oz	230	1	25
Hot Popcorn Chicken	1 pkg (3 oz)	290	2	35
Nuggets	3 oz	240	1	35
Nuggets Chicken & Cheddar	2.7 oz	280	1	25
Nuggets Chicken & Mozzarella	6 (2.8 oz)	210	2	10
Nuggets Southern Fried	6 (4.5 oz)	340	2	45
Nuggets Sweet & Sour	6 (4.5 oz)	320	2	45
Patties	1 (2.5 oz)	180	tr	25
Patties Southern Fried	1 (2.5 oz)	190	tr	25
Skinless Fried	1 serv (3 oz)	210	2	55
Skinless Fried Honey BBQ	1 serv (3 oz)	210	2	55
Southern Fried	1 serv (3 oz)	270	1	65
Tenders	3 pieces (3 oz)	260	2	25
Tenders Southern Fried	3 pieces (3 oz)	260	1	15
Wings Hot & Spicy	4 pieces (5 oz)	230	1	85
Country Skillet				
Chicken Chunks	5 (3.1 oz)	270	1	20
Chicken Nuggets	10 (3.3 oz)	280	1	24
Chicken Patties	2.5 oz	190	1	20
Southern Fried Chicken Chunks	5 (3.1 oz)	250	1	20
Southern Fried Chicken Patties	1 (2.5 oz)	190	1	20

FOOD	PORTION	CALS.	FIB.	CHOL.
Empire				
Nuggets	5 (3 oz)	180	1	15
Stix	4 (3.1 oz)	180	2	25
Ozark Valley				
Nuggets	4 (2.9 oz)	210	2	25
Patties	1 (3 oz)	210	1	30
Sensible Chef				
Fried Breast	1 (3 oz)	200	2	55
Tyson				
BBQ Breast Fillets	3 oz	110	—	50
Boneless Breasts	3.5 oz	210	—	80
Boneless Skinless Breast	3.5 oz	130	—	55
Boneless Skinless Thighs	3.5 oz	200	—	105
Breast Chunks	3 oz	240	—	30
Breast Fillets	3 oz	190	—	25
Breast Patties	2.6 oz	220	—	35
Chick'n Cheddar	2.6 oz	220	—	40
Chick'n Chunks	2.6 oz	220	—	35
Cordon Bleu Mini	1	90	—	17
Diced	3 oz	130	—	70
Drums & Thighs	3.5 oz	270	—	130
Grilled Sandwich	3.5 oz	200	—	32
Hors D'Oeuvres Mesquite Chunks	3.5 oz	100	—	45
Hot BBQ Breast Tenders	2.75 oz	110	—	45
Mesquite Breast Fillets	2.75 oz	100	—	50
Mesquite Breast Strips	2.75 oz	100	—	50
Mesquite Breast Tenders	2.75 oz	110	—	55
Microwave Chunks BBQ Sandwich	4 oz	230	—	30
Roasted Breast Fillets	1 oz	50	—	15
Roasted Breasts	1 oz	50	—	15
Roasted Drumsticks	1 oz	50	—	40
Roasted Half Chicken	1 oz	60	—	30
Roasted Thighs	1 oz	70	—	40
Roasted Whole Chicken	1 oz	60	—	30
Skinless Breast Tenders	3.5 oz	120	—	50
Southern Fried Breast Fillets	3 oz	220	—	25
Southern Fried Breast Patties	2.6 oz	220	—	35
Southern Fried Chick'n Chunks	2.6 oz	220	—	35
Thick & Crispy Patties	2.6 oz	220	—	40
READY-TO-EAT				
chicken roll light meat	2 oz	90	—	28
chicken roll light meat	1 pkg (6 oz)	271	—	85

FOOD	PORTION	CALS.	FIB.	CHOL.
poultry salad sandwich spread	1 tbsp (13 g)	109	—	4
poultry salad sandwich spread	1 oz	238	—	9
Banquet				
Breast Tenders Fat Free	3 (3.2 oz)	130	2	30
Carl Buddig				
Chicken	1 oz	50	0	20
Chicken By George				
Cajun	1 breast (4 oz)	120	0	55
Caribbean Grill	1 breast (4 oz)	150	0	55
Garlic & Herb	1 breast (4 oz)	120	0	50
Italian Bleu Cheese	1 breast (4 oz)	130	0	60
Lemon Herb	1 breast (4 oz)	120	0	50
Lemon Oregano	1 breast (4 oz)	130	0	50
Mesquite Barbecue	1 breast (4 oz)	120	0	50
Mustard Dill	1 breast (4 oz)	140	0	65
Roasted	1 breast (4 oz)	110	0	55
Teriyaki	1 breast (4 oz)	130	0	50
Tomato Herb With Basil	1 breast (4 oz)	140	0	60
Empire				
Barbecue Whole	5 oz	280	0	110
Battered & Breaded Cutlets	1 (3.3 oz)	200	2	25
Battered & Breaded Fried Breasts	3 oz	170	tr	45
Battered & Breaded Nuggets	5 (3 oz)	200	1	30
Bologna	3 slices (1.8 oz)	200	0	40
Fried Drum & Thigh	3 oz	240	2	80
Falls				
BBQ	3 oz	150	—	75
Healthy Choice				
Deli-Thin Oven Roasted Breast	6 slices (2 oz)	45	0	25
Deli-Thin Smoked Breast	6 slices (2 oz)	60	0	30
Fresh-Trak Oven Roasted Breast	1 slice (1 oz)	30	0	15
Oven Roasted Breast	1 slice (1 oz)	25	0	15
Smoked Breast	1 slice (1 oz)	35	0	15
Hebrew National				
Deli Thin Oven Roasted	1.8 oz	45	—	20
Louis Rich				
Deluxe Oven Roasted Breast	1 slice (1 oz)	40	0	15
Hickory Smoked Breast	1 slice (1 oz)	30	0	15
Oven Roasted Breast	1 slice (1 oz)	40	0	15
Mr. Turkey				
Deli Cuts Hardwood Smoked	3 slices	30	—	13
Deli Cuts Oven Roasted	3 slices	25	—	15

FOOD	PORTION	CALS.	FIB.	CHOL.
Oscar Mayer				
Deli-Thin Honey Glazed Breast	4 slices (1.8 oz)	60	0	25
Free Oven Roasted Breast	4 slices (1.8 oz)	45	—	25
Healthy Favorites Oven Roasted Breast	4 slices (1.8 oz)	40	0	25
Lunchables Chicken/Monterey Jack	1 pkg (4.5 oz)	350	1	75
Lunchables Deluxe Chicken/ Turkey	1 pkg (5.1 oz)	380	1	70
Lunchables Dessert Chocolate Pudding/Chicken/Jack	1 pkg (6.2 oz)	370	0	55
Smoked Breast	1 slice (1 oz)	25	—	15
Perdue				
Cornish Hen Dark Meat Cooked	3 oz	200	—	130
Cornish Hen Split White Meat Roasted	½ hen (6.5 oz)	200	0	115
Nuggets Chicken & Cheese	5 (3 oz)	220	2	95
Nuggets Chik-Tac-Toe Cooked	5 (3 oz)	200	2	35
Nuggets Football Basketball Baseball	4 (3 oz)	230	—	35
Nuggets Original	5 (3 oz)	200	2	35
Nuggets Star & Drumstick	4 (3 oz)	200	2	35
Original Tenderloins Cooked	3 oz	160	2	65
Original Cutlets Cooked	1 (3.5 oz)	230	2	40
Oven Roasted Breast	1 (5 oz)	190	0	115
Oven Roasted Drumsticks	2 (2.5 oz)	100	0	95
Oven Roasted Half Dark Meat	3 oz	170	0	110
Oven Roasted Half White Meat	3 oz	140	0	80
Oven Roasted Thighs	1 (3 oz)	170	0	105
Oven Roasted Whole Chicken Dark Meat	3 oz	170	0	110
Oven Roasted Whole Chicken White Meat	3 oz	140	0	60
Perdue Done It! Nuggets Original	1 (0.67 oz)	48	—	7
Short Cuts Italian	3 oz	110	0	55
Short Cuts Lemon Pepper	3 oz	110	0	60
Short Cuts Mesquite	3 oz	110	0	50
Short Cuts Oven Roasted	3 oz	110	0	55
Wings Barbecued	3 oz	200	1	105
Wings Hot & Spicy	3 oz	190	1	110
Tyson				
Roasted Drumsticks w/ Skin	2 (3.8 oz)	220	—	150

FOOD	PORTION	CALS.	FIB.	CHOL.
Wampler Longacre				
Breast	1 oz	35	—	15
Chef's Select Breast	1 oz	35	—	15
Premium Oven Roasted Breast	1 oz	50	—	20
Roll	1 oz	65	—	25
Roll Sliced	1 slice (0.8 oz)	50	—	20
Weaver				
Roasted Wings	1 oz	70	—	45
Weight Watchers				
Roasted & Smoked Breast	2 slices (¾ oz)	25	—	15
Roasted Ham	2 slices (¾ oz)	25	—	10
TAKE-OUT				
boneless breaded & fried w/ barbecue sauce	6 pieces (4.6 oz)	330	—	61
boneless breaded & fried w/ honey	6 pieces (4 oz)	339	—	61
boneless breaded & fried w/ mustard sauce	6 pieces (4.6 oz)	323	—	62
boneless breaded & fried w/ sweet & sour sauce	6 pieces (4.6 oz)	346	—	61
breast & wing breaded & fried	2 pieces (5.7 oz)	494	—	149
drumstick breaded & fried	2 pieces (5.2 oz)	430	—	165
oven roasted breast of chicken	2 oz	60	—	25
thigh breaded & fried	2 pieces (5.2 oz)	430	—	165

CHICKEN DISHES

(*see also* CHICKEN SUBSTITUTES, DINNER)

CANNED

FOOD	PORTION	CALS.	FIB.	CHOL.
Dinty Moore				
Microwave Cup Chicken & Dumpling	1 cup (7.5 oz)	200	1	35
Stew	1 cup (8.5 oz)	220	2	40
FROZEN				
Croissant Pocket				
Stuffed Sandwich Chicken Broccoli & Cheddar	1 piece (4.5 oz)	300	5	35
Hot Pocket				
Stuffed Sandwich Chicken & Cheddar With Broccoli	1 (4.5 oz)	300	tr	30
Jimmy Dean				
Grilled Breast Sandwich	1 (5.5 oz)	330	1	70
Lean Pockets				
Stuffed Sandwich Chicken Fajita	1 (4.5 oz)	260	3	40

FOOD	PORTION	CALS.	FIB.	CHOL.
Lean Pockets (CONT.)				
Stuffed Sandwich Chicken Parmesan	1 (4.5 oz)	260	1	25
Stuffed Sandwich Glazed Chicken Supreme	1 (4.5 oz)	240	1	30
Luigino's				
Chicken A La King With Noodles	1 pkg (8 oz)	240	2	60
Noodles With Chicken Peas & Carrots	1 pkg (8 oz)	300	2	50
Noodles With Chicken Peas & Carrots	1 cup (6.3 oz)	260	2	40
Sweet & Sour Chicken With Rice	1 pkg (8 oz)	300	2	20
MicroMagic				
Chicken Sandwich	1 pkg (4.5 oz)	390	—	35
Weight Watchers				
Chicken, Broccoli & Cheese Pocket Sandwich	1 (5 oz)	250	1	25
Grilled Chicken Sandwich	1 (4 oz)	210	2	20
White Castle				
Grilled Chicken Sandwich	2 (4 oz)	250	5	20
Grilled Chicken Sandwich w/ Sauce	2 (4.8 oz)	290	5	20
READY-TO-EAT				
Spreadables				
Chicken Salad	¼ can	100	—	16
Wampler Longacre				
Cacciatore	1 serv (4 oz)	118	—	40
Salad	1 oz	70	—	15
Salad Lite	1 oz	45	—	10
Smokey Barbecue	1 serv (4 oz)	175	—	65
Sweet N Sour	1 serv (4 oz)	106	—	25
Szechwan With Peanuts	1 serv (4 oz)	112	—	22
SHELF-STABLE				
Dinty Moore				
Stew	1 cup (7.5 oz)	180	2	30
Lunch Bucket				
Light'n Healthy Chicken Fiesta	1 pkg (7.5 oz)	170	—	10
Top Shelf				
Chicken Cacciatore	1 bowl (10 oz)	210	3	45
Chicken Acapulco Fiesta Chicken	1 bowl (10 oz)	420	2	70

FOOD	PORTION	CALS.	FIB.	CHOL.
Top Shelf (CONT.)				
Chicken Ala King	1 bowl (10 oz)	380	2	45
Glazed Breast Of Chicken	1 bowl (10 oz)	200	2	50
TAKE-OUT				
chicken & dumplings	¾ cup	256	tr	109
chicken & noodles	1 cup	365	—	103
chicken a la king	1 cup	470	—	221
chicken cacciatore	¾ cup	394	2	99
chicken paprikash	1½ cups	296	—	90
fillet sandwich plain	1	515	—	60
fillet sandwich w/ cheese lettuce mayonnaise & tomato	1	632	—	76

CHICKEN SUBSTITUTES

Harvest Direct				
TVP Poultry Chunks	3.5 oz	280	18	0
TVP Poultry Ground	3.5 oz	280	18	0
Jaclyn's				
Salsa Chicken Style Dinner	11.5 oz	325	—	0
Sesame Chicken Style Dinner	11.5 oz	345	—	0
LaLoma				
Chicken Supreme not prep	¼ cup (16 g)	50	—	0
Chik Nuggets	5 nuggets (85 g)	270	—	0
Fried Chicken	1 piece (57 g)	180	—	0
Fried Chicken w/ Gravy	2 pieces (85 g)	140	—	0
Soy Is Us				
Chicken Not!	½ cup (1.75 oz)	140	9	0
White Wave				
Meatless Sandwich Slices	2 slices (1.6 oz)	80	0	0

CHICKPEAS

CANNED				
chickpeas	1 cup	285	—	0
Allen				
Garbanzo	½ cup (4.4 oz)	120	8	0
East Texas Fair				
Garbanzo	½ cup (4.4 oz)	120	8	0
Eden				
Organic	½ cup (4.1 oz)	110	4	0
Goya				
Spanish Style	7.5 oz	150	9	0
Green Giant				
Garbanzo	½ cup	90	5	0
Hanover				
Chickpeas	½ cup	100	—	0

FOOD	PORTION	CALS.	FIB.	CHOL
Old El Paso				
Garbanzo	½ cup (4.6 oz)	120	7	0
Progresso				
Chick Peas	½ cup (4.6 oz)	120	7	0
S&W				
Garbanzo Lite 50% Less Salt	½ cup	110	—	0
Garbanzo Premium Large	½ cup	110	—	0
Garbanzo Water Pack	½ cup	105	—	0
DRIED				
cooked	1 cup	269	—	0
Bean Cuisine				
Garbanzo	½ cup	115	5	0

CHICORY

FOOD	PORTION	CALS.	FIB.	CHOL
greens raw chopped	½ cup	21	—	0
root raw	1 (2.1 oz)	44	—	0
roots raw cut up	½ cup (1.6 oz)	33	—	0
witloof head raw	1 (1.9 oz)	9	—	0
witloof raw	½ cup (1.6 oz)	8	—	0

CHILI
CANNED

FOOD	PORTION	CALS.	FIB.	CHOL
chili w/ beans	1 cup	286	—	43
Allen				
Mexican Chili Beans	½ cup (4.5 oz)	120	8	0
Armour				
Chili No Beans	1 cup (8.7 oz)	470	—	85
Chili With Beans	1 cup (8.9 oz)	440	—	50
Chili With Beans Hot	1 cup (8.9 oz)	440	—	50
Chili With Beans Western Style	1 cup (8.8 oz)	460	—	60
Brown Beauty				
Mexican Chili Beans	½ cup (4.5 oz)	120	8	0
Chi-Chi's				
San Antonio	1 cup (8.5 oz)	240	6	60
Del Monte				
Sauce	1 tbsp (0.6 oz)	20	0	0
Gebhardt				
Hot With Beans	1 cup	470	6	65
Plain	1 cup	530	1	70
With Beans	1 cup	495	6	92
Hain				
Spicy Tempeh	7½ oz	160	—	0
Spicy Vegetarian	7½ oz	160	—	0
Spicy Vegetarian Reduced Sodium	7½ oz	170	—	0

FOOD	PORTION	CALS.	FIB.	CHOL.
Hain (CONT.)				
Spicy With Chicken	7½ oz	130	—	40
Health Valley				
Mild Vegetarian With Beans	5 oz	160	12	0
Mild Vegetarian With Beans No Salt Added	5 oz	160	12	0
Mild Vegetarian With Lentils	5 oz	140	7	0
Mild Vegetarian With Lentils No Salt Added	5 oz	140	7	0
Spicy Vegetarian With Beans	5 oz	160	12	0
Hormel				
Chunky With Beans	1 cup (8.7 oz)	270	7	35
Hot No Beans	1 cup (8.2 oz)	210	3	35
Hot With Beans	1 cup (8.7 oz)	270	7	35
No Beans	1 cup (8.2 oz)	210	3	35
Turkey With Beans	1 cup (8.7 oz)	210	5	35
Turkey No Beans	1 cup (8.2 oz)	190	3	75
Vegetarian	1 cup (8.7 oz)	200	7	0
With Beans	1 cup (8.7 oz)	270	7	35
Hunt's				
Chili Beans	½ cup (4.5 oz)	87	6	0
Just Rite				
Hot With Beans	4 oz	195	1	33
With Beans	4 oz	200	1	33
Without Beans	4 oz	180	tr	41
Old El Paso				
Chili With Beans	1 cup (8 oz)	200	6	30
S&W				
Chili Beans	½ cup	130	—	0
Chili Makin's Original	½ cup	100	—	0
Van Camp's				
Chilee Beanee Weenee	1 can (8 oz)	240	9	35
Chili With Beans	1 cup (8.9 oz)	350	7	45
DRIED				
powder	1 tsp	8	—	0
Gebhardt				
Chili Powder	1 tsp	15	tr	0
Chili Quik Seasoning	1 tsp	10	tr	0
Hain				
Hot Chili	¼ pkg	30	—	0
Medium Chili	¼ pkg	30	—	0
Mild Chili	¼ pkg	30	—	0
Nile Spice				
Chili'n Beans Original	1 pkg	150	6	0

FOOD	PORTION	CALS.	FIB.	CHOL.
Nile Spice (CONT.)				
Chili'n Beans Spicy	1 pkg	150	6	0
Old El Paso				
Chili Seasoning Mix	1 tbsp (0.3 oz)	25	1	0
Watkins				
Chili Seasoning	1¼ tsp (4 g)	15	0	0
Powder	¼ tsp (0.5 g)	0	0	0
FROZEN				
Lean Cuisine				
Three Bean	1 pkg (9 oz)	210	7	10
Lightlife				
Chili	4.3 oz	110	—	0
Luigino's				
Chili-Mac	1 pkg (8 oz)	230	3	25
Stouffer's				
With Beans	1 pkg (8.75 oz)	270	8	35
Tabatchnick				
Vegetarian	7.5 oz	210	10	0
SHELF-STABLE				
Lunch Bucket				
Chili With Beans	1 pkg (7.5 oz)	300	—	45
Micro Cup Meals				
Chili Mac	1 cup (7.5 oz)	200	2	25
Chili No Beans	1 cup (7.5 oz)	290	3	65
Chili With Beans	1 cup (7.5 oz)	250	6	50
Chili With Beans	1 cup (10.4 oz)	410	12	75
Hot Chili With Beans	1 cup (7.5 oz)	250	6	50
Wampler Longacre				
Turkey	1 serv (4 oz)	118	—	32
TAKE-OUT				
con carne w/ beans	8.9 oz	254	—	133

CHINESE CABBAGE
(see CABBAGE)

CHINESE FOOD
(see ORIENTAL FOOD)

CHINESE PRESERVING MELON

cooked	½ cup	11	—	0

CHIPS
(see also POPCORN, PRETZELS, SNACKS)

CORN

barbecue	1 oz	148	1	0
barbecue	1 bag (7 oz)	1036	10	0

FOOD	PORTION	CALS.	FIB.	CHOL.
cones plain	1 oz	145	—	0
onion	1 oz	142	—	0
plain	1 oz	153	1	0
plain	1 bag (7 oz)	1067	9	0
puffs cheese	1 oz	157	tr	1
puffs cheese	1 bag (8 oz)	1256	2	9
twists cheese	1 oz	157	tr	1
twists cheese	1 bag (8 oz)	1256	2	9
Energy Food Factory				
Corn Pops Fat Free	½ oz	50	1	0
Corn Pops Nacho	½ oz	50	1	0
Corn Pops Original	½ oz	50	1	0
Fritos				
Chili Cheese	34 pieces (1 oz)	160	1	0
Chips	34 pieces (1 oz)	150	1	0
Crisp 'N Thin	18 pieces (1 oz)	160	1	0
Dip Size	13 pieces (1 oz)	150	1	0
Non-Stop Nacho Cheese	34 pieces (1 oz)	150	1	tr
Rowdy Rustlers Bar-B-Q	34 pieces (1 oz)	150	1	0
Wild 'N Mild	32 pieces (1 oz)	160	1	0
Health Valley				
Chips	1 oz	160	1	0
No Salt Added	1 oz	160	1	0
With Cheddar Cheese	1 oz	160	1	2
Lance				
BBQ	1 pkg (50 g)	260	—	0
Chips	1 pkg (50 g)	270	—	0
Planters				
Corn Chips	34 chips (1 oz)	170	2	0
King Size	17 chips (1 oz)	160	2	0
Snacks To Go	1 pkg (1.5 oz)	240	3	0
Snyder's				
BBQ	1 oz	160	2	0
Chips	1 oz	160	2	0
Wise				
Corn Crunchies	1 oz	160	—	0
Crispy Corn	1 oz	160	—	0
Crispy Corn Nacho Cheese	1 oz	160	—	0
Dipsy Doodles	1 pkg (1.5 oz)	240	1	0
MULTIGRAIN				
Sunchips				
Chips	12 pieces (1 oz)	150	—	0
French Onion	12 pieces (1 oz)	140	—	tr

FOOD	PORTION	CALS.	FIB.	CHOL.
POTATO				
barbecue	1 bag (7 oz)	971	—	0
barbecue	1 oz	139	—	0
light	1 bag (6 oz)	801	—	0
light	1 oz	134	—	0
potato	1 oz	152	1	0
potato	1 pkg (8 oz)	1217	8	0
potato	1 oz	152	—	0
potato	1 bag (8 oz)	1217	—	0
sour cream & onion	1 bag (7 oz)	1051	—	14
sour cream & onion	1 oz	150	—	2
sticks	½ cup (0.6 oz)	94	1	0
sticks	1 oz	148	1	0
sticks	1 pkg (1 oz)	148	—	0
sticks	½ cup	94	—	0
Barrel O' Fun				
Barbeque	1 oz	145	0	0
Chips	1 oz	150	0	0
Sour Cream & Onion	1 oz	150	0	0
Butterfield				
Sticks	1 pkg (1.7 oz)	250	3	1
Sticks	⅔ cup (1 oz)	150	2	0
Cape Cod				
Chips	19 chips (1 oz)	150	1	0
Cottage Fries				
No Salt Added	1 oz	160	—	0
Energy Food Factory				
Potato Pops Au Gratin	½ oz	60	1	<5
Potato Pops Fat Free	½ oz	50	1	0
Potato Pops Herb & Garlic	½ oz	50	1	0
Potato Pops Mesquite	½ oz	50	1	0
Potato Pops Original	½ oz	50	1	0
Potato Pops Salt N' Vinegar	½ oz	50	1	0
Health Valley				
Country Ripple	1 oz	160	1	0
Country Ripple No Salt Added	1 oz	160	1	0
Dip Chips	1 oz	160	1	0
Dip Chips No Salt Added	1 oz	160	1	0
Natural	1 oz	160	1	0
Natural No Salt Added	1 oz	160	1	0
Kelly's				
Bar-B-Q	1 oz	150	1	0
Chips	1 oz	150	2	0
Crunchy	1 oz	150	2	0

FOOD	PORTION	CALS.	FIB.	CHOL.
Kelly's (CONT.)				
Rippled	1 oz	150	2	0
Sour Cream n' Onion	1 oz	150	1	0
Unsalted	1 oz	150	—	0
Lance				
BBQ	1 pkg (32 g)	190	—	0
Cajun Style	1 pkg (32 g)	160	—	0
Chips	1 pkg (32 g)	190	—	0
Hot Fries	1 pkg (28 g)	160	—	0
Ripple	1 pkg (32 g)	190	—	0
Sour Cream & Onion	1 pkg (32 g)	190	—	0
Lay's				
Bar-B-Q	17 pieces (1 oz)	150	1	0
Cheddar Cheese	17 pieces (1 oz)	150	1	tr
Chips	17 pieces (1 oz)	150	1	0
Crunch Tators	16 pieces (1 oz)	150	1	0
Crunch Tators Amazin' Cajun	16 pieces (1 oz)	150	—	0
Crunch Tators Hoppin' Jalapeno	16 pieces (1 oz)	140	1	0
Crunch Tators Mighty Mesquite	16 pieces (1 oz)	150	—	0
Crunch Tators Supreme Sour Cream	16 pieces (1 oz)	150	—	0
Flamin' Hot	17 pieces (1 oz)	150	1	0
Kansas City Style Bar-B-Q	17 pieces (1 oz)	150	1	0
Salt & Vinegar	17 pieces (1 oz)	150	1	0
Sour Cream & Onion	17 pieces (1 oz)	160	1	tr
Tangy Ranch	17 pieces (1 oz)	160	1	0
Unsalted	17 pieces (1 oz)	150	1	0
Louise's				
"1g" Mesquite BBQ	1 oz	110	2	0
"1g" Original	1 oz	110	2	0
70% Less Fat Mesquite BBQ	1 oz	110	2	0
70% Less Fat Original	1 oz	110	2	0
Fat-Free Maui Onion	1 oz	110	2	0
Fat-Free Mesquite BBQ	1 oz	110	2	0
Fat-Free No Salt	1 oz	110	2	0
Fat-Free Original	1 oz	110	2	0
Fat-Free Vinegar & Salt	1 oz	110	2	0
Mr. Phipps				
Tater Crisps Bar-B-Que	21 (1 oz)	130	1	0
Tater Crisps Original	23 (1 oz)	120	1	0
Tater Crisps Sour Cream 'n Onion	22 (1 oz)	130	1	0
New York Deli				
Chips	1 oz	160	—	0

FOOD	PORTION	CALS.	FIB.	CHOL.
Pringles				
BBQ	14 chips (1 oz)	150	—	0
Cheez-ums	14 chips (1 oz)	150	—	1
Original	14 chips (1 oz)	160	—	0
Ranch	14 chips (1 oz)	150	—	0
Ridges Cheddar & Sour Cream	12 chips (1 oz)	150	—	0
Ridges Mesquite BBQ	12 chips (1 oz)	150	—	0
Ridges Original	12 chips (1 oz)	150	—	0
Right BBQ	16 chips (1 oz)	140	—	0
Right Original	16 chips (1 oz)	140	—	0
Right Ranch	16 chips (1 oz)	140	—	0
Right Sour Cream 'N Onion	16 chips (1 oz)	140	—	0
Rippled Original	10 chips (1 oz)	160	—	0
Sour Cream N'Onion	14 chips (1 oz)	160	—	1
Ruffles				
Cheddar Cheese & Sour Cream	18 chips (1 oz)	160	1	tr
Chips	18 chips (1 oz)	150	1	0
Light	18 chips (1 oz)	130	1	0
Light Sour Cream & Onion	18 chips (1 oz)	130	1	tr
Mesquite Grille B-B-Q	18 chips (1 oz)	160	1	0
Monterey Jack Cheese Attack	18 chips (1 oz)	160	1	tr
Ranch	18 chips (1 oz)	160	1	0
Sour Cream & Onion	18 chips (1 oz)	160	1	tr
Snyder's				
BBQ	1 oz	150	1	0
Cheddar Bacon	1 oz	150	1	0
Chips	1 oz	150	1	0
Coney Island	1 oz	150	1	0
Grilled Steak & Onion	1 oz	150	1	0
Hot Buffalo Wings	1 oz	150	1	0
Kosher Dill	1 oz	150	1	0
No Salt	1 oz	150	1	0
Salt & Vinegar	1 oz	150	1	0
Sausage Pizza	1 oz	150	1	0
Sour Cream & Onion	1 oz	150	1	0
Sour Cream & Onion Unsalted	1 oz	150	1	0
State Line				
Chips	1 pkg (0.5 oz)	80	tr	0
Suprimos				
Cheddar & Jack	1 oz	140	—	tr
Cool Onion	1 oz	140	—	tr
Weight Watchers				
Barbecue Curls	1 pkg (0.5 oz)	60	1	0

FOOD	PORTION	CALS.	FIB.	CHOL.
Wise				
Natural	1 oz	160	—	0
Ridgies Barbecue	1 oz	150	—	0
TORTILLA				
nacho	1 oz	141	2	0
nacho	1 bag (8 oz)	1131	12	0
nacho light	1 bag (6 oz)	757	—	0
nacho light	1 oz	126	—	0
plain	1 bag (7.5 oz)	1067	14	0
plain	1 oz	142	2	0
ranch	1 oz	139	—	0
ranch	1 bag (7 oz)	969	—	1
Barrel O' Fun				
Nacho	1 oz	140	1	0
Tostada Yellow	1 oz	140	0	0
White	1 oz	140	0	0
Doritos				
Lightly Salted	16 chips (1 oz)	150	2	0
Frito Lay				
Salsa 'N Cheese	16 (1 oz)	150	2	0
Guiltless Gourmet				
Baked	22-26 chips (1 oz)	110	1	0
Hain				
Sesame	1 oz	140	—	0
Sesame Cheese	1 oz	160	—	<5
Sesame No Salt Added	1 oz	140	—	0
Taco Style	1 oz	160	—	<5
La FAMOUS				
No Salt Added	1 oz	140	—	0
Tortilla	1 oz	140	—	0
Lance				
Jalapeno Cheese	1 pkg (1⅛ oz)	160	—	0
Nacho	1 pkg (32 g)	160	—	0
Louise's				
95% Fat-Free	1 oz	120	1	0
Mr. Phipps				
Nacho	28 (1 oz)	130	3	0
Original	28 (1 oz)	130	3	0
Old El Paso				
NACHIPS	9 chips (1 oz)	150	2	0
White Corn	11 chips (1 oz)	140	1	0
Santitas				
Cantina Style	1 oz	140	2	0
Cantina Style Fajita	1 oz	140	2	0

FOOD	PORTION	CALS.	FIB.	CHOL.
Santitas (CONT.)				
Chips	1 oz	140	2	0
Strips	1 oz	140	2	0
Snyder's				
Chips	1 oz	140	2	0
Enchilada	1 oz	140	2	0
Nacho Cheese	1 oz	140	2	0
No Salt	1 oz	140	2	0
Ranch	1 oz	140	2	0
Tostitos				
Baked	1 oz	110	2	0
Baked Cool Ranch	1 oz	130	2	0
Baked Unsalted	1 oz	110	2	0
Bite Size	16 pieces (1 oz)	150	2	0
Chips	11 pieces (1 oz)	140	2	0
Restaurant Style Lime 'N Chili	7 pieces (1 oz)	150	2	0
Restaurant Style White Corn	7 pieces (1 oz)	150	2	0
Tyson				
Nacho Cheese	1 oz	140	—	0
Ranch Flavor	1 oz	140	—	0
Traditional	1 oz	140	—	0
Unsalted	1 oz	140	—	0
Wise				
Bravos	1 oz	150	—	0
VEGETABLE				
taro	10 (0.8 oz)	115	—	0
taro	1 oz	141	—	0
Eden				
Vegetable Chips	50 (1 oz)	130	0	0
Wasabi Chip Hot & Spicy	50 (1 oz)	130	0	0
Hain				
Carrot Chips No Salt Added	1 oz	150	0	0
Health Valley				
Carrot Lites	0.5 oz	75	tr	0
Terra Chips				
Sweet Potato	1 oz	140	1	0
Sweet Potato Spiced	1 oz	140	3	0
Taro Spiced	1 oz	130	2	0
Vegetable	1 oz	140	3	0
Top Banana				
Plantain Chips	1 oz	150	—	0

CHITTERLINGS

pork simmered	3 oz	258	—	122

FOOD	PORTION	CALS.	FIB.	CHOL.

CHIVES
freeze-dried	1 tbsp	1	—	0
fresh chopped	1 tbsp	1	—	0
fresh chopped	1 tsp	0	—	0

CHOCOLATE
(see also CANDY, CAROB, COCOA, ICE CREAM TOPPINGS, MILK DRINKS)

BAKING
baking	1 oz	145	—	0
grated unsweetened	1 cup (4.6 oz)	690	18	0
liquid unsweetened	1 oz	134	—	0
squares unsweetened	1 square (1 oz)	148	4	0
Hershey				
Premium Unsweetened	1 oz	190	—	0
Nestle				
Premier White	½ oz	80	—	<5

CHIPS
milk chocolate	1 cup (6 oz)	862	—	38
semisweet	60 pieces (1 oz)	136	—	0
semisweet	1 cup (6 oz)	804	—	0
Baker's				
Big Milk Chocolate	¼ cup	239	—	8
Chips	1 oz	143	—	5
Semi-Sweet	¼ cup	197	—	tr
Hershey				
Milk Chocolate	1 oz	150	—	10
Semi-Sweet	¼ cup (1.5 oz)	220	—	0
Semi-Sweet Miniature	¼ cup (1.5 oz)	220	—	0
M&M's				
Baking Bits Milk Chocolate	0.5 oz	70	0	5
Baking Bits Semi-Sweet	0.5 oz	70	1	0

MIX
powder	2-3 heaping tsp	75	—	0
powder as prep w/ whole milk	9 oz	226	—	33
Hershey				
Chocolate Milk Mix	3 tbsp	90	—	0

CHOCOLATE MILK
(see CHOCOLATE, COCOA, MILK DRINKS, MILKSHAKE)

CHOCOLATE SYRUP
syrup	1 cup	653	—	0
syrup	2 tbsp	82	—	0
syrup as prep w/ whole milk	9 oz	232	—	33
Estee				
Choco-Syp	2 tbsp (1.2 oz)	50	—	0

FOOD	PORTION	CALS.	FIB.	CHOL.
Hershey				
Syrup	2 tbsp	80	—	0
Marzetti				
Syrup	2 tbsp	40	0	0
Red Wing				
Syrup	2 tbsp (1.4 oz)	110	0	0
CHUTNEY				
apple cranberry	1 tbsp	16	—	0
coconut	¼ cup	74	2	0
Sonoma				
Dried Tomato	1 tbsp (0.7 g)	35	0	0
CILANTRO				
fresh	¼ cup	1	—	0
Watkins				
Dried	¼ tsp (0.5 oz)	0	0	0
CINNAMON				
ground	1 tsp	6	—	0
Watkins				
Ground	¼ tsp (0.5 g)	0	0	0
CISCO				
smoked	3 oz	151	—	27
smoked	1 oz	50	—	9
CLAMS				
CANNED				
meat only	1 cup	236	—	107
meat only	3 oz	126	—	57
American Original				
Quahogs	4 oz	66	—	16
Progresso				
Creamy Clam	½ cup (4.2 oz)	100	0	10
Minced	¼ cup (2 oz)	25	0	10
Red Clam	½ cup (4.4 oz)	80	1	5
White Clam Sauce	½ cup (4.4 oz)	120	0	15
FRESH				
cooked	3 oz	126	—	57
cooked	20 sm	133	—	60
raw	20 sm (180 g)	133	—	60
raw	9 lg (180 g)	133	—	60
raw	3 oz	63	—	29
FROZEN				
Gorton's				
Microwave Crunchy Clam Strips	3.5 oz	330	—	30

FOOD	PORTION	CALS.	FIB.	CHOL.
Mrs. Paul's				
Fried	2½ oz	200	—	15
HOME RECIPE				
breaded & fried	3 oz	171	—	52
breaded & fried	20 sm	379	—	115
TAKE-OUT				
breaded & fried	¾ cup	451	—	87

CLOVES
ground	1 tsp	7	—	0

COCOA
(see also CHOCOLATE)

FOOD	PORTION	CALS.	FIB.	CHOL.
hot cocoa	1 cup	218	—	33
powder unsweetened	1 tbsp (5 g)	11	2	0
powder unsweetened	1 cup (3 oz)	197	29	0
Carnation				
Hot Cocoa 70 Calorie	3 tsp (21 g)	70	—	2
Hot Cocoa Milk Chocolate	1 pkg or 4 heaping tsp (1 oz)	110	—	2
Hot Cocoa Natural Mint	1 pkg or 4 heaping tsp (1 oz)	110	—	2
Hot Cocoa Rich Chocolate	1 pkg or 4 heaping tsp (1 oz)	110	—	2
Hot Cocoa Rich Chocolate w/ Marshmallows	1 pkg or 4 heaping tsp (1 oz)	110	—	2
Hot Cocoa Sugar Free Mint	1 pkg or 4 heaping tsp (15 g)	50	—	2
Hot Cocoa Sugar Free Rich Chocolate	1 pkg or 4 heaping tsp (15 g)	50	—	2
Hershey				
Cocoa	⅓ cup (1 oz)	120	—	0
European Cocoa	1 oz	90	—	0
Hills Bros.				
Hot Cocoa	6 oz	110	—	0
Hot Cocoa Sugar Free	6 oz	60	—	0
Nestle				
Cocoa	1 tbsp	15	2	0
Swiss Miss				
Cocoa Diet	6 oz	20	0	1
Hot Cocoa Bavarian Chocolate	6 oz	110	0	2
Hot Cocoa Double Rich	6 oz	110	0	0
Hot Cocoa Milk Chocolate	6 oz	110	0	5

FOOD	PORTION	CALS.	FIB.	CHOL.
Swiss Miss (CONT.)				
Hot Cocoa Milk Chocolate	1 serv	110	1	1
Hot Cocoa Mini-Marshmallow	1 serv	109	1	1
Hot Cocoa Rich Chocolate	1 serv	110	1	1
Hot Cocoa Sugar Free	1 serv	67	1	1
Hot Cocoa Sugar Free Milk Chocolate	1 serv	49	1	tr
Hot Cocoa Sugar Free Mini-Marshmallow	1 serv	51	1	1
Hot Cocoa White Chocolate	1 serv	109	tr	1
Hot Cocoa With Mini Marshmallows	6 oz	110	0	5
Hot Cocoa Lite	1 serv	74	2	tr
Lite as prep	6 oz	70	0	1
Sugar Free With Sugar Free Marshmallows as prep	6 oz	50	0	2
Sugar Free as prep	6 oz	60	0	2
Ultra Slim-Fast				
Hot Cocoa as prep w/ water	8 oz	190	5	8
Weight Watchers				
Cocoa	1 pkg	60	—	5
COCONUT				
coconut water	1 cup	46	—	0
coconut water	1 tbsp	3	—	0
cream canned	1 tbsp	36	—	0
cream canned	1 cup	568	—	0
dried sweetened flaked	1 cup	351	—	0
dried sweetened flaked	7 oz pkg	944	—	0
dried sweetened flaked canned	1 cup	341	—	0
dried sweetened shredded	7 oz pkg	997	—	0
dried sweetened shredded	1 cup	466	—	0
dried toasted	1 oz	168	—	0
dried unsweetened	1 oz	187	—	0
fresh	1 piece (1½ oz)	159	4	0
fresh shredded	1 cup	283	7	0
milk canned	1 tbsp	30	—	0
milk canned	1 cup	445	—	0
milk frozen	1 cup	486	—	0
milk frozen	1 tbsp	30	—	0
Baker's				
Angel Flake Toasted	⅓ cup	212	—	0
Premium Shred	⅓ cup	135	—	0
COD				
CANNED				
atlantic	3 oz	89	—	47

FOOD	PORTION	CALS.	FIB.	CHOL.
atlantic	1 can (11 oz)	327	—	171
DRIED				
atlantic	3 oz	246	—	129
FRESH				
atlantic cooked	1 fillet (6.3 oz)	189	—	99
atlantic cooked	3 oz	89	—	47
atlantic raw	3 oz	70	—	37
pacific baked	3 oz	95	—	43
roe raw	3½ oz	130	—	360
FROZEN				
Mrs. Paul's				
Light Fillets	1 fillet	240	—	50
Van De Kamp's				
Lightly Breaded Fillets	1 (4 oz)	220	0	35

COFFEE

(*see also* COFFEE BEVERAGES, COFFEE SUBSTITUTES)

FOOD	PORTION	CALS.	FIB.	CHOL.
INSTANT				
decaffeinated	1 rounded tsp (1.8 g)	4	—	0
regular	1 rounded tsp	4	—	0
regular as prep	6 oz	4	—	0
regular w/ chicory	1 rounded tsp	6	—	0
regular w/ chicory as prep	6 oz	6	—	0
REGULAR				
brewed	6 oz	4	—	0
Folgers				
Colombian Supreme	1 tbsp	16	—	0
Custom Roast	1 tbsp	16	—	0
Decaffeinated	1 tbsp	17	—	0
French Roast	1 tbsp	16	—	0
Gourmet Supreme	1 tbsp	16	—	0
Instant	1 tsp	8	—	0
Instant Decaffeinated	1 tsp	8	—	0
Singles	1 bag	21	—	0
Singles Decaffeinated	1 bag	21	—	0
Special Roast	1 tbsp	16	—	0
Vacuum Pack	1 tbsp	16	—	0
Maryland Club				
Ground	1 tbsp	16	—	0
TAKE-OUT				
cafe au lait	1 cup (8 fl oz)	77	—	17
cafe brulot	1 cup (4.8 fl oz)	48	—	0
cappuccino	1 cup (8 fl oz)	77	—	17

FOOD	PORTION	CALS.	FIB.	CHOL.
coffee con leche	1 cup (8 fl oz)	77	—	17
espresso	1 cup (3 fl oz)	2	—	0
irish coffee	1 serv (9 fl oz)	107	—	12
mocha	1 mug (9.6 fl oz)	202	—	40

COFFEE BEVERAGES
(see also COFFEE SUBSTITUTES*)*

General Foods

International Coffee Cafe Amaretto	6 oz	51	—	tr
International Coffee Cafe Francais	6 oz	55	—	tr
International Coffee Cafe Irish Creme	6 oz	55	—	tr
International Coffee Cafe Vienna	6 oz	59	—	tr
International Coffee Irish Mocha Mint	6 oz	51	—	tr
International Coffee Orange Cappuccino	6 oz	59	—	tr
International Coffee Sugar Free Cafe Francais	6 oz	35	—	tr
International Coffee Sugar Free Cafe Irish Creme	6 oz	31	—	tr
International Coffee Sugar Free Cafe Vienna	6 oz	29	—	tr
International Coffee Sugar Free Irish Mocha Mint	6 oz	28	—	tr
International Coffee Sugar Free Orange Cappuccino	6 oz	29	—	tr
International Coffee Sugar Free Suisse Mocha	6 oz	29	—	tr
International Coffee Suisse Mocha	6 oz	53	—	tr

Starbucks

Frappuccino	1 bottle (9.5 fl oz)	190	0	12

COFFEE SUBSTITUTES

powder	1 tsp	9	—	0
powder as prep	6 oz	9	—	0
powder as prep w/ milk	6 oz	121	—	25
Kava				
Instant	1 tsp	2	—	0
Natural Touch				
Kaffree Roma	1 tsp	6	—	0

FOOD	PORTION	CALS.	FIB.	CHOL.
Pero				
Instant Grain Beverage	1 tsp (1.5 g)	5	—	0
Postum				
Instant	6 oz	11	—	0
Instant Coffee Flavored	6 oz	11	—	0

COFFEE WHITENERS
(*see also* MILK SUBSTITUTES)

FOOD	PORTION	CALS.	FIB.	CHOL.
liquid nondairy frzn	1 tbsp (0.5 oz)	20	—	0
powder nondairy	1 tsp	11	—	0
Coffee-Mate				
Liquid	1 tbsp (0.5 fl oz)	16	—	0
Powder	1 tsp (2 g)	10	—	0
Hood				
Non Dairy	1 tbsp (0.5 oz)	20	0	0
International Delight				
Amaretto	1 tbsp (0.6 fl oz)	45	0	0
Cinnamon Hazelnut	1 tbsp (0.6 fl oz)	45	0	0
Irish Creme	1 tbsp (0.6 fl oz)	45	0	0
No Fat Amaretto	1 tbsp (0.5 fl oz)	30	0	0
No Fat French Vanilla Royale	1 tbsp (0.5 fl oz)	30	0	0
No Fat Hawaiian Macadamia	1 tbsp (0.5 fl oz)	30	0	0
No Fat Irish Creme	1 tbsp (0.5 fl oz)	30	0	0
Suisse Chocolate Mocha	1 tbsp (0.6 fl oz)	45	0	0
Mocha Mix				
Fat-Free	1 tbsp (0.5 fl oz)	10	0	0
Lite	1 tbsp (0.5 fl oz)	10	0	0
Lite	4 fl oz	80	0	0
Original	1 tbsp (0.5 fl oz)	20	0	0
Signature Flavors French Vanilla	1 tbsp (0.5 fl oz)	35	—	0
Signature Flavors Irish Creme	1 tbsp (0.5 fl oz)	35	—	0
Signature Flavors Kahlua	1 tbsp (0.5 fl oz)	35	—	0
Signature Flavors Mauna Loa Macadamia Nut	1 tbsp (0.5 fl oz)	35	—	0
N-Rich Creamer				
Whitener	1 tsp	10	0	0

COLESLAW
(*see* CABBAGE)

COLLARDS
CANNED
Allen

FOOD	PORTION	CALS.	FIB.	CHOL.
Collards	½ cup (4.1 oz)	30	3	0

FOOD	PORTION	CALS.	FIB.	CHOL.
Sunshine				
Collards	½ cup (4.1 oz)	30	3	0
FRESH				
cooked	½ cup	17	—	0
raw chopped	½ cup	6	—	0
FROZEN				
chopped cooked	½ cup	31	—	0

COOKIES

(*see also* BROWNIE, CAKE, DOUGHNUTS, PIE)

HOME RECIPE

FOOD	PORTION	CALS.	FIB.	CHOL.
chocolate chip as prep w/ butter	1 (0.42 oz)	78	—	11
chocolate chip as prep w/ margarine	1 (0.56 oz)	78	—	5
macaroons	1 (0.8 oz)	97	—	0
oatmeal	1 (0.5 oz)	67	—	5
oatmeal w/ raisins	1 (0.52 oz)	65	—	5
peanut butter	1 (0.7 oz)	95	—	6
shortbread as prep w/ butter	1 (0.38 oz)	60	—	10
shortbread as prep w/ margarine	1 (0.38 oz)	60	—	0
sugar as prep w/ butter	1 (0.49 oz)	66	—	12
sugar as prep w/ margarine	1 (0.49 oz)	66	—	4
MIX				
chocolate chip	1 (0.56 oz)	79	—	7
oatmeal	1 (0.6 oz)	74	tr	7
oatmeal raisin	1 (0.6 oz)	74	tr	7
Betty Crocker				
Date Bar Classic Dessert	1	60	—	0
Estee				
Chocolate Chip	3	130	0	0
READY-TO-EAT				
animal crackers	1 box (2.4 oz)	299	—	11
chocolate chip	1 box (1.9 oz)	233	—	12
chocolate chip low fat	1 (0.25 oz)	45	—	0
chocolate chip low sugar low sodium	1 (0.24 oz)	31	—	0
chocolate chip soft-type	1 (0.5 oz)	69	tr	0
chocolate wafer	1 (0.2 oz)	26	—	0
chocolate wafer cookie crumbs	½ cup (5.9 oz)	728	—	0
gingersnaps	1 (0.24 oz)	29	—	0
graham	1 square (0.24 oz)	30	—	0
graham chocolate covered	1 (0.49 oz)	68	—	0
graham cracker crumbs	½ cup (4.4 oz)	540	3	0
graham honey	1 (0.24 oz)	30	tr	0

FOOD	PORTION	CALS.	FIB.	CHOL.
ladyfingers	1 (0.38 oz)	40	—	40
molasses	1 (0.5 oz)	65	—	0
oatmeal	1 (0.52 oz)	71	tr	0
oatmeal	1 (0.6 oz)	81	1	0
oatmeal raisin	1 (0.6 oz)	81	1	0
oatmeal raisin low sugar no sodium	1 (0.24 oz)	31	—	0
peanut butter sandwich	1 (0.5 oz)	67	—	0
peanut butter soft-type	1 (0.5 oz)	69	tr	0
raisin soft-type	1 (0.5 oz)	60	—	0
shortbread	1 (0.28 oz)	40	—	2
shortbread pecan	1 (0.49 oz)	79	tr	5
sugar	1 (0.52 oz)	72	—	8
sugar low sugar sodium free	1 (0.24 oz)	30	—	0
sugar wafers w/ creme filling	1 (0.12 oz)	18	—	0
sugar wafers w/ creme filling sugar free sodium free	1 (0.14 oz)	20	—	0
vanilla sandwich	1 (0.35 oz)	48	tr	0
Archway				
Almond Crescents	2 (0.8 oz)	100	tr	<5
Apple N'Raisin	1 (1.1 oz)	130	1	<5
Apricot Filled	1 (1 oz)	110	tr	5
Bells And Stars	3 (1 oz)	150	tr	5
Blueberry Filled	1 (1 oz)	110	tr	5
Carrot Cake	1 (1 oz)	120	0	<5
Cherry Filled	1 (1 oz)	110	tr	10
Cherry Nougat	3 (1 oz)	150	0	0
Chocolate Chip	1 (1 oz)	130	0	tr
Chocolate Chip & Toffee	1 (1 oz)	140	tr	<5
Chocolate Chip Bag	3 (0.9 oz)	130	0	10
Chocolate Chip Drop	1 (1 oz)	140	tr	10
Chocolate Chip Ice Box	1 (1 oz)	140	0	5
Chocolate Chip Mini	12 (1.1 oz)	150	0	5
Cinnamon Snaps	12 (1.1 oz)	150	0	5
Coconut Macaroon	1 (0.8 oz)	90	2	0
Cookie Jar Hermits	1 (1 oz)	110	tr	<5
Dark Chocolate	1 (1 oz)	110	tr	<5
Dutch Chocolate	1 (1 oz)	120	0	<5
Fig Bars Low Fat	2 (1.1 oz)	100	1	0
Frosty Lemon	1 (1 oz)	120	0	0
Frosty Orange	1 (1 oz)	120	1	0
Fruit And Honey Bar	1 (1 oz)	110	tr	5
Fruit Bar No Fat	1 (1 oz)	90	0	0
Fruit Cake	1 (1.1 oz)	140	2	0

FOOD	PORTION	CALS.	FIB.	CHOL.
Archway (CONT.)				
Fudge Nut Bar	1 (1 oz)	110	tr	<5
Fun Chip Mini	12 (1.1 oz)	140	0	5
Gingersnaps	5 (1.1 oz)	130	0	0
Granola No Fat	1 (0.5 oz)	50	tr	0
Holiday Pak	3 (1.1 oz)	150	tr	<5
Iced Gingerbread	3 (1.1 oz)	140	0	5
Iced Molasses	1 (1 oz)	110	tr	0
Iced Oatmeal	1 (1 oz)	120	1	<5
Lemon Snaps	12 (1.1 oz)	150	0	5
New Orleans Cake	1 (1 oz)	110	tr	<5
Nutty Nougat	3 (1.1 oz)	160	0	0
Oatmeal	1 (0.9 oz)	110	tr	<5
Oatmeal Apple Filled	1 (1 oz)	110	0	<5
Oatmeal Date Filled	1 (1 oz)	110	tr	<5
Oatmeal Mini	12 (1.1 oz)	150	1	5
Oatmeal Pecan	1 (1 oz)	120	1	<5
Oatmeal Raisin	1 (1 oz)	110	tr	<5
Oatmeal Raisin Bran	1 (1 oz)	110	tr	<5
Old Fashioned Molasses	1 (1 oz)	120	0	5
Old Fashioned Windmill	1 (0.7 oz)	100	0	0
Party Treats	3 (1.1 oz)	140	0	15
Peanut Butter	1 (1 oz)	140	tr	10
Peanut Butter & Chip	3 (0.9 oz)	130	0	10
Peanut Butter N' Chips	1 (1 oz)	140	tr	10
Peanut Butter Nougat	3 (1.1 oz)	160	1	0
Pecan Crunch	6 (1.1 oz)	150	0	10
Pecan Ice Box	1 (1 oz)	140	0	10
Pecan Malted Nougat	3 (1.1 oz)	160	2	0
Pfeffernusse	2 (1.3 oz)	140	tr	0
Pineapple Filled	1 (0.9 oz)	100	1	5
Raisin Oatmeal	1 (1 oz)	130	1	5
Raisin Oatmeal Bag	3 (1 oz)	130	1	10
Raspberry Filled	1 (1 oz)	110	tr	5
Rocky Road	1 (1 oz)	130	tr	10
Ruth's Golden Oatmeal	1 (1 oz)	120	tr	<5
Select Assortment	3 (0.9 oz)	130	0	10
Soft Molasses Drop	1 (1 oz)	110	1	<5
Soft Sugar	1 (1 oz)	110	0	5
Strawberry Filled	1 (1 oz)	110	tr	<5
Sugar	1 (1 oz)	120	0	<5
Vanilla Wafer	5 (1.1 oz)	130	0	5
Wedding Cakes	3 (1.1 oz)	160	0	0

FOOD	PORTION	CALS.	FIB.	CHOL.
Bakery Wagon				
Apple Walnut Raisin	1	100	1	0
Cobbler Apple Cranberry Fat Free	1	70	1	0
Cobbler Apple Fat Free	1	70	1	0
Cobbler Mixed Fruit Fat Free	1	70	1	0
Cobbler Raspberry Fat Free	1	70	1	0
Ginger Snaps	5	160	1	0
Honey Fruit Bars	1	100	1	5
Iced Molasses	1	100	1	2
Iced Molasses Mini	3	130	1	0
Oatmeal Apple Filled	1	90	1	0
Oatmeal Chocolate Chunk	1	100	1	0
Oatmeal Date Filled	1	90	1	0
Oatmeal Raspberry Filled	1	100	1	0
Oatmeal Soft	1	100	1	0
Oatmeal Walnut Raisin	1	100	1	0
Vanilla Wafers Cholesterol Free	6	130	1	0
Baking On The Lite Side				
Oatmeal Crunchy	2 (0.6 oz)	60	0	0
Raspberry Linzer	1 (0.6 oz)	55	0	0
Barnum's				
Animal Crackers	12 (1.1 oz)	140	1	0
Biscos				
Sugar Wafers	8 (1 oz)	140	tr	0
Waffle Cremes	4 (1.2 oz)	180	tr	0
Cadbury				
Fingers	3	85	tr	2
Chip-A-Roos				
Cookies	3 (1.3 oz)	190	1	0
Chips Ahoy!				
Bite Size Chocolate Chip	14 (1.1 oz)	170	tr	0
Chewy Chocolate Chip	3 (1.3 oz)	170	tr	<5
Chunky Chocolate Chip	1 (0.5 oz)	80	tr	10
Real Chocolate Chip	3 (1.1 oz)	160	1	0
Reduced Fat	3 (1.1 oz)	150	1	0
Sprinkled Real Chocolate Chip	3 (1.3 oz)	170	tr	0
Striped Chocolate Chip	1 (0.5 oz)	80	tr	0
Cookie Lover's				
Blue Ribbon Brownies	1 (0.8 oz)	90	0	11
Classic Shortbread	1 (0.8 oz)	110	0	15
Dutch Chocolate Chip	1 (0.8 oz)	90	0	14
Fancy Peanut Butter	1 (0.8 oz)	100	0	7
Grahams Cinnamon Honey	2 (1 oz)	110	1	0

FOOD	PORTION	CALS.	FIB.	CHOL.
Cookie Lover's (CONT.)				
Grahams Honey	2 (1 oz)	100	1	0
Old-Time Raisin	1 (0.8 oz)	90	0	15
Delacre				
Cookie Assortment	4 (1.1 oz)	130	1	8
Drake's				
Chocolate Chip	2 (1 oz)	140	—	0
Chocolate-Chocolate Chip	2 (1 oz)	130	—	0
Coconut	2 (1 oz)	130	—	0
Coconut Macaroon	1 (1 oz)	135	—	0
Hermit	1 (2 oz)	230	—	10
Oatmeal	2 (1 oz)	120	—	0
Oatmeal Creme	1 (2 oz)	240	—	2
Peanut Butter Wafers	1 (2.25 oz)	324	—	0
Dutch Mill				
Chocolate Chip	3 (1.1 oz)	160	1	0
Coconut Macaroons	3 (1 oz)	120	0	0
Oatmeal Raisin	3 (1 oz)	130	1	0
Estee				
Chocolate Chip	4 (1.1 oz)	150	tr	0
Coconut	4 (1 oz)	140	tr	0
Creme Wafers Chocolate	7 (1.1 oz)	160	tr	0
Creme Wafers Lemon	5 (1.2 oz)	170	0	0
Creme Wafers Peanut Butter	5 (1.2 oz)	170	0	0
Creme Wafers Triple Decker Banana Split	3 (0.9 oz)	140	0	0
Creme Wafers Triple Decker Chocolate Caramel & Peanut Butter	3 (0.9 oz)	140	0	0
Creme Wafers Vanilla	7 (1.1 oz)	160	0	0
Creme Wafers Vanilla & Strawberry	5 (1.2 oz)	170	0	0
Fig Bars Apple Low Fat	2 (1 oz)	100	3	0
Fig Bars Cranberry Low Fat	2 (1 oz)	100	3	0
Fig Bars Low Fat	2 (1 oz)	100	3	0
Fudge	4 (1 oz)	150	1	0
Lemon	4 (1 oz)	140	tr	0
Oatmeal Raisin	4 (1 oz)	130	1	0
Sandwich Chocolate	3 (1.2 oz)	160	1	0
Sandwich Original	3 (1.2 oz)	160	1	0
Sandwich Peanut Butter	3 (1.2 oz)	160	1	0
Sandwich Vanilla	3 (1.2 oz)	160	tr	0
Shortbread Reduced Fat	4 (1 oz)	130	tr	0
Vanilla	4 (1 oz)	140	tr	0

FOOD	PORTION	CALS.	FIB.	CHOL.
Freihofer's				
Chocolate Chip	2 (0.9 oz)	120	1	10
Frito Lay				
Peanut Butter Bar	1.75 oz	270	—	0
Frookie				
7-Grain Oatmeal	1	45	—	0
Animal Frackers	6	60	—	0
Apple Cinnamon Oat Bran	1 lg	120	—	0
Apple Cinnamon Oat Bran	1	45	—	0
Apple Fruitins	1	60	—	0
Chocolate Chip	1	45	—	0
Chocolate Chip	1 lg	120	—	0
Chocolate Chip Mint	1	45	—	0
Fig Fruitins	1	60	—	0
Ginger Spice	1	45	—	0
Mandarin Chocolate Chip	1	45	—	0
Oat Bran Muffin	1	45	—	0
Oat Bran Muffin	1 lg	120	—	0
Oatmeal Raisin	1 lg	120	—	0
Oatmeal Raisin	1	45	—	0
General Mills				
Dunkaroos	1 pkg (1 oz)	130	—	0
Girl Scout				
Chalet Cremes Sugar Free	4 (1 oz)	150	1	0
Do-si-dos	3 (1.2 oz)	170	1	0
Samoas	2 (1 oz)	160	2	0
Snaps	7 (1.1 oz)	130	1	0
Striped Chocolate Chip	3 (1.2 oz)	180	1	0
Tagalongs	2 (0.9 oz)	150	2	0
Thin Mints	4 (1 oz)	140	1	0
Trefoils	5 (1.1 oz)	160	1	0
Golden Fruit				
Apple	1 (0.7 oz)	80	tr	0
Cranberry	1 (0.7 oz)	70	tr	0
Cranberry Low Fat	1 (0.7 oz)	70	tr	0
Raisin	1 (0.7 oz)	80	tr	0
Grandma's				
Animal Cookies Candied	5 (1 oz)	140	—	0
Chocolate Chip	2 (2.75 oz)	370	—	5
Chocolate Chip Rich'N Chewy	3 (1 oz)	140	—	5
Fudge Chocolate Chip	2 (2.75 oz)	350	—	5
Grab Cookie Bits Chocolate	8 (1 oz)	140	—	0
Grab Cookie Bits Peanut Butter	8 (1 oz)	140	—	0
Grab Cookie Bits Vanilla	8 (1 oz)	140	—	5

FOOD	PORTION	CALS.	FIB.	CHOL.
Grandma's (CONT.)				
Oatmeal Apple Spice	2 (2.75 oz)	330	—	10
Old Time Molasses	2 (2.75 oz)	320	—	5
Peanut Butter	2 (2.75 oz)	410	—	10
Raisin Soft	2 (2.75 oz)	320	—	10
Health Valley				
Amaranth Cookies	1	70	2	0
Fancy Fruit Chunks Apricot Almond	2	90	2	0
Fancy Fruit Chunks Date Pecan	2	90	2	0
Fancy Fruit Chunks Raisin Oat Bran	2	70	2	0
Fancy Fruit Chunks Tropical Fruit	2	90	2	0
Fancy Peanut Chunks	2	90	2	0
Fat Free Apple Spice	3	75	3	0
Fat Free Apricot Delight	3	75	3	0
Fat Free Date Delight	3	75	3	0
Fat Free Hawaiian Fruit	3	75	3	0
Fat Free Jumbos Apple Raisin	1	70	3	0
Fat Free Jumbos Raisin	1	70	3	0
Fat Free Jumbos Raspberry	1	70	3	0
Fat Free Raisin Oatmeal	3	75	3	0
Fiber Jumbos Blueberry Nut	1	100	3	0
Fiber Jumbos Chunky Pecan	1	100	3	0
Fiber Jumbos Raisin Nut	1	100	3	0
Fruit & Fitness	5	200	6	0
Fruit Jumbos Almond Date	1	70	1	0
Fruit Jumbos Oat Bran	1	70	2	0
Fruit Jumbos Raisin Nut	1	70	1	0
Fruit Jumbos Tropical Fruit	1	70	2	0
Graham Amaranth	7	110	3	0
Graham Honey	7	100	2	0
Graham Oat Bran	7	120	5	0
Honey Jumbos Crisp Cinnamon	1	70	1	0
Honey Jumbos Crisp Peanut Butter	1	70	1	0
Honey Jumbos Fancy Oat Bran	2	130	4	0
Oat Bran Animal Cookies	7	110	3	0
Oat Bran Fruit & Nut	2	110	3	0
The Great Tofu	2	90	4	0
The Great Wheat Free	2	80	3	0
Heyday				
Caramel & Peanut	1 (0.8 oz)	110	tr	0

FOOD	PORTION	CALS.	FIB.	CHOL.
Heyday (cont.)				
Fudge	1 (0.8 oz)	110	tr	0
Honey Maid				
Cinnamon Grahams	10 (1.1 oz)	140	1	0
Honey Grahams	8 (1 oz)	120	1	0
Hydrox				
Original	3	150	1	0
Reduced Fat	3 (1.1 oz)	130	1	0
Keebler				
Buttercup	3	70	—	0
Chocolate Fudge Sandwich	1	80	—	0
Commodore	1	60	—	0
Cookies Mates	2	50	—	0
French Vanilla Creme	1	80	—	0
Graham Honey Fiber Enriched	2	90	—	0
Graham Kitchen Rich	2	60	—	0
Homeplate	1	60	—	1
Keebies	1	80	—	0
Krisp Kreem Wafers	2	50	—	0
Old Fashion Chocolate Chip	1	80	—	0
Old Fashion Double Fudge	1	80	—	0
Old Fashion Oatmeal	1	80	—	0
Old Fashion Peanut Butter	1	80	—	0
Old Fashion Sugar	1	80	—	0
Pitter Patter	1	90	—	0
Vanilla Wafers	4	80	—	1
La Choy				
Fortune	1	15	tr	0
Lance				
Choc-O-Lunch	1 pkg (37 g)	180	—	0
Choc-O-Mint	1 pkg (35 g)	180	—	0
Chocolate Chip Fudge	1 (28 g)	130	—	5
Chocolate Chip Soft	1 (28 g)	130	—	5
Coated Graham	1 pkg (50 g)	200	—	0
Fig Bar	1 pkg (42 g)	150	—	0
Lem-O-Lunch	1 pkg (48 g)	240	—	0
Lemon Nekot	1 pkg (42 g)	220	—	5
Malt	1 pkg (35 g)	190	—	0
Nut-O-Lunch	1 oz	140	—	0
Oatmeal	1 (57 g)	130	—	0
Peanut Butter Creme Filled Wafer	1 pkg (50 g)	240	—	0
Van-O-Lunch	1 pkg (37 g)	180	—	0

FOOD	PORTION	CALS.	FIB.	CHOL.
Little Debbie				
Animal	1 pkg (1.5 oz)	190	0	0
Caramel Cookie Bars	1 pkg (1.2 oz)	160	1	0
Chocolate Chip Chewy	1 pkg (2 oz)	370	1	10
Chocolate Chip Crisp	1 pkg (1.5 oz)	210	1	5
Cookie Wreaths	1 pkg (0.6 oz)	90	0	0
Creme Filled Chocolate	1 pkg (1.2 oz)	180	1	0
Creme Filled Chocolate	1 pkg (1.8 oz)	260	1	0
Easter Puffs	1 pkg (1.2 oz)	140	0	0
Figaroos	1 pkg (1.5 oz)	160	3	0
Figaroos	1 pkg (2 oz)	200	2	0
Fudge Macaroons	1 pkg (1 oz)	140	1	0
Ginger	1 pkg (0.7 oz)	90	1	5
Oatmeal Crisp	1 pkg (1.5 oz)	210	1	5
Oatmeal Lights	1 pkg (1.3 oz)	140	1	0
Oatmeal Raisin	1 pkg (2.7 oz)	320	2	0
Peanut Butter	1 pkg (1.5 oz)	210	1	5
Peanut Butter & Jelly Sandwich	1 pkg (1.1 oz)	130	1	0
Peanut Butter Bars	1 pkg (1.9 oz)	270	1	0
Peanut Clusters	1 pkg (1.4 oz)	190	1	0
Pecan Spinwheels	1 pkg (1 oz)	110	1	0
Pecan Shortbread	1 pkg (1.5 oz)	220	0	5
Lorna Doone				
Cookies	4 (1 oz)	140	tr	5
LU				
Chocolatiers	4 (1.1 oz)	170	2	0
Chocolatiers Dipped	3 (1 oz)	170	1	0
Le Petit Ecolier Dark Chocolate	2 (0.9 oz)	130	1	5
Little Schoolboy Milk Chocolate	2 (0.9 oz)	130	0	5
Marie Lu	3 (1.2 oz)	170	1	5
Truffle Lu	4 (1.2 oz)	180	1	0
Mallomars				
Cookies	2 (0.9 oz)	120	1	0
Mallopuffs				
Cookies	1 (0.6 oz)	70	tr	0
Manischewitz				
Macaroons Chocolate	2 (0.9 oz)	90	4	0
Mother's				
Almond Shortbread	3	180	1	0
Butter	5	140	—	10
Checkerboard Wafers	8	150	1	0
Chocolate Chip	2	160	0	10
Chocolate Chip Angel	3	180	1	0
Chocolate Chip Bag	4	140	1	2

FOOD	PORTION	CALS.	FIB.	CHOL.
Mother's (CONT.)				
Chocolate Chip Parade	4	130	1	0
Circus Animals	6	140	0	0
Cocadas	5	150	2	5
Cookie Parade	4	140	2	0
Dinosaur Grrrahams	2	130	—	0
Double Fudge	3	170	2	0
Duplex Creme	3	170	1	0
English Tea	2	180	1	0
Fig Bar	2	130	0	0
Fig Bar Fat Free	1	70	1	0
Fig Bar Whole Wheat	2	130	3	0
Fig Bar Whole Wheat Fat Free	1	70	1	0
Flaky Flix Fudge	2	140	2	0
Flaky Flix Vanilla	2	140	1	0
Frosted Holiday	4	130	0	0
Fudge Bowl Crowns	2	140	1	0
Fudge Bowl Nuggets	2	140	1	0
Gaucho Peanut Butter	2	190	2	0
Gingerbread Man	6	140	1	5
Iced Oatmeal	2	120	1	0
Iced Oatmeal Bag	4	120	1	0
Iced Raisin	2	180	1	0
MLB Double Header Duplex	3	170	1	5
Macaroon	2	150	2	0
Marias	3	170	1	5
North Poles	2	140	0	0
Oatmeal	2	110	1	0
Oatmeal Chocolate Chip	2	120	1	0
Oatmeal Raisin	5	150	2	5
Oatmeal Walnut Chocolate Chip	2	130	1	0
Pecan Goldens	2	170	5	0
Rainbow Wafers	8	150	1	0
Striped Shortbread	3	170	1	0
Sugar	2	140	1	0
Taffy	2	180	2	0
Triplet Assortment	2	140	1	0
Vanilla Wafers	6	150	1	4
Walnut Fudge	2	130	1	0
Zoo Pals	14	140	1	0
Mystic Mint				
Cookies	1 (0.5 oz)	90	0	0
Nabisco				
Brown Edge Wafers	5 (1 oz)	140	tr	<5

FOOD	PORTION	CALS.	FIB.	CHOL.
Nabisco (CONT.)				
Bugs Bunny Chocolate Graham	13 (1.1 oz)	140	1	0
Bugs Bunny Cinnamon Graham	13 (1.1 oz)	140	tr	0
Bugs Bunny Graham	13 (1.1 oz)	140	1	0
Cameo	2 (1 oz)	130	tr	0
Chocolate Grahams	3 (1.1 oz)	160	1	0
Chocolate Chip Snaps	7 (1.1 oz)	150	tr	0
Chocolate Snaps	7 (1.1 oz)	140	1	0
Cookie Break	3 (1.1 oz)	160	tr	0
Danish Imported	5 (1.1 oz)	170	1	0
Family Favorites Fudge Covered Grahams	3 (1 oz)	140	1	0
Family Favorites Fudge Striped Shortbread	3 (1.1 oz)	160	1	0
Family Favorites Oatmeal	1 (0.5 oz)	80	tr	0
Family Favorites Vanilla Sandwich	3 (1.2 oz)	170	0	0
Famous Chocolate Wafers	5 (1.1 oz)	140	1	<5
Ginger Snaps Old Fashioned	4 (1 oz)	120	tr	0
Grahams	8 (1 oz)	120	1	0
Marshmallow Puffs	1 (0.75 oz)	90	0	0
Marshmallow Twirls	1 (1 oz)	130	tr	0
Nilla Wafers	8 (1.1 oz)	140	0	5
Pecan Passion	1 (0.5 oz)	90	0	<5
Pinwheels	1 (1 oz)	130	tr	0
National				
Arrowroot	1 (5 g)	20	tr	0
Newtons				
Apple Fat Free	2 (1 oz)	100	1	0
Cranberry Fat Free	2 (1 oz)	100	1	0
Fig	2 (1.1 oz)	110	1	0
Fig Fat Free	1 (1 oz)	100	2	0
Raspberry Fat Free	2 (1 oz)	100	tr	0
Strawberry Fat Free	2 (1 oz)	100	tr	0
Nutter Butter				
Bites Peanut Butter Sandwich	10 (1.1 oz)	150	1	<5
Peanut Butter Sandwich	2 (1 oz)	130	1	<5
Peanut Creme Patties	5 (1.1 oz)	160	1	0
Oreo				
Cookies	3 (1.2 oz)	160	1	0
Double Stuf	2 (1 oz)	140	tr	0
Fudge Covered	1 (0.75 oz)	110	tr	0
Halloween Treats	2 (1 oz)	140	1	0
Reduced Fat	3 (1.2 oz)	140	1	0

FOOD	PORTION	CALS.	FIB.	CHOL.
Oreo (CONT.)				
White Fudge Covered	1 (0.75 oz)	110	tr	0
Pally				
Butter	4 (0.88 oz)	100	—	7
Pepperidge Farm				
Beacon Hill Chocolate Chocolate Walnut	1	120	—	5
Blondie Chocolate Chip Fat Free	1 (1.4 oz)	120	tr	0
Bordeaux	2	70	0	0
Brownie Chocolate Nut	2	110	—	<5
Brownie Nut Large	1	140	—	5
Brussels	2	110	0	0
Brussels Mint	2	130	—	0
Butter Chessman	2	90	—	10
Cappucino	1	50	—	<5
Capri	1	80	—	0
Chantilly	1	80	—	<5
Chesapeake Chocolate Chunk Pecan	1	120	1	5
Cheyenne Peanut Butter Milk Chocolate Chunk	1	110	1	5
Chocolate Chip	2	100	0	5
Chocolate Chip Large	1	130	—	5
Chocolate Chunk Pecan	1	70	—	12
Dakota Milk Chocolate Oatmeal	1	110	1	5
Date Pecan	2	110	—	10
Fruit Filled Apricot-Raspberry	2	100	—	10
Fruit Filled Strawberry	2	100	—	10
Geneva	2	130	—	0
Gingerman	2	70	—	5
Hazelnut	2	110	—	0
Irish Oatmeal	2	90	—	5
Lemon Nut Crunch	2	110	—	<5
Lido	1	90	—	<5
Linzer	1	120	—	<5
Milano	2	120	—	15
Mint Milano	2	150	—	5
Molasses Crisps	2	70	—	0
Nantucket Chocolate Chunk	1	120	1	5
Nassau	1	80	—	<5
Oatmeal Large	1	120	—	5
Oatmeal Raisin	2	110	—	10
Old Fashioned Chocolate Chip	2	100	0	5
Orange Milano	2	150	—	5

FOOD	PORTION	CALS.	FIB.	CHOL.
Pepperidge Farm (CONT.)				
Orleans	3	90	—	0
Orleans Sandwich	2	120	—	0
Pecan Shortbread	1	70	—	0
Pirouettes Chocolate Laced	2	70	—	<5
Pirouettes Original	2	70	—	<5
Raisin Bran	2	110	—	<5
Ripple Milk Chocolate Fat Free	1 (0.6 oz)	60	tr	0
Santa Fe Oatmeal Raisin	1	100	1	<5
Sausalito Milk Chocolate Macadamia	1	120	0	5
Shortbread	2	150	—	<5
Sugar	2	100	—	10
Tahiti	1	90	—	5
Zurich	1	60	—	0
Ritz				
Chocolate Covered	3 (1 oz)	150	1	0
Sargento				
MooTown Snackers Cookies & Creme Honey Graham Sticks & Vanilla Creme w/ Sprinkle	1 pkg (1.1 oz)	140	0	0
MooTown Snackers Cookies & Creme Vanilla Sticks & Chocolate Fudge Creme	1 pkg (1.1 oz)	140	0	0
SnackWell's				
Fat Free Cinnamon Grahams	20 (1 oz)	110	1	0
Fat Free Devil's Food	1 (0.5 oz)	50	tr	0
Fat Free Double Fudge	1 (0.5 oz)	50	tr	0
Golden Devil's Food	1 (0.5 oz)	50	0	0
Reduced Fat Chocolate Chip	13 (1 oz)	130	1	0
Reduced Fat Chocolate Sandwich With Chocolate Creme	2 (0.9 oz)	100	1	0
Reduced Fat Oatmeal Raisin	2 (1 oz)	110	1	0
Reduced Fat Vanilla Sandwich	2 (0.9 oz)	110	1	0
Social Tea				
Cookies	6 (1 oz)	120	tr	5
Stella D'Oro				
Almond Toast Mandel	1	60	—	tr
Angel Bars	1	80	—	tr
Angel Wings	1	70	—	1
Angelica Goodies	1	110	—	tr
Anginetti	1	30	—	tr

FOOD	PORTION	CALS.	FIB.	CHOL.
Stella D'Oro (CONT.)				
Anisette Sponge	1	50	—	tr
Anisette Toast	1	50	—	tr
Anisette Toast Jumbo	1	110	—	tr
Apple Pastry Low Sodium	1	80	—	>5
Breakfast Treats	1	100	—	tr
Castelets Chocolate	1	60	—	tr
Chinese Dessert Cookies	1	170	—	tr
Como Delight	1	150	—	1
Deep Night Fudge	1	65	—	2
Dutch Apple Bars	1	110	—	1
Egg Biscuits Low Sodium	3	120	—	40
Egg Biscuits Sugared	1	80	—	1
Egg Jumbo	1	50	—	tr
Fruit Delight Apple Cinnamon Fat Free	1	70	—	0
Fruit Delight Peach Apricot Fat Free	1	70	—	0
Fruit Delight Raspberry Fat Free	1	70	—	0
Fruit Slices	1	60	—	tr
Fruit Slices Fat Free	1	50	—	0
Golden Bars	1	110	—	tr
Holiday Rings & Stars	1	47	—	0
Holiday Trinkets	1	40	—	tr
Hostess Assortment	1	40	—	tr
Indulgente Cashew Biscottini	1 (1.1 oz)	150	tr	10
Kichel Low Sodium	21	150	—	80
Lady Stella Assortment	1	40	—	tr
Margherite Chocolate	1	70	—	tr
Margherite Vanilla	1	70	—	tr
Peach Apricot Pastry Sodium Free	1	80	—	>5
Pfeffernusse Spice Drops	1	40	—	tr
Prune Pastry Dietetic	1	90	—	>5
Roman Egg Biscuits	1	140	—	tr
Royal Nuggets	1	2	—	tr
Sesame Regina	1	50	—	tr
Swiss Fudge	1	70	—	tr
Sunshine				
Almond Crescents	4 (1.1 oz)	150	tr	0
Animal Crackers	1 box (2 oz)	260	1	0
Animal Crackers	14 (1.1 oz)	140	tr	0
Classics Chocolate Chip With Pecans	1 (0.7 oz)	110	tr	3

FOOD	PORTION	CALS.	FIB.	CHOL.
Sunshine (CONT.)				
Classics Chocolate Chip With Walnuts	1 (0.7 oz)	100	1	5
Classics Premier Chocolate Chip	1 (0.7 oz)	100	tr	5
Dixie Vanilla	2 (0.9 oz)	120	tr	0
Fig Bars	2 (1 oz)	110	1	0
Fudge Family Bears Vanilla	2 (1 oz)	140	tr	0
Fudge Mint Patties	2 (0.8 oz)	130	tr	0
Fudge Striped Shortbread	3 (1.1 oz)	160	1	0
Ginger Snaps	7 (1 oz)	130	tr	0
Grahams Cinnamon	2 (1.1 oz)	140	tr	0
Grahams Fudge Dipped	4 (1.2 oz)	170	1	0
Grahams Honey	2 (1 oz)	120	1	0
Grahamy Bears	1 pkg (2 oz)	260	2	0
Grahamy Bears	10 (1.1 oz)	140	1	0
Iced Gingerbread	5 (1 oz)	130	tr	5
Iced Oatmeal	2 (0.9 oz)	120	tr	0
Jingles	6 (1.1 oz)	150	tr	0
Lemon Coolers	5 (1 oz)	140	tr	0
Mini Chocolate Chip Cookies	5 (1.1 oz)	160	tr	0
Mini Fudge Royals	15 (1.1 oz)	160	1	0
Oatmeal Chocolate Chip	3 (1.3 oz)	170	2	0
Oatmeal Country Style	3 (1.2 oz)	170	1	0
School House Cookies	20 (1.1 oz)	140	tr	0
Sugar Wafers Chocolate	3 (0.9 oz)	130	tr	0
Sugar Wafers Peanut Butter	4 (1.1 oz)	170	1	0
Sugar Wafers Vanilla	3 (0.9 oz)	130	tr	0
Tru Blu Chocolate	1 (0.6 oz)	80	tr	0
Tru Blu Lemon	1 (0.6 oz)	80	tr	0
Tru Blu Vanilla	1 (0.5 oz)	80	tr	0
Vanilla Wafers	7 (1.1 oz)	150	tr	3
Vienna Fingers	2 (1 oz)	140	tr	0
Tastykake				
Chocolate Chip Bar	1 (43 g)	190	1	5
Chocolate Chunk Macadamia Nut	1 pkg (56 g)	310	2	40
Fudge Bar	1 (50 g)	200	1	5
Oatmeal Raisin Bar	1 (50 g)	210	1	15
Soft'n Chewy Chocolate Chip	1 (39 g)	170	1	10
Soft'n Chewy Chocolate Chocolate Chip	1 (32 g)	170	1	5
Soft'n Chewy Oatmeal Raisin	1 (39 g)	160	1	5
Vanilla Sugar Wafer	1 (6 g)	36	0	0

FOOD	PORTION	CALS.	FIB.	CHOL.
Teddy Grahams				
Chocolate	24 (1 oz)	140	1	0
Cinnamon	24 (1 oz)	140	1	0
Honey	24 (1 oz)	140	1	0
Tree Of Life				
Creme Supremes	2 (0.9 oz)	120	1	0
Creme Supremes Mint	2 (0.9 oz)	120	1	0
Fat Free Classic Carrot Cake	1 (0.8 oz)	60	1	0
Fat Free Devil's Food Chocolate	1 (0.8 oz)	70	1	0
Fat Free Golden Oatmeal Raisin	1 (0.8 oz)	70	1	0
Fat Free Harvest Fruit & Nut	1 (0.8 oz)	70	1	0
Fat Free Toasted Almond Butter	1 (0.8 oz)	70	1	0
Fruit Bars Apple Spice	2 (1.3 oz)	120	2	0
Fruit Bars Fat Free Fig	1 (0.8 oz)	70	2	0
Fruit Bars Fat Free Peach Apricot	1 (0.8 oz)	70	1	0
Fruit Bars Fat Free Wildberry	1 (0.8 oz)	70	2	0
Fruit Bars Fig	2 (1.3 oz)	120	3	0
Fruit Bars Peach Apricot	2 (1.3 oz)	120	2	0
Honey-Sweet Colossal Carrot Cake	1 (0.8 oz)	110	1	0
Honey-Sweet Lemon Burst	1 (0.8 oz)	110	1	0
Honey-Sweet Oh-So-Oatmeal	1 (0.8 oz)	110	1	0
Honey-Sweet Pecans-A-Plenty	1 (0.8 oz)	125	1	0
Monster Fat Free Carrot Cake	¼ cookie (0.9 oz)	60	1	0
Monster Fat Free Devil's Food Chocolate	¼ cookie (0.9 oz)	80	2	0
Monster Fat Free Gingerbread	¼ cookie (0.9 oz)	80	2	0
Monster Fat Free Maple Pecan	¼ cookie (0.9 oz)	90	2	0
Royal Vanilla	2 (0.9 oz)	120	0	0
Small World Animal Grahams	7 (1 oz)	120	3	0
Small World Chocolate Chip	7 (1 oz)	120	3	0
Soft-Bake Chocolate Chip	1 (0.8 oz)	125	1	0
Soft-Bake Double Fudge	1 (0.8 oz)	110	2	0
Soft-Bake Maui Macaroon	1 (0.8 oz)	135	2	0
Soft-Bake Oatmeal	1 (0.8 oz)	115	2	0
Soft-Bake Peanut Butter	1 (0.8 oz)	125	1	0
Wheat-Free American Oatmeal	1 (0.8 oz)	90	1	0
Wheat-Free California Carob	1 (0.8 oz)	105	6	0
Wheat-Free Georgia Peanut Butter	1 (0.8 oz)	95	1	0
Wheat-Free Mountain Maple Walnut	1 (0.8 oz)	100	6	0

FOOD	PORTION	CALS.	FIB.	CHOL.
Vienna Fingers				
Low Fat	2 (1 oz)	130	tr	0
Weight Watchers				
Apple Raisin Bar	1 (0.75 oz)	70	2	0
Chocolate Chip	2 (1.06 oz)	140	1	0
Chocolate Sandwich	2 (1.06 oz)	140	1	0
Fruit Filled Fig	1 (0.7 oz)	70	0	0
Fruit Filled Raspberry	1 (0.7 oz)	70	0	0
Oatmeal Raisin	2 (1.06 oz)	120	1	0
Vanilla Sandwich	2 (1.06 oz)	140	1	0
REFRIGERATED				
chocolate chip	1 (0.42 oz)	59	—	3
chocolate chip unbaked	1 oz	126	—	7
oatmeal	1 (0.4 oz)	56	—	3
oatmeal raisin	1 (0.4 oz)	56	—	3
peanut butter	1 (0.4 oz)	60	—	4
peanut butter dough	1 oz	130	—	8
sugar	1 (0.42 oz)	58	—	4
sugar dough	1 oz	124	—	8
Pillsbury				
Chocolate Chip	1	70	—	5
Oatmeal Raisin	1	60	—	0
Peanut Butter	1	70	—	5
Sugar	1	70	—	5
TAKE-OUT				
biscotti with nuts chocolate dipped	1 (1.3 oz)	117	1	18
CORIANDER				
leaf dried	1 tsp	2	—	0
leaf fresh	¼ cup	1	—	0
seed	1 tsp	5	—	0
CORN				
(*see also* BRAN, CEREAL, CORNMEAL, FLOUR)				
CANNED				
cream style	½ cup	93	—	0
w/ red & green peppers	½ cup	86	—	0
white	½ cup	66	—	0
yellow	½ cup	66	1	0
Del Monte				
Cream Style Golden	½ cup (4.4 oz)	90	2	0
Cream Style Golden 50% Less Salt	½ cup (4.4 oz)	90	2	0
Cream Style Golden No Salt Added	½ cup (4.4 oz)	90	2	0

FOOD	PORTION	CALS.	FIB.	CHOL.
Del Monte (CONT.)				
Cream Style Supersweet Golden	½ cup (4.4 oz)	60	2	0
Cream Style White	½ cup (4.4 oz)	100	2	0
Whole Kernel Golden	½ cup (4.4 oz)	90	3	0
Whole Kernel Golden Supersweet 50% Less Salt	½ cup (4.4 oz)	60	3	0
Whole Kernel Golden Supersweet No Salt Added	½ cup (4.4 oz)	60	3	0
Whole Kernel Golden Supersweet No Sugar	½ cup (4.4 oz)	60	3	0
Whole Kernel Golden Supersweet Vacuum Packed	½ cup (3.7 oz)	70	3	0
Whole Kernel Golden Supersweet Vacuum Packed No Salt Added	½ cup (3.7 oz)	70	3	0
Whole Kernel White Sweet	½ cup (4.4 oz)	80	2	0
Green Giant				
50% Less Salt No Sugar Added	½ cup	50	2	0
Corn	½ cup	70	2	0
Cream Style	½ cup	100	2	0
Deli Corn	½ cup	80	2	0
Golden Kernel 50% Less Salt	½ cup	70	2	0
Golden Vacuum Packed	½ cup	80	2	0
Mexi Corn	½ cup	80	2	0
No Salt No Sugar	½ cup	80	2	0
Sweet Select	½ cup	60	2	0
White Vacuum Packed	½ cup	80	2	0
Ka-Me				
Baby	½ cup (4.5 oz)	20	2	0
Stir Fry	½ cup (4.5 oz)	20	2	0
Owatonna				
Cream Style	½ cup	100	—	0
Whole Kernel In Brine	½ cup	90	—	0
Whole Kernel Vacuum Pack	½ cup	100	—	0
S&W				
Cream Style Premium Homestyle	½ cup	105	—	0
Whole Kernel Tender Young	½ cup	90	—	0
Whole Kernel Water Pack	½ cup	80	—	0
Seneca				
Cream Style	½ cup	80	1	0
Whole Kernel	½ cup	90	2	0

FOOD	PORTION	CALS.	FIB.	CHOL.
Seneca (CONT.)				
Whole Kernel Natural Pack	½ cup	80	2	0
DRIED				
Goya				
Giant White	⅓ cup (1.6 oz)	160	4	0
FRESH				
on-the-cob w/ butter cooked	1 ear	155	—	6
white cooked	½ cup	89	—	0
white raw	½ cup	66	—	0
yellow cooked	1 ear (2.7 oz)	83	—	0
yellow cooked	½ cup	89	—	0
yellow raw	½ cup	66	—	0
yellow raw	1 ear (3 oz)	77	—	0
FROZEN				
cooked	½ cup	67	—	0
on-the-cob cooked	1 ear (2.2 oz)	59	—	0
Birds Eye				
Big Ears	1 ear	160	—	0
In Butter Sauce	½ cup	90	2	5
Little Ears	2 ears	130	—	0
On The Cob	1 ear	120	—	0
Polybag Cut	½ cup	80	2	0
Polybag Deluxe Tender Sweet	½ cup	80	2	0
Sweet	½ cup	80	2	0
Green Giant				
Cream Style	½ cup	110	3	0
Harvest Fresh Niblets	½ cup	80	2	0
Harvest Fresh White Shoepeg	½ cup	90	2	0
In Butter Sauce	½ cup	100	—	5
Nibblers Corn On The Cob	2 ears	120	2	0
Niblet Ears	1 ear	120	2	0
Niblets	½ cup	90	2	0
One Serve Niblets In Butter Sauce	1 pkg	120	3	5
One Serve On The Cob	1 pkg	120	2	0
Super Sweet Nibblers Corn On The Cob	2 ears	90	2	0
Super Sweet Niblet Ears	1 ear	90	2	0
Super Sweet Niblet Select	½ cup	60	2	0
White In Butter Sauce	½ cup	100	2	5
White Select	½ cup	90	2	0
Hanover				
White Shoepeg	½ cup	80	—	0
White Sweet	½ cup	80	—	0

FOOD	PORTION	CALS.	FIB.	CHOL.
Hanover (CONT.)				
Yellow Sweet	½ cup	80	—	0
Mrs. Paul's				
Fritters	2	240	—	10
Ore Ida				
Cob Corn	1 ear (6.1 oz)	180	4	0
Cob Corn Mini-Gold	1 ear (3.1 oz)	90	2	0
Stouffer's				
Souffle	½ cup (2.4 oz)	170	1	65
Tree Of Life				
Corn	⅔ cup (3.2 oz)	80	1	0
SHELF-STABLE				
Pantry Express				
Golden Whole Kernel	½ cup	60	1	0
TAKE-OUT				
fritters	1 (1 oz)	62	1	12
scalloped	½ cup	258	—	47

CORN CHIPS
(*see* CHIPS)

CORNISH HENS

CORNMEAL

FOOD	PORTION	CALS.	FIB.	CHOL.
corn grits cooked	1 cup	146	—	0
corn grits uncooked	1 cup	579	—	0
degermed	1 cup	506	7	0
self-rising degermed	1 cup	489	—	0
whole grain	1 cup	442	13	0
Albers				
White	3 tbsp	110	tr	0
Yellow	3 tbsp	110	tr	0
Arrowhead				
Yellow	¼ cup (1.2 oz)	120	3	0
Aunt Jemima				
White	3 tbsp	102	1	0
Yellow	3 tbsp	102	1	0
Quaker				
White	3 tbsp	102	1	0
Yellow	3 tbsp	102	1	0
MIX				
Arrowhead				
Corn Bread	¼ cup (1.2 oz)	120	4	0
Golden Dipt				
Corny Dog Batter Mix	1 oz	100	—	0

FOOD	PORTION	CALS.	FIB.	CHOL.
Golden Dipt (CONT.)				
Hush Puppy Deluxe Mix	1¼ oz	120	—	0
Hush Puppy Jalapeno Mix	1¼ oz	120	—	0
Hush Puppy With Onion	1¼ oz	120	—	0
Hodgson Mill				
Yellow	¼ cup (1 oz)	100	3	0
Yellow Self Rising	¼ cup (1 oz)	90	3	0
Kentucky Kernal				
White Corn Meal Mix	¼ cup (1 oz)	100	2	0
Miracle Maize				
Complete as prep	1 piece (1.5 oz)	193	2	0
Country Style as prep	1 piece 2 in x 2 in (1.8 oz)	230	2	0
Sweet as prep	1 piece 2 in x 2 in (1.8 oz)	236	1	0
Stone-Buhr				
Yellow Corn Meal	¼ cup (1 oz)	100	1	0
READY-TO-EAT				
Aurora				
Polenta	½ cup (5 oz)	110	1	0
TAKE-OUT				
hush puppies	5 (2.7 oz)	256	4	135
hush puppies	1 (0.75 oz)	74	1	10
CORNSALAD				
raw	1 cup	12	—	0
CORNSTARCH				
cornstarch	⅓ cup	164	tr	0
Argo				
Cornstarch	1 tbsp (8 g)	30	—	0
Cornstarch	1 cup (128 g)	460	—	0
Hodgson Mill				
Cornstarch	2 tsp (0.4 oz)	35	—	0
Kingsford's				
Cornstarch	1 cup (128 g)	460	—	0
Cornstarch	1 tbsp (8 g)	30	—	0
COTTAGE CHEESE				
creamed	1 cup (7.4 oz)	217	—	31
creamed	4 oz	117	—	17
creamed w/ fruit	4 oz	140	—	13
dry curd	1 cup (5.1 oz)	123	—	10
dry curd	4 oz	96	—	8
lowfat 1%	4 oz	82	—	5

FOOD	PORTION	CALS.	FIB.	CHOL.
lowfat 1%	1 cup (7.9 oz)	164	—	10
lowfat 2%	4 oz	101	—	9
lowfat 2%	1 cup (7.9 oz)	203	—	19
Axelrod				
Nonfat	½ cup (4.4 oz)	90	0	10
Breakstone				
2% Fat Large Curd	½ cup (4.2 oz)	90	0	15
2% Fat Small Curd	½ cup (4.2 oz)	90	0	15
4% Fat Large Curd	½ cup (4.2 oz)	120	0	25
4% Fat Small Curd	½ cup (4.2 oz)	120	0	25
Dry Curd ½% Fat	¼ cup (1.9 oz)	45	0	5
Cabot				
Cottage Cheese	4 oz	120	—	17
Light	4 oz	90	—	5
Friendship				
California Style	½ cup (4 oz)	115	0	25
Lowfat No Salt Added	½ cup (4 oz)	90	0	10
Lowfat Pineapple	½ cup (4 oz)	120	0	10
Lowfat 1%	½ cup (4 oz)	90	0	10
Nonfat	½ cup (4 oz)	80	0	0
Nonfat Plus Peach	½ cup (4 oz)	110	0	0
Pot Style	½ cup (4 oz)	90	0	15
With Pineapple	½ cup (4 oz)	140	0	15
Hood				
1% Fat	½ cup (4 oz)	90	0	10
1% Fat Chive & Onion	½ cup (4 oz)	90	0	10
1% Fat No Salt Added	½ cup (4 oz)	90	0	10
1% Fat Pepper & Herb	½ cup (4 oz)	90	0	10
1% Fat Pineapple Cherry	½ cup (4 oz)	110	0	10
4% Fat	½ cup (4 oz)	120	0	25
4% Fat Chive	½ cup (4 oz)	130	0	25
4% Fat Pineapple	½ cup (4 oz)	130	0	20
Nonfat	½ cup (4 oz)	80	0	5
Nonfat Pineapple	½ cup (4 oz)	110	0	<5
Knudsen				
1.5% Fat Peach	4 oz	110	0	10
1.5% Fat Pineapple	4 oz	110	0	15
1.5% Fat Strawberry	4 oz	110	0	10
1.5% Fat Tropical Fruit	4 oz	120	0	10
2% Fat Small Curd	½ cup (4.2 oz)	100	0	15
4% Fat Large Curd	½ cup (4.5 oz)	130	0	30
4% Fat Small Curd	½ cup (4.3 oz)	120	0	25
Free	½ cup (4.3 oz)	80	0	10

FOOD	PORTION	CALS.	FIB.	CHOL.
Lactaid				
1%	4 oz	72	—	4
Light N'Lively				
1% Fat	½ cup (4 oz)	80	0	15
1% Fat Garden Salad	½ cup (4.2 oz)	90	0	15
1% Fat Peach & Pineapple	½ cup (4.3 oz)	120	0	10
Free	½ cup (4.4 oz)	80	0	10
Sealtest				
2% Fat Small Curd	½ cup (4.2 oz)	90	0	15
4% Fat Large Curd	½ cup (4.2 oz)	120	0	25
4% Fat Small Curd	½ cup (4.2 oz)	120	0	25
Viva				
Nonfat	½ cup	70	—	5
Weight Watchers				
1%	½ cup	90	0	5
2%	½ cup	90	0	15

COTTONSEED

kernels roasted	1 tbsp	51	—	0

COUGH DROPS

FOOD	PORTION	CALS.	FIB.	CHOL.
Halls				
Cough Drops	1 (3.8 g)	15	—	0
Plus	1 (4.7 g)	18	—	0
With Vitamin C	1 (3.8 g)	14	—	0
Lifesavers				
Menthol	2 (0.5 oz)	60	—	0

COUSCOUS

FOOD	PORTION	CALS.	FIB.	CHOL.
cooked	½ cup	101	—	0
dry	½ cup	346	—	0
Casbah				
Almond Chicken Vegetarian	1 pkg (1.5 oz)	160	tr	0
Asparagus Au Gratin Organic	1 pkg (1.5 oz)	150	1	<5
Cheddar Broccoli	1 pkg (1.3 oz)	130	tr	<5
Hearty Harvest Zestful Organic as prep	1 pkg (10 fl oz)	180	2	0
Moroccan Stew	1 pkg (2 oz)	180	1	0
Pilaf as prep	1 cup	200	tr	0
Tomato Parmesan	1 pkg (1.8 oz)	170	2	<5
Kitchen Del Sol				
Aegean Citrus as prep	½ cup (1.1 oz)	110	1	0
Moroccan Ginger as prep	½ cup (1.1 oz)	120	1	0
Spicy Vegetable as prep	½ cup (1.1 oz)	120	1	0
Tomato & Olive	½ cup (1.1 oz)	120	1	0

FOOD	PORTION	CALS.	FIB.	CHOL.
Near East				
as prep	1¼ cup	260	2	0
COWPEAS				
catjang dried cooked	1 cup	200	—	0
common canned	1 cup	184	—	0
frozen cooked	½ cup	112	—	0
leafy tips chopped cooked	1 cup	12	—	0
leafy tips raw chopped	1 cup	10	—	0
CRAB				
CANNED				
blue	3 oz	84	—	76
blue	1 cup	133	—	120
FRESH				
alaska king cooked	1 leg (4.7 oz)	129	—	72
alaska king cooked	3 oz	82	—	45
alaska king raw	1 leg (6 oz)	144	—	72
alaska king raw	3 oz	71	—	35
blue cooked	3 oz	87	—	85
blue cooked	1 cup	138	—	135
blue raw	3 oz	74	—	66
blue raw	1 crab (0.7 oz)	18	—	16
dungeness raw	3 oz	73	—	50
dungeness raw	1 crab (5.7 oz)	140	—	97
queen steamed	3 oz	98	—	60
FROZEN				
Mrs. Paul's				
Deviled Crab	1 cake	180	—	20
Deviled Crab Miniatures	3½ oz	240	—	20
READY-TO-EAT				
crab cakes	1 cake (2.1 oz)	93	—	90
TAKE-OUT				
baked	1 (3.8 oz)	160	—	184
cake	1 (2 oz)	160	—	82
soft-shell fried	1 (4.4 oz)	334	—	45
CRACKER CRUMBS				
cracker meal	1 cup (4 oz)	440	—	0
Golden Dipt				
Cracker Meal	1 oz	100	—	0
Honey Maid				
Graham Cracker	0.5 oz	70	tr	0
Keebler				
Cracker Meal	1 cup	100	—	0

FOOD	PORTION	CALS.	FIB.	CHOL.
Keebler (CONT.)				
Graham Crumbs	1 cup	520	—	0
Zesty Meal	1 cup	85	—	0
Kellogg's				
Corn Flake Crumbs	2 tbsp (0.4 oz)	40	0	0
Lance				
Cracker Meal	1 oz	100	—	0
Nabisco				
Nilla Cookie Crumbs	2 tbsp (0.5 oz)	70	tr	<5
Oreo				
Cookie Crumbs	2 tbsp (0.5 oz)	80	1	0
Premium				
Fat Free Cracker Crumbs	¼ cup (1 oz)	100	1	0
Ritz				
Cracker Crumbs	⅓ cup (1 oz)	140	1	0
Sunshine				
Graham	3 tbsp (0.6 oz)	80	tr	0

CRACKERS
(*see also* CRACKER CRUMBS)

FOOD	PORTION	CALS.	FIB.	CHOL.
cheese	1 (1 in sq) (1 g)	5	—	0
cheese	14 (½ oz)	71	—	2
cheese low sodium	1 (1 in sq) (1 g)	5	—	0
cheese low sodium	14 (½ oz)	71	—	2
cheese w/ peanut butter filling	1 (0.24 oz)	34	tr	0
crispbread rye	1 (0.35 oz)	37	2	0
melba toast plain	1 (5 g)	19	tr	0
melba toast pumpernickel	1 (5 g)	19	tr	0
melba toast rye	1 (5 g)	19	tr	0
melba toast wheat	1 (5 g)	19	tr	0
oyster cracker	1 (1 g)	4	tr	0
rye w/ cheese filling	1 (0.24 oz)	34	—	1
rye wafers plain	1 (0.9 oz)	84	—	0
rye wafers seasoned	1 (0.8 oz)	84	—	0
saltines	1 (3 g)	13	tr	0
saltines fat free low sodium	3 (0.5 oz)	59	—	0
saltines fat free low sodium	6 (1 oz)	118	—	0
saltines low salt	1 (3 g)	13	tr	0
snack cracker	1 (3 g)	15	tr	0
snack cracker low salt	1 (3 g)	15	tr	0
snack cracker w/ cheese filling	1 (7 g)	33	—	0
soup cracker	1 (1 g)	4	tr	0
wheat w/ cheese filling	1 (0.24 oz)	35	—	1
wheat w/ peanut butter filling	1 (0.24 oz)	35	—	0

FOOD	PORTION	CALS.	FIB.	CHOL.
wheat thins	1 (2 g)	9	—	0
wheat thins	7 (0.5 oz)	67	1	0
wheat thins low salt	7 (0.5 oz)	67	1	0
whole wheat	1 (4 g)	18	—	0
whole wheat low salt	1 (4 g)	18	—	0
Adrienne's				
Gourmet Flatbread Caraway & Rye	2	20	—	<5
Gourmet Flatbread Classic Island	2	20	—	<5
Gourmet Flatbread Slightly Onion	2	20	—	<5
Gourmet Flatbread Ten Grain	2	20	1	0
American Heritage				
Sesame	9 (1.1 oz)	160	1	0
Wheat & Bran	9 (1 oz)	140	2	0
Better Cheddars				
Crackers	22 (1 oz)	70	tr	<5
Low Sodium	22 (1 oz)	150	tr	<5
Reduced Fat	24 (1 oz)	140	tr	<5
Burns & Ricker				
Bagel Crisps Garlic	5 (1 oz)	100	1	0
Cheez-It				
Crackers	27 (1 oz)	160	tr	0
Crackers	1 pkg (2 oz)	290	2	3
Crackers	1 pkg (1.5 oz)	220	1	3
Hot & Spicy	1 pkg (1.5 oz)	220	1	0
Hot & Spicy	26 (1 oz)	160	1	0
Low Sodium	27 (1 oz)	160	tr	0
Party Mix	½ cup (1 oz)	140	1	0
Reduced Fat	30 (1 oz)	130	tr	0
White Cheddar	1 pkg (1.5 oz)	220	tr	3
White Cheddar	26 (1 oz)	160	tr	3
Crown Pilot				
Crackers	1 (0.5 oz)	70	tr	0
Devonsheer				
Melba Rounds Garlic	½ oz	56	1	0
Melba Rounds Honey Bran	½ oz	52	1	0
Melba Rounds Onion	½ oz	51	1	0
Melba Rounds Plain	½ oz	53	1	0
Melba Rounds Plain Unsalted	½ oz	52	1	0
Melba Rounds Rye	½ oz	53	1	0
Melba Rounds Sesame	½ oz	57	1	0

FOOD	PORTION	CALS.	FIB.	CHOL.
Eden				
Brown Rice	5 (1 oz)	120	2	0
Escort				
Crackers	3 (0.5 oz)	70	—	0
Estee				
Unsalted	1 (0.5 oz)	70	0	0
Frito Lay				
Cheese Filled	6 (1.5 oz)	210	—	5
Cracker Snacks Cheddar	13-16 (1 oz)	70	—	0
Cracker Snacks Zesty Italian	13-16 (1 oz)	70	—	0
Peanut Butter Filled	6 (1.5 oz)	210	—	0
Harvest Crisps				
5 Grain	13 (1.1 oz)	130	1	0
Oat	13 (1.1 oz)	140	1	0
Health Valley				
Herb Stoned Wheat	13	55	2	0
Herb Stoned Wheat No Salt	13	55	2	0
Rice Bran	7	130	2	0
Sesame Stoned Wheat	13	55	2	0
Sesame Stoned Wheat No Salt Added	13	55	2	0
Seven Grain Vegetable Stoned Wheat	13	55	2	0
Seven Grain Vegetable Stoned Wheat No Salt Added	13	55	2	0
Stoned Wheat	13	55	2	0
Stoned Wheat No Salt Added	13	55	2	0
Healthy Choice				
Bread Crisps Garlic Herb	11 (1 oz)	110	2	0
Hi Ho				
Butter Flavored	9 (1.1 oz)	160	tr	3
Cracked Pepper	9 (1.1 oz)	160	tr	3
Crackers	9	160	tr	0
Low Salt	9 (1.1 oz)	160	tr	0
Multi Grain	9 (1.1 oz)	160	1	0
Reduced Fat	10 (1.1 oz)	140	tr	0
Whole Wheat	9 (1.1 oz)	150	2	0
J.J. Flats				
Breadflats Caraway	1	52	1	tr
Breadflats Caraway And Salt	1	51	1	tr
Breadflats Cinnamon	1	53	1	tr
Breadflats Flavorall	1	52	1	tr
Breadflats Garlic	1	52	1	tr
Breadflats Oat Bran	1	49	2	0

FOOD	PORTION	CALS.	FIB.	CHOL.
J.J. Flats (CONT.)				
Breadflats Onion	1	53	1	tr
Breadflats Plain	1	53	1	tr
Breadflats Poppy	1	53	1	tr
Breadflats Sesame	1	55	1	tr
Kavli				
Crackers	1 piece	40	2	0
Keebler				
Club	2	30	—	0
Melba Toast Garlic	2	25	—	0
Melba Toast Long	2	30	—	0
Melba Toast Onion	2	25	—	0
Melba Toast Plain	2	25	—	0
Melba Toast Sesame	2	25	—	0
Oyster Crackers Large	26	80	—	0
Oyster Crackers Small	50	80	—	0
Snack Crackers Toasted Rye	2	30	—	0
Snack Crackers Toasted Sesame	2	30	—	0
Snack Crackers Toasted Wheat	2	30	—	0
Toasted Snack Bacon	2	30	—	0
Toasted Snack Onion	2	30	—	0
Toasted Snack Pumpernickel	2	30	—	0
Wholegrain Wheat	2	30	—	0
Krispy				
Cracked Pepper	5 (0.5 oz)	60	tr	0
Fat Free	5 (0.5 oz)	60	tr	0
Mild Cheddar	5 (0.5 oz)	60	tr	0
Original	5 (0.5 oz)	60	tr	0
Soup & Oyster Crackers	17 (0.5 oz)	60	tr	0
Unsalted Tops	5 (0.5 oz)	60	tr	0
Whole Wheat	5 (0.5 oz)	60	tr	0
Lance				
Bonnie	1 pkg (34 g)	160	—	5
Captain Wafers	2	30	—	0
Captain Wafers Very Low Sodium	2	30	—	0
Captain Wafers w/ Cream Cheese & Chives	1 pkg (37 g)	170	—	0
Cheese-On-Wheat	1 pkg (37 g)	180	—	5
Lanchee	1 pkg (35 g)	180	—	5
Melba Toast Oblong	2	30	—	0
Melba Toast Plain	2	20	—	0
Melba Toast Round Garlic	2	20	—	0

FOOD	PORTION	CALS.	FIB.	CHOL.
Lance (CONT.)				
Melba Toast Round Onion	2	20	—	0
Melba Toast Sesame	2	25	—	0
Nekot	1 pkg (42 g)	210	—	5
Nip-Chee	1 pkg (37 g)	180	—	5
Oyster Crackers	1 pkg (14 g)	70	—	0
Peanut Butter Wheat	1 pkg (37 g)	190	—	0
Rye Twins	2	30	—	0
Rye-Chee	1 pkg (41 g)	190	—	5
Saltines	2	25	—	0
Saltines Slug Pack	4 crackers	50	—	0
Sesame Twins	2	40	—	0
Toastchee	1 pkg (39 g)	190	—	5
Toasty	1 pkg (35 g)	180	—	0
Wheat Twins	2	30	—	0
Wheatswafer	2	30	—	0
Lavash				
Bread Crisp Original	2 (0.5 oz)	60	—	0
Bread Crisp Sesame	2 (0.5 oz)	60	—	0
Little Debbie				
Cheese Crackers With Peanut Butter	1 pkg (1.4 oz)	210	1	0
Cheese Crackers With Peanut Butter	1 pkg (0.9 oz)	140	1	0
Toasty Crackers With Peanut Butter	1 pkg (0.9 oz)	140	1	0
Toasty Crackers With Peanut Butter	1 pkg (1.4 oz)	200	1	0
Wheat Crackers With Cheddar Cheese	1 pkg (0.9 oz)	140	0	5
Manischewitz				
Tam Tams	10	147	—	0
Tam Tams No Salt	10	138	—	0
Tams Garlic	10	153	—	0
Tams Onion	10	150	—	0
Tams Wheat	10	150	—	0
McCrackens				
Cracker Crisp Country Butter	1 oz	140	—	tr
Cracker Crisp Sour Cream & Chives	1 oz	140	—	tr
Cracker Crisp Tangy Cheddar	1 oz	140	—	tr
Cracker Crisp Toasted Wheat	1 oz	140	—	0
NABS				
Cheese Peanut Butter Sandwich	6 (1.4 oz)	190	1	0

FOOD	PORTION	CALS.	FIB.	CHOL.
NABS (CONT.)				
Peanut Butter Toast Sandwich	6 (1.4 oz)	190	1	0
Nabisco				
Bacon Flavored	15 (1.1 oz)	160	tr	0
Chicken In A Biskit	14 (1 oz)	160	tr	0
Garden Crisps	15 (1 oz)	130	1	0
Oat Thins	18 (1 oz)	140	2	0
Royal Lunch	1 (0.4 oz)	50	0	0
Swiss	15 (1 oz)	140	tr	0
Tid-Bit Cheese	32 (1 oz)	150	tr	0
Vegetable Thins	14 (1.1 oz)	160	1	0
Wheat Thins Original	16 (1 oz)	140	2	0
Wheat Thins Reduced Fat	18 (1 oz)	120	2	0
Zings!	1 pkg (1.8 oz)	240	2	0
Nips				
Cheese	29 (1 oz)	150	tr	0
Old London				
Melba Toast Pumpernickel	½ oz	54	1	0
Melba Toast Rye	½ oz	52	—	0
Melba Toast Sesame	½ oz	55	1	0
Melba Toast Sesame Unsalted	½ oz	55	1	0
Melba Toast Wheat	½ oz	51	1	0
Melba Toast White	½ oz	51	1	0
Melba Toast White Unsalted	½ oz	51	1	0
Melba Toast Whole Grain	½ oz	52	1	0
Melba Toast Whole Grain Unsalted	½ oz	53	1	0
Rounds Bacon	½ oz	53	1	0
Rounds Garlic	½ oz	56	1	0
Rounds Onion	½ oz	52	1	0
Rounds Rye	½ oz	52	—	0
Rounds Sesame	½ oz	56	1	0
Rounds White	½ oz	48	1	0
Rounds Whole Grain	½ oz	54	1	0
Oysterettes				
Crackers	19 (0.5 oz)	60	tr	0
Partners				
Walla Walla Sweet Onion Preservative Free	0.5 oz	65	tr	3
Pepperidge Farm				
Butter Thins	4	70	0	<5
Cracked Wheat	3	100	1	0
Crispy Graham	4	70	—	0
English Water Biscuits	4	70	0	0

FOOD	PORTION	CALS.	FIB.	CHOL.
Pepperidge Farm (CONT.)				
Flutters Garden Herb	¾ oz	100	—	0
Flutters Golden Sesame	¾ oz	110	—	0
Flutters Original Butter	¾ oz	100	—	5
Flutters Toasted Wheat	¾ oz	110	—	0
Garden Vegetable	5	60	—	0
Goldfish Cheddar Cheese	1 pkg (1½ oz)	190	1	5
Goldfish Cheddar Cheese	1 oz	120	1	5
Goldfish Cheese Thins	4	50	0	0
Goldfish Original	1 oz	130	1	0
Goldfish Parmesan Cheese	1 oz	120	1	<5
Goldfish Pizza Flavored	1 oz	130	1	<5
Goldfish Pretzel	1 oz	110	1	0
Hearty Wheat	4	100	1	0
Multi Grain	4	70	—	0
Sesame	4	80	2	0
Snack Mix Classic	1 oz	140	1	0
Snack Mix Lightly Smoked	1 oz	150	1	0
Snack Sticks Cheese	8	130	1	0
Snack Sticks Pretzel	8	120	1	0
Snack Sticks Pumpernickel	8	140	1	0
Snack Sticks Sesame	8	140	1	0
Spicy Lightly Smoked	1 oz	140	1	<5
Toasted Rice	4	60	—	0
Toasted Wheat With Onion	4	80	0	0
Planters				
Cheese Peanut Butter Sandwiches	1 pkg (1.4 oz)	190	1	0
Toast Peanut Butter Sandwiches	1 pkg (1.4 oz)	190	1	0
Premium				
Saltine Bits	34 (1 oz)	150	tr	0
Saltine Fat Free	5 (0.5 oz)	50	0	0
Saltine Low Sodium	5 (0.5 oz)	60	tr	0
Saltine Original	5 (0.5 oz)	60	tr	0
Saltine Unsalted Tops	5 (0.5 oz)	60	tr	0
Soup & Oyster	23 (0.5 oz)	60	tr	0
Ralston				
Oat Bran Krisp	2	60	3	0
Ritz				
Bits	48 (1 oz)	160	1	0
Bits Sandwiches With Peanut Butter	13 (1 oz)	150	1	0

FOOD	PORTION	CALS.	FIB.	CHOL.
Ritz (CONT.)				
Bits Sanwiches With Real Cheese	14 (1.1 oz)	160	1	5
Crackers	5 (0.5 oz)	80	tr	0
Low Sodium	5 (0.5 oz)	80	tr	0
Sandwiches With Real Cheese	1 pkg (1.4 oz)	210	1	5
Rykrisp				
Natural	2	40	4	0
Seasoned	2	45	3	0
Seasoned Twindividuals	2	45	3	0
Sesame	2	50	3	0
Ryvita				
Crisp Bread Dark Finn Crisp	2	38	—	0
Crisp Bread Dark Rye	1	26	—	0
Crisp Bread Dark w/ Caraway Seeds Finn Crisp	2	38	—	0
Crisp Bread High Fiber	1	23	—	0
Crisp Bread Light Rye	1	26	—	0
Crisp Bread Toasted Sesame Rye	1	31	—	0
Snackbread High Fiber	1	14	—	0
Snackbread Original Wheat	1	20	—	0
Sesmark				
Brown Rice	15 (1 oz)	120	tr	0
Cheese Thins	15 (1 oz)	130	tr	0
Rice Thins Original	15 (1 oz)	130	tr	0
Rice Thins Teriyaki Flavored	13 (1 oz)	130	tr	0
Savory Thins Original	15 (1 oz)	125	1	0
Sesame Thins Cheddar	9 (1 oz)	150	3	0
Sesame Thins Garlic	9 (1 oz)	150	3	0
Sesame Thins Original	9 (1 oz)	150	2	0
Sesame Thins Unsalted	11 (1 oz)	150	3	0
SnackWell's				
Cracked Pepper	7 (0.5 oz)	60	tr	0
Fat Free Wheat	5 (0.5 oz)	60	1	0
Reduced Fat Cheese	38 (1 oz)	130	1	0
Reduced Fat Classic Golden	6 (0.5 oz)	60	0	0
Salsa Cheddar	32 (1 oz)	120	1	0
Snorkles				
Cheddar	56 (1 oz)	140	1	5
Sociables				
Crackers	7 (0.5 oz)	80	tr	0
Sunshine				
Saltines Cracked Pepper	5 (0.5 oz)	60	tr	0

FOOD	PORTION	CALS.	FIB.	CHOL.
Town House				
Crackers	2	35	—	0
Tree Of Life				
Bite Size Fat Free Corn & Salsa	12	60	0	0
Bite Size Fat Free Cracked Pepper	12	55	0	0
Bite Size Fat Free Garden Vegetable	12	55	0	0
Bite Size Fat Free Garlic & Herb	12	55	0	0
Bite Size Fat Free Soya Nut	12	60	0	0
Bite Size Fat Free Toasted Onion	12	60	0	0
Bite Size Fat Free Whole Wheat	12	60	2	0
Fat Free Oyster	40 (0.5 oz)	60	0	0
Saltine Cracked Pepper Fat Free	4 (0.5 oz)	60	1	0
Saltine Fat Free	4 (0.5 oz)	50	0	0
Triscuit				
Crackers	7 (1.1 oz)	140	4	0
Deli-Style Rye	7 (1.1 oz)	140	4	0
Garden Herb	6 (1 oz)	130	3	0
Low Sodium	7 (1.1 oz)	150	3	0
Reduced Fat	8 (1.1 oz)	130	4	0
Wheat 'n Bran	7 (1.1 oz)	140	4	0
Tuscany				
Pita Crisps	1 oz	90	—	0
Pita Crisps Sesame	1 oz	96	—	0
Toast	1 oz	95	—	0
Toast Pepato	1 oz	93	—	0
Toast Pesto	1 oz	96	—	3
Toast Tomato	1 oz	95	—	0
Twigs				
Sesame & Cheese Sticks	15 (1 oz)	150	tr	0
Uneeda Biscuit				
Unsalted Tops	2 (0.5 oz)	60	tr	0
Venus				
Armenian Thin Bread	2 (0.9 oz)	100	—	0
Bran Wafers Salt Free	5 (0.5 oz)	60	2	0
Corn Crackers Salt Free	5 (0.5 oz)	60	2	0
Cracked Wheat Wafers Salt Free	5 (0.5 oz)	60	—	0
Cracker Bread	5 (0.5 oz)	60	—	0
Hors D'oeuvre	3 (0.5 oz)	60	—	0
Oat Bran Wafers	5 (0.5 oz)	60	2	0
Oat Bran Wafers Salt Free	5 (0.5 oz)	60	1	0

FOOD	PORTION	CALS.	FIB.	CHOL.
Venus (CONT.)				
Old Brussels Cheddar Waferettes	5 (0.5 oz)	80	—	1
Old Brussels Jalapeno Waferettes	5 (0.5 oz)	80	1	1
Rye Wafers Low Salt	5 (0.5 oz)	60	—	0
Stoned Wheat Wafers Bite Size	7 (0.5 oz)	60	—	0
Water Crackers Fat Free	5 (0.5 oz)	55	—	0
Wheat Wafers Low Salt	5 (0.5 oz)	60	1	0
Waldorf				
Sodium Free	2	30	—	0
Wasa				
Crisp	3 (0.5 oz)	50	2	0
Crisp'N Light Sourdough Rye	3 (0.6 oz)	60	1	0
Crisp'N Light Wheat	2 (0.5 oz)	50	1	0
Crispbread Cinnamon Toast	1 (0.6 oz)	60	1	0
Crispbread Fiber Rye	1 (0.4 oz)	30	2	0
Crispbread Gluten & Wheat Free Corn	1 (0.4 oz)	40	0	0
Crispbread Hearty Rye	1 (0.5 oz)	45	2	0
Crispbread Light Rye	1 (0.3 oz)	25	1	0
Crispbread Multi Grain	1 (0.5 oz)	45	2	0
Crispbread Organic Rye	1 (0.3 oz)	25	1	0
Crispbread Sodium Free Rye	1 (0.3 oz)	30	2	0
Crispbread Sourdough Rye	1 (0.4 oz)	35	1	0
Crispbread Toasted Wheat	1 (0.5 oz)	50	1	0
Crispbread Whole Wheat	1 (0.5 oz)	50	1	0
Waverly				
Crackers	5 (0.5 oz)	70	0	0
Wheat Thins				
Low Salt	16 (1 oz)	140	2	0
Multi-Grain	17 (1 oz)	130	2	0
Wheatsworth				
Stone Ground	5 (0.5 oz)	80	1	0
Zesta				
Saltine	2	25	—	0
Saltine Unsalted Top	2	25	—	0
Zwieback				
Crackers	1 (8 g)	35	tr	0

CRANBERRIES
CANNED

cranberry sauce sweetened	½ cup	209	—	0

FOOD	PORTION	CALS.	FIB.	CHOL.
Ocean Spray				
CranFruit Cranberry Orange Sauce	2 oz	100	—	0
CranFruit Cranberry Raspberry Sauce	2 oz	100	—	0
CranFruit Cranberry Strawberry Sauce	2 oz	100	—	0
Cranberry Sauce Jellied	2 oz	90	—	0
Whole Berry Sauce	2 oz	90	—	0
S&W				
Cranberry Sauce Jellied Old Fashioned	½ cup	90	—	0
Cranberry Sauce Whole Berry Old Fashioned	½ cup	90	—	0
DRIED				
Ocean Spray				
Craisins	⅓ cup (1.4 oz)	130	2	0
FRESH				
chopped	1 cup	54	—	0
Ocean Spray				
Fresh	½ cup	25	—	0

CRANBERRY BEANS
CANNED

FOOD	PORTION	CALS.	FIB.	CHOL.
cranberry beans	1 cup	216	—	0
DRIED				
cooked	1 cup	240	—	0
Bean Cuisine				
Dried	½ cup	115	5	0

CRANBERRY JUICE

FOOD	PORTION	CALS.	FIB.	CHOL.
cocktail	1 cup	147	—	0
cranberry juice cocktail	6 oz	108	—	0
cranberry juice cocktail low calorie	6 oz	33	—	0
cranberry juice cocktail frzn	12 oz can	821	—	0
cranberry juice cocktail frzn as prep	6 oz	102	—	0
After The Fall				
Cape Cod Cranberry	1 bottle (10 oz)	130	—	0
Cranberry Ginger Ale	1 can (12 oz)	140	0	0
Apple & Eve				
Juice	6 fl oz	100	—	0
Ocean Spray				
Cocktail	8 fl oz	140	0	0

FOOD	PORTION	CALS.	FIB.	CHOL.
Ocean Spray (CONT.)				
Cocktail Reduced Calorie	8 fl oz	50	0	0
Lightstyle Low Calorie Cranberry Juice Cocktail	8 fl oz	40	0	0
Seneca				
Cocktail frzn as prep	8 fl oz	140	0	0
Snapple				
Cranberry Royal	10 fl oz	150	—	0
Tree Of Life				
Concentrate	8 tsp (1.4 oz)	110	—	0
Tropicana				
Twister Ruby Red	1 bottle (10 fl oz)	150	—	0
Twister Ruby Red	8 fl oz	120	—	0
Veryfine				
Drink	8 oz	160	—	0

CRAYFISH

(*see also* LOBSTER)

cooked	3 oz	97	—	151
raw	3 oz	76	—	118
raw	8	24	—	37

CREAM

(*see also* SOUR CREAM, SOUR CREAM SUBSTITUTES, WHIPPED TOPPINGS)

LIQUID

half & half	1 tbsp (0.5 oz)	20	—	6
half & half	1 cup (8.5 oz)	315	—	89
heavy whipping	1 tbsp (0.5 oz)	52	—	21
light coffee	1 cup (8.4 oz)	496	—	159
light coffee	1 tbsp (0.5 oz)	29	—	10
light whipping	1 tbsp (0.5 oz)	44	—	17
Farmland				
Half & Half	2 tbsp	40	0	0
Light Cream	2 tbsp	30	0	0
Hood				
Half & Half	2 tbsp (1 oz)	40	0	15
Heavy	1 tbsp (0.5 oz)	50	0	20
Light	1 tbsp (0.5 oz)	30	0	10
Whipping Cream	1 tbsp (0.5 oz)	45	0	20
Parmalat				
Half & Half	2 tbsp (1 oz)	40	0	15

WHIPPED

heavy whipping	1 cup (4.1 oz)	411	—	163
light whipping	1 cup (4.2 oz)	345	—	132

FOOD	PORTION	CALS.	FIB.	CHOL.
CREAM CHEESE				
cream cheese	1 oz	99	—	31
cream cheese	1 pkg (3 oz)	297	—	93
Alpine Lace				
Fat Free Garden Vegetable	2 tbsp (1 oz)	30	0	3
Fat Free Garlic & Herbs	2 tbsp (1 oz)	30	0	3
Breakstone				
Temp-Tee Whipped	3 tbsp (1.2 oz)	110	0	30
Fleur De Lait				
Bermuda Onion & Chives	2 tbsp (0.9 oz)	90	0	30
Cinnamon Raisin	2 tbsp (0.9 oz)	90	0	25
Date Nut Rum	2 tbsp (0.9 oz)	90	0	30
Fresh Cut Garden Vegetable	2 tbsp (0.9 oz)	80	0	30
Garden Vegetable	2 tbsp (0.9 oz)	80	0	30
Garlic & Spice	2 tbsp (0.9 oz)	90	0	30
Herb & Spice	2 tbsp (0.9 oz)	90	0	30
Irish Creme	2 tbsp (0.9 oz)	100	0	30
Lemon	2 tbsp (0.9 oz)	90	0	25
Lox	2 tbsp (0.9 oz)	90	0	30
Mandarin Orange	2 tbsp (0.9 oz)	90	0	30
Peach	2 tbsp (0.9 oz)	90	0	25
Pineapple	2 tbsp (0.9 oz)	90	0	30
Plain	2 tbsp (1 oz)	100	0	35
Strawberry	2 tbsp (0.9 oz)	90	0	30
Toasted Onion	2 tbsp (0.9 oz)	90	0	30
Wildberry	2 tbsp (0.9 oz)	90	0	25
Fresh Cut				
Bac'n & Horseradish	2 tbsp (0.9 oz)	90	0	30
Bermuda Onion & Chives	2 tbsp (0.9 oz)	90	0	30
Date Nut & Rum	2 tbsp (0.9 oz)	90	0	30
Garlic & Spice	2 tbsp (0.9 oz)	90	0	35
Herb & Spice	2 tbsp (0.9 oz)	90	0	30
Lox	2 tbsp (0.9 oz)	90	0	30
Peaches & Cream	2 tbsp (0.9 oz)	90	0	25
Strawberry	2 tbsp (0.9 oz)	90	0	30
Friendship				
NY Style Reduced Fat	2 tbsp (1 oz)	50	0	10
Healthy Choice				
Herbs & Garlic	2 tbsp (1 oz)	25	—	<5
Plain	2 tbsp (1 oz)	25	—	<5
Strawberry	2 tbsp (1 oz)	30	—	<5
Heluva Good Cheese				
Cream Cheese	1 tbsp (1 oz)	100	0	30

FOOD	PORTION	CALS.	FIB.	CHOL.
Philadelphia				
Free	1 oz	25	0	<5
Free Soft	2 tbsp (1.2 oz)	30	0	<5
Light Soft	2 tbsp (1.1 oz)	70	0	15
Regular	1 oz	100	0	30
Soft	2 tbsp (1 oz)	100	0	30
Soft Herb & Garlic	2 tbsp (1.1 oz)	110	0	30
Soft Olive & Pimento	2 tbsp (1.1 oz)	100	0	30
Soft Pineapple	2 tbsp (1.1 oz)	100	0	30
Soft Smoked Salmon	2 tbsp (1.1 oz)	100	0	30
Soft Strawberries	2 tbsp (1.1 oz)	100	0	30
Soft With Chives & Onions	2 tbsp (1.1 oz)	110	0	30
Whipped	3 tbsp (1.1 oz)	110	0	35
Whipped Smoked Salmon	3 tbsp (1.1 oz)	100	0	30
With Chives	1 oz	90	0	30
With Pimentos	1 oz	90	0	30
Ultra Delight				
Cheddar Cream Cheese	2 tbsp (0.9 oz)	60	1	20
Chive	2 tbsp (0.9 oz)	60	1	20
Garlic	2 tbsp (0.9 oz)	60	1	20
Mixed Berry	2 tbsp (0.9 oz)	70	1	20
Nacho	2 tbsp (0.9 oz)	60	1	20
Salsa	2 tbsp (0.9 oz)	60	1	20
Shrimp	2 tbsp (0.9 oz)	60	1	30
Strawberry	2 tbsp (0.9 oz)	60	1	20
Vegetable	2 tbsp (0.9 oz)	50	1	20
Weight Watchers				
Light	2 tbsp	40	0	10

CREAM CHEESE SUBSTITUTES

Tofutti				
Better Than Cream Cheese French Onion	1 oz	80	—	0
Better Than Cream Cheese Herb & Chive	1 oz	80	—	0
Better Than Cream Cheese Plain	1 oz	80	—	0

CREAM OF TARTAR

cream of tartar	1 tsp	8	—	0

CREPES

basic crepe unfilled	1	75	—	55

CRESS

(see also WATERCRESS*)*

garden cooked	½ cup	16	—	0
garden raw	½ cup	8	—	0

FOOD	PORTION	CALS.	FIB.	CHOL.
CROAKER				
atlantic breaded & fried	3 oz	188	—	71
atlantic raw	3 oz	89	—	52
CROISSANT				
Rudy's Farm				
Ham & Swiss Sandwich	1 (3.4 oz)	310	1	25
TAKE-OUT				
w/ egg & cheese	1	369	—	216
w/ egg cheese & bacon	1	413	—	215
w/ egg cheese & ham	1	475	—	213
w/ egg cheese & sausage	1	524	—	216
CROUTONS				
plain	1 cup (1 oz)	122	2	0
Arnold				
Crispy Cheddar Romano	½ oz	64	tr	3
Crispy Cheese Garlic	½ oz	60	tr	0
Crispy Fine Herbs	½ oz	50	1	0
Crispy Italian	½ oz	60	tr	0
Crispy Onion & Garlic	½ oz	60	—	0
Crispy Seasoned	½ oz	60	—	0
Brownberry				
Caesar Salad	½ oz	62	1	tr
Cheddar Cheese	½ oz	63	tr	3
Onion & Garlic	½ oz	60	tr	1
Seasoned	½ oz	59	1	1
Toasted	½ oz	56	tr	0
Pepperidge Farm				
Cheddar & Romano Cheese	½ oz	60	—	0
Cheese & Garlic	½ oz	70	—	0
Onion & Garlic	½ oz	70	—	0
Seasoned	½ oz	70	—	0
Sour Cream & Chive	½ oz	70	—	0
CUCUMBER				
FRESH				
raw	1 (11 oz)	38	3	0
raw sliced	½ cup (1.8 oz)	7	1	0
JARRED				
Rosoff's				
Salad	3 slices (1 oz)	12	—	0
Schorr's				
Cucumber Garden Salad	3 slices (1 oz)	12	—	0
TAKE-OUT				
cucumber salad	3.5 oz	50	—	0

FOOD	PORTION	CALS.	FIB.	CHOL.
CUMIN				
seed	1 tsp	8	—	0
CURRANTS				
black fresh	½ cup	36	—	0
zante dried	½ cup	204	—	0
CUSK				
fillet baked	3 oz	106	—	50
CUSTARD				
HOME RECIPE				
baked	½ cup (5 oz)	148	—	123
baked	1 recipe 4 serv (19.8 oz)	549	—	491
flan	1 recipe 10 serv (53.7 oz)	2206	—	1408
MIX				
as prep w/ 2% milk	½ cup (4.7 oz)	148	—	74
as prep w/ 2% milk	1 recipe 4 serv (18.7 oz)	595	—	297
flan as prep w/ 2% milk	1 recipe 4 serv (18.7 oz)	542	—	57
flan as prep w/ 2% milk	½ cup (4.7 oz)	135	—	9
flan as prep w/ whole milk	1 recipe 4 serv (18.7 oz)	600	—	66
flan as prep w/ whole milk	½ cup (4.7 oz)	150	—	17
Jell-O				
Flan	½ cup	151	—	17
Golden Egg Americana as prep	½ cup	160	—	81
READY-TO-EAT				
Kozy Shack				
Flan	1 pkg (4 oz)	150	0	40
TAKE-OUT				
baked	½ cup (5 oz)	148	—	123
flan	½ cup (5.4 oz)	220	—	140
zabaglione	½ cup (57.2 g)	135	0	213
CUTTLEFISH				
steamed	3 oz	134	—	190
DANDELION GREENS				
fresh cooked	½ cup	17	—	0
raw chopped	½ cup	13	—	0
DANISH PASTRY				
FROZEN				
Morton				
Honey Buns	1 (2.28 oz)	250	2	0

FOOD	PORTION	CALS.	FIB.	CHOL.
Morton (CONT.)				
Honey Buns Mini	1 (1.23 oz)	160	tr	0
Sara Lee				
Apple Danish Twist	1 slice (1.9 oz)	190	—	10
Apple Free & Light	1 slice (2 oz)	130	—	0
Cheese Danish Twist	1 slice (1.9 oz)	200	—	15
Raspberry Danish Twist	1 slice (1.9 oz)	200	—	15
READY-TO-EAT				
plain ring	1 (12 oz)	1305	—	292
Hostess				
Apple	1 (3.8 oz)	400	2	20
Apple Fruit Roll	1 (2 oz)	180	1	<5
Coffee Cake Raspberry	1 (1.2 oz)	110	tr	<5
REFRIGERATED				
Pillsbury				
Caramel Danish w/ Nuts	1	160	—	0
Cinnamon Raisin Danish w/ Icing	1	150	—	0
Orange Danish w/ Icing	1	150	—	0
TAKE-OUT				
almond	1 (4¼ in) (2.3 oz)	280	2	30
cheese	1 (3 oz)	353	—	20
cinnamon	1 (3 oz)	349	—	28
cinnamon nut	1 (4¼ in) (2.3 oz)	280	2	30
fruit	1 (3.3 oz)	335	—	19
raisin nut	1 (4¼ in) (2.3 oz)	280	2	30

DATES

FOOD	PORTION	CALS.	FIB.	CHOL.
DRIED				
chopped	1 cup	489	—	0
deglet noor	10	240	—	0
whole	10	228	—	0
Bordo				
Diced	2 oz	203	—	0
Dole				
Chopped	½ cup	230	—	0
Pitted	½ cup	280	—	0
Dromedary				
Chopped	¼ cup	130	—	0
Pitted	5	100	—	0
Sonoma				
Dried	5-6 (1.4 oz)	110	5	0

DEER

(*see* VENISON)

DELI MEATS/COLD CUTS

(*see also* CHICKEN, HAM, MEAT SUBSTITUTES, TURKEY)

FOOD	PORTION	CALS.	FIB.	CHOL.
barbecue loaf pork & beef	1 oz	49	—	11

FOOD	PORTION	CALS.	FIB.	CHOL.
beerwurst beef	1 slice (2¾ in x ¹⁄₁₆ in)	20	—	4
beerwurst beef	1 slice (4 in x ⅛ in)	75	—	13
beerwurst pork	1 slice (2¾ in x ¹⁄₁₆ in)	14	—	4
beerwurst pork	1 slice (4 in x ⅛ in)	55	—	13
berliner pork & beef	1 oz	65	—	13
blood sausage	1 oz	95	—	30
bologna beef	1 oz	88	—	16
bologna beef & pork	1 oz	89	—	16
bologna pork	1 oz	70	—	17
braunschweiger pork	1 oz	102	—	44
braunschweiger pork	1 slice (2½ in x ¼ in)	65	—	28
corned beef loaf	1 oz	43	—	13
dutch brand loaf pork & beef	1 oz	68	—	13
headcheese pork	1 oz	60	—	23
honey loaf pork & beef	1 oz	36	—	10
honey roll sausage beef	1 oz	42	—	12
lebanon bologna beef	1 oz	60	—	20
liver cheese pork	1 oz	86	—	49
liverwurst pork	1 oz	92	—	45
luncheon meat beef	1 oz	87	—	18
luncheon meat pork & beef	1 oz	100	—	15
luncheon meat pork canned	1 oz	95	—	18
luncheon sausage pork & beef	1 oz	74	—	18
luxury loaf pork	1 oz	40	—	10
mortadella beef & pork	1 oz	88	—	16
mother's loaf pork	1 oz	80	—	13
new england sausage pork & beef	1 oz	46	—	14
olive loaf pork	1 oz	67	—	11
peppered loaf pork & beef	1 oz	42	—	13
pickle & pimiento loaf pork	1 oz	74	—	10
picnic loaf pork & beef	1 oz	66	—	11
salami cooked beef & pork	1 oz	71	—	18
salami hard pork & beef	1 slice (⅓ oz)	42	—	8
salami hard pork & beef	1 pkg (4 oz)	472	—	89
sandwich spread pork & beef	1 tbsp	35	—	6
sandwich spread pork & beef	1 oz	67	—	11
summer sausage thuringer cervelat	1 oz	98	—	19
Carl Buddig				
Beef	1 oz	40	0	20
Corned Beef	1 oz	40	0	20
Pastrami	1 oz	40	0	20

FOOD	PORTION	CALS.	FIB.	CHOL.
DiLusso				
Genoa	1 oz	100	0	25
Hansel n' Gretel				
Healthy Deli Bologna Beef & Pork	1 oz	41	—	9
Healthy Deli Cooked Corn Beef	1 oz	35	—	11
Healthy Deli Italian Roast Beef	1 oz	31	—	16
Healthy Deli Pastrami Round	1 oz	34	—	14
Healthy Deli Regular Roast Beef	1 oz	30	—	13
Healthy Deli St Paddy's Corned Beef	1 oz	24	—	7
Healthy Choice				
Bologna	1 slice (1 oz)	30	0	15
Bologna Beef	1 slice (1 oz)	35	0	10
Deli-Thin Bologna	4 slices (1.8 oz)	60	0	25
Well-Pack Bologna	1 slice (1 oz)	30	0	15
Hebrew National				
Bologna Beef	2 oz	180	—	40
Bologna Beef Reduced Fat	2 oz	130	—	35
Bologna Lean Chub	2 oz	90	—	25
Bologna Midget	2 oz	180	—	40
Deli Pastrami	2 oz	80	—	30
Deli Express Corned Beef	2 oz	80	—	35
Deli Express Tongue Sliced	2 oz	120	—	50
Salami Beef	2 oz	170	—	40
Salami Beef Reduced Fat	2 oz	110	—	30
Salami Lean Chub	2 oz	90	—	30
Salami Midget	2 oz	170	—	40
Homeland				
Hard Salami	1 oz	110	0	35
Hormel				
Liverwurst Spread	4 tbsp (2 oz)	130	0	70
Pepperoni Chunk	1 oz	140	0	35
Pepperoni Sliced	15 slices (1 oz)	140	0	35
Pepperoni Twin	1 oz	140	0	35
Pillow Pack Genoa Salami	4 slices (1.1 oz)	120	0	30
Pillow Pack Pepperoni	16 slices (1 oz)	140	0	35
Pillow Pack Pepperoni	1 oz	140	0	35
Jones				
Liver Sausage	1 slice	80	—	43
Liver Sausage Chub	1 slice	80	—	43
Jordan's				
Healthy Trim 95% Fat Free Macaroni & Cheese Loaf	2 slices (1.6 oz)	50	0	15

FOOD	PORTION	CALS.	FIB.	CHOL.

Jordan's (CONT.)

FOOD	PORTION	CALS.	FIB.	CHOL.
Healthy Trim 95% Fat Free Olive Loaf	2 slices (1.6 oz)	50	0	15
Healthy Trim 95% Fat Free Pickle & Pepper Loaf	2 slices (1.6 oz)	50	0	15
Healthy Trim 97% Fat Free Corned Beef	2 slices (1.6 oz)	45	0	30
Healthy Trim Low Fat Cooked Salami	3 slices (2 oz)	70	0	25
Healthy Trim Low Fat German Brand Bologna	3 slices (2 oz)	70	0	25

Oscar Mayer

FOOD	PORTION	CALS.	FIB.	CHOL.
Bologna Beef	1 slice (1 oz)	90	0	15
Bologna Garlic	1 slice (1.4 oz)	110	0	30
Bologna Light	1 slice (1 oz)	60	0	15
Bologna Light Beef	1 slice (1 oz)	60	0	10
Bologna Pork & Chicken & Beef	1 slice (1 oz)	90	0	20
Bologna Wisconsin Made Ring	2 oz	140	0	35
Braunschweiger	1 slice (1 oz)	100	0	50
Braunschweiger	2 oz	190	0	100
Braunschweiger German Brand	2 oz	200	0	90
Cotto Salami	2 slices (1.6 oz)	100	0	35
Cotto Salami Beef	2 slices (1.6 oz)	90	0	35
Free Bologna	2 slices (1.6 oz)	35	—	15
Genoa Salami	3 slices (1 oz)	100	0	25
Hard Salami	3 slices (1 oz)	100	0	25
Head Cheese	1 slice (1 oz)	50	0	25
Healthy Favorites Bologna	2 slices (1.6 oz)	45	0	15
Honey Loaf	1 slice (1 oz)	35	0	15
Liver Cheese	1 slice (1.3 oz)	120	0	80
Lunchables Bologna/American	1 pkg (4.5 oz)	450	0	85
Lunchables Deluxe Turkey/Ham	1 pkg (5.1 oz)	360	1	60
Lunchables Dessert Jello/ Honey Turkey/Cheddar	1 pkg (5.7 oz)	320	tr	50
Lunchables Fun Pack Bologna/ Wild Cherry	1 pkg (11.2 oz)	530	tr	60
Lunchables Fun Pack Ham/Fruit Punch	1 pkg (11.2 oz)	450	tr	50
Lunchables Ham/Swiss	1 pkg (4.5 oz)	320	0	60
Lunchables Pepperoni/ American	1 pkg (4.5 oz)	480	0	95
Lunchables Salami/American	1 pkg (4.5 oz)	430	0	80
Luncheon Loaf Spiced	1 slice (1 oz)	70	0	20
New England Brand Sausage	2 slices (1.6 oz)	60	0	25

FOOD	PORTION	CALS.	FIB.	CHOL.
Oscar Mayer (CONT.)				
Old Fashioned Loaf	1 slice (1 oz)	60	0	15
Olive Loaf	1 slice (1 oz)	70	0	20
Peppered Loaf	1 slice (1 oz)	39	—	14
Pickle And Pimiento Loaf	1 slice (1 oz)	70	0	20
Salami For Beer	2 slices (1.6 oz)	110	0	30
Salami Machaich Brand Beef	2 slices (1.6 oz)	120	0	30
Sandwich Spread	2 oz	140	0	20
Summer Sausage	2 slices (1.6 oz)	140	0	40
Summer Sausage Beef	2 slices (1.6 oz)	140	0	35
Russer				
Bologna	2 oz	180	—	30
Bologna Beef	2 oz	180	—	30
Bologna Garlic	2 oz	180	—	30
Bologna Italian Brand Sweet Red Pepper	2 oz	180	—	30
Bologna Jalapeno Pepper	2 oz	170	—	25
Bologna Wunderbar German Brand	2 oz	190	—	20
Braunschweiger	2 oz	170	—	90
Cooked Salami	2 oz	120	—	50
Dutch Brand	2 oz	130	—	25
Hot Cooked Salami	2 oz	110	—	45
Italian Brand Loaf	2 oz	130	—	25
Jalapeno Loaf With Monterey Jack Cheese	2 oz	160	—	25
Kielbasa Loaf	2 oz	120	—	35
Light Bologna	2 oz	120	—	30
Light Bologna Beef	2 oz	120	—	30
Light Braunschweiger	2 oz	120	—	60
Light Old Fashioned Loaf	2 oz	90	—	30
Light P&P Loaf	2 oz	100	—	30
Light Salami Cooked	2 oz	90	—	40
Olive Loaf	2 oz	160	—	20
P&P Loaf	2 oz	160	—	25
Pepper Loaf	2 oz	90	—	30
Polish Loaf	2 oz	140	—	25
Sara Lee				
Pastrami Beef	2 oz	100	1	25
Peppered Beef	2 oz	70	—	25
Shofar				
Salami Beef	2 oz	160	0	40
Spam				
Less Salt	2 oz	170	0	40

FOOD	PORTION	CALS.	FIB.	CHOL.
Spam (CONT.)				
Lite	2 oz	110	0	45
Original	2 oz	170	0	40
Underwood				
Liverwurst	2.08 oz	180	—	90
Weight Watchers				
Bologna	2 slices (¾ oz)	35	—	15
TAKE-OUT				
corned beef	2 oz	70	—	40
corned beef brisket	2 oz	90	—	35
submarine w/ salami ham cheese lettuce tomato onion & oil	1	456	—	35

DIETING AIDS

(*see* NUTRITIONAL SUPPLEMENTS)

DILL

seed	1 tsp	6	—	0
sprigs fresh	5	0	—	0
sprigs fresh	1 cup	4	—	0
weed dry	1 tsp	3	—	0
Watkins				
Liquid Spice	1 tbsp (0.5 oz)	120	0	0

DINNER

(*see also* ORIENTAL FOOD, PASTA DINNERS, POT PIE, SPANISH FOOD)

FROZEN

Armour

Classics Chicken Parmigiana	1 meal (10.75 oz)	360	7	45
Classics Chicken & Noodles	1 meal (11 oz)	280	6	60
Classics Chicken Mesquite	1 meal (9.5 oz)	280	5	65
Classics Chicken w/ Wine & Mushroom	1 meal (10 oz)	260	4	50
Classics Glazed Chicken	1 meal (10.75 oz)	280	4	55
Classics Meatloaf	1 meal (11.25 oz)	300	7	65
Classics Salisbury Steak	1 meal (11.25 oz)	330	4	50
Classics Swedish Meatballs	1 meal (10 oz)	300	4	40
Classics Turkey and Dressing	1 meal (11.25 oz)	270	5	60
Classics Veal Parmigiana	1 meal (11.25 oz)	400	5	65
Classics Lite Beef Pepper	1 meal (11 oz)	210	5	60
Classics Lite Chicken Burgundy	1 meal (10 oz)	210	4	45
Classics Lite Salisbury Steak	1 meal (11.5 oz)	260	6	55
Classics Lite Shrimp Creole	1 meal (10 oz)	220	16	20
Classics Lite Sweet & Sour Chicken	1 meal (11 oz)	220	4	30

FOOD	PORTION	CALS.	FIB.	CHOL.
Banquet				
BBQ Style Chicken	1 meal (9 oz)	320	3	60
Beef	1 meal (9 oz)	240	12	70
Chicken Parmigiana	1 pkg (9.5 oz)	290	3	50
Chicken & Dumplings	1 meal (10 oz)	260	16	35
Chicken Fried Steak	1 pkg (10 oz)	400	4	30
Chicken Nuggets	1 pkg (6.75 oz)	410	11	45
Extra Helping All White Chicken	1 meal (18 oz)	820	8	95
Extra Helping Chicken Parmigiana	1 meal (19 oz)	650	9	65
Extra Helping Chicken Fried Steak	1 meal (18.5 oz)	800	6	55
Extra Helping Fried Chicken	1 meal (18 oz)	790	8	110
Extra Helping Meatloaf	1 meal (19 oz)	650	10	85
Extra Helping Mexican Style	1 meal (22 oz)	820	20	50
Extra Helping Salisbury Steak	1 meal (19 oz)	740	11	75
Extra Helping Southern Fried Chicken	1 meal (17.5 oz)	750	9	120
Extra Helping Turkey Dinner	1 meal (18.8 oz)	560	7	75
Family Entree Beef Stew	1 serv (8.13 oz)	160	4	25
Family Entree Chicken Parmigiana	1 serv (4.67 oz)	240	2	20
Family Entree Chicken & Dumplings	1 serv (7.47 oz)	290	2	2
Family Entree Gravy & Sliced Turkey	1 serv (4.8 oz)	100	tr	25
Family Entree Gravy w/ Charbroiled Beef	1 serv (4.67 oz)	180	2	25
Family Entree Onion Gravy w/ Beef	1 serv (4.67 oz)	180	2	20
Family Entree Salisbury Steak	1 serv (4.67 oz)	200	2	25
Family Entree Veal Parmigiana	1 serv (4.67 oz)	230	2	20
Family Entrees Gravy & Sliced Beef	1 serv (5.6 oz)	100	tr	40
Fried Chicken	1 meal (9 oz)	470	6	105
Gravy w/ Beef Patty	1 pkg (9.5 oz)	300	2	35
Hot Sandwich Toppers Chicken Ala King	1 pkg (4.5 oz)	100	1	40
Hot Sandwich Toppers Creamed Chipped Beef	1 pkg (4 oz)	100	0	25
Hot Sandwich Toppers Gravy & Sliced Beef	1 pkg (4 oz)	70	tr	25
Hot Sandwich Toppers Gravy & Sliced Turkey	1 pkg (5 oz)	90	tr	30

FOOD	PORTION	CALS.	FIB.	CHOL.
Banquet (CONT.)				
Hot Sandwich Toppers Salisbury Steak	1 pkg (5 oz)	220	2	25
Hot Sandwich Toppers Sloppy Joe	1 meal (4 oz)	140	1	25
Meatloaf	1 meal (9.5 oz)	280	2	40
Mexican Style Combo Meal	1 pkg (11 oz)	380	9	15
Mexican Style Meal	1 pkg (11 oz)	340	10	15
Oriental Style Chicken	1 pkg (9 oz)	260	4	40
Salisbury Steak	1 meal (9.5 oz)	310	2	35
Southern Fried Chicken Meal	1 pkg (8.75 oz)	260	4	85
Turkey	1 meal (9.25 oz)	270	3	45
Veal Parmagiana	1 pkg (9 oz)	530	7	25
Western Style Meal	1 meal (9.5 oz)	210	5	30
White Meat Chicken Meal	1 pkg (8.75 oz)	470	2	100
Birds Eye				
Easy Recipe Beef Burgundy not prep	½ pkg	120	4	0
Easy Recipe Beef Fajitas not prep	½ pkg	80	3	0
Budget Gourmet				
Beef Cantonese	1 meal (9.1 oz)	270	—	40
Beef Stroganoff	1 meal (8.75 oz)	260	—	50
Chicken And Egg Noodles	1 meal (10 oz)	440	—	90
Chicken Au Gratin	1 meal (9.1 oz)	230	—	40
Chicken Breast Parmigiana	1 pkg (11 oz)	270	—	50
Chicken Marsala	1 meal (9 oz)	260	—	90
Chicken With Fettucini	1 meal (10 oz)	400	—	85
Chinese Style Vegetables & Chicken	1 meal (10 oz)	280	—	10
French Recipe Chicken	1 meal (10 oz)	220	—	40
Glazed Turkey	1 meal (9 oz)	260	—	30
Ham & Asparagus Au Gratin	1 meal (8.7 oz)	300	—	50
Herbed Chicken Breast With Fettucini	1 pkg (11 oz)	240	—	45
Italian Style Vegetables & Chicken	1 meal (10.25 oz)	310	—	30
Mandarin Chicken	1 meal (10 oz)	240	—	40
Mesquite Chicken Breast	1 pkg (11 oz)	250	—	40
Orange Glazed Chicken	1 meal (9 oz)	270	—	25
Oriental Beef	1 meal (10 oz)	290	—	30
Oriental Chicken With Vegetables	1 meal (9 oz)	280	—	20
Pepper Steak With Rice	1 meal (10 oz)	300	—	35

FOOD	PORTION	CALS.	FIB.	CHOL.
Budget Gourmet (CONT.)				
Pot Roast Beef	1 meal (10.5 oz)	230	—	60
Roast Chicken With Homestyle Gravy	1 meal (11 oz)	280	—	35
Roast Sirloin Supreme	1 meal (9 oz)	320	—	85
Sirloin Salisbury Steak	1 meal (9 oz)	220	—	25
Sirloin Salisbury Steak	1 meal (11 oz)	280	—	40
Sirloin Cheddar Melt	1 meal (9.4 oz)	380	—	85
Sirloin Of Beef In Herb Sauce	1 meal (9.5 oz)	250	—	30
Sirloin Of Beef In Wine Sauce	1 pkg (11 oz)	280	—	25
Sirloin Tips And Country Vegetables	1 meal (10 oz)	290	—	40
Special Recipe Sirloin Of Beef	1 meal (11 oz)	250	—	60
Stuffed Turkey Breast	1 pkg (11 oz)	250	—	35
Swedish Meatballs With Noodles	1 meal (10 oz)	590	—	145
Sweet And Sour Chicken	1 meal (10 oz)	340	—	30
Teriyaki Beef	1 pkg (10.75 oz)	260	—	30
Teriyaki Chicken Breast	1 meal (11 oz)	300	—	30
Healthy Choice				
Beef & Peppers Cantonese	1 meal (11.5 oz)	270	5	35
Beef Pepper Steak Oriental	1 meal (9.5 oz)	250	3	35
Beef Tips Francais	1 meal (9.5 oz)	280	4	30
Beef Tips With Sauce	1 meal (11 oz)	290	5	40
Chicken Cantonese	1 meal (11.25 oz)	210	5	30
Chicken Parmigiana	1 meal (11.5 oz)	300	6	35
Chicken & Vegetables Marsala	1 meal (11.5 oz)	220	3	30
Chicken Bangkok	1 meal (9.5 oz)	270	5	45
Chicken Dijon	1 meal (11 oz)	280	9	30
Chicken Imperial	1 meal (9 oz)	230	3	40
Chicken Picante	1 meal (11.25 oz)	220	6	35
Chicken Teriyaki	1 meal (12.25 oz)	270	5	40
Classics Beef Broccoli Beijing	1 meal (12 oz)	330	5	20
Classics Cacciatore Chicken	1 meal (12.5 oz)	260	6	25
Classics Chicken Fransesca	1 meal (12.5 oz)	360	5	30
Classics Country Inn Roast Turkey	1 meal (10 oz)	250	6	30
Classics Ginger Chicken Hunan	1 meal (12.6 oz)	350	5	25
Classics Mesquite Beef Barbecue	1 meal (11 oz)	310	6	45
Classics Salisbury Steak	1 meal (11 oz)	260	5	30
Classics Sesame Chicken Shanghai	1 meal (12 oz)	310	5	30
Classics Shrimp & Vegetables Maria	1 meal (12.5 oz)	260	5	35

FOOD	PORTION	CALS.	FIB.	CHOL.
Healthy Choice (CONT.)				
Country Glazed Chicken	1 meal (8.5 oz)	200	3	30
Country Herb Chicken	1 meal (11.5 oz)	270	6	35
Country Roast Turkey With Mushroom	1 meal (8.5 oz)	220	3	25
Country Turkey & Pasta	1 meal (12.6 oz)	300	6	35
Homestyle Turkey With Vegetables	1 meal (9.5 oz)	260	3	35
Honey Mustard Chicken	1 meal (9.5 oz)	260	4	30
Lemon Pepper Fish	1 meal (10.7 oz)	290	7	25
Mandarin Chicken	1 meal (10 oz)	280	4	25
Mesquite Chicken Barbecue	1 meal (10.5 oz)	320	6	35
Shrimp Marinara	1 meal (10.5 oz)	220	5	50
Smoky Chicken Barbecue	1 meal (12.75 oz)	380	7	50
Southwestern Glazed Chicken	1 meal (12.5 oz)	300	6	45
Sweet & Sour Chicken	1 meal (11.5 oz)	310	5	50
Traditional Beef Tips	1 meal (11.25 oz)	260	6	40
Traditional Breast Of Turkey	1 meal (10.5 oz)	280	7	45
Traditional Meat Loaf	1 meal (12 oz)	320	7	35
Traditional Salisbury Steak	1 meal (11.5 oz)	320	7	45
Yankee Pot Roast	1 meal (11 oz)	280	5	45
Kid Cuisine				
Chicken Sandwiche	1 pkg (9.43 oz)	480	4	20
Chicken Nuggets	1 pkg (9.1 oz)	440	5	30
Fish Sticks	1 pkg (8.25 oz)	370	4	15
Fried Chicken	1 pkg (10.1 oz)	440	5	40
Hot Dogs w/ Buns	6.7 oz	450	—	40
Macaroni & Beef	1 pkg (9.6 oz)	370	5	30
Le Menu				
Entree LightStyle Chicken A La King	8¼ oz	240	—	30
Entree LightStyle Chicken Dijon	8 oz	240	—	40
Entree LightStyle Empress Chicken	8¼ oz	210	—	30
Entree LightStyle Glazed Turkey	8¼ oz	260	—	35
Entree LightStyle Herb Roast Chicken	7¾ oz	260	—	45
Entree LightStyle Swedish Meatballs	8 oz	260	—	40
Entree LightStyle Traditional Turkey	8 oz	200	—	25
LightStyle Glazed Chicken Breast	10 oz	230	—	55
LightStyle Herb Roasted Chicken	10 oz	240	—	70

FOOD	PORTION	CALS.	FIB.	CHOL.
Le Menu (CONT.)				
LightStyle Salisbury Steak	10 oz	280	—	35
LightStyle Sliced Turkey	10 oz	210	—	30
LightStyle Turkey Divan	10 oz	260	—	60
LightStyle Veal Marsala	10 oz	230	—	75
Lean Cuisine				
Baked Chicken	1 meal (8 oz)	240	3	35
Beef Pot Roast	1 meal (9 oz)	210	3	40
Chicken Italiano	1 pkg (9 oz)	270	3	40
Chicken & Vegetables	1 meal (10.5 oz)	240	5	35
Chicken A L'Orange	1 meal (8 oz)	260	1	40
Chicken In Peanut Sauce	1 pkg (9 oz)	280	3	45
Chicken In Honey Barbecue Sauce	1 pkg (8.75 oz)	250	6	50
Chicken Marsala	1 meal (8.1 oz)	180	5	60
Chicken Oriental	1 pkg (9 oz)	260	3	30
Chicken Parmesan	1 meal (10.9 oz)	220	5	50
Chicken Pie	1 meal (9.5 oz)	320	3	35
Fiesta Chicken	1 pkg (8.5 oz)	240	3	45
Fish Divan	1 pkg (10.4 oz)	210	3	65
Glazed Chicken	1 meal (8.5 oz)	240	2	60
Homestyle Turkey	1 pkg (9.4 oz)	230	3	50
Honey Mustard Chicken	1 pkg (7.5 oz)	250	4	32
Meatloaf	1 pkg (9.4 oz)	270	4	55
Oriental Beef	1 meal (9 oz)	250	4	30
Roasted Turkey Breast	1 pkg (9.75 oz)	290	3	25
Salisbury Steak With Macaroni & Cheese	1 meal (9.5 oz)	200	2	60
Stuffed Cabbage	1 meal (9.5 oz)	220	5	25
Swedish Meatballs	1 pkg (9.1 oz)	290	3	55
Sweet & Sour Chicken	1 pkg (10.4 oz)	260	3	45
Turkey Pie	1 pkg (9.5 oz)	300	3	50
Life Choice				
Garden Potato Casserole	1 meal (13.4 oz)	160	9	5
Morton				
Breaded Chicken Pattie	1 meal (6.75 oz)	280	4	20
Chicken Nugget	1 meal (7 oz)	320	3	30
Fried Chicken	1 meal (9 oz)	420	4	85
Meatloaf	1 meal (9 oz)	250	5	20
Mexican	1 meal (10 oz)	260	8	5
Salisbury Steak	1 meal (9 oz)	210	3	20
Turkey	1 meal (9 oz)	230	5	35
Veal Parmagiana	1 meal (8.75 oz)	280	4	20
Western	1 meal (9 oz)	290	6	25

FOOD	PORTION	CALS.	FIB.	CHOL.
Patio				
Chili	1 cup (8 oz)	260	4	55
Ranchera	1 pkg (13 oz)	410	14	25
Stouffer's				
Chicken A La King	1 pkg (9.5 oz)	320	3	55
Chicken Divan	1 pkg (8 oz)	210	1	65
Creamed Chicken	1 pkg (6.5 oz)	280	1	80
Creamed Chipped Beef	½ cup (4.5 oz)	150	1	40
Creamed Chipped Beef Over Country Biscuit	1 pkg (9 oz)	460	3	70
Escalloped Chicken & Noodles	1 pkg (10 oz)	440	2	80
Green Pepper Steak	1 pkg (10.5 oz)	330	3	35
Ham & Asparagus Bake	1 pkg (9.5 oz)	520	2	75
Homestyle Beef Pot Roast	1 pkg (8.9 oz)	270	4	40
Homestyle Breaded Chicken Tenders	1 pkg (6.8 oz)	380	4	50
Homestyle Chicken Parmigiana	1 pkg (10.9 oz)	320	4	75
Homestyle Chicken & Noodles	1 pkg (10 oz)	310	2	80
Homestyle Chicken Monterey	1 pkg (9.4 oz)	410	4	75
Homestyle Fish Filet With Macaroni & Cheese	1 pkg (9 oz)	430	2	70
Homestyle Fried Chicken	1 pkg (7.1 oz)	330	3	55
Homestyle Meatloaf	1 pkg (9.9 oz)	380	3	80
Homestyle Roast Turkey	1 pkg (7.9 oz)	280	1	40
Homestyle Salisbury Steak	1 pkg (9.6 oz)	370	—	50
Homestyle Sliced Beef & Potatoes	1 pkg (8.1 oz)	270	2	45
Homestyle Veal Parmigiana	1 pkg (11.9 oz)	420	6	75
Homestyle Baked Chicken	1 pkg (8.9 oz)	270	2	75
Lunch Express Chicken With Garden Vegetables	1 pkg (9.9 oz)	340	2	30
Lunch Express Mandarin Chicken	1 pkg (9.75 oz)	270	2	30
Lunch Express Mexican Style Rice With Chicken	1 pkg (9 oz)	270	3	20
Lunch Express Oriental Beef	1 pkg (6.2 oz)	260	4	20
Lunch Express Stir-Fry Rice & Chicken	1 pkg (9 oz)	280	3	15
Stuffed Pepper	1 pkg (10 oz)	200	1	25
Swedish Meatballs	1 pkg (9.25 oz)	440	3	85
Tyson				
Beef Champignon	1 pkg (10.5 oz)	370	—	51
Chicken Picante	1 pkg (9 oz)	250	—	50
Chicken Supreme	1 pkg (9 oz)	230	—	51

FOOD	PORTION	CALS.	FIB.	CHOL.
Tyson (CONT.)				
Francais	1 pkg (9.5 oz)	280	—	54
Glazed Chicken With Sauce	1 pkg (9.25 oz)	240	—	44
Grilled Chicken	1 pkg (7.75 oz)	220	—	55
Grilled Italian Chicken	1 pkg (9 oz)	210	—	40
Healthy Portions BBQ Chicken	1 pkg (12.5 oz)	400	—	50
Healthy Portions Chicken Marinara	1 pkg (13.75 oz)	340	—	45
Healthy Portions Herb Chicken	1 pkg (13.75 oz)	340	—	50
Healthy Portions Italian Style Chicken	1 pkg (13.75 oz)	310	—	50
Healthy Portions Mesquite Chicken	1 pkg (13.25 oz)	330	—	45
Healthy Portions Salsa Chicken	1 pkg (13.75 oz)	370	—	45
Healthy Portions Sesame Chicken	1 pkg (13.5 oz)	400	—	45
Honey Roasted Chicken	1 pkg (9 oz)	220	—	48
Kiev	1 pkg (9.25 oz)	450	—	78
Marsala	1 pkg (9 oz)	200	—	52
Mexquite	1 pkg (9 oz)	320	—	55
Picatta	1 pkg (9 oz)	200	—	60
Roasted Chicken	1 pkg (9 oz)	200	—	42
Turkey With Gravy	1 pkg (9.5 oz)	320	—	35
Ultra Slim-Fast				
Beef Pepper Steak	12 oz	270	0	45
Chicken Fettucini	12 oz	380	1	65
Chicken & Vegetable	12 oz	290	4	30
Country Style Vegetable & Beef Tips	12 oz	230	4	45
Mesquite Chicken	12 oz	360	5	65
Roasted Chicken In Mushroom Sauce	12 oz	280	0	55
Shrimp Creole	12 oz	240	5	80
Shrimp Marinara	12 oz	290	0	70
Sweet & Sour Chicken	12 oz	330	0	45
Turkey Medallions In Herb Sauce	12 oz	280	0	40
Weight Watchers				
Barbecue Glazed Chicken	1 pkg (7.4 oz)	190	1	20
Chicken Mirabella	1 pkg (9.2 oz)	170	6	20
Chicken Parmigiana	1 pkg (9.1 oz)	230	2	50
Chicken Cordon Bleu	1 pkg (9 oz)	220	3	20
Chicken Marsala	1 pkg (9 oz)	150	6	25
Fiesta Chicken	1 pkg (8.5 oz)	220	2	25

FOOD	PORTION	CALS.	FIB.	CHOL.
Weight Watchers (CONT.)				
Fried Filet Of Fish	1 pkg (7.7 oz)	230	2	25
Grilled Salisbury Steak	1 pkg (8.5 oz)	250	4	30
Honey Mustard Chicken	1 pkg (8.5 oz)	200	6	30
Lemon Herb Chicken Picante	1 pkg (8.5 oz)	190	3	25
Roast Glazed Chicken	1 pkg (8.9 oz)	200	4	15
Roast Turkey Medallions	1 pkg (8.5 oz)	190	2	20
Shrimp Marinara	1 pkg (9 oz)	190	4	40
Southern Fried Chicken	1 pkg (8 oz)	280	1	65
Stuffed Turkey Breast	1 pkg (8.75 oz)	240	1	20
Swedish Meatballs	1 pkg (9 oz)	280	3	30
Tex-Mex Chicken	1 pkg (8.3 oz)	260	1	35
SHELF-STABLE				
My Own Meal				
Beef Stew	1 pkg (10 oz)	260	4	55
Chicken Mediterranean	1 pkg (10 oz)	270	4	45
Chicken Noodles	1 pkg (10 oz)	270	3	65
Chicken & Black Beans	1 pkg (10 oz)	240	6	40
Old World Stew	1 pkg (10 oz)	310	3	55
DIP				
Breakstone				
Sour Cream Bacon & Onion	2 tbsp (1.1 oz)	60	0	20
Sour Cream Chesapeake Clam	2 tbsp (1.1 oz)	50	0	30
Sour Cream French Onion	2 tbsp (1.1 oz)	50	0	20
Sour Cream Jalapeno Cheddar	2 tbsp (1.1 oz)	60	0	15
Sour Cream Toasted Onion	2 tbsp (1.1 oz)	50	0	20
Chi-Chi's				
Fiesta Bean	2 tbsp (0.9 oz)	35	1	0
Fiesta Cheese	2 tbsp (0.9 oz)	40	0	10
Durkee				
Sour Cream as prep	2 tbsp	25	0	0
Frito Lay				
Cheddar Cheese	1 oz	45	—	6
French Onion	1 oz	50	—	12
Jalapeno Bean	1 oz	30	—	0
Picante Sauce	1 oz	10	—	0
Guiltless Gourmet				
Black Bean Mild	1 oz	25	1	0
Black Bean Spicy	1 oz	25	1	0
Pinto Bean	1 oz	25	1	0
Hain				
Hot Bean	4 tbsp	70	—	5
Mexican Bean	4 tbsp	60	—	5

FOOD	PORTION	CALS.	FIB.	CHOL.
Hain (CONT.)				
Onion Bean	4 tbsp	70	—	5
Taco Dip & Sauce	4 tbsp	25	—	5
Heluva Good Cheese				
Bacon Horseradish	2 tbsp (1.1 oz)	60	0	20
Clam	2 tbsp (1.1 oz)	50	0	20
French Onion	2 tbsp (1.1 oz)	50	0	20
Homestyle Onion	2 tbsp (1.1 oz)	60	0	20
Light French Onion	2 tbsp (1.1 oz)	35	0	10
Light Jalapeno Cheddar	2 tbsp (1.1 oz)	40	0	10
Ranch	2 tbsp (1.1 oz)	60	0	20
Knudsen				
Nacho Cheese	2 tbsp (1.1 oz)	60	0	15
Sour Cream Bacon & Onion	2 tbsp (1.1 oz)	60	0	20
Sour Cream French Onion	2 tbsp (1.1 oz)	50	0	20
Kraft				
Avocado	2 tbsp (1.1 oz)	60	0	0
Bacon & Horseradish	2 tbsp (1.1 oz)	60	0	0
Clam	2 tbsp (1.1 oz)	60	0	0
French Onion	2 tbsp (1.1 oz)	60	0	0
Green Onion	2 tbsp (1.1 oz)	60	0	0
Jalapeno	2 tbsp (1.1 oz)	60	0	0
Jalapeno Cheese	2 tbsp (1.1 oz)	60	0	15
Premium Bacon & Horseradish	2 tbsp (1.1 oz)	50	0	15
Premium Bacon & Onion	2 tbsp (1.1 oz)	60	0	15
Premium Blue Cheese	2 tbsp (1.1 oz)	45	0	10
Premium Clam	2 tbsp (1.1 oz)	45	0	10
Premium Creamy Cucumber	2 tbsp (1.1 oz)	50	0	15
Premium Creamy Onion	2 tbsp (1.1 oz)	45	0	10
Premium French Onion	2 tbsp (1.1 oz)	50	0	10
Premium Nacho Cheese	2 tbsp (1.1 oz)	60	0	15
Ranch	2 tbsp (1.1 oz)	60	0	0
Louise's				
Fat Free Honey Mustard	1 oz	40	0	0
Fat Free Sour Cream & Onion	1 oz	25	0	0
Fat Free White Cheese Peppercorn	1 oz	25	0	0
Marzetti				
Blue Cheese Veggie	2 tbsp	200	0	20
Lemon Dill Veggie	2 tbsp	140	0	25
Light Ranch Veggie	2 tbsp	60	1	10
Ranch Veggie	2 tbsp	140	0	25
Sour Cream & Onion	2 tbsp	130	0	25
Southwestern Veggie	2 tbsp	130	0	25

FOOD	PORTION	CALS.	FIB.	CHOL.
Marzetti (CONT.)				
Spinach Veggie	2 tbsp	130	0	20
Old El Paso				
Black Bean	2 tbsp (1 oz)	20	1	0
Cheese 'n Salsa Medium	2 tbsp (1 oz)	40	0	<5
Cheese 'n Salsa Mild	2 tbsp (1 oz)	40	0	<5
Chunky Salsa Medium	2 tbsp (1 oz)	15	1	0
Chunky Salsa Mild	2 tbsp (1 oz)	15	1	0
Jalapeno	2 tbsp (1 oz)	30	2	<5
Sealtest				
French Onion	2 tbsp (1.1 oz)	50	0	20
Snyder's				
Mustard Pretzel	2 tbsp (1.2 oz)	90	1	20
Wise				
Jalapeno Bean	2 tbsp	25	—	0
Taco	2 tbsp	12	—	0
DOCK				
fresh cooked	3½ oz	20	—	0
raw chopped	½ cup	15	—	0
DOGFISH				
raw	3½ oz	193	—	74
DOLPHINFISH				
fresh baked	3 oz	93	—	80
fresh fillet baked	5.6 oz	174	—	149
DOUGHNUTS				
(*see also* DUNKIN' DONUTS)				
cake type unsugared	1 (1.6 oz)	198	1	18
creme filled	1 (3 oz)	307	—	20
french cruller glazed	1 (1.4 oz)	169	—	5
honey bun	1 (2.1 oz)	242	1	4
jelly	1 (3 oz)	289	—	22
old fashioned	1 (1.6 oz)	198	1	18
sugared	1 (1.6 oz)	192	1	14
wheat glazed	1 (1.6 oz)	162	—	9
wheat sugared	1 (1.6 oz)	162	—	9
yeast glazed	1 (2.1 oz)	242	1	4
Drake's				
Old Fashion Donuts	1 (1.7 oz)	182	—	10
Powdered Sugar Donut Delites	7 (2.5 oz)	300	—	16
Dutch Mill				
Cider	1 (2.1 oz)	240	1	15
Cinnamon	1 (1.8 oz)	210	1	15

FOOD	PORTION	CALS.	FIB.	CHOL.
Dutch Mill (cont.)				
Donut Holes Double-Dipped Chocolate	3 (1.4 oz)	220	0	5
Donut Holes Shootin' Stars	3 (1.4 oz)	190	0	5
Double-Dipped Chocolate	1 (2.1 oz)	280	1	15
Glazed	1 (2.1 oz)	250	1	15
Glazed Chocolate	1 (2.4 oz)	270	1	15
Plain	1 (1.8 oz)	210	1	15
Sugared	1 (1.8 oz)	220	1	15
Earth Grains				
Cinnamon Apple	1	310	—	25
Devil's Food	1	330	—	20
Glazed Old Fashioned	1	310	—	20
Powdered Old Fashioned	1	290	—	20
Freihofer's				
Assorted	1 (2 oz)	270	0	10
Hostess				
Assorted Regular	1 (1.6 oz)	200	tr	10
Cinnamon Family Pack	1 (1 oz)	110	tr	5
Cinnamon Swirl	1 (1.6 oz)	180	tr	<5
Crumb Regular	1 (1 oz)	130	tr	5
Frosted Regular	1 (1.4 oz)	180	1	5
Gem Donettes Cinnamon	6 (3 oz)	320	1	10
Gem Donettes Frosted	6 (3 oz)	390	2	10
Gem Donettes Frosted Strawberry Filled	3 (3 oz)	240	1	<5
Gem Donettes Powdered	6 (3 oz)	350	1	10
Gem Donettes Powdered Strawberry Filled	3 (3 oz)	210	tr	<5
Glazed Party	1 (2.3 oz)	260	1	5
Jumbo Frosted	1 (2 oz)	260	1	10
Jumbo Plain	1 (1.1 oz)	140	tr	10
Jumbo Powdered	1 (1.3 oz)	160	tr	5
Mini Chocolate	5 (2 oz)	220	1	35
O's Raspberry Filled Powdered	1 (2.2 oz)	230	tr	5
Old Fashioned Glazed	1 (2.1 oz)	250	tr	15
Old Fashioned Glazed Honey Wheat	1 (2.1 oz)	250	1	25
Old Fashioned Plain	1 (1.5 oz)	170	tr	10
Plain Regular	1 (1 oz)	120	tr	5
Powdered Family Pack	1 (1 oz)	110	1	5
Little Debbie				
Donut Sticks	1 pkg (1.6 oz)	210	1	5
Donut Sticks	1 pkg (2.5 oz)	320	1	10

FOOD	PORTION	CALS.	FIB.	CHOL.
Little Debbie (CONT.)				
Donut Sticks	1 pkg (3 oz)	390	1	10
Donut Sticks	1 pkg (2 oz)	250	1	5
Tastykake				
Cinnamon	1 (47 g)	180	1	10
Frosted Rich	1 (57 g)	260	3	10
Frosted Rich Mini	1 (14 g)	44	1	5
Honey Wheat	1 (57 g)	210	1	10
Honey Wheat Mini	1 (12 g)	40	0	5
Orange Glazed	1 (57 g)	210	1	10
Plain	1 (47 g)	190	1	10
Powdered Sugar	1 (46 g)	180	1	24
Powdered Sugar Mini	1 (12 g)	40	0	5

DRESSING
(*see* STUFFING/DRESSING)

DRINK MIXERS
(*see also* MINERAL/BOTTLED WATER, SODA)

FOOD	PORTION	CALS.	FIB.	CHOL.
whiskey sour mix	2 oz	55	—	0
whiskey sour mix as prep	3.6 oz	169	—	0
Bacardi				
Margarita Mix w/o liquor	8 fl oz	100	—	0
Pina Colada	8 fl oz	140	—	0
Rum Runner	8 fl oz	140	—	0
Strawberry Daiquiri w/o liquor	8 fl oz	140	—	0
Canada Dry				
Collins Mixer	8 fl oz	120	0	0
Sour Mixer	8 fl oz	90	0	0
Libby				
Bloody Mary Mix	6 oz	40	—	0
McIlhenny				
Tabasco Bloody Mary Mix	8 fl oz	56	1	0
Schweppes				
Collins Mixer	8 fl oz	100	0	0
Tabasco				
Bloody Mary Mix Extra Spicy	8 fl oz	58	2	0

DRUM

FOOD	PORTION	CALS.	FIB.	CHOL.
freshwater fillet baked	5.4 oz	236	—	126
freshwater baked	3 oz	130	—	70

DUCK
FRESH

FOOD	PORTION	CALS.	FIB.	CHOL.
w/ skin roasted	1 cup (4.9 oz)	472	0	118
w/ skin w/ bone leg roasted	3 oz	184	—	97

FOOD	PORTION	CALS.	FIB.	CHOL.
w/ skin w/o bone breast roasted	3 oz	172	—	116
w/o skin roasted	1 cup (4.9 oz)	281	0	125
w/o skin w/ bone leg braised	1 cup (6.1 oz)	310	—	183
w/o skin w/o bone breast broiled	1 cup (6.1 oz)	244	—	249
wild w/ skin raw	½ duck (9.5 oz)	571	—	216

DURIAN
fresh	3½ oz	141	—	0

EEL
fresh cooked	1 fillet (5.6 oz)	375	—	257
fresh cooked	3 oz	200	—	137
raw	3 oz	156	—	107

EGG
(see also EGG DISHES, EGG SUBSTITUTES)

CHICKEN
fried w/ margarine	1	91	—	211
frozen	1 cup	363	—	1033
frozen	1	75	—	213
hard cooked	1	77	—	213
hard cooked chopped	1 cup	210	—	578
poached	1	74	—	212
raw	1	75	—	213
scrambled plain	2	200	—	400
scrambled w/ whole milk & margarine	1 cup	365	—	774
scrambled w/ whole milk & margarine	1	101	—	215
white only	1	17	—	0
white only	1 cup	121	—	0

EggsPlus
Fresh	1 (1.8 oz)	70	0	215

OTHER POULTRY
duck raw	1 (2.5 oz)	130	0	619
quail raw	1 (9 g)	14	—	76
turkey raw	1 (2.7 oz)	135	—	737

EGG DISHES
FROZEN
Chefwich
Cheese Omelet	5 oz	380	—	130
Ham & Cheese Omelet	5 oz	340	—	140
Sausage & Cheese Omelet	5 oz	400	—	130
Western Style Omelet	5 oz	350	—	100

FOOD	PORTION	CALS.	FIB.	CHOL.
Quaker				
Scrambled Eggs & Sausage With Hash Browns	1 pkg (5.7 oz)	290	—	212
Scrambled Eggs & Sausage With Pancakes	1 pkg (5.2 oz)	270	—	180
Scrambled Eggs Cheddar Cheese & Fried Potatoes	1 pkg (5.9 oz)	250	—	176
Weight Watchers				
Classic Omelet Sandwich	1 (3.8 oz)	220	1	0
Garden Omelet Sandwich	1 (3.6 oz)	220	2	15
Handy Ham & Cheese Omelet	1 (4 oz)	230	3	35
TAKE-OUT				
deviled	2 halves	145	—	280
salad	½ cup	307	—	562
sandwich w/ cheese	1	340	—	291
sandwich w/ cheese & ham	1	348	—	245
EGG ROLLS				
(*see also* ORIENTAL FOOD)				
egg roll wrapper fresh	1	83	—	3
Chun King				
Chicken	8 (4.4 oz)	270	4	10
Pork & Shrimp	8 (4.4 oz)	290	4	15
Shrimp	8 (4.4 oz)	260	4	10
Empire				
Large	1 (3 oz)	190	2	2
Miniature	6 (4.8 oz)	280	4	0
La Choy				
Almond Chicken Restaurant Style	1 (3 oz)	170	3	5
Chicken Mini	14 (7.25 oz)	430	6	15
Chicken Restaurant Style	1 (3 oz)	170	4	10
Lobster Mini	14 (7.25 oz)	410	9	0
Meat & Shrimp Mini	15 (3.75 oz)	240	3	10
Mu Sho Pork Restaurant Style	1 (3 oz)	190	2	15
Pork Restaurant Style	1 (3 oz)	150	—	7
Pork & Shrimp Mini	14 (7.25 oz)	430	7	15
Shrimp Mini	14 (7.25 oz)	410	7	10
Shrimp Restaurant Style	1 (3 oz)	150	3	10
Sweet & Sour Restaurant Style	1 (3 oz)	180	3	5
Lo-An				
White Meat Chicken	1 (2.7 oz)	140	1	10
Luigino's				
Chicken	1 pkg (6 oz)	360	2	25

FOOD	PORTION	CALS.	FIB.	CHOL.
Luigino's (CONT.)				
Pork & Shrimp	1 pkg (6 oz)	340	3	25
Shrimp	1 pkg (6 oz)	350	4	20
Sweet & Sour Chicken	1 pkg (6 oz)	400	4	25
Sweet & Sour Pork	1 pkg (6 oz)	360	4	15
Szechwan Vegetable	1 pkg (6 oz)	350	3	10
TAKE-OUT				
lobster	1 (4.8 oz)	270	6	0
meat & shrimp	1 (4.8 oz)	320	4	10
pork & shrimp	1 (5 oz)	300	7	15
shrimp	1 (3 oz)	170	5	<5
spicy pork	1 (3 oz)	200	3	5
vegetable	1 (3 oz)	170	4	0
EGG SUBSTITUTES				
frozen	¼ cup	96	—	1
frozen	1 cup	384	—	5
liquid	1½ oz	40	—	tr
liquid	1 cup (8.8 oz)	211	—	3
powder	0.35 oz	44	—	57
powder	0.7 oz	88	—	113
Egg Beaters				
Eggs Substitute	¼ cup	25	0	0
Omelette Cheese	½ cup	110	—	5
Omelette Vegetable	½ cup	50	—	0
Egg Watchers				
Egg Substitute	2 oz	50	—	0
Healthy Choice				
Cholesterol Free	¼ cup (2 oz)	25	0	0
Second Nature				
No Cholesterol	2 fl oz	60	—	0
No Fat	2 fl oz	40	—	0
No Fat With Garden Vegetables	2.5 fl oz	40	—	0
Simply Eggs				
Egg Substitute	1.75 fl oz	35	1	30
EGGNOG				
eggnog	1 cup	342	—	149
eggnog	1 qt	1368	—	596
eggnog flavor mix as prep w/ milk	9 oz	260	—	33
Hood				
Fat Free	4 fl oz	100	0	<5
Golden	4 fl oz	180	0	65
Light	4 fl oz	120	0	40

FOOD	PORTION	CALS.	FIB.	CHOL.
Hood (cont.)				
Select	4 fl oz	210	0	80
EGGPLANT				
CANNED				
Progresso				
Appetizer	2 tbsp (1 oz)	30	2	0
FRESH				
cubed cooked	½ cup	13	—	0
raw cut up	½ cup (1.4 oz)	11	—	0
slices cooked	4 (7 oz)	38	—	0
whole peeled raw	1 (1 lb)	117	—	0
FROZEN				
Mrs. Paul's				
Parmigiana	5 oz	240	—	15
TAKE-OUT				
baba ghannouj	¼ cup	55	—	0
caponata	2 tbsp (1 oz)	30	—	0
ELDERBERRIES				
fresh	1 cup	105	—	0
ELDERBERRY JUICE				
elderberry	3½ oz	38	—	0
ELK				
roasted	3 oz	124	—	62
ENDIVE				
fresh	3½ oz	9	2	0
raw chopped	½ cup	4	—	0
ENERGY BARS				
(*see* BREAKFAST BAR, CEREAL BARS, NUTRITIONAL SUPPLEMENTS)				
ENGLISH MUFFIN				
FROZEN				
Weight Watchers				
Sandwich	1 (4 oz)	230	3	20
HOME RECIPE				
cinnamon raisin	1	186	—	0
english muffin	1	158	—	0
honey bran	1	153	—	0
whole wheat	1	167	—	1
READY-TO-EAT				
apple cinnamon	1	138	—	0
granola	1	155	—	0
mixed grain	1	155	—	0

FOOD	PORTION	CALS.	FIB.	CHOL.
plain	1	134	—	0
plain toasted	1	133	—	0
raisin cinnamon	1	138	—	0
sourdough	1	134	—	0
wheat	1	127	—	0
whole wheat	1	134	4	0
Arnold				
Extra Crisp	1	130	1	0
Sourdough	1	130	1	0
Matthew's				
9 Grain & Nut	1	140	5	0
Cinnamon Raisin	1	160	4	0
Golden White	1	140	1	0
Whole Wheat	1	150	4	0
Pepperidge Farm				
Cinnamon Apple	1	140	—	0
Cinnamon Chip	1	160	—	0
Cinnamon Raisin	1	150	—	0
Plain	1	140	—	0
Sourdough	1	135	—	0
Roman Meal				
English Muffin	1 (2.2 oz)	135	3	0
Tastykake				
Cinnamon Raisin	1 (64 g)	150	—	0
English Muffin	1 (57 g)	130	—	0
Sourdough	1 (57 g)	130	—	0
Thomas'				
Oat Bran	1	116	3	0
Sandwich Size	1 (92 g)	210	2	0
Wonder				
English Muffin	1 (2 oz)	120	1	0
Raisin Rounds	1 (2.1 oz)	150	2	0
Sourdough	1 (2 oz)	120	1	0
REFRIGERATED				
Roman Meal				
English Muffin	½ muffin (1.1 oz)	66	1	0
Honey Nut Oat Bran	½ muffin (1.1 oz)	81	1	0
TAKE-OUT				
w/ butter	1	189	—	13
w/ cheese & sausage	1	394	—	58
w/ egg cheese & bacon	1	487	—	274
w/ egg cheese & canadian bacon	1	383	—	234
EPPAW				
raw	½ cup	75	—	0

FOOD	PORTION	CALS.	FIB.	CHOL.

FALAFEL
MIX
Casbah

as prep	5	130	2	0

Near East

as prep	2½ patties	230	5	0

TAKE-OUT

falafel	3 (1.8 oz)	170	—	0
falafel	1 (1.2 oz)	57	—	0

FAST FOODS
(*see individual names in Part Two*)

FAT
(*see also* BUTTER, BUTTER BLENDS, BUTTER SUBSTITUTES, MARGARINE, OIL)

beef cooked	1 oz	193	—	27
beef suet	1 oz	242	—	19
beef tallow	1 tbsp (13 g)	115	—	14
chicken	1 cup	1846	—	174
chicken	1 tbsp	115	—	11
cocoa butter	1 tbsp	120	—	0
duck	1 tbsp (13 g)	115	0	13
goose	1 tbsp	115	—	13
lamb new zealand raw	1 oz	182	—	25
lard	1 cup (205 g)	1849	—	195
lard	1 tbsp (13 g)	115	—	12
pork backfat	1 oz	230	—	16
pork cooked	1 oz	200	—	26
pork cured	1 oz	164	—	19
pork cured roasted	1 oz	167	—	24
salt pork	1 oz	212	—	25
shortening	1 tbsp	113	—	0
shortening	1 cup	1812	—	0
turkey	1 tbsp	115	—	13

Crisco

Butter Flavor	1 tbsp	110	—	0
Shortening	1 tbsp	110	—	0
Shortening	1 tbsp (0.4 oz)	110	—	0
Sticks	1 tbsp (0.4 oz)	110	0	0
Sticks Butter Flavor	1 tbsp (0.4 oz)	110	0	0

Empire

Chicken Fat Rendered	1 tbsp (0.5 oz)	120	0	10

FOOD	PORTION	CALS.	FIB.	CHOL.
Wesson				
Shortening	1 tbsp	100	0	0
FAT SUBSTITUTES				
Soy Is Us				
Fat Not! Organic	3 tbsp	66	4	0
FAVA BEANS				
CANNED				
Progresso				
Fava Beans	½ cup (4.6 oz)	110	5	0
FEIJOA				
fresh	1 (1.75 oz)	25	—	0
puree	1 cup	119	—	0
FENNEL				
fresh bulb	1 (8.2 oz)	72	—	0
fresh sliced	1 cup	27	—	0
seed	1 tsp	7	—	0
FENUGREEK				
seed	1 tsp	12	—	0
FIBER				
Delta				
Natural Fiber	½ cup (1 oz)	20	20	0
FIGS				
CANNED				
in heavy syrup	3	75	—	0
in light syrup	3	58	—	0
water pack	3	42	—	0
S&W				
Kadota Figs Whole Fancy	½ cup	100	—	0
DRIED				
california	½ cup (3.5 oz)	200	17	0
cooked	½ cup	140	—	0
whole	10	477	17	0
Sonoma				
White Misson	3-4 (1.4 oz)	110	5	0
FRESH				
fig	1 med	50	—	0
FISH				
(*see also* FISH SUBSTITUTES, INDIVIDUAL NAMES, SUSHI)				
CANNED				
Holmes				
Finest Kippered Snacks drained	1 can (3.2 oz)	135	0	60

FOOD	PORTION	CALS.	FIB.	CHOL.
Port Clyde				
Fish Steaks In Louisiana Hot Sauce	1 can (3.75 oz)	150	0	80
Fish Steaks In Mustard Sauce	1 can (3.75 oz)	140	0	70
Fish Steaks In Soybean Oil With Hot Chilies drained	1 can (3.3 oz)	155	0	80
Fish Steaks In Soybean Oil drained	1 can (3.3 oz)	220	0	115
FROZEN				
breaded fillet	1 (2 oz)	155	—	64
sticks	1 stick (1 oz)	76	—	31
Gorton's				
Crispy Batter Dipped Fillets	2	290	—	35
Crispy Batter Sticks	4	260	—	25
Crunchy Fillets	2	230	—	40
Crunchy Sticks	4	210	—	25
Light Recipe Lightly Breaded Fish Fillets	1 fillet	180	—	30
Light Recipe Tempura Fillets	1 fillet	200	—	30
Microwave Entree Fillets In Herb Butter	1 pkg	190	—	90
Microwave Fillets	2	340	—	30
Microwave Larger Cut Fillets	1	320	—	35
Microwave Sticks	6	340	—	35
Potato Crisp Fillets	2	300	—	30
Potato Crisp Sticks	4	260	—	25
Kineret				
Fish Sticks	5 pieces (4 oz)	280	1	20
Mrs. Paul's				
Entree Light Seafood Dijon	8¾ oz	200	—	60
Entree Light Seafood Florentine	8 oz	220	—	95
Entree Light Seafood Mornay	9 oz	230	—	80
Fish Cakes	2	190	—	20
Fish Fillets Batter Dipped	2 fillets	330	—	60
Fish Fillets Crispy Crunchy	2 fillets	220	—	22
Fish Fillets Crunchy Batter	2 fillets	280	—	22
Fish Sticks Crispy Crunchy	4 sticks	190	—	25
In Butter Sauce Light Fillet	1 fillet	140	—	40
Portions Battered Fish	2 portions	300	—	33
Portions Crispy Crunchy Breaded Fish	2 portions	230	—	25
Seafood Platter Combination	9 oz	600	—	85
Sticks Battered Fish	4 sticks	210	—	25
Sticks Crispy Crunchy Breaded Fish	4 sticks	140	—	20

FOOD	PORTION	CALS.	FIB.	CHOL.
Van De Kamp's				
Battered Fish Fillets	1 (2.6 oz)	180	0	20
Battered Fish Nuggets	8 (4 oz)	280	0	25
Battered Fish Portions	2 pieces (5 oz)	350	0	35
Battered Fish Sticks	6 (4 oz)	260	0	30
Breaded Fillets	2 (3.5 oz)	280	0	35
Breaded Fish Portions	3 pieces (4.5 oz)	330	0	35
Breaded Fish Sticks	6 (4 oz)	290	0	35
Breaded Mini Fish Sticks	13 (3.3 oz)	250	0	30
Crisp & Healthy Breaded Fillets	2 (3.5 oz)	150	0	30
Crisp & Healthy Fish Sticks	6 (4 oz)	180	0	25
Fish 'n Fries	1 pkg (6.6 oz)	380	2	25
MIX				
Golden Dipt				
Beer Batter Fry	1 oz	100	—	0
Cajun Style Fish Fry	⅔ oz	60	—	0
Fish & Chips Batter Mix	1¼ oz	120	—	0
Fish Fry	⅔ oz	60	—	0
Seafood Frying Mix	⅔ oz	60	—	0
Tempura Batter Mix	1 oz	100	—	0
TAKE-OUT				
jamaican brown fish stew	1 serv	426	2	84
sandwich w/ tartar sauce & cheese	1	524	—	68

FISH SUBSTITUTES
LaLoma

Ocean Platter mix not prep	¼ cup (16 g)	50	—	0

FLAXSEED
Arrowhead

Flaxseed	3 tbsp (1 oz)	140	6	0
Stone-Buhr				
Flaxseed	3 tbsp (1 oz)	150	5	0

FLOUNDER
FRESH

cooked	1 fillet (4.5 oz)	148	—	86
cooked	3 oz	99	—	58
FROZEN				
Gorton's				
Microwave Entree Stuffed	1 pkg	350	—	120
Mrs. Paul's				
Crunchy Batter Fillets	2 fillets	220	—	40
Light Fillets	1 fillet	240	—	50

FOOD	PORTION	CALS.	FIB.	CHOL.
Van De Kamp's				
Lightly Breaded Fillets	1 (4 oz)	230	0	40
Natural Fillets	1 (4 oz)	110	0	45
TAKE-OUT				
battered & fried	3.2 oz	211	—	31
breaded & fried	3.2 oz	211	—	31
FLOUR				
corn masa	1 cup	416	—	0
corn whole grain	1 cup	422	8	0
cottonseed lowfat	1 oz	94	—	0
peanut defatted	1 cup	196	—	0
peanut defatted	1 oz	92	—	0
peanut lowfat	1 cup	257	—	0
potato	1 cup (6.3 oz)	628	—	0
rice brown	1 cup	574	4	0
rice white	1 cup	578	2	0
rye dark	1 cup	415	—	0
rye light	1 cup	374	7	0
rye medium	1 cup	361	7	0
sesame lowfat	1 oz	95	—	0
triticale whole grain	1 cup	440	9	0
white all-purpose	1 cup	455	2	0
white bread	1 cup	495	—	0
white cake	1 cup	395	—	0
white self-rising	1 cup	442	—	0
whole wheat	1 cup	407	8	0
Arrowhead				
Kamut	¼ cup (1.2 oz)	110	4	0
Pastry	⅓ cup (1.1 oz)	100	3	0
Rye Whole Grain	¼ cup (1.6 oz)	160	6	0
Spelt	¼ cup (1.2 oz)	100	5	0
Teff	¼ cup (1.4 oz)	140	5	0
Unbleached White	⅓ cup (1.6 oz)	160	0	0
Whole Grain Wheat	¼ cup (1.6 oz)	160	7	0
Whole Wheat	¼ cup (1.2 oz)	130	4	0
Aunt Jemima				
Self-Rising	3 tbsp	90	1	0
Ballard				
All Purpose	1 cup	400	—	0
Self-Rising	1 cup	380	—	0
Ceresota				
All Purpose	1 cup	390	—	0
Whole Wheat	1 cup	400	—	0

FOOD	PORTION	CALS.	FIB.	CHOL.
General Mills				
Drifted Snow	1 cup	400	—	0
Softasilk	¼ cup	100	—	0
Gold Medal				
La Pina	1 cup	390	—	0
Heckers				
All Purpose	1 cup	390	—	0
Whole Wheat	1 cup	400	—	0
Hodgson Mill				
50/50 Flour	¼ cup (1 oz)	100	2	0
Best For Bread	¼ cup (1 oz)	100	1	0
Buckwheat	⅓ cup (1.6 oz)	160	2	0
Oat Bran Blend	¼ cup (1 oz)	110	3	0
Oat Bran Flour	¼ cup (1 oz)	110	3	0
Rye	¼ cup (1 oz)	90	5	0
Seasoned Flour	¼ cup (1 oz)	90	0	0
White	¼ cup (1 oz)	100	3	0
Whole Wheat	¼ cup (1 oz)	100	3	0
King Arthur				
All Purpose Unbleached	¼ cup (1 oz)	100	tr	0
Pillsbury				
All Purpose Best	1 cup	400	—	0
Bohemian Style Rye and Wheat Best	1 cup	400	—	0
Bread Best	1 cup	400	—	0
Rye Medium Best	1 cup	400	—	0
Self-Rising Best	1 cup	380	—	0
Shake & Blend Best	2 tbsp	50	—	0
Unbleached Best	1 cup	400	—	0
Whole Wheat Best	1 cup	400	—	0
Red Band				
All-Purpose	1 cup	390	—	0
Self-Rising	1 cup	380	—	0
Stone Ground Mills				
White Unbleached Organic	¼ cup (1.4 oz)	130	1	0
Whole Wheat 100% Stone Ground	3 tbsp (1 oz)	90	3	0
White Deer				
All-Purpose	1 cup	400	—	0
Wondra				
Flour	1 cup	400	—	0

FRANKFURTER
(*see* HOT DOG)

FRENCH BEANS
dried cooked	1 cup	228	—	0

FOOD	PORTION	CALS.	FIB.	CHOL.

FRENCH FRIES
(*see* POTATO)

FRENCH TOAST
FROZEN

french toast	1 slice (2 oz)	126	2	48
Aunt Jemima				
Cinnamon Swirl	2 pieces (4.1 oz)	240	2	90
Slices	2 pieces (4.1 oz)	240	1	80
Downyflake				
French Toast	2 slices	270	—	73
Healthy Starts				
French Toast With LeanLinks	6.5 oz	400	—	0
Quaker				
French Toast Sticks & Syrup	1 pkg (5.2 oz)	400	—	64
French Toast Wedges & Sausage	1 pkg (5.3 oz)	360	—	96
HOME RECIPE				
as prep w/ 2% milk	1 slice	149	—	75
as prep w/ whole milk	1 slice	151	—	75
TAKE-OUT				
w/ butter	2 slices	356	—	117

FROG'S LEGS

frog leg as prep w/ seasoned flour & fried	1 (0.8 oz)	70	—	12

FROSTING
(*see* CAKE)

FRUCTOSE
Estee

Fructose	1 tsp (4 g)	15	—	0
Packet	1 pkg (3 g)	10	—	0

FRUIT DRINKS
(*see also* LEMONADE)
FROZEN

citrus juice drink as prep	1 cup	114	—	0
citrus juice drink not prep	1 can (12 fl oz)	684	—	0
fruit punch as prep w/water	1 cup	113	—	0
fruit punch not prep	1 can (12 fl oz)	678	—	0
limeade	1 can (6 oz)	408	—	0
limeade as prep w/ water	1 cup	102	—	0
Bright & Early				
Fruit Punch	8 fl oz	130	—	0

FOOD	PORTION	CALS.	FIB.	CHOL.
Dole				
100% Juice Blend Country Raspberry as prep	8 fl oz	140	0	0
100% Juice Blend Orchard Peach as prep	8 fl oz	140	0	0
Mountain Cherry 100% Juice Blend as prep	8 fl oz	120	0	0
Pineapple Grapefruit as prep	8 fl oz	130	0	0
Pineapple Orange as prep	8 fl oz	120	0	0
Pineapple Orange Banana as prep	8 fl oz	130	0	0
Pineapple Orange Guava as prep	8 fl oz	120	0	0
Pineapple Passion Banana as prep	8 fl oz	120	0	0
Tropical Fruit as prep	8 fl oz	140	0	0
Five Alive				
Berry Citrus	8 fl oz	120	—	0
Citrus	8 fl oz	120	—	0
Tropical Citrus	8 fl oz	120	—	0
Minute Maid				
Berry Punch	8 fl oz	130	—	0
Citrus Punch	8 fl oz	120	—	0
Fruit Punch	8 fl oz	120	—	0
Limeade	8 fl oz	100	—	0
Pineapple Orange	8 fl oz	120	—	0
Tropical Punch	8 fl oz	120	—	0
Seneca				
Cranberry-Apple Juice Cocktail frzn as prep	8 fl oz	140	0	0
Raspberry-Cranberry Juice Cocktail frzn as prep	8 fl oz	140	0	0
Tree Top				
Apple Citrus as prep	6 oz	90	—	0
Apple Cranberry as prep	6 oz	100	—	0
Apple Grape as prep	6 oz	100	—	0
Apple Pear as prep	6 oz	90	—	0
Apple Raspberry as prep	6 oz	80	—	0
MIX				
fruit punch as prep w/water	9 oz	97	—	0
Crystal Light				
Berry Blend Sugar Free	8 oz	3	—	0
Fruit Punch Sugar Free	8 oz	3	—	0
Lemon-Lime	8 oz	4	—	0

FOOD	PORTION	CALS.	FIB.	CHOL.
Crystal Light (CONT.)				
Tropic Quencher	8 oz	5	—	0
Kool-Aid				
Lemon-Lime	8 oz	98	—	0
Purplesaurus Rex	8 oz	98	—	0
Rainbow Punch	8 oz	98	—	0
Sharkleberry Fin	8 oz	98	—	0
Sugar Free Berry Blue	8 oz	3	—	0
Sugar Free Berry Punch	8 oz	3	—	0
Sugar Free Purplesaurus Rex	8 oz	3	—	0
Sugar Free Rainbow Punch	8 oz	4	—	0
Sugar Free Sharkleberry Fin	8 oz	3	—	0
Sugar Free Tropical Punch	8 oz	3	—	0
Sugar Sweetened Mountain Berry Punch	8 oz	98	—	0
Sugar Sweetened Purplesaurus Rex	8 oz	84	—	0
Sugar Sweetened Rainbow Punch	8 oz	84	—	0
Sugar Sweetened Sharkleberry Fin	8 oz	84	—	0
Sugar Sweetened Sunshine Punch	8 oz	83	—	0
Sugar Sweetened Surfin' Berry Punch	8 oz	79	—	0
Sugar Sweetened Tropical Punch	8 oz	84	—	0
Tropical Punch	8 oz	98	—	0
Unsweetened Berry Blue	8 oz	98	—	0
READY-TO-DRINK				
cranberry apple drink	6 fl oz	123	—	0
cranberry apricot drink	6 fl oz	118	—	0
fruit punch	6 fl oz	87	—	0
orange grapefruit juice	8 fl oz	107	—	0
orange & apricot	8 fl oz	128	—	0
pineapple & grapefruit	8 fl oz	117	—	0
pineapple & orange drink	8 fl oz	125	—	0
After The Fall				
Amaretto Almond	1 can (12 oz)	170	0	0
American Pie Cherry	1 can (12 oz)	190	0	0
Apple Apricot	1 cup (8 oz)	100	0	0
Apple Raspberry	1 bottle (10 oz)	110	—	0
Apple Strawberry	1 bottle (10 oz)	120	—	0
Banana Casablanca	1 bottle (10 oz)	120	—	0

FOOD	PORTION	CALS.	FIB.	CHOL.
After The Fall (CONT.)				
Berrymeister	1 can (12 oz)	160	0	0
Cranberry Meets Raspberry	1 bottle (10 oz)	120	—	0
Georgia Peach Blend	1 bottle (10 oz)	130	—	0
Mango Montage	1 bottle (10 oz)	140	—	0
Maui Grove	1 bottle (10 oz)	120	—	0
Nantucket Ginger Ale	1 can (12 oz)	140	0	0
Orange Icicle Cream	1 can (12 oz)	170	0	0
Oregon Berry	1 bottle (10 oz)	130	—	0
Passion Of The Islands	1 bottle (10 oz)	125	—	0
Peach Vanilla	1 can (12 oz)	170	0	0
Strawberry Vanilla	1 can (12 oz)	160	0	0
Twist O' Strawberry	1 can (12 oz)	190	0	0
Vanilla Bean Cream	1 can (12 oz)	170	0	0
Apple & Eve				
Apple Cranberry	6 fl oz	80	—	0
Apple Grape	6 fl oz	120	—	0
Cranberry Grape	6 fl oz	100	—	0
Fruit Punch	6 fl oz	78	—	0
Raspberry Cranberry	6 fl oz	90	—	0
BAMA				
Fruit Punch	8.45 fl oz	130	—	0
Boku				
White Grape Raspberry	16 fl oz	120	—	0
Chiquita				
Orange Banana	6 fl oz	90	—	0
Crystal Geyser				
Juice Squeeze Citrus Grape	1 bottle (12 fl oz)	145	—	0
Juice Squeeze Orange & Passion Fruit	1 bottle (12 fl oz)	130	—	0
Juice Squeeze Passion Fruit & Mango	1 bottle (12 fl oz)	125	—	0
Juice Squeeze Wild Berry	1 bottle (12 fl oz)	130	—	0
Dole				
Pineapple Orange	6 fl oz	90	—	0
Pineapple Orange Banana	6 fl oz	100	—	0
Pineapple Orange Guava	6 fl oz	100	—	0
Pineapple Passion Banana	6 fl oz	100	—	0
Five Alive				
Citrus	1 bottle (16 fl oz)	120	—	0
Citrus	6 fl oz	90	—	0
Citrus	1 can (11.5 fl oz)	170	—	0
Citrus Chilled	8 fl oz	120	—	0

FOOD	PORTION	CALS.	FIB.	CHOL.
Fresh Samantha				
Banana Strawberry	1 cup (8 oz)	148	2	0
Beta Yet	1 cup (8 oz)	98	2	0
Carrot Orange	1 cup (8 oz)	107	1	0
Colossal C	1 cup (8 oz)	116	2	0
Desperately Seeking C	1 cup (8 oz)	129	3	0
Protein Blast	1 cup (8 oz)	156	2	0
Spirulina Fruit Blend	1 cup (8 oz)	129	2	0
Strawberry Orange	1 cup (8 oz)	120	1	0
The Big Bang	1 cup (8 oz)	97	2	0
Hawaiian Punch				
Fruit Juicy Red	6 fl oz	90	—	0
Island Fruit Cocktail	6 fl oz	90	—	0
Lite Fruit Juicy Red	6 fl oz	60	—	0
Tropical Fruits	6 fl oz	90	—	0
Very Berry	6 fl oz	90	—	0
Wild Fruit	6 fl oz	90	—	0
Hi-C				
Boppin Berry Box	8.45 fl oz	140	—	0
Boppin' Berry	8 fl oz	130	—	0
Double Fruit Box	8.45 fl oz	130	—	0
Double Fruit Cooler	8 fl oz	130	—	0
Ecto Cooler	8 fl oz	130	—	0
Ecto Cooler	1 can (11.5 fl oz)	180	—	0
Ecto Cooler Box	8.45 fl oz	130	—	0
Fruit Punch	8 fl oz	130	—	0
Fruit Punch	1 can (11.5 fl oz)	190	—	0
Fruit Punch Box	8.45 fl oz	140	—	0
Fruity Bubble Gum	8 fl oz	120	—	0
Fruity Bubble Gum Box	8.45 fl oz	130	—	0
Hula Punch	8 fl oz	120	—	0
Hula Punch	1 can (11.5 fl oz)	170	—	0
Hula Punch Box	8.45 fl oz	120	—	0
Jammin' Apple Box	8.45 fl oz	130	—	0
Stompin' Banana Berry	8 fl oz	130	—	0
Stompin' Banana Berry Box	8.45 fl oz	130	—	0
Wild Berry	8 fl oz	120	—	0
Wild Berry Box	8.45 fl oz	130	—	0
Hood				
Natural Blenders Apple Cranberry Raspberry	1 cup (8 oz)	130	—	0
Natural Blenders Apple Grape Cherry	1 cup (8 oz)	130	—	0
Natural Blenders Apple Peach Pear	1 cup (8 oz)	120	—	0

FOOD	PORTION	CALS.	FIB.	CHOL.
Hood (CONT.)				
Natural Blenders Apple Wild Blueberry Strawberry	1 cup (8 oz)	120	—	0
Natural Blenders Pineapple Orange Kiwi	1 cup (8 oz)	120	—	0
Juice Works				
Appleberry	6 fl oz	100	—	0
Juicy Juice				
Apple Grape	1 box (8.45 fl oz)	120	—	0
Berry	1 box (8.45 fl oz)	130	—	0
Berry	1 bottle (6 fl oz)	90	—	0
Punch	1 box (8.45 fl oz)	140	—	0
Punch	1 bottle (6 fl oz)	100	—	0
Tropical	1 bottle (6 fl oz)	110	—	0
Tropical	1 box (8.45 fl oz)	150	—	0
Kern's				
Apple Strawberry Nectar	6 fl oz	110	—	0
Apricot Pineapple Nectar	6 fl oz	110	—	0
Banana Pineapple Nectar	6 fl oz	110	—	0
Coconut Pineapple Nectar	6 fl oz	140	—	0
Orange Banana Nectar	6 fl oz	110	—	0
Strawberry Banana Nectar	6 fl oz	110	—	0
Tropical Nectar	6 fl oz	110	—	0
Kool-Aid				
Koolers Sharkleberry Fin	1 pkg (8.45 fl oz)	140	—	0
Libby				
Strawberry Banana Nectar	1 can (11.5 fl oz)	220	—	0
Mauna La'i				
Island Guava Hawaiian Guava Fruit Juice Drink	8 fl oz	130	0	0
Mango & Hawaiian Guava Fruit Juice Drink	8 fl oz	130	0	0
Paradise Guava Hawaiian Guava & Passion Fruit Juice Drink	8 fl oz	130	0	0
Minute Maid				
Berry Punch Box	8.45 fl oz	130	—	0
Berry Punch Chilled	8 fl oz	130	—	0
Citrus Punch Chilled	8 fl oz	130	—	0
Fruit Punch Box	8.45 fl oz	120	—	0
Fruit Punch Chilled	8 fl oz	120	—	0
Juices To Go Citrus Punch	1 can (11.5 fl oz)	180	—	0
Juices To Go Citrus Punch	1 bottle (10 fl oz)	160	—	0
Juices To Go Concord Punch	1 can (11.5 fl oz)	180	—	0

FOOD	PORTION	CALS.	FIB.	CHOL.
Minute Maid (CONT.)				
Juices To Go Concord Punch	1 bottle (10 fl oz)	160	—	0
Juices To Go Concord Punch	1 bottle (16 fl oz)	130	—	0
Juices To Go Fruit Punch	1 bottle (10 fl oz)	160	—	0
Juices To Go Fruit Punch	1 can (11.5 fl oz)	180	—	0
Juices To Go Fruit Punch	1 bottle (16 fl oz)	120	—	0
Juices To Go Orange Blend	1 can (11.5 fl oz)	170	—	0
Juices To Go Orange Blend	1 bottle (10 fl oz)	150	—	0
Naturals Apple Cranberry	8 fl oz	170	—	0
Naturals Concord Medley	8 fl oz	130	—	0
Naturals Fruit Medley	8 fl oz	120	—	0
Naturals Tropical Medley	8 fl oz	120	—	0
Tropical Punch Box	8.45 fl oz	130	—	0
Tropical Punch Chilled	8 fl oz	120	—	0
Mott's				
Apple Cranberry Blend	10 fl oz	180	0	0
Apple Cranberry From Concentrate as prep	8 fl oz	120	0	0
Apple Grape From Concentrate as prep	8 fl oz	120	0	0
Apple Raspberry Blend	10 fl oz	140	0	0
Apple Raspberry From Concentrate	8.45 fl oz	120	0	0
Fruit Basket Apple Raspberry Juice Cocktail as prep	8 fl oz	130	0	0
Fruit Basket Tropical Blend Juice Cocktail as prep	8 fl oz	120	0	0
Fruit Punch From Concentrate	8.45 fl oz	120	0	0
Fruit Punch From Concentrate	10 fl oz	170	0	0
Grape Apple	10 fl oz	170	0	0
Pineapple Orange	10 fl oz	170	0	0
Ocean Spray				
Cran.Blueberry	8 fl oz	160	0	0
Cran.Cherry	6 fl oz	160	0	0
Cran.Grape	8 fl oz	170	0	0
Cran.Raspberry	8 fl oz	140	0	0
Cran.Raspberry Reduced Calorie	8 fl oz	50	0	0
Cran.Strawberry	8 fl oz	140	tr	0
Cranapple	8 fl oz	160	tr	0
Cranapple Reduced Calorie	8 fl oz	50	0	0
Cranicot	8 fl oz	160	0	0
Crantastic	8 fl oz	150	0	0
Fruit Punch	8 fl oz	130	0	0

FOOD	PORTION	CALS.	FIB.	CHOL.
Ocean Spray (CONT.)				
Lightstyle Low Calorie Cran.Grape	8 fl oz	40	0	0
Lightstyle Low Calorie Cran.Raspberry	8 fl oz	40	0	0
Refreshers Juice Drink Citrus Cranberry	8 fl oz	140	0	0
Refreshers Juice Drink Citrus Peach	8 fl oz	120	0	0
Refreshers Juice Drink Orange Cranberry	8 fl oz	130	0	0
Ruby Red & Tangerine Grapefruit Juice Cocktail	8 fl oz	130	0	0
Odwalla				
Boyzenberry Mango	8 fl oz	140	2	0
C Monster	16 fl oz	300	4	0
Fruitshake Blackberry	8 fl oz	160	3	0
Guanaba Dabba Doo!	8 fl oz	130	0	0
Raspberry Smoothie	8 fl oz	140	2	0
Strawberry Banana Smoothie	8 fl oz	100	2	0
Pek				
Mango Guava Ecstasy	1 bottle (20 fl oz)	110	0	0
Passionate Peach Grapefruit	8 fl oz	110	0	0
S&W				
Apricot Pineapple Nectar	6 fl oz	120	—	0
Apricot Pineapple Nectar Diet	6 fl oz	80	—	0
Sipps				
Fruit Punch	8.45 oz	130	—	0
Lemon Lime Cooler	8.45 oz	130	—	0
Mixed Berry	8.45 oz	130	—	0
Sunshine Punch	8.45 oz	130	—	0
Smucker's				
Apple Cranberry	8 oz	120	—	0
Orange Banana	8 oz	120	—	0
Snapple				
Diet Kiwi Strawberry	8 fl oz	13	—	0
Fruit Punch	8 fl oz	120	—	0
Kiwi Strawberry Cocktail	8 fl oz	130	—	0
Melonberry Cocktail	8 fl oz	120	—	0
Vitamin Supreme	10 fl oz	150	—	0
Squeezit				
Berry B. Wild	1 (6.75 fl oz)	90	—	0
Chucklin' Cherry	1 (6.75 fl oz)	90	—	0
Grumpy Grape	1 (6.75 fl oz)	90	—	0

FOOD	PORTION	CALS.	FIB.	CHOL.
Squeezit (CONT.)				
Mean Green Puncher	1 (6.75 fl oz)	90	—	0
Silly Billy Strawberry	1 (6.75 fl oz)	90	—	0
Smarty Arty Orange	1 (6.75 fl oz)	90	—	0
Sunny Delight				
Drink	6 fl oz	90	—	0
Tang				
Mixed Fruit	8.45 fl oz	137	—	0
Tree Top				
Apple Citrus	6 fl oz	90	—	0
Apple Cranberry	6 fl oz	100	—	0
Apple Grape	6 fl oz	100	—	0
Apple Pear	6 fl oz	90	—	0
Apple Raspberry	6 fl oz	80	—	0
Tropicana				
Berry Punch	8 fl oz	120	—	0
Citrus Punch	1 bottle (10 fl oz)	180	—	0
Citrus Punch	8 fl oz	140	—	0
Cranberry Punch	1 can (11.5 fl oz)	200	—	0
Cranberry Punch	1 bottle (10 fl oz)	170	—	0
Cranberry Punch	8 fl oz	140	—	0
Fruit Punch	8 fl oz	130	—	0
Fruit Punch	1 can (11.5 fl oz)	170	—	0
Fruit Punch	1 bottle (10 fl oz)	150	—	0
Fruit Punch	1 container (10 fl oz)	160	—	0
Orange Pineapple	8 fl oz	110	—	0
Orange Pineapple	1 bottle (10 fl oz)	130	—	0
Pineapple Punch	1 bottle (10 fl oz)	160	—	0
Pineapple Punch	8 fl oz	120	—	0
Season's Best Cranberry Medley	8 fl oz	120	—	0
Tropics Apple Cranberry Kiwi	8 fl oz	120	—	0
Tropics Orange Strawberry Banana	8 fl oz	110	—	0
Tropics Orange Kiwi Passion	8 fl oz	100	—	0
Tropics Orange Peach Mango	8 fl oz	110	—	0
Tropics Orange Pineapple	8 fl oz	110	—	0
Tropics Pineapple Passion	8 fl oz	120	—	0
Twister Apple Raspberry Blackberry	1 bottle (10 fl oz)	150	—	0
Twister Apple Raspberry Blackberry	1 can (11.5 fl oz)	180	—	0
Twister Apple Raspberry Blackberry	8 fl oz	120	—	0

FOOD	PORTION	CALS.	FIB.	CHOL.
Tropicana (CONT.)				
Twister Cranberry Raspberry Strawberry	1 bottle (10 fl oz)	160	—	0
Twister Cranberry Raspberry Strawberry	8 fl oz	120	—	0
Twister Light Cranberry Raspberry Strawberry	8 fl oz	45	—	0
Twister Light Cranberry Raspberry Strawberry	1 container (10 fl oz)	50	—	0
Twister Light Orange Cranberry	1 container (10 fl oz)	35	—	0
Twister Light Orange Cranberry	8 fl oz	30	—	0
Twister Light Orange Cranberry	1 container (10 fl oz)	35	—	0
Twister Light Orange Raspberry	1 container (10 fl oz)	45	—	0
Twister Light Orange Raspberry	8 fl oz	35	—	0
Twister Light Orange Strawberry Banana	1 container (10 fl oz)	45	—	0
Twister Light Orange Strawberry Banana	1 container (10 fl oz)	45	—	0
Twister Orange Cranberry	1 container (10 fl oz)	140	—	0
Twister Orange Cranberry	8 fl oz	120	—	0
Twister Orange Cranberry	1 bottle (10 fl oz)	140	—	0
Twister Orange Peach	8 fl oz	120	—	0
Twister Orange Peach	1 can (11.5 fl oz)	160	—	0
Twister Orange Peach	1 bottle (10 fl oz)	140	—	0
Twister Orange Raspberry	8 fl oz	120	—	0
Twister Orange Raspberry	1 bottle (10 fl oz)	140	—	0
Twister Orange Strawberry Banana	1 container (10 fl oz)	140	—	0
Twister Strawberry Banana	1 bottle (10 fl oz)	140	—	0
Twister Strawberry Banana	8 fl oz	120	—	0
Twister Strawberry Banana	1 can (11.5 fl oz)	160	—	0
Twister Strawberry Guava	1 bottle (10 fl oz)	140	—	0
Twister Strawberry Guava	8 fl oz	110	—	0
Veryfine				
Apple Cherryberry	8 fl oz	130	—	0
Apple Cranberry	8 fl oz	130	—	0
Apple Raspberry	8 fl oz	110	—	0
Fruit Punch	8 fl oz	130	—	0
Guava Strawberry	8 fl oz	120	—	0
Lemon & Lime	8 fl oz	120	—	0

FOOD	PORTION	CALS.	FIB.	CHOL.
Veryfine (CONT.)				
Papaya Punch	8 fl oz	120	—	0
Passionfruit Orange	8 fl oz	110	—	0
Pineapple Orange	8 fl oz	130	—	0
White House				
Apple Cherry	6 fl oz	90	0	0

FRUIT MIXED
(see also individual names)
CANNED

FOOD	PORTION	CALS.	FIB.	CHOL.
fruit cocktail in heavy syrup	½ cup	93	—	0
fruit cocktail juice pack	½ cup	56	—	0
fruit cocktail water pack	½ cup	40	—	0
fruit salad in heavy syrup	½ cup	94	—	0
fruit salad in light syrup	½ cup	73	—	0
fruit salad juice pack	½ cup	62	—	0
fruit salad water pack	½ cup	37	—	0
mixed fruit in heavy syrup	½ cup	92	—	0
tropical fruit salad in heavy syrup	½ cup	110	—	0
Del Monte				
Fruit Cocktail Fruit Naturals	½ cup (4.4 oz)	60	1	0
Fruit Cocktail In Heavy Syrup	½ cup (4.5 oz)	100	1	0
Fruit Cocktail Lite	½ cup (4.4 oz)	60	1	0
Lite Mixed Fruits Chunky	½ cup (4.4 oz)	60	1	0
Mixed Fruits Chunky Fruit Naturals	½ cup (4.4 oz)	60	1	0
Mixed Fruits Chunky In Heavy Syrup	½ cup (4.5 oz)	100	1	0
Snack Cups Mixed Fruit Fruit Naturals	1 serv (4.5 oz)	60	1	0
Snack Cups Mixed Fruit Fruit Naturals EZ-Open Lid	1 serv (4.5 oz)	60	1	0
Snack Cups Mixed Fruit In Heavy Syrup	1 serv (4.5 oz)	100	1	0
Snack Cups Mixed Fruit In Heavy Syrup EZ-Open Lid	1 serv (4.2 oz)	90	1	0
Snack Cups Mixed Fruit Lite	1 serv (4.5 oz)	60	1	0
Snack Cups Mixed Fruit Lite EZ-Open Lid	1 serv (4.5 oz)	60	1	0
Dole				
Tropical Fruit Salad	½ cup	70	—	0
Hunt's				
Fruit Cocktail	½ cup (4.5 oz)	90	1	0
Libby				
Chunky Mixed Lite	½ cup (4.3 oz)	60	1	0

FOOD	PORTION	CALS.	FIB.	CHOL.
Libby (CONT.)				
Fruit Cocktail Lite	½ cup (4.3 oz)	60	1	0
S&W				
Chunky Mixed Diet	½ cup	40	—	0
Chunky Mixed Natural Style	½ cup	90	—	0
Chunky Mixed Unsweetened	½ cup	40	—	0
Fruit Cocktail Diet	½ cup	40	—	0
Fruit Cocktail Heavy Syrup	½ cup	90	—	0
Fruit Cocktail Natural Lite	½ cup	60	—	0
Fruit Cocktail Natural Style	½ cup	90	—	0
Fruit Cocktail Unsweetened	½ cup	40	—	0
DRIED				
mixed	11 oz pkg	712	—	0
Del Monte				
Mixed	⅓ cup (1.4 oz)	110	5	0
Planters				
Fruit'n Nut Mix	1 oz	140	2	0
Sonoma				
Diced	⅓ cup (1.4 oz)	120	3	0
Mixed Fruit	5–8 pieces (1.4 oz)	120	3	0
FROZEN				
mixed fruit sweetened	1 cup	245	—	0
Big Valley				
Burst O' Berries	⅔ cup (4.9 oz)	70	3	0
California Tropics	⅔ cup (4.9 oz)	60	2	0
Cup A Fruit	1 pkg (4 oz)	50	2	0
Mixed	4.9 oz	60	2	0
Birds Eye				
Mixed Fruit	½ cup	120	1	0
Dole				
Applesauce Strawberry	1 pkg (4 oz)	60	1	0
FRUIT SNACKS				
fruit leather	1 bar (0.8 oz)	81	—	0
fruit leather pieces	1 pkg (0.9 oz)	92	—	0
fruit leather pieces	1 oz	97	—	0
fruit leather rolls	1 lg (0.7 oz)	73	—	0
fruit leather rolls	1 sm (0.5 oz)	49	—	0
Betty Crocker				
String Thing Berry 'N Blue	1 pkg (0.7 oz)	80	—	0
String Thing Cherry	1 pkg (0.7 oz)	80	—	0
String Thing Strawberry	1 pkg (0.7 oz)	80	—	0
Brock				
Beauty & The Beast	1 pkg (0.9 oz)	90	—	0

FOOD	PORTION	CALS.	FIB.	CHOL.
Brock (CONT.)				
Cinderella	1 pkg (0.9 oz)	90	—	0
Dinosaurs	1 pkg (0.9 oz)	90	—	0
Ninja Trolls	1 pkg (0.9 oz)	90	—	0
Sharks	1 pkg (0.9 oz)	90	—	0
Del Monte				
Sierra Trail Mix	¼ cup (1.2 oz)	150	3	0
Sierra Trail Mix	1 pkg (1 oz)	120	2	0
Sierra Trail Mix	1 pkg (0.9 oz)	110	2	0
Health Valley				
Bakes Apple	1 bar	100	3	0
Bakes Date	1 bar	100	3	0
Bakes Raisin	1 bar	100	3	0
Fat Free Fruit Bars 100% Organic Apple	1 bar	140	4	0
Fat Free Fruit Bars 100% Organic Apricot	1 bar	140	4	0
Fat Free Fruit Bars 100% Organic Date	1 bar	140	4	0
Fat Free Fruit Bars 100% Organic Raisin	1 bar	140	4	0
Fruit & Fitness Bars	2 bars	200	5	0
Oat Bran Bakes Apricot	1 bar	100	2	0
Oat Bran Bakes Fig & Nut	1 bar	110	2	0
Oat Bran Jumbo Fruit Bars Almond & Date	1 bar	170	7	0
Oat Bran Jumbo Fruit Bars Raisin & Cinnamon	1 bar	160	6	0
Rice Bran Jumbo Fruit Bars Almond & Date	1 bar	160	4	0
Sonoma				
Trail Mix	¼ cup (1.4 oz)	160	2	0
Sovex				
Fruit Bites Jungle Pals	1 pkg (0.9 oz)	90	—	0
Stretch Island				
Fruit Leather Berry Blackberry	2 pieces (1 oz)	90	3	0
Fruit Leather Chunky Cherry	2 pieces (1 oz)	90	2	0
Fruit Leather Great Grape	2 pieces (1 oz)	90	2	0
Fruit Leather Organic Apple	2 pieces (1 oz)	90	2	0
Fruit Leather Organic Grape	2 pieces (1 oz)	90	2	0
Fruit Leather Organic Raspberry	2 pieces (1 oz)	90	2	0
Fruit Leather Rare Raspberry	2 pieces (1 oz)	90	2	0
Fruit Leather Snappy Apple	2 pieces (1 oz)	90	3	0

FOOD	PORTION	CALS.	FIB.	CHOL.
Stretch Island (CONT.)				
Fruit Leather Tangy Apricot	2 pieces (1 oz)	90	2	0
Fruit Leather Truly Tropical	2 pieces (1 oz)	90	1	0
Sunbelt				
Fruit Boosters Apple	1 (1.3 oz)	130	0	0
Fruit Boosters Blueberry	1 (1.3 oz)	130	1	0
Fruit Boosters Strawberry	1 (1.3 oz)	130	0	0
Fruit Jammers	1 (1 oz)	100	0	0
Sunkist				
Fruit Roll Apple	1 (0.7 oz)	70	1	0
Fruit Roll Apricot	1 (0.5 oz)	70	2	0
Fruit Roll Apricot	1	76	0	0
Fruit Roll Cherry	1 (0.7 oz)	70	2	0
Fruit Roll Cherry	1 (0.5 oz)	50	1	0
Fruit Roll Fruit Punch	1 (0.7 oz)	70	2	0
Fruit Roll Grape	1	76	0	0
Fruit Roll Grape	1 (0.5 oz)	50	1	0
Fruit Roll Grape	1 (0.7 oz)	80	2	0
Fruit Roll Raspberry	1 (0.7 oz)	70	1	0
Fruit Roll Raspberry	1 (0.5 oz)	45	1	0
Fruit Roll Strawberry	1 (0.7 oz)	70	2	0
Fruit Roll Strawberry	1	74	0	0
Fruit Roll Strawberry	1 (0.5 oz)	45	1	0
Weight Watchers				
Apple	1 pkg (0.5 oz)	50	2	0
Apple Chips	1 pkg (0.75 oz)	70	3	0
Cinnamon	1 pkg (0.5 oz)	50	2	0
Peach	1 pkg (0.5 oz)	50	2	0
Strawberry	1 pkg (0.5 oz)	50	2	0

GARBANZOS
(*see* CHICKPEAS)

GARLIC

clove	1	4	—	0
powder	1 tsp	9	—	0
Watkins				
Garlic & Chive Seasoning	1 tbsp (7 g)	25	0	5
Garlic Lover's Herb Blend	¼ tsp (0.5 oz)	0	0	0
Liquid Spice	1 tbsp (0.5 oz)	120	0	0

GEFILTE FISH

sweet	1 piece (1.5 oz)	35	—	12

GELATIN
MIX

low calorie	½ cup	8	0	0

FOOD	PORTION	CALS.	FIB.	CHOL.
mix artificially sweetened as prep	1 pkg 4 serv (16.5 oz)	33	—	0
mix artificially sweetened as prep	½ cup (4.1 oz)	8	—	0
mix as prep	1 pkg 4 serv (19 oz)	319	—	0
mix as prep	½ cup (4.7 oz)	80	—	0
mix not prep	1 pkg (3 oz)	324	—	0
mix w/ fruit as prep	½ cup (3.7 oz)	73	—	0
mix w/ fruit as prep	1 pkg 8 serv (19 oz)	588	—	0
D-Zerta				
Cherry	½ cup	8	—	0
Lemon	½ cup	8	—	0
Lime	½ cup	9	—	0
Orange	½ cup	8	—	0
Raspberry	½ cup	8	—	0
Strawberry	½ cup	8	—	0
Emes				
Kosher-Jel	½ cup (4 fl oz)	60	—	0
Kosher-Jel Plain	1 tbsp (7 g)	21	1	0
Jell-O				
Apricot	½ cup	82	0	0
Black Cherry	½ cup	82	tr	0
Black Raspberry	½ cup	82	tr	0
Blackberry	½ cup	82	tr	0
Cherry Sugar Free	½ cup	9	—	0
Concord Grape	½ cup	82	0	0
Hawaiian Pineapple Sugar Free	½ cup	8	—	0
Lemon	½ cup	82	0	0
Lemon Sugar Free	½ cup	8	—	0
Lime	½ cup	82	tr	0
Lime Sugar Free	½ cup	9	—	0
Mixed Fruit	½ cup	82	tr	0
Mixed Fruit Sugar Free	½ cup	8	—	0
Orange	½ cup	82	tr	0
Orange Sugar Free	½ cup	8	—	0
Peach Sugar Free	½ cup	8	—	0
Raspberry Sugar Free	½ cup	8	—	0
Strawberry Banana Sugar Free	½ cup	9	—	0
Strawberry Sugar Free	½ cup	9	—	0
Triple Berry Sugar Free	½ cup	8	—	0
Wild Strawberry	½ cup	81	tr	0
Royal				
Apple	½ cup	80	—	0
Blackberry	½ cup	80	—	0
Cherry	½ cup	80	—	0

FOOD	PORTION	CALS.	FIB.	CHOL.
Royal (CONT.)				
Cherry Sugar Free	½ cup	8	—	0
Concord Grape	½ cup	80	—	0
Fruit Punch	½ cup	80	—	0
Lemon	½ cup	80	—	0
Lemon-Lime	½ cup	80	—	0
Lime	½ cup	80	—	0
Lime Sugar Free	½ cup	8	—	0
Mixed Berry	½ cup	80	—	0
Orange	½ cup	80	—	0
Orange Sugar Free	½ cup	10	—	0
Peach	½ cup	80	—	0
Pineapple	½ cup	80	—	0
Raspberry	½ cup	80	—	0
Raspberry Sugar Free	½ cup	8	—	0
Strawberry	½ cup	80	—	0
Strawberry Banana Sugar Free	½ cup	8	—	0
Strawberry Orange	½ cup	80	—	0
Strawberry Sugar Free	½ cup	8	—	0
Tropical Fruit	½ cup	80	—	0
READY-TO-EAT				
Del Monte				
Gel Snack Cups Blue Berry	1 serv (3.5 oz)	70	tr	0
Gel Snack Cups Cherry	1 serv (3.5 oz)	70	tr	0
Gel Snack Cups Orange	1 serv (3.5 oz)	70	tr	0
Gel Snack Cups Strawberry	1 serv (3.5 oz)	70	tr	0
Hunt's				
Snack Pack Juicy Gels Cherry	1 (4 oz)	100	0	0
Snack Pack Juicy Gels Lemon Lime	1 (4 oz)	100	0	0
Snack Pack Juicy Gels Mixed Fruit	1 (4 oz)	100	0	0
Snack Pack Juicy Gels Orange	1 (4 oz)	100	0	0
Snack Pack Juicy Gels Strawberry	1 (4 oz)	100	0	0
Kozy Shack				
Gel Treat Cherry	1 pkg (4 oz)	100	1	0
Gel Treat Lemon Lime	1 pkg (4 oz)	100	1	0
Gel Treat Orange	1 pkg (4 oz)	100	1	0
Gel Treat Strawberry	1 pkg (4 oz)	100	1	0
Gel Treat Sugar Free Orange	1 pkg (4 oz)	10	1	0
Gel Treat Sugar Free Strawberry	1 pkg (4 oz)	10	1	0
GIBLETS				
capon simmered	1 cup (5 oz)	238	—	629

FOOD	PORTION	CALS.	FIB.	CHOL.
chicken floured & fried	1 cup (5 oz)	402	—	647
chicken simmered	1 cup (5 oz)	228	—	570
turkey simmered	1 cup (5 oz)	243	—	606
GINGER				
ground	1 tsp (1.8 g)	6	—	0
root fresh	¼ cup	17	—	0
root fresh	5 slices	8	—	0
root fresh sliced	¼ cup	17	—	0
Ka-Me				
Crystallized Slices	5 pieces (1 oz)	100	1	0
Sliced	20 pieces (0.5 oz)	0	0	0
GINKGO NUTS				
canned	1 oz	32	—	0
dried	1 oz	99	—	0
raw	1 oz	52	—	0
GIZZARDS				
chicken simmered	1 cup (5 oz)	222	—	281
turkey simmered	1 cup (5 oz)	236	—	336
GOAT				
roasted	3 oz	122	—	64
GOOSE				
w/ skin roasted	6.6 oz	574	—	172
w/ skin roasted	½ goose (1.7 lbs)	2362	—	708
w/o skin roasted	5 oz	340	—	138
w/o skin roasted	½ goose (1.3 lbs)	1406	—	569
GOOSEBERRIES				
canned in light syrup	½ cup	93	—	0
fresh	1 cup	67	—	0
GRANOLA				
BARS				
almond	1 (0.8 oz)	117	—	0
almond	1 (1 oz)	140	—	0
chewy chocolate coated chocolate chip	1 (1 oz)	132	1	1
chewy chocolate coated chocolate chip	1 (1.25 oz)	165	1	2
chewy chocolate coated peanut butter	1 (1 oz)	144	—	3
chewy chocolate coated peanut butter	1 (1.3 oz)	187	—	4
chewy raisin	1 (1 oz)	127	1	0

FOOD	PORTION	CALS.	FIB.	CHOL.
chewy raisin	1 (1.5 oz)	191	2	0
chocolate chip	1 (1 oz)	124	1	0
chocolate chip	1 (0.8 oz)	103	1	0
chocolate chip chewy	1 (1.5 oz)	178	2	1
chocolate chip chewy	1 (1 oz)	119	1	0
chocolate chip graham & marshmallow chewy	1 (1 oz)	121	1	0
nut & raisin chewy	1 (1 oz)	129	2	0
peanut	1 (1 oz)	136	—	0
peanut	1 (0.8 oz)	113	1	0
peanut butter	1 (0.8 oz)	114	—	0
peanut butter	1 (1 oz)	137	—	0
peanut butter chewy	1 (1 oz)	121	1	0
peanut butter & chocolate chip chewy	1 (1 oz)	122	1	0
plain	1 (1 oz)	134	2	0
plain	1 (0.9 oz)	115	1	0
plain chewy	1 (1 oz)	126	1	0
Carnation				
Chocolate Chunk	1 (1.26 oz)	140	1	0
Honey & Oats	1 (1.26 oz)	130	1	0
Fi-Bar				
Coconut	1	120	6	0
Peanut Butter	1	130	6	0
General Mills				
Nature Valley Cinnamon	1	120	1	0
Nature Valley Oat Bran Honey Graham	1	110	1	0
Nature Valley Oats N'Honey	1	120	1	0
Nature Valley Peanut Butter	1	120	1	0
Nature Valley Rice Bran Cinnamon Graham	1	90	1	0
Grist Mill				
Chewy Apple Cinnamon	1 (1 oz)	120	1	0
Chewy Chocolate Chip	1 (1 oz)	130	1	0
Chewy Chunky Nut & Raisin	1 (1 oz)	130	1	0
Chewy Peanut Butter	1 (1 oz)	130	1	0
Chewy Peanut Butter Chocolate	1 (1 oz)	130	2	0
Chocolate Snack Chocolate Chip	1 (1.2 oz)	180	1	5
Chocolate Snack Nutty Fudge	1 (1.3 oz)	190	2	5
Crunchy Cinnamon	1 (0.8 oz)	110	1	0
Crunchy Oats 'N Honey	1 (0.8 oz)	110	1	0

FOOD	PORTION	CALS.	FIB.	CHOL.
Hershey				
Chocolate Covered Cocoa Creme	1 (1.2 oz)	180	—	5
Chocolate Covered Peanut Butter	1 (1.2 oz)	180	—	5
Kellogg's				
Low Fat Crunchy Almond & Brown Sugar	1 (0.7 oz)	80	1	0
Low Fat Crunchy Apple Spice	1 (0.7 oz)	80	1	0
Low Fat Crunchy Cinnamon Raisin	1 (0.7 oz)	80	1	0
Kudos				
Chocolate Chunk	1 (0.7 oz)	90	1	0
Chocolate Coated Chocolate Chip	1 (1 oz)	120	1	5
Chocolate Coated Milk & Cookies	1 (1 oz)	130	1	5
Chocolate Coated Nutty Fudge	1 (1 oz)	130	1	5
Chocolate Coated Peanut Butter	1 (1 oz)	130	1	5
Low Fat Blueberry	1 (0.7 oz)	90	1	0
Low Fat Strawberry	1 (0.7 oz)	80	1	0
Quaker				
Chewy Chocolate Chip	1	128	1	tr
Chewy Chunky Nut & Raisin	1	131	2	tr
Chewy Cinnamon Raisin	1	128	1	tr
Chewy Honey & Oats	1	125	1	tr
Chewy Peanut Butter	1	128	1	tr
Chewy Peanut Butter Chocolate Chip	1	131	1	tr
Dipps Caramel Nut	1	148	1	2
Dipps Chocolate Chip	1	139	1	1
Dipps Peanut Butter	1	170	1	2
Sunbelt				
Chewy Chocolate Chip	1 (1.25 oz)	160	2	0
Chewy Chocolate Chip	1 (1.8 oz)	220	2	0
Chewy Oats & Honey	1 (1 oz)	130	1	0
Chewy Oats & Honey	1 (1.7 oz)	210	2	0
Chewy With Almonds	1 (1 oz)	130	2	0
Chewy With Almonds	1 (1.5 oz)	190	2	0
Chewy With Raisins	1 (1.2 oz)	150	2	0
Fudge Dipped Chewy Chocolate Chip	1 (1.5 oz)	190	2	0
Fudge Dipped Chewy Macaroo	1 bar (2 oz)	280	3	0
Fudge Dipped Chewy Macaroo	1 (1.4 oz)	200	2	0

FOOD	PORTION	CALS.	FIB.	CHOL.
Sunbelt (CONT.)				
Fudge Dipped Chewy With Peanuts	1 bar (1.5 oz)	210	2	0
Fudge Dipped Chewy With Peanuts	1 (2 oz)	270	2	0
CEREAL				
Erewhon				
Honey Almond	1 oz	130	—	0
Maple	1 oz	130	—	0
Spiced Apple	1 oz	130	—	0
Sunflower Crunch	1 oz	130	—	0
With Bran	1 oz	130	4	0
General Mills				
Nature Valley Cinnamon & Raisin	⅓ cup (1 oz)	120	1	0
Nature Valley Fruit & Nut	⅓ cup (1 oz)	130	1	0
Nature Valley Toasted Oat	⅓ cup (1 oz)	130	1	0
Good Shepherd				
Crunchy	1 oz	130	2	0
Honey Almond	1 oz	120	2	0
Organic 5 Grain Muesli	1 oz	160	3	0
Organic Brown Rice	1 oz	130	4	0
Organic Wheat Free	1 oz	90	2	0
Organic Wheat Free Apple Cinnamon	1 oz	125	3	0
Organic Wheat Free Blueberry Amaranth	1 oz	110	2	0
Organic Wheat Free Strawberry Amaranth	1 oz	110	2	0
Grist Mill				
Low-Fat With Raisins	⅔ cup (1.9 oz)	220	3	0
Kellogg's				
Low Fat	½ cup (1.9 oz)	210	3	0
Low Fat With Raisins	⅔ cup (1.9 oz)	210	3	0
Stone-Buhr				
Hot Apple	⅓ cup (1.6 oz)	153	5	0
Sun Country				
100% Natural With Almonds	¼ cup	130	1	0
100% Natural With Raisins & Dates	¼ cup	123	2	0
With Raisins	¼ cup	125	2	0
Sunbelt				
Banana Nut	1.9 oz	250	4	1
Fruit & Nut	1.9 oz	230	4	1

FOOD	PORTION	CALS.	FIB.	CHOL.
Sunbelt (CONT.)				
Low Fat	1.9 oz	200	4	0
Uncle Roy's				
Cashew Raisin	½ cup (1.6 oz)	180	3	0
Fat Free Apple Cinnamon	½ cup (1.6 oz)	175	3	0
Fat Free Wild Cherry	½ cup (1.6 oz)	175	3	0
Fruit & Nut	½ cup (1.6 oz)	175	3	0
Low Fat Berries Jubilee	½ cup (1.6 oz)	175	3	0
Low Fat Crispy	½ cup (1.4 oz)	160	3	0
Low Fat Luscious Raspberry	½ cup (1.6 oz)	175	3	0
Low Fat True Blueberry	½ cup (1.6 oz)	175	3	0
Maple Date Nut	½ cup (1.6 oz)	180	3	0
Nut Butter & Almonds	½ cup (1.6 oz)	195	3	0
Organic Golden Honey	½ cup (1.6 oz)	190	3	0
Organic Maple Nut'N Rice	½ cup (1.4 oz)	170	3	0
Organic Maple Raisin	½ cup (1.6 oz)	190	3	0

GRANOLA BARS

(*see* CEREAL BARS, NUTRITIONAL SUPPLEMENTS)

GRAPE JUICE

FOOD	PORTION	CALS.	FIB.	CHOL.
bottled	1 cup	155	—	0
frzn sweetened as prep	1 cup	128	—	0
frzn sweetened not prep	6 oz	386	—	0
grape drink	6 oz	84	—	0
BAMA				
Juice	8.45 fl oz	120	—	0
Bright & Early				
Frozen	8 fl oz	140	—	0
Hawaiian Punch				
Drink	6 oz	90	—	0
Hi-C				
Box	8.45 fl oz	130	—	0
Drink	1 can (11.5 fl oz)	180	—	0
Drink	8 fl oz	130	—	0
Juice Works				
Drink	6 oz	100	—	0
Juicy Juice				
Drink	1 bottle (6 fl oz)	90	—	0
Drink	1 box	130	—	0
Kool-Aid				
Drink	8 oz	98	—	0
Sugar Free	8 oz	3	—	0
Sugar Sweetened	8 oz	80	—	0

FOOD	PORTION	CALS.	FIB.	CHOL.
Minute Maid				
Chilled	8 fl oz	130	—	0
Grape Punch frzn	8 fl oz	130	—	0
Punch Chilled	8 fl oz	130	—	0
Mott's				
Drink	10 fl oz	170	0	0
Fruit Basket Cocktail as prep	8 fl oz	130	0	0
S&W				
Concord Unsweetened	6 oz	100	—	0
Seneca				
Blush Grape Juice frzn as prep	8 fl oz	170	0	0
Fortified With Vitamin C frzn as prep	8 fl oz	170	0	0
Sweetened frzn as prep	8 fl oz	140	0	0
White Grape Juice frzn as prep	8 fl oz	140	0	0
Sippin' Pak				
100% Pure	8.45 fl oz	130	—	0
Sipps				
Juice	8.45 oz	130	—	0
Snapple				
Grapeade	8 fl oz	120	—	0
Tang				
Fruit Box	8.45 oz	131	—	0
Tree Top				
Juice	6 oz	120	—	0
Sparkling Juice	6 oz	120	—	0
Tropicana				
Season's Best	8 fl oz	160	—	0
Veryfine				
100%	8 oz	153	—	0
Grape Drink	8 oz	130	—	0

GRAPE LEAVES

Cedar's				
Grape Leaves Stuffed With Rice	6 pieces (4.9 oz)	180	8	0

GRAPEFRUIT
CANNED

juice pack	½ cup	46	—	0
unsweetened	1 cup	93	—	0
water pack	½ cup	44	—	0
S&W				
Sections In Light Syrup	½ cup	80	—	0
Sections Natural Style	½ cup	40	—	0
Sections Unsweetened	½ cup	40	—	0

FOOD	PORTION	CALS.	FIB.	CHOL.
FRESH				
pink	½	37	1	0
pink sections	1 cup	69	1	0
red	½	37	—	0
red sections	1 cup	69	—	0
white	½	39	1	0
white sections	1 cup	76	1	0
Chiquita				
Ruby Red	½ fruit	40	—	0
Dole				
Grapefruit	½	50	6	0
Ocean Spray				
Pink	½ med	50	—	0
White	½ med	45	—	0
GRAPEFRUIT JUICE				
fresh	1 cup	96	—	0
frzn as prep	1 cup	102	—	0
frzn not prep	6 oz	302	—	0
sweetened	1 cup	116	—	0
After The Fall				
Pink	1 bottle (10 oz)	100	—	0
Crystal Geyser				
Juice Squeeze	1 bottle (12 fl oz)	150	—	0
Del Monte				
Juice	8 fl oz	100	1	0
Fresh Samantha				
Juice	1 cup (8 oz)	101	tr	0
Hood				
Select	1 cup (8 oz)	100	—	0
Minute Maid				
Frozen	8 fl oz	100	—	0
Juices To Go	1 can (11.5 fl oz)	140	—	0
Juices To Go	1 bottle (16 fl oz)	100	—	0
Juices To Go	1 bottle (10 fl oz)	120	—	0
Juices To Go Pink Cocktail	1 bottle (16 fl oz)	110	—	0
Juices To Go Pink Cocktail	1 bottle (10 fl oz)	140	—	0
Juices To Go Pink Cocktail	8 fl oz	160	—	0
Mott's				
From Concentrate as prep	8 fl oz	120	0	0
Ocean Spray				
100% Juice	8 oz	100	tr	0
Lightstyle Low Calorie Pink Cocktail	8 fl oz	40	0	0

FOOD	PORTION	CALS.	FIB.	CHOL.
Ocean Spray (CONT.)				
Pink Juice Cocktail	8 oz	110	0	0
Ruby Red Drink	8 oz	130	0	0
Odwalla				
Juice	8 fl oz	90	—	0
S&W				
Unsweetened	6 oz	80	—	0
Snapple				
Juice	10 fl oz	110	—	0
Pink Grapefruit Cocktail	8 fl oz	120	—	0
Tree Of Life				
Juice	8 fl oz	100	0	0
Tree Top				
Juice	6 oz	80	—	0
Tropicana				
Juice	1 container (6 fl oz)	80	—	0
Juice	8 fl oz	90	—	0
Ruby Red	8 fl oz	100	—	0
Ruby Red	1 container (10 fl oz)	120	—	0
Season's Best	1 can (11.5 fl oz)	120	—	0
Season's Best	1 bottle (7 fl oz)	80	—	0
Season's Best	8 fl oz	90	—	0
Season's Best	1 bottle (10 fl oz)	110	—	0
Twister Light Pink	8 fl oz	40	—	0
Twister Light Pink	1 container (10 fl oz)	50	—	0
Twister Pink	1 container (10 fl oz)	140	—	0
Twister Pink	1 can (11.5 fl oz)	160	—	0
Twister Pink	8 fl oz	110	—	0
Veryfine				
100%	8 oz	101	—	0
Pink	8 oz	120	—	0

GRAPES

CANNED

FOOD	PORTION	CALS.	FIB.	CHOL.
thompson seedless in heavy syrup	½ cup	94	—	0
thompson seedless water pack	½ cup	48	—	0
S&W				
Thompson Seedless Premium	½ cup	100	—	0
FRESH				
grapes	10	36	tr	0

FOOD	PORTION	CALS.	FIB.	CHOL.
Dole				
Grapes	1½ cup	85	2	0
GRAVY				
(*see also* SAUCE)				
CANNED				
au jus	1 cup	38	—	1
beef	1 cup	124	—	7
beef	1 can (10 oz)	155	—	9
chicken	1 cup	189	—	5
mushroom	1 cup	120	—	0
turkey	1 cup	122	—	5
Gravymaster				
Seasoning	¼ tsp	3	—	0
Rudy's Farm				
Sausage Gravy	¼ cup (2 oz)	50	0	10
MIX				
au jus as prep w/ water	1 cup	32	—	1
brown as prep w/ water	1 cup	75	—	2
chicken as prep	1 cup	83	—	3
mushroom as prep	1 cup	70	—	1
onion as prep w/ water	1 cup	77	—	tr
pork as prep	1 cup	76	—	3
turkey as prep	1 cup	87	—	3
Durkee				
Au Jus as prep	¼ cup	5	0	0
Brown as prep	¼ cup	10	0	0
Brown Herb as prep	¼ cup	15	0	0
Brown Mushroom as prep	¼ cup	15	0	0
Brown Onion as prep	¼ cup	15	0	0
Chicken as prep	¼ cup	20	0	0
Country as prep	¼ cup	35	0	0
Homestyle as prep	¼ cup	15	0	0
Mushroom as prep	¼ cup	15	0	0
Onion as prep	¼ cup	10	0	0
Pork as prep	¼ cup	10	0	0
Sausage as prep	¼ cup	35	0	0
Swiss Steak as prep	¼ cup	15	0	0
Turkey as prep	¼ cup	20	0	0
French's				
Au Jus as prep	¼ cup	5	0	0
Brown as prep	¼ cup	10	0	0
Chicken as prep	¼ cup	25	0	0
Country as prep	¼ cup	35	0	0

FOOD	PORTION	CALS.	FIB.	CHOL.
French's (CONT.)				
Herb Brown as prep	¼ cup	15	0	0
Homestyle as prep	¼ cup	10	0	0
Mushroom as prep	¼ cup	10	0	0
Onion, as prep	¼ cup	15	0	0
Pork as prep	¼ cup	10	0	0
Sausage as prep	¼ cup	35	0	0
Turkey as prep	¼ cup	20	0	0
Hain				
Brown	¼ pkg	16	—	0
Pillsbury				
Brown	¼ cup	15	—	0
Home Style	¼ cup	15	—	0
Weight Watchers				
Brown as prep	¼ cup	5	0	0
Brown With Mushrooms as prep	¼ cup	10	0	0
Brown With Onion as prep	¼ cup	10	0	0
Chicken as prep	¼ cup	10	0	0

GREAT NORTHERN BEANS
CANNED

FOOD	PORTION	CALS.	FIB.	CHOL.
great northern	1 cup	300	14	0
Allen				
Great Northern	½ cup (4.5 oz)	100	7	0
Green Giant				
Great Northern	½ cup	80	5	0
Hanover				
Great Northern	½ cup	110	—	0
Trappey				
With Sausage	½ cup (4.5 oz)	100	7	0
DRIED				
cooked	1 cup	210	—	0
Bean Cuisine				
Dried	½ cup	115	5	0

GREEN BEANS
CANNED

FOOD	PORTION	CALS.	FIB.	CHOL.
green beans	½ cup	13	1	0
italian	½ cup	13	1	0
italian low sodium	½ cup	13	1	0
low sodium	½ cup	13	1	0
Allen				
Cut	½ cup (4.2 oz)	30	3	0
Cut No Added Salt	½ cup (4.2 oz)	15	2	0

FOOD	PORTION	CALS.	FIB.	CHOL.
Allen (CONT.)				
French Style	½ cup (4.2 oz)	25	2	0
Italian	½ cup (4.2 oz)	35	3	0
Shell Outs	½ cup (4.5 oz)	30	2	0
Alma				
Cut	½ cup (4.2 oz)	30	3	0
Crest Top				
Cut	½ cup (4.2 oz)	30	3	0
Del Monte				
Cut	½ cup (4.3 oz)	20	2	0
Cut 50% Less Salt	½ cup (4.3 oz)	20	2	0
Cut Italian	½ cup (4.3 oz)	30	3	0
Cut No Salt Added	½ cup (4.3 oz)	20	2	0
French Style	½ cup (4.3 oz)	20	2	0
French Style 50% Less Salt	½ cup (4.3 oz)	20	2	0
French Style No Salt Added	½ cup (4.3 oz)	20	2	0
French Style Seasoned	½ cup (4.3 oz)	20	2	0
Whole	½ cup (4.3 oz)	20	2	0
GaBelle				
Cut	½ cup (4.2 oz)	30	3	0
Green Giant				
Almondine	½ cup	45	2	0
Cut	½ cup	16	1	0
French	½ cup	16	1	0
Kitchen Sliced	½ cup	16	1	0
Hanover				
Cut	½ cup	20	—	0
Owatonna				
Cut	½ cup	20	—	0
French	½ cup	20	—	0
S&W				
Cut Water Pack	½ cup	20	—	0
Cut Premium Blue Lake	½ cup	20	—	0
Dilled	½ cup	60	—	0
French Style Premium Blue Lake	½ cup	20	—	0
Green Beans & Wax Beans	½ cup	20	—	0
Whole Fancy Stringless	½ cup	20	—	0
Whole Vertical Pack	½ cup	20	—	0
Seneca				
Cut	½ cup	20	2	0
Cuts Natural Pack	½ cup	25	2	0
French	½ cup	20	2	0
French Natural Pack	½ cup	25	2	0

FOOD	PORTION	CALS.	FIB.	CHOL.
Seneca (CONT.)				
Whole	½ cup	20	2	0
Sunshine				
Cut	½ cup (4.2 oz)	30	3	0
Italian	½ cup (4.2 oz)	35	3	0
FRESH				
cooked	½ cup	22	—	0
raw	½ cup	17	1	0
FROZEN				
cooked	½ cup	18	—	0
italian cooked	½ cup	18	—	0
Birds Eye				
Cut	½ cup	25	2	0
Farm Fresh Whole	¾ cup	30	2	0
French Cut	½ cup	25	2	0
In Sauce French Green Beans	½ cup	50	2	0
With Toasted Almonds				
Italian	½ cup	30	3	0
Polybag Cut	½ cup	25	2	0
Polybag Deluxe Whole	½ cup	20	2	0
Polybag French Cut	½ cup	25	2	0
Whole Deluxe	½ cup	45	2	0
Green Giant				
Cut	½ cup	16	1	0
Cut In Butter Sauce	½ cup	30	2	5
Green Beans	½ cup	14	2	0
One Serve In Butter Sauce	1 pkg	60	3	5
Hanover				
Cut	½ cup	20	—	0
French Style Blue Lake	½ cup	25	—	0
Italian Cut	½ cup	35	—	0
Whole Blue Lake	½ cup	30	—	0
Southland				
Cut Beans	3 oz	25	—	0
French	3 oz	25	—	0
Stouffer's				
Green Bean Mushroom	½ cup (1.9 oz)	130	2	10
Casserole				
Tree Of Life				
Green Beans	⅔ cup (2.8 oz)	25	2	0
SHELF-STABLE				
Pantry Express				
Cut	½ cup	12	1	0
GREENS				
CANNED				
Allen				
Mixed	½ cup (4.2 oz)	30	4	0

FOOD	PORTION	CALS.	FIB.	CHOL.
Sunshine				
Mixed	½ cup (4.2 oz)	30	4	0
GROUNDCHERRIES				
fresh	½ cup	37	—	0
GROUPER				
cooked	3 oz	100	—	40
cooked	1 fillet (7.1 oz)	238	—	95
raw	3 oz	78	—	31
GUANABANA JUICE				
Libby				
Nectar	1 can (11.5 fl oz)	210	—	0
GUAVA				
fresh	1	45	—	0
guava sauce	½ cup	43	—	0
GUAVA JUICE				
Kern's				
Nectar	6 fl oz	110	—	0
Libby				
Nectar	6 oz	110	—	0
Nectar	1 can (11.5 fl oz)	220	—	0
Snapple				
Guava Mania	8 fl oz	110	—	0
GUINEA HEN				
w/o skin raw	½ hen (9.3 oz)	292	—	166
HADDOCK				
FRESH				
cooked	1 fillet (5.3 oz)	168	—	110
cooked	3 oz	95	—	63
raw	3 oz	74	—	49
roe raw	3½ oz	130	—	360
FROZEN				
Gorton's				
Microwave Entree Haddock In Lemon Butter	1 pkg	360	—	100
Mrs. Paul's				
Crunchy Batter Fillets	2 fillets	190	—	25
Light Fillets	1 fillet	220	—	45
Van De Kamp's				
Battered Fillets	2 (4 oz)	260	0	30
Breaded Fillets	2 (3.5 oz)	280	0	25
Lightly Breaded Fillets	1 (4 oz)	220	0	30

FOOD	PORTION	CALS.	FIB.	CHOL.
SMOKED				
smoked	1 oz	33	—	21
smoked	3 oz	99	—	65
HALIBUT				
FRESH				
atlantic & pacific cooked	3 oz	119	—	35
atlantic & pacific cooked	½ fillet (5.6 oz)	223	—	65
atlantic & pacific raw	3 oz	93	—	27
greenland baked	3 oz	203	—	50
greenland baked	5.6 oz	380	—	94
FROZEN				
Van De Kamp's				
Battered Fillets	3 (4 oz)	300	0	20
HALVA				
(see SESAME)				
HAM				
(see also HAM DISHES, PORK, TURKEY)				
boneless 11% fat	3 oz	151	—	50
boneless extra lean roasted	3 oz	140	—	48
canned 13% fat	1 oz	54	—	11
canned 13% fat	3 oz	192	—	52
canned extra lean	1 oz	41	—	11
canned extra lean	3 oz	142	—	34
canned extra lean 4% fat	3 oz	116	—	25
center slice lean & fat	4 oz	229	—	61
chopped	1 oz	65	—	15
chopped canned	1 oz	68	—	14
ham & cheese loaf	1 oz	73	—	16
ham & cheese spread	1 tbsp	37	—	9
ham & cheese spread	1 oz	69	—	17
ham salad spread	1 tbsp	32	—	6
ham salad spread	1 oz	61	—	10
minced	1 oz	75	—	20
patties uncooked	1 (2.3 oz)	206	—	46
patties grilled	1 patty (2 oz)	203	—	43
sliced extra lean 5% fat	1 oz	37	—	13
sliced regular 11% fat	1 oz	52	—	16
steak boneless extra lean	1 oz	35	—	13
whole lean & fat roasted	3 oz	207	—	52
whole lean only roasted	3 oz	133	—	47
Alpine Lace				
Boneless Cooked	2 oz	60	0	25

FOOD	PORTION	CALS.	FIB.	CHOL.
Armour				
Chopped Ham canned	2 oz	120	—	35
Deviled Ham canned	1 pkg (3 oz)	200	—	60
Golden Star Boneless	1 oz	33	—	13
Golden Star Canned	1 oz	32	—	11
Lower Salt 93% Fat Free	1 oz	35	—	14
Lower Salt Boneless	1 oz	34	—	13
Star Boneless	1 oz	41	—	15
Star Canned	1 oz	34	—	11
Star Speedy Cut	1 oz	44	—	15
1877 Boneless	1 oz	42	—	42
Black Label				
Chopped	2 oz	140	0	30
Carl Buddig				
Ham	1 oz	50	0	20
Honey Ham	1 oz	50	—	30
Hansel n' Gretel				
Baked Virginia	1 oz	34	—	12
Black Forest	1 oz	32	—	16
Cappy	1 oz	31	—	11
Cooked Fresh	1 oz	33	—	13
Deluxe	1 oz	31	—	12
Honey Valley	1 oz	31	—	10
Jalapeno	1 oz	25	—	11
Lessalt	1 oz	30	—	13
Lessalt Virginia	1 oz	32	—	13
Light AM	1 oz	27	—	11
Travane	1 oz	31	—	15
Healthy Choice				
Baked Cooked	3 slices (2.2 oz)	70	0	30
Cooked	3 slices (2.2 oz)	70	0	30
Deli-Thin Baked Cooked With Natural Juices	6 slices (2 oz)	60	0	25
Deli-Thin Cooked	6 slices (2 oz)	60	0	30
Deli-Thin Honey With Natural Juices	6 slices (2 oz)	60	0	25
Deli-Thin Smoked With Natural Juices	6 slices (2 oz)	60	0	25
Fresh-Trak Cooked	1 slice (1 oz)	30	0	10
Fresh-Trak Honey	1 slice (1 oz)	30	0	15
Honey Boneless	3 oz	100	0	40
Smoked	3 slices (2.2 oz)	70	0	30
Variety Pack Regular	3 slices (2.2 oz)	70	0	30

FOOD	PORTION	CALS.	FIB.	CHOL.
Hormel				
Black Label Canned (refrigerated)	3 oz	100	0	40
Black Label Canned (shelf-stable)	3 oz	110	0	45
Canned Chunk	2 oz	90	0	30
Cure 81 Half Ham	3 oz	100	0	45
Curemaster	3 oz	80	0	40
Deli Cooked	1 oz	29	—	11
Deviled Ham	4 tbsp (2 oz)	150	0	40
Ham & Cheese Patties	1 patty (2 oz)	190	0	45
Light & Lean	3 oz	90	0	35
Light & Lean 97	3 oz	90	0	35
Light & Lean 97 Cuts	16 pieces (1 oz)	35	0	15
Light & Lean 97 Sliced	1 slice (1 oz)	25	0	15
Patties	1 patty (2 oz)	180	0	35
Primissimo Prosciutti	1 oz	70	0	25
Spread	4 tbsp (2 oz)	100	0	40
Supreme Cut Canned	1 oz	31	—	14
Jones				
Family Ham	1 slice	40	—	14
Ham Slices	1 slice	30	—	21
Jordan's				
Healthy Trim 97% Fat Free Cooked	1 slice (1 oz)	30	0	10
Healthy Trim 97% Fat Free EZ Serve	1 slice (1 oz)	30	0	15
Healthy Trim 97% Fat Free Virginia	1 slice (1 oz)	30	0	15
Krakus				
Ham	1 oz	25	—	25
Louis Rich				
Carving Board Baked With Natural Juices	2 slices (1.6 oz)	45	0	25
Carving Board Carved Thin Honey With Natural Juices	6 slices (2.1 oz)	70	0	35
Carving Board Honey With Natural Juices	2 slices (1.6 oz)	50	0	25
Carving Board Smoked Cooked With Natural Juices	1 slice (1.6 oz)	50	0	25
Dinner Slices Baked	1 slice (3.3 oz)	80	0	40
Mr. Turkey				
Deli Cuts Honey Cured	3 slices	35	—	20

FOOD	PORTION	CALS.	FIB.	CHOL.
Oscar Mayer				
Baked	3 slices (2.2 oz)	60	0	30
Boiled	3 slices (2.2 oz)	60	0	30
Chopped	1 slice (1 oz)	50	0	15
Deli-Thin Boiled	4 slices (1.8 oz)	50	0	25
Deli-Thin Honey Ham	4 slices (1.8 oz)	60	0	25
Deli-Thin Smoked	4 slices (1.8 oz)	50	0	25
Dinner Slice	3 oz	90	0	45
Dinner Steaks	1 (2 oz)	60	0	30
Ham & Cheese Loaf	1 slice (1 oz)	70	0	20
Healthy Favorites Baked	4 slices (1.8 oz)	50	0	25
Healthy Favorites Honey Ham	4 slices (1.8 oz)	50	0	25
Healthy Favorites Smoked Cooked	4 slices (1.8 oz)	50	0	25
Honey Ham	3 slices (2.2 oz)	70	0	30
Lower Sodium	3 slices (2.2 oz)	70	0	30
Lunchables Cookies/Ham/ Swiss	1 pkg (4.2 oz)	360	tr	50
Lunchables Dessert Chocolate Pudding/Ham/American	1 pkg (6.2 oz)	390	tr	55
Lunchables Ham/Cheddar	1 pkg (4.5 oz)	340	0	75
Lunchables Ham/Garden Vegetable Cheese	1 pkg (4.5 oz)	380	1	45
Lunchables Honey Ham/Herb & Chive Cheese	1 pkg (4.5 oz)	390	1	45
Smoked Cooked	3 slices (2.2 oz)	60	0	30
Russer				
Baked	2 oz	70	—	30
Canadian Brand Maple	2 oz	70	—	30
Chopped	2 oz	130	—	30
Cooked Ham	2 oz	60	—	30
Ham & Cheese Loaf	2 oz	120	—	30
Honey & Maple Cured	2 oz	70	—	30
Honey Cured	2 oz	60	—	30
Hot	2 oz	70	—	30
Light Cooked	2 oz	60	—	30
Light Smoked	2 oz	60	—	30
Smoked Virginia	2 oz	70	—	30
Spiced	2 oz	160	—	30
Sara Lee				
Bavarian Brand Baked	2 oz	80	—	40
Bavarian Brand Baked Honey	2 oz	80	—	40
Golden Cure Smoked	2 oz	80	—	30
Honey Ham	2 oz	60	—	25

FOOD	PORTION	CALS.	FIB.	CHOL.
Sara Lee (CONT.)				
Honey Roasted	2 oz	90	—	30
Spreadables				
Ham Salad	¼ can	100	—	24
Underwood				
Deviled	2.08 oz	220	—	50
Deviled Light	2.08 oz	120	—	35
Deviled Smoked	2.08 oz	190	—	65
Weight Watchers				
Deli Thin Oven Roasted	5 slices (⅓ oz)	12	—	5
Deli Thin Oven Roasted Honey Ham	5 slices (⅓ oz)	12	—	5
Deli Thin Premium Smoked	5 slices (⅓ oz)	12	—	5
Oven Roasted Honey Ham	2 slices (¾ oz)	25	—	15
Oven Roasted Smoked	2 slices (¾ oz)	25	—	15
Premium Cooked	2 slices (¾ oz)	25	—	15

HAM DISHES
FROZEN

FOOD	PORTION	CALS.	FIB.	CHOL.
Croissant Pocket				
Stuffed Sandwich Ham & Cheddar	1 piece (4.5 oz)	360	5	45
Hot Pocket				
Stuffed Sandwich Ham & Cheese	1 (4.5 oz)	340	4	45
Weight Watchers				
Ham & Cheese Pocket Sandwich	1 (5 oz)	240	5	10
Hickory Smoked Ham & Cheddar Pretzel Sandwich	1 (4 oz)	260	3	10

TAKE-OUT

FOOD	PORTION	CALS.	FIB.	CHOL.
croquettes	1 (3.1 oz)	217	tr	77
salad	½ cup	287	tr	237
sandwich w/ cheese	1	353	—	58

HAMBURGER
(*see also* BEEF)
FROZEN

FOOD	PORTION	CALS.	FIB.	CHOL.
Jimmy Dean				
Burger	1 (2 oz)	220	0	40
Flame Broiled Cheeseburger	1 (6.3 oz)	540	1	80
Mini Cheeseburger	2 (3 oz)	270	1	35
Kid Cuisine				
Beef Patty Sandwich w/ Cheese	1 (8.5 oz)	410	4	15

FOOD	PORTION	CALS.	FIB.	CHOL.
MicroMagic				
Cheeseburger	1 pkg (4.75 oz)	450	—	80
Hamburger	1 pkg (4 oz)	350	—	55
Rudy's Farm				
Mild Burger	1 (3 oz)	360	0	65
White Castle				
Cheeseburger	2 (3.6 oz)	310	6	30
Hamburger	2 (3.2 oz)	270	5	20
TAKE-OUT				
double patty w/ bun	1 reg	544	—	99
double patty w/ ketchup mayonnaise onion pickle tomato & bun	1 reg	649	—	94
double patty w/ cheese ketchup mayonnaise mustard pickle tomato & bun	1 lg	706	—	141
double patty w/ ketchup mustard mayonnaise onion pickle tomato & bun	1 lg	540	—	122
double patty w/ ketchup mustard onion pickle & bun	1 reg	576	—	102
double patty w/ cheese & bun	1 reg	457	—	110
double patty w/ cheese & double bun	1 reg	461	—	80
double patty w/ cheese ketchup mayonnaise onion pickle tomato & bun	1 reg	416	—	60
single patty w/ bacon cheese ketchup mustard onion pickle & bun	1 lg	609	—	112
single patty w/ bun	1 reg	275	—	36
single patty w/ bun	1 lg	400	—	71
single patty w/ cheese ham ketchup mayonnaise pickle tomato & bun	1 lg	745	—	122
single patty w/ ketchup mustard mayonnaise onion pickle tomato & bun	1 reg	279	—	26
single patty w/ cheese & bun	1 lg	608	—	96
single patty w/ cheese & bun	1 reg	320	—	50
triple patty w/ ketchup mustard pickle & bun	1 lg	693	—	142
triple patty w/ cheese & bun	1 lg	769	—	161

FOOD	PORTION	CALS.	FIB.	CHOL.
HAZELNUTS				
dried blanched	1 oz	191	—	0
dried unblanched	1 oz	179	—	0
dry roasted unblanched	1 oz	188	—	0
oil roasted unblanched	1 oz	187	2	0
Crumpy				
Chocolate Hazelnut Spread	1 tbsp (0.5 oz)	80	0	0
HEART				
beef simmered	3 oz	148	—	164
chicken simmered	1 cup (5 oz)	268	—	350
lamb braised	3 oz	158	—	212
pork braised	1 heart (4.3 oz)	191	—	285
turkey simmered	1 cup (5 oz)	257	—	327
veal braised	3 oz	158	—	150
HEARTS OF PALM				
canned	1 cup (5.1 oz)	41	—	0
canned	1 (1.2 oz)	9	—	0
HERBAL TEA				
(*see* TEA/HERBAL TEA)				
HERBS/SPICES				
(*see also individual names*)				
curry powder	1 tsp	6	—	0
poultry seasoning	1 tsp	5	—	0
pumpkin pie spice	1 tsp	6	—	0
Ac'cent				
Flavor Enhancer	½ tsp	5	0	0
Herbal All Purpose Seasoning	½ tsp	0	0	0
Golden Dipt				
All Purpose Seafood	¼ tsp	2	—	0
Blackened Redfish	¼ tsp	2	—	0
Broiled Fish	¼ tsp	2	—	0
Cajun Style Shrimp & Crab	¼ tsp	2	—	0
Lemon Pepper Seafood	¼ tsp	8	—	0
Ka-Me				
Five Spice Powder	¼ tsp (1 g)	0	0	0
Lawry's				
Seasoning Blend Sloppy Joe	1 pkg	126	1	0
McIlhenny				
Crab Boil	3 oz	378	32	4
Mrs. Dash				
Extra Spicy	⅛ tsp (0.02 oz)	2	—	0
Garlic & Herb	⅛ tsp (0.02 oz)	2	—	tr

FOOD	PORTION	CALS.	FIB.	CHOL.
Mrs. Dash (cont.)				
Lemon & Herb	⅛ tsp (0.02 oz)	2	—	0
Low Pepper No Garlic	⅛ tsp (0.02 oz)	2	—	0
Original Blend	⅛ tsp (0.02 oz)	2	—	0
Table Blend	⅛ tsp (0.02 oz)	2	—	0
Watkins				
Apple Bake Seasoning	¼ tsp (0.5 g)	0	0	0
Barbecue Spice	¼ tsp (0.5 g)	0	0	0
Bean Soup Seasoning	¾ tsp (2 g)	5	0	0
Beef Jerky Seasoning	2 tsp (6 g)	15	0	0
Chicken Seasoning	½ tsp (1 g)	0	0	0
Cole Slaw Seasoning	½ tsp (1.5 g)	5	0	0
Egg Sensations	1 tsp (3 g)	10	0	0
Fajita Seasoning	½ tsp (3 g)	10	0	0
Grill Seasoning	¼ tsp (1 g)	0	0	0
Ground Beef Seasoning	⅛ tsp (0.5 g)	0	0	0
Italian Blend	1 tsp (3 g)	1	0	0
Meat Tenderizer	⅛ tsp (0.5 g)	0	0	0
Meatloaf Seasoning	½ tsp (5 g)	15	0	0
Mexican Blend	½ tbsp (4 g)	15	0	0
Omelet & Souffle Seasoning	¾ tsp (2 g)	5	0	0
Oriental Ginger Garlic Liquid Spice Blend	1 tbsp (0.5 oz)	120	0	0
Potato Salad Seasoning	¼ tsp (1 g)	0	0	0
Pumpkin Pie Spice	¼ tsp (0.5 g)	0	0	0
Smokehouse Liquid Blend	1 tbsp (0.5 oz)	120	0	0
Soup & Vegetable Seasoning	¼ tsp (0.5 g)	0	0	0
Spanish Seasoning Blend	¼ tsp (2 g)	0	0	0
HERRING				
FRESH				
atlantic cooked	3 oz	172	—	65
atlantic cooked	1 fillet (5 oz)	290	—	110
atlantic raw	3 oz	134	—	51
pacific baked	3 oz	213	—	84
pacific fillet baked	5.1 oz	360	—	142
roe raw	3½ oz	130	—	360
READY-TO-EAT				
atlantic kippered	1 fillet (1.4 oz)	87	—	33
atlantic pickled	½ oz	39	—	2
HICKORY NUTS				
dried	1 oz	187	—	0
HOMINY				
CANNED				
canned	½ cup	57	—	0

FOOD	PORTION	CALS.	FIB.	CHOL.
Allen				
Golden	½ cup (4.5 oz)	120	4	0
Mexican	½ cup (4.5 oz)	120	3	0
White	½ cup (4.5 oz)	100	4	0
Uncle William				
Golden	½ cup (4.5 oz)	120	4	0
Mexican	½ cup (4.5 oz)	120	3	0
White	½ cup (4.5 oz)	100	4	0
Van Camp's				
Golden	½ cup (4.3 oz)	80	1	0
White	½ cup (4.3 oz)	80	1	0
HONEY				
honey	1 cup (11.9 oz)	1031	—	0
honey	1 tbsp (0.7 oz)	64	—	0
Burleson's				
Clover	1 tbsp	60	0	0
Creamed	1 tbsp	60	0	0
Natural	1 tbsp	60	0	0
Pure	1 tbsp	60	0	0
Raw	1 tbsp	60	0	0
Rocky Mountain Clover	1 tbsp	60	0	0
Golden Blossom				
Honey	1 tsp	20	—	0
Tree Of Life				
Alfalfa	1 tbsp (0.7 oz)	60	—	0
Avocado	1 tbsp (0.7 oz)	60	—	0
Buckwheat	1 tbsp (0.7 oz)	60	—	0
Clover	1 tbsp (0.7 oz)	60	—	0
Honeybear Wildflower	1 tbsp (0.7 oz)	60	—	0
Orange	1 tbsp (0.7 oz)	60	—	0
Tupelo	1 tbsp (0.7 oz)	60	—	0
Wildflower	1 tbsp (0.7 oz)	60	—	0
HONEYDEW				
FRESH				
cubed	1 cup	60	—	0
wedge	1/10	46	—	0
Chiquita				
Fresh	1 cup	70	—	0
Dole				
Honeydew	1/10	50	1	0
FROZEN				
Big Valley				
Balls	¾ cup (4.9 oz)	45	1	0

FOOD	PORTION	CALS.	FIB.	CHOL.
HORSE				
roasted	3 oz	149	—	58
HORSERADISH				
Gold's				
Hot	1 tsp	4	—	0
Red	1 tsp	4	—	0
White	1 tsp	4	—	0
Hebrew National				
White	1 tbsp	7	—	0
Heluva Good Cheese				
Horseradish	1 tsp (5 g)	0	—	0
Ka-Me				
Wasabi Powder	¼ tsp (1 g)	0	0	0
Kraft				
Cream Style	1 tsp (0.2 oz)	0	0	0
Horseradish Mustard	1 tsp (0.2 oz)	0	0	0
Prepared	1 tsp (0.2 oz)	0	0	0
Rosoff's				
Red	1 tbsp (0.5 oz)	8	—	0
White	1 tbsp (0.5 oz)	7	—	0
Sauceworks				
Horseradish	1 tsp (0.2 oz)	20	0	<5
Schorr's				
Red	1 tbsp (0.5 oz)	8	—	0
White	1 tbsp (0.5 oz)	7	—	0
HOT CAKES				
(*see* PANCAKES)				
HOT COCOA				
(*see* COCOA)				
HOT DOG				
(*see also* MEAT SUBSTITUTES, SAUSAGE, SAUSAGE SUBSTITUTES)				
CHICKEN				
chicken	1 (1.5 oz)	116	—	45
Empire				
Hot Dog	1 (2 oz)	100	0	70
Health Valley				
Weiners	1	96	0	49
Wampler Longacre				
Chicken	1 (2 oz)	130	—	65
Chicken	1 (1.6 oz)	110	—	50
MEAT				
beef	1 (2 oz)	180	—	35

FOOD	PORTION	CALS.	FIB.	CHOL.
beef	1 (1.5 oz)	142	—	27
beef & pork	1 (2 oz)	183	—	29
beef & pork	1 (1.5 oz)	144	—	22
pork cheesefurter smokie	1 (1.5 oz)	141	—	29
Armour				
Lower Salt Jumbo	1	170	—	30
Lower Salt Jumbo Beef	1	170	—	30
Star Jumbo	1	190	—	30
Star Jumbo Beef	1	190	—	30
Chefwich				
Chili Dog	5 oz	380	—	27
Healthy Choice				
Beef	1 (1.8 oz)	60	0	20
Bunsize	1 (2 oz)	70	0	20
Franks	1 (1.6 oz)	50	0	15
Jumbo	1 (2 oz)	70	0	20
Hebrew National				
Beef	1 (1.7 oz)	150	—	30
Cocktail Beef	6 (1.8 oz)	160	—	35
Dinner Beef	1 (4 oz)	350	—	75
Reduced Fat Beef	1 (1.7 oz)	120	—	25
Hormel				
Big 8	1 (2 oz)	170	0	35
Light & Lean 97	1 (1.6 oz)	45	0	15
Light & Lean 97 Beef	1 (1.6 oz)	45	—	10
Jordan's				
Healthy Trim Low Fat	1 (1.8 oz)	70	0	25
Healthy Trim Low Fat Skinless	1 (1.8 oz)	70	0	25
Nathan's				
Natural Casing Franks	1	158	—	43
Skinless Franks	1	176	—	53
Oscar Mayer				
Beef	1 (1.6 oz)	150	0	25
Big & Juicy Deli Style Beef	1 (2.7 oz)	250	0	50
Big & Juicy Hot 'N Spicy	1 (2.7 oz)	220	0	45
Big & Juicy Original	1 (2.7 oz)	240	0	45
Big & Juicy Original Beef	1 (2.7 oz)	230	0	45
Big & Juicy Quarter Pound Beef	1 (4 oz)	350	0	65
Big & Juicy Smokie Links	1 (2.7 oz)	200	0	50
Bun-Length Beef	1 (2 oz)	180	0	35
Cheese	1 (1.6 oz)	150	0	35
Free	1 (1.8 oz)	40	—	15
Healthy Favorites Turkey & Beef	1 (2 oz)	60	0	25
Light Beef	1 (2 oz)	110	0	25

FOOD	PORTION	CALS.	FIB.	CHOL.
Oscar Mayer (CONT.)				
Wieners Bun-Length Pork & Turkey	1 (2 oz)	180	0	35
Wieners Little	6 (2 oz)	170	0	35
Wieners Pork & Turkey	1 (1.6 oz)	150	0	30
Wieners Light Pork Turkey Beef	1 (2 oz)	110	0	35
Russer				
Lil'Salt Deli Franks	1 (2.67 oz)	160	—	40
Shofar				
Kosher Beef	1 (1.8 oz)	150	0	20
Kosher Beef Reduced Fat Reduced Sodium	1 (1.8 oz)	120	0	25
Wrangler				
Beef	1 (2 oz)	170	0	40
Cheese	1 (2 oz)	170	0	40
Smoked	1 (2 oz)	170	0	40
TAKE-OUT				
corndog	1	460	—	79
w/ bun chili	1	297	—	51
w/ bun plain	1	242	—	44
TURKEY				
turkey	1 (1.5 oz)	102	—	48
Empire				
Hot Dog	1 (2 oz)	90	0	35
Health Valley				
Weiners	1	96	0	35
Louis Rich				
Bun Length	1 (2 oz)	110	0	50
Turkey	1 (1.6 oz)	90	0	40
Turkey	1 (1.5 oz)	80	0	40
Turkey Cheese	1 (1.6 oz)	90	0	40
Mr. Turkey				
Bun Size	1	130	—	50
Cheese	1	140	—	50
Hot Dog	1	110	—	40
Wampler Longacre				
Turkey	1 (2 oz)	130	—	60
Turkey	1 (1.6 oz)	110	—	45
HUMMUS				
hummus	⅓ cup	140	—	0
hummus	1 cup	420	—	0
Casbah				
Mix as prep	¼ cup	120	1	0

FOOD	PORTION	CALS.	FIB.	CHOL.
Cedar's				
No Salt Added Hommus Tahini	2 tbsp (1 oz)	50	3	0

HYACINTH BEANS

dried cooked	1 cup	228	—	0

ICE CREAM AND FROZEN DESSERTS

(*see also* ICES AND ICE POPS, PUDDING POPS, SHERBET, YOGURT FROZEN)

FOOD	PORTION	CALS.	FIB.	CHOL.
chocolate	½ cup (4 fl oz)	143	—	22
dixie cup chocolate	1 (3.5 fl oz)	125	—	20
dixie cup strawberry	1 (3.5 fl oz)	112	—	17
dixie cup vanilla	1 (3.5 fl oz)	116	—	25
freeze dried ice cream chocolate strawberry & vanilla	1 pkg (0.75 oz)	158	1	1
french vanilla soft serve	½ gal	3014	—	1226
french vanilla soft serve	½ cup (4 fl oz)	185	—	78
strawberry	½ cup (4 fl oz)	127	—	19
vanilla	½ cup (4 fl oz)	132	—	29
vanilla light	½ cup (2.3 oz)	92	—	9
vanilla rich	½ cup (2.6 oz)	178	—	45
vanilla soft serve	½ cup	111	—	10
vanilla 10% fat	½ gal	2153	—	476
vanilla 16% fat	½ gal	2805	—	256
vanilla light	½ gal	1469	—	146
vanilla light	1 cup	184	—	18
vanilla light soft serve	½ gal	1787	—	106
vanilla light soft serve	1 cup	223	—	13
3 Musketeers				
Single Chocolate	1 (2 fl oz)	160	0	20
Single Vanilla	1 (2 fl oz)	160	0	15
Snack Chocolate	1 (0.72 fl oz)	60	0	5
Snack Vanilla	1 (0.72 fl oz)	60	0	5
Avari				
Creme Glace All Flavors	1 oz	10	—	0
Ben & Jerry's				
Banana Walnut	½ cup (3.9 oz)	290	1	75
Butter Pecan	½ cup (3.9 oz)	310	1	100
Cherry Garcia	½ cup (3.7 oz)	240	0	80
Cherry Vanilla	½ cup (3.9 oz)	240	0	85
Chocolate Chip Cookie Dough	½ cup (3.7 oz)	270	0	80
Chocolate Fudge Brownie	½ cup (3.7 oz)	250	2	50
Chunky Monkey	½ cup (3.7 oz)	280	1	70
Coconut Almond	½ cup (3.7 oz)	260	1	80
Coconut Almond Fudge Chip	½ cup (3.8 oz)	320	2	75
Coffee Almond Fudge	½ cup (3.7 oz)	290	2	75

FOOD	PORTION	CALS.	FIB.	CHOL.
Ben & Jerry's (CONT.)				
Coffee Toffee Crunch	½ cup (3.7 oz)	280	0	80
English Toffee Crunch	½ cup (4 oz)	310	0	90
Mint Chocolate Cookie	½ cup (3.8 oz)	260	1	80
New York Super Fudge Chunk	½ cup (3.7 oz)	290	2	50
No Fat Strawberry	½ cup (3.3 oz)	140	0	0
No Fat Vanilla Fudge Swirl	½ cup (3.1 oz)	150	0	0
Peanut Butter Cup	½ cup (4.1 oz)	370	2	75
Pop Chocolate Chip Cookie Dough	1 (4.1 oz)	450	1	60
Pop English Toffee Crunch	1 (3.7 oz)	340	0	75
Pop Vanilla	1 (3.9 oz)	360	0	75
Rain Forest Crunch	½ cup (3.7 oz)	300	0	85
Smooth Aztec Harvest Coffee	½ cup (3.8 oz)	230	0	90
Smooth Deep Dark Chocolate	½ cup (3.9 oz)	260	2	55
Smooth Double Chocolate Fudge	½ cup (4.1 oz)	280	3	55
Smooth Mocho Fudge	½ cup (4 oz)	270	1	85
Smooth Vanilla	½ cup (3.8 oz)	230	0	95
Smooth Vanilla Bean	½ cup (3.8 oz)	230	0	95
Smooth Vanilla Caramel Fudge	½ cup (4.1 oz)	280	1	95
Smooth White Russian	½ cup (3.8 oz)	240	0	90
Vanilla	½ cup (3.7 oz)	230	0	95
Wavy Gravy	½ cup (4.1 oz)	330	2	80
Bon Bons				
Vanilla With Milk Chocolate Coating	8 pieces	330	0	20
Vanilla With Milk Chocolate Coating	5 pieces	200	0	10
Borden				
Fat Free Black Cherry	½ cup	90	—	0
Fat Free Chocolate	½ cup	100	—	0
Fat Free Peach	½ cup	90	—	0
Fat Free Strawberry	½ cup	90	—	0
Fat Free Vanilla	½ cup	90	—	0
Bounty				
Cherry/Dark	1 (0.84 fl oz)	70	0	5
Coconut/Dark	1 (0.84 fl oz)	70	0	5
Coconut/Milk	1 (0.84 fl oz)	70	0	5
Bresler's				
All Flavors Ice Cream	3.5 oz	230	—	36
All Flavors Royale Cremes	4 oz	260	—	48
All Flavors Royale Lites	4 oz	217	—	0

FOOD	PORTION	CALS.	FIB.	CHOL.
Breyers				
Bar Vanilla	1 (2.7 oz)	250	tr	50
Bar Vanilla Carmel w/ Chocolate Brittle Coating	1 (2.7 oz)	260	0	45
Bar Vanilla With Chocolate Coating	1 (2.6 oz)	230	0	50
Butter Almond	½ cup	170	0	35
Butter Pecan	½ cup (2.6 oz)	180	0	35
Cherry Vanilla	½ cup	150	0	30
Chocolate	½ cup (2.6 oz)	160	1	30
Chocolate Chip	½ cup (2.5 oz)	170	0	35
Chocolate Chip Cookie Dough	½ cup (2.5 oz)	190	0	40
Chocolate Chocolate Chip	½ cup (2.5 oz)	180	1	25
Chocolate Peanut Butter Twirl	½ cup (2.6 oz)	220	1	25
Coffee	½ cup (2.6 oz)	150	0	35
Cookies n'Cream	½ cup (2.6 oz)	170	0	30
Deluxe Rocky Road	½ cup (2.5 oz)	190	1	25
French Vanilla	(2.5 oz)	170	0	105
Light Brownie Marble Fudge	½ cup (2.6 oz)	150	tr	30
Light Chocolate	½ cup (2.4 oz)	130	tr	30
Light Chocolate Fudge Twirl	½ cup (2.6 oz)	140	1	25
Light Heavenly Hash	½ cup (2.4 oz)	150	tr	25
Light Rocky Road Deluxe	½ cup (2.4 oz)	150	tr	25
Light Strawberry	½ cup (2.4 oz)	120	0	30
Light Toffee Fudge Parfait	½ cup (2.6 oz)	150	tr	35
Light Vanilla	½ cup (2.4 oz)	130	0	35
Light Vanilla Chocolate Strawberry	½ cup (2.4 oz)	120	0	30
Mint Chocolate Chip	½ cup (2.6 oz)	170	0	35
Mocha Almond Fudge	½ cup (2.7 oz)	190	1	30
Peach	½ cup (2.6 oz)	130	0	25
Reduced Fat Chocolate Chocolate Chip	½ cup (2.4 oz)	150	tr	25
Reduced Fat Heavenly Hash	½ cup (2.4 oz)	150	tr	25
Reduced Fat Mocha Almond Fudge	½ cup (2.5 oz)	160	tr	30
Reduced Fat Praline Almond Crunch	½ cup (2.4 oz)	140	tr	35
Reduced Fat Swiss Almond Fudge Twirl	½ cup (2.5 oz)	160	tr	30
Sandwich Vanilla	1 (2.8 oz)	250	1	25
Strawberry	½ cup (2.6 oz)	130	0	25
Toffee Bar Crunch	½ cup (2.5 oz)	180	0	40
Vanilla	½ cup (2.6 oz)	150	0	35

FOOD	PORTION	CALS.	FIB.	CHOL.
Breyers (CONT.)				
Vanilla Caramel Praline	½ cup (2.6 oz)	190	0	35
Vanilla Chocolate	½ cup (2.5 oz)	160	0	35
Vanilla Chocolate Strawberry	½ cup (2.5 oz)	150	0	30
Vanilla Fudge Twirl	½ cup (2.6 oz)	160	tr	35
Vanilla Peanut Butter Fudge Sundae	½ cup (2.5 oz)	170	0	35
Butterfinger				
Bar	1 (2.5 oz)	170	0	15
Nuggets	8	340	0	20
Carnation				
Berry Swirl Bar Raspberry	1 bar	70	—	10
Berry Swirl Bar Strawberry	1 bar	70	—	9
Cheesecake Bar Original	1 bar	120	—	12
Cheesecake Bar Strawberry	1 bar	125	—	10
Chocolate Malted Bar	1 bar	70	—	19
Creamy Lites Bar Chocolate	1 bar	50	—	8
Creamy Lites Bar Strawberry	1 bar	50	—	7
Sundae Cup Strawberry	1 (3.3 oz)	200	0	30
Cool 'N Creamy				
Amarello With Chocolate Swirl	1 bar	62	—	1
Chocolate Vanilla	1 bar	54	—	1
Double Chocolate Fudge	1 bar	55	—	1
Orange Vanilla	1 bar	31	—	tr
Cool Creations				
Cookies & Cream Sandwich	1 (3.5 oz)	240	1	15
Mini Sandwich	1 (2.3 oz)	110	0	10
DoveBar				
Almond	1 (3.67 fl oz)	335	0	35
Bite Size Almond Praline	1 (0.75 fl oz)	80	0	7
Bite Size Cherry Royale	1 (0.75 fl oz)	70	0	8
Bite Size Classic Vanilla	1 (0.75 fl oz)	70	0	8
Bite Size French Vanilla	1 (0.75 fl oz)	70	0	15
Bite Size Mint Supreme	1 (0.75 fl oz)	80	0	7
Caramel Pecan	1 (3.67 fl oz)	350	0	35
Chocolate Milk Chocolate	1 (3.8 fl oz)	340	0	40
Coffee Cashew	1 (3.67 fl oz)	335	0	35
Crunchy Cookie	1 (3.8 fl oz)	340	0	40
Peanut	1 (3.8 fl oz)	380	0	40
Single Vanilla/Dark	1 (2 fl oz)	200	0	20
Vanilla Dark Chocolate	1 (3.8 fl oz)	340	0	45
Vanilla Milk Chocolate	1 (3.8 fl oz)	340	0	40
Drumstick				
Cone Chocolate	1 (4.6 oz)	340	2	25

FOOD	PORTION	CALS.	FIB.	CHOL.
Drumstick (CONT.)				
Cone Chocolate Dipped	1 (4.6 oz)	340	1	25
Cone Vanilla	1 (4.6 oz)	350	2	20
Cone Vanilla Caramel	1 (4.6 oz)	360	6	25
Cone Vanilla Fudge	1 (4.6 oz)	370	2	20
Edy's				
American Dream Chocolate	3 oz	90	—	0
American Dream Chocolate Chip	3 oz	100	—	0
American Dream Cookies'N'Cream	3 oz	100	—	0
American Dream Mocha Almond Fudge	3 oz	110	—	0
American Dream Rocky Road	3 oz	110	—	0
American Dream Strawberry	3 oz	70	—	0
American Dream Toasted Almond	3 oz	110	—	0
American Dream Vanilla	3 oz	80	—	0
American Dream Vanilla Chocolate Strawberry	3 oz	80	—	0
Light Almond Praline	4 oz	140	—	15
Light Banana-Politan	4 oz	110	—	15
Light Butter Pecan	4 oz	140	—	15
Light Cafe Au Lait	4 oz	110	—	15
Light Candy Bar	4 oz	140	—	15
Light Chocolate Chip	4 oz	120	—	15
Light Chocolate Fudge Mousse	4 oz	130	—	15
Light Cookies'N'Cream	4 oz	120	—	15
Light Dreamy Caramel Cream	4 oz	140	—	15
Light Malt Ball 'N' Fudge	4 oz	140	—	15
Light Marble Fudge	4 oz	120	—	15
Light Mocha Almond Fudge	4 oz	140	—	15
Light Peanut Butter & Chocolate	4 oz	130	—	15
Light Raspberry Truffle	4 oz	110	—	15
Light Rocky Road	4 oz	130	—	15
Light Strawberry	4 oz	110	—	15
Light Vanilla	4 oz	100	—	15
Vanilla Chocolate Strawberry	4 oz	110	—	15
Flintstones				
Cool Cream	1 (2.75 oz)	90	0	5
Push-Up	1 (2.75 oz)	100	0	5
Friendly's				
Black Raspberry	½ cup	150	0	30

FOOD	PORTION	CALS.	FIB.	CHOL.
Friendly's (CONT.)				
Chocolate Almond Chip	½ cup	170	0	35
Forbidden Chocolate	½ cup	150	0	30
Fudge Nut Brownie	½ cup	200	0	25
Heath English Toffee	½ cup (2.7 oz)	190	0	30
Purely Pistachio	½ cup	160	0	35
Vanilla	½ cup	150	0	35
Vanilla Chocolate Strawberry	½ cup	150	tr	30
Vienna Mocha Chunk	½ cup	180	0	30
Frusen Gladje				
Butter Pecan	½ cup	280	—	60
Chocolate	½ cup	240	—	75
Chocolate Chocolate Chip	½ cup	270	—	55
Strawberry	½ cup	230	—	65
Swiss Chocolate Candy Almond	½ cup	270	—	55
Vanilla	½ cup	230	—	65
Vanilla Swiss Almond	½ cup	270	—	60
Good Humor				
Banana Bob	1 (3 fl oz)	155	0	5
Bar Classic Toasted Almond	1 (3.1 fl oz)	170	1	10
Bar Classic Vanilla	1 (3.1 fl oz)	190	0	15
Bar Classic Almond	1 (3.1 fl oz)	210	1	15
Bar Sidewalk Sundae	1	280	2	15
Bubble O'Bill	1 (3.6 fl oz)	170	1	15
Chip Burrrger	1 (4.7 oz)	320	1	20
Chip Sandwich	1 (4.7 fl oz)	320	1	20
Choco Taco	1 (4.4 fl oz)	320	1	20
Chocolate Eclair Classic	1 (3.1 fl oz)	170	1	15
Classic Candy Center Crunch Vanilla	1	280	0	15
Colonel Crunch Chocolate	1 (3.1 oz)	160	1	10
Colonel Crunch Strawberry	1 (3.1 oz)	170	0	10
Combo Cup	1 (6.2 fl oz)	200	1	35
Cone Olde Nut Sundae	1 (3.9 oz)	230	2	5
Cone Sidewalk Sundae	1 (4.2 oz)	270	1	10
Creamee Burrrger	1 (4.7 oz)	310	1	20
Crunch Classic Candy Center	1 (3.1 fl oz)	260	1	10
Far Frog	1 (3.6 fl oz)	150	1	20
Fun Box Ice Cream Sandwich	1 (3.1 fl oz)	160	1	10
King Cone	1 (5.7 fl oz)	300	2	25
King Cone Classic Vanilla	1 (4.8 oz)	300	1	20
King Cone Strawberry	1 (5.7 oz)	250	1	25
Light Chocolate Chocolate Chip	½ cup (2.4 oz)	130	tr	10
Light Chocolate Chip	½ cup (2.4 oz)	130	0	10

FOOD	PORTION	CALS.	FIB.	CHOL.
Good Humor (CONT.)				
Light Coffee	½ cup (2.4 oz)	110	0	15
Light Cookies N'Cream	½ cup (2.4 oz)	130	0	10
Light Heavenly Hash	½ cup (2.4 oz)	140	tr	10
Light Praline Almond Crunch	½ cup (2.4 oz)	130	0	15
Light Toffee Bar Crunch	½ cup (2.4 oz)	130	0	15
Light Vanilla	½ cup (2.4 oz)	110	0	15
Light Vanilla Chocolate Strawberry	½ cup (2.4 oz)	110	0	10
Light Vanilla Fudge	½ cup (2.6 oz)	120	0	15
Magnum Almond	1 (4.2 fl oz)	270	5	30
Magnum Chocolate	1 (4.2 fl oz)	260	2	30
Number One Bar	1 (4.1 fl oz)	190	1	15
Popsicle Ice Cream Bar	1 (3.1 fl oz)	160	1	15
Popsicle Ice Cream Sandwich	1 (3.6 fl oz)	190	1	15
Sandwich Classic Chip Cookie	1 (4.1 fl oz)	300	1	18
Sandwich Giant Neapolitan	1 (5.2 fl oz)	260	1	20
Sandwich Giant Vanilla	1 (5.2 fl oz)	240	1	20
Sandwich Ice Cream	1	190	1	15
Sandwich Sidewalk Sundae	1 (3.1 oz)	160	1	10
Sandwich Sprinkle	1 (3.1 fl oz)	180	1	10
Strawberry Shortcake Bar Classic	1 (3.1 fl oz)	160	1	10
Sundae Twist Cup	1	160	0	10
Toffee Taco	1 (4.4 fl oz)	300	1	15
Viennetta Chocolate	1 (4.2 fl oz)	160	1	10
Viennetta Vanilla	1 (4.2 fl oz)	160	0	20
WWF Bar	1 (3.7 fl oz)	200	1	15
X-Men Bar	1 (3 fl oz)	150	0	15
Haagen-Dazs				
Baileys Original Irish Cream	½ cup (3.6 oz)	280	0	110
Brownies A La Mode	½ cup (3.7 oz)	280	0	100
Butter Pecan	½ cup (3.7 oz)	320	tr	105
Cappuccino Commotion	½ cup (3.6 oz)	310	1	100
Caramel Cone Explosion	½ cup (3.6 oz)	310	tr	95
Chocolate	½ cup (3.7 oz)	270	1	115
Chocolate Chocolate Chip	½ cup (3.7 oz)	300	2	100
Coffee	½ cup (3.7 oz)	270	0	120
Cookie Dough Dynamo	½ cup (3.6 oz)	300	0	95
Cookies & Cream	½ cup (3.6 oz)	270	0	110
DiSaronno Amaretto	½ cup (3.6 oz)	260	0	95
Macadamia Brittle	½ cup (3.7 oz)	300	0	110
Multi Pack Bars Caramel Cone Explosion	1 (3.1 oz)	330	tr	60

FOOD	PORTION	CALS.	FIB.	CHOL.
Haagen-Dazs (CONT.)				
Multi Pack Bars Chocolate & Dark Chocolate	1 (3.2 oz)	320	3	70
Multi Pack Bars Coffee & Almond Crunch	1 (3 oz)	290	tr	80
Multi Pack Bars Iced Cappuccino Explosion	1 (2.9 oz)	290	tr	70
Multi Pack Bars Triple Brownie Overload	1 (3 oz)	320	1	80
Multi Pack Bars Vanilla & Almonds	1 (3 oz)	300	1	70
Multi Pack Bars Vanilla & Dark Chocolate	1 (3.2 oz)	320	4	70
Multi Pack Bars Vanilla & Milk Chocolate	1 (3 oz)	280	0	75
Peanut Butter Burst	½ cup (3.6 oz)	330	1	95
Rum Raisin	½ cup (3.7 oz)	270	0	110
Single Pack Bars Caramel Cone Explosion	1 (3.3 oz)	350	tr	65
Single Pack Bars Chocolate & Dark Chocolate	1 (3.9 oz)	400	4	85
Single Pack Bars Coffee & Almond Crunch	1 (3.7 oz)	360	1	100
Single Pack Bars Cookie Dough Dynamo	1 (3.5 oz)	380	1	65
Single Pack Bars Iced Cappuccino	1 (3.4 oz)	330	tr	80
Single Pack Bars Triple Brownie Overload	1 (3.5 oz)	380	1	95
Single Pack Bars Vanilla & Almonds	1 (3.7 oz)	370	1	90
Single Pack Bars Vanilla & Dark Chocolate	1 (3.9 oz)	400	4	85
Single Pack Bars Vanilla & Milk Chocolate	1 (3.5 oz)	330	tr	90
Strawberry	½ cup (3.7 oz)	250	tr	95
Strawberry Cheesecake Craze	½ cup (3.7 oz)	290	tr	100
Triple Brownie Overload	½ cup (3.5 oz)	300	0	90
Vanilla	½ cup (3.7 oz)	270	0	120
Vanilla Fudge	½ cup (3.7 oz)	280	0	105
Vanilla Swiss Almond	½ cup (3.7 oz)	310	1	105
Healthy Choice				
Black Forest	½ cup (2.5 oz)	120	1	5
Bordeaux Cherry Chocolate Chip	½ cup (2.5 oz)	110	tr	<5

FOOD	PORTION	CALS.	FIB.	CHOL.
Healthy Choice (CONT.)				
Butter Pecan Crunch	½ cup (2.5 oz)	120	1	<5
Cappuccino Chocolate Chunk	½ cup (2.5 oz)	120	1	10
Cookies 'N Cream	½ cup (2.5 oz)	120	tr	<5
Double Fudge Swirl	½ cup (2.5 oz)	120	1	<5
Fudge Brownie	½ cup (2.5 oz)	120	2	5
Malt Caramel Cone	½ cup (2.5 oz)	120	1	10
Mint Chocolate Chip	½ cup (2.5 oz)	120	tr	<5
Peanut Butter Cookie Dough 'N Fudge	½ cup (2.5 oz)	120	tr	<5
Praline & Caramel	½ cup (2.5 oz)	130	tr	<5
Rocky Road	½ cup (2.5 oz)	140	2	<5
Vanilla	½ cup	100	1	5
Heath				
Bar	1 (2.5 oz)	160	0	15
Nuggets	8	180	0	25
Heaven				
Sundae Bars Chocolate Fudge	1 bar	150	—	7
Sundae Bars Vanilla Fudge	1 bar	150	—	7
Vanilla Caramel Nut	1 bar	225	—	9
Vanilla Nut Fudge	1 bar	222	—	9
Hood				
Bar Orange Cream	1 bar (1.8 oz)	90	0	5
Bar Vanilla	1 bar (1.6 oz)	160	0	15
Caramel Butterscotch Blast	½ cup (2.3 oz)	160	0	25
Chocolate	½ cup (2.3 oz)	140	0	30
Chocolate Chip	½ cup (2.3 oz)	160	0	30
Chocolate Eclair	1 bar (1.6 oz)	150	0	5
Christmas Tree	½ cup (2.3 oz)	140	0	30
Coffee	½ cup (2.3 oz)	140	0	30
Cookie Dough Delight	½ cup (2.3 oz)	160	0	30
Cookies N Cream	½ cup (2.3 oz)	160	0	30
Cooler Cups	1 (2.1 oz)	80	0	<5
Crispy Bar	1 (1.9 oz)	180	0	20
Egg Nog	½ cup (2.3 oz)	130	0	25
Fabulous Fudge & Peanut Butter Swirled Fudge Bars	1 bar (2.1 oz)	110	0	10
Fabulous Fudgies Assorted Bars	1 bar (2.1 oz)	100	0	10
Fat Free Chocolate Passion	½ cup (2.5 oz)	100	0	0
Fat Free Classic Harlequin	½ cup (2.5 oz)	100	0	0
Fat Free Double Brownie Sundae	½ cup (2.5 oz)	120	0	0
Fat Free Heavenly Hash	½ cup (2.5 oz)	120	0	0

FOOD	PORTION	CALS.	FIB.	CHOL.
Hood (CONT.)				
Fat Free Mississippi Mud Pie	½ cup (2.5 oz)	130	0	0
Fat Free Praline Pecan Delight	½ cup (2.5 oz)	120	0	0
Fat Free Raspberry Blush	½ cup (2.5 oz)	120	0	0
Fat Free Super Strawberry Swirl	½ cup (2.5 oz)	100	0	0
Fat Free Vanilla Fudge Twist	½ cup (2.5 oz)	120	0	0
Fat Free Very Vanilla	½ cup (2.5 oz)	100	0	0
Fudge Bars	1 bar (2.7 oz)	100	0	0
Grasshopper Pie	½ cup (2.3 oz)	160	0	25
Heavenly Hash	½ cup (2.3 oz)	140	0	20
Hendrie's Cherry Chocolate Dips	1 bar (1.3 oz)	120	0	15
Hoodsie Cup Vanilla & Chocolate	1 (1.7 oz)	100	0	20
Light Almond Praline Delight	½ cup (2.4 oz)	110	0	15
Light Brownie Nut Sundae	½ cup (2.4 oz)	140	0	10
Light Caribbean Coffee Royale	½ cup (2.4 oz)	110	0	15
Light Chocolate Almond Chip Sundae	½ cup (2.4 oz)	140	0	10
Light Chocolate Chocolate Chip Cookie Dough	½ cup (2.4 oz)	140	0	15
Light Cookies N Cream	½ cup (2.4 oz)	130	0	15
Light Heath Toffee Chunk Swirl	½ cup (2.4 oz)	140	0	15
Light Heavenly Hash	½ cup (2.4 oz)	130	0	10
Light Maple Sugar Shack	⅓ cup (2.4 oz)	130	0	10
Light Massachusetts Mud Pie	½ cup (2.4 oz)	140	0	10
Light Raspberry Swirl	½ cup (2.4 oz)	120	0	10
Light Strawberry Supreme	½ cup (2.4 oz)	110	0	15
Light Triple Nut Cluster Sundae	½ cup (2.4 oz)	140	0	10
Light Vanilla	½ cup (2.4 oz)	110	0	15
Light Vanilla Chocolate Strawberry	½ cup (2.4 oz)	110	0	15
Low Fat No Sugar Added Caramel Swirl	½ cup (2.4 oz)	120	0	10
Low Fat No Sugar Added Chocolate Supreme	½ cup (2.4 oz)	120	0	10
Low Fat No Sugar Added Mocha Fudge	½ cup (2.4 oz)	110	0	10
Low Fat No Sugar Added Raspberry Swirl	½ cup (2.4 oz)	110	0	10
Low Fat No Sugar Added Vanilla	½ cup (2.4 oz)	100	0	10
Maple Walnut	½ cup (2.3 oz)	160	0	30
Rockets	1 (2 oz)	120	1	20

FOOD	PORTION	CALS.	FIB.	CHOL.
Hood (CONT.)				
Sandwich Light	1 (2.2 oz)	160	1	10
Sandwich Vanilla	1 (2.2 oz)	180	1	20
Sports Bar	1 (2.9 oz)	250	0	25
Spumoni	½ cup (2.3 oz)	140	0	30
Strawberry	½ cup (2.3 oz)	130	0	30
Super Sortment Chocolate & Banana Fudge Bar	1 bar (2.1 oz)	100	0	10
Super Sortment Root Beer Float & Orange Cream Bar	1 bar (1.5 oz)	70	0	10
Vanilla	½ cup (2.3 oz)	140	0	30
Vanilla Chocolate Patchwork	½ cup (2.3 oz)	140	0	30
Vanilla Chocolate Strawberry	½ cup (2.3 oz)	140	0	30
Vanilla Fudge	½ cup (2.3 oz)	140	0	25
Klondike				
Almond Bar	1 (5.2 fl oz)	310	3	25
Caramel Crunch	1 (5.2 fl oz)	300	tr	30
Chocolate Chocolate Bar	1 (5.2 fl oz)	280	tr	20
Coffee Bar	1 (5.2 fl oz)	290	0	15
Dark Chocolate Bar	1 (5.2 fl oz)	290	tr	30
Gold Bar	1 (5.2 fl oz)	340	1	34
Krispy Bar	1 (5.2 fl oz)	300	0	25
Krunch	1 (3.1 fl oz)	200	1	20
Lite Bar	1 (2.3 fl oz)	110	1	5
Lite Bar Caramel	1 (2.4 fl oz)	120	1	5
Movie Bites Chocolate	8 pieces (4.6 fl oz)	340	1	25
Movie Bites Vanilla	8 pieces (4.6 fl oz)	320	1	25
Original Bar	1 (5.2 fl oz)	290	0	15
Sandwich Chocolate	1 (5.2 fl oz)	270	2	20
Sandwich Lite	1 (2.9 fl oz)	100	1	5
Sandwich Vanilla	1 (5.2 fl oz)	250	1	20
Mars				
Almond Bar	1 (1.85 fl oz)	210	0	15
Milky Way				
Single Chocolate/Milk	1 (2 fl oz)	210	0	20
Snack Chocolate/Milk	1 (0.72 fl oz)	70	0	5
Snack Vanilla/Dark	1 (0.72 fl oz)	70	0	5
Mocha Mix				
Berry Berry Berry	½ cup	140	0	0
Dutch Chocolate	½ cup (2.3 oz)	140	0	0
Mocha Almond Fudge	½ cup (2.3 oz)	150	0	0
Neapolitan	½ cup (2.3 oz)	140	0	0
Strawberry Swirl	½ cup (2.3 oz)	140	0	0
Vanilla	½ cup (2.3 oz)	140	0	0

FOOD	PORTION	CALS.	FIB.	CHOL.
Nestle Crunch				
Chocolate	1 bar (3 oz)	200	0	15
Cones	1 (4.6 oz)	300	2	25
Crunch King	1 (4 oz)	270	0	20
Nuggets	8 pieces	140	0	10
Reduced Fat	1 (2.5 oz)	130	0	5
Vanilla	1 bar (3 oz)	200	0	15
Rice Dream				
Bar Chocolate	1	270	—	0
Bar Chocolate Nutty	1	330	—	0
Bar Strawberry	1	260	—	0
Bar Vanilla	1	275	—	0
Bar Vanilla Nutty	1	330	—	0
Cappuccino	½ cup	130	—	0
Carob	½ cup	130	—	0
Carob Almond	½ cup	140	—	0
Carob Chip	½ cup	140	—	0
Carob Chip Mint	½ cup	140	—	0
Cocoa Marble Fudge	½ cup	140	—	0
Dream Pie Chocolate	1	380	—	0
Dream Pie Mint	1	380	—	0
Dream Pie Mocha	1	380	—	0
Dream Pie Vanilla	1	380	—	0
Lemon	½ cup	130	—	0
Peanut Butter Fudge	½ cup	160	—	0
Strawberry	½ cup	130	—	0
Vanilla	½ cup	130	—	0
Vanilla Fudge	½ cup	140	—	0
Vanilla Swiss Almond	½ cup	140	—	0
Wildberry	½ cup	130	—	0
Sealtest				
American Glory	½ cup (2.4 oz)	130	0	25
Butter Pecan	½ cup (2.4 oz)	160	0	30
Candy Cane Crunch	½ cup (2.4 oz)	150	0	25
Chocolate	½ cup (2.4 oz)	140	0	25
Chocolate Butter Pecan	½ cup (2.4 oz)	150	0	30
Chocolate Chip	½ cup (2.4 oz)	150	0	30
Coconut Chocolate	½ cup (2.4 oz)	160	tr	25
Coffee	½ cup (2.4 oz)	140	0	30
Cupid's Scoops	½ cup (2.5 oz)	140	0	25
Dessert Bar Free Chocolate Fudge	1	90	—	0
Dessert Bar Free Vanilla Strawberry Swirl	1	80	—	0

FOOD	PORTION	CALS.	FIB.	CHOL.
Sealtest (CONT.)				
Dessert Bar Free Vanilla Fudge	1	80	—	0
Free Black Cherry	½ cup	100	—	0
Free Chocolate	½ cup	100	—	0
Free Peach	½ cup	100	—	0
Free Strawberry	½ cup	100	—	0
Free Vanilla	½ cup	100	—	0
Free Vanilla Fudge Royale	½ cup	100	—	0
Free Vanilla Strawberry Royale	½ cup	100	—	0
French Vanilla	½ cup (2.4 oz)	140	0	60
Fudge Royale	½ cup (2.5 oz)	150	0	25
Heavenly Hash	½ cup (2.4 oz)	150	tr	25
Maple Walnut	½ cup (2.4 oz)	160	0	30
Strawberry	½ cup (2.4 oz)	130	0	25
Triple Chocolate Passion	½ cup (2.5 oz)	160	tr	25
Vanilla	½ cup (2.4 oz)	140	0	30
Vanilla Chocolate Strawberry	½ cup (2.4 oz)	140	0	25
Vanilla With Orange Sherbet	½ cup (2.7 oz)	130	0	20
Simple Pleasures				
Chocolate	4 oz	140	—	10
Chocolate Caramel Sundae Light	4 oz	90	—	15
Chocolate Chip	4 oz	150	—	15
Chocolate Light	4 oz	80	—	15
Coffee	4 oz	120	—	15
Cookies n' Cream	4 oz	150	—	10
Mint Chocolate Chip	4 oz	150	—	5
Peach	4 oz	120	—	10
Pecan Praline	4 oz	140	—	5
Rum Raisin	4 oz	130	—	15
Strawberry	4 oz	120	—	10
Toffee Crunch	4 oz	130	—	10
Vanilla	4 oz	120	—	15
Vanilla Fudge Swirl Light	4 oz	90	—	15
Vanilla Light	4 oz	80	—	15
Snickers				
Single	1 (2 fl oz)	220	0	15
Snack	1 (1 fl oz)	110	0	5
Starbucks				
Frappuccino	1 bar (2.8 oz)	110	0	10
Tofu Ice Creme				
Carob	4 fl oz	190	—	0
Vanilla	4 fl oz	190	—	0

FOOD	PORTION	CALS.	FIB.	CHOL.
Tofutti				
Frutti Vanilla Apple Orchard	4 fl oz	100	—	0
Turkey Hill				
Black Cherry	½ cup (2.3 oz)	140	0	25
Butter Pecan	½ cup (2.3 oz)	170	0	30
Choco Mint Chip	½ cup (2.3 oz)	160	0	30
Cookies 'N Cream	½ cup (2.3 oz)	160	0	30
Lite Butter Pecan	½ cup (2.3 oz)	130	0	15
Lite Choco Mint Chip	½ cup (2.3 oz)	140	0	15
Lite Cookies 'N Cream	½ cup (2.3 oz)	130	0	15
Lite Vanilla & Chocolate	½ cup (2.3 oz)	110	0	15
Lite Vanilla Bean	½ cup (2.3 oz)	110	0	15
Neapolitan	½ cup (2.3 oz)	150	0	30
Rocky Road	½ cup (2.3 oz)	170	0	30
Tin Roof Sundae	½ cup (2.3 oz)	160	0	30
Vanilla	½ cup (2.3 oz)	140	0	30
Vanilla & Chocolate	½ cup (2.3 oz)	150	0	30
Vanilla Bean	½ cup (2.3 oz)	140	0	30
Ultra Slim-Fast				
Bar Fudge	1	90	2	0
Bar Vanilla Cookie Crunch	1	90	1	0
Chocolate	4 oz	100	2	0
Chocolate Fudge	4 oz	120	2	0
Peach	4 oz	100	2	0
Pralines & Caramel	4 oz	120	2	0
Sandwich Vanilla	1	140	1	0
Sandwich Vanilla Chocolate	1	140	1	0
Sandwich Vanilla Oatmeal	1	150	3	0
Vanilla	4 oz	90	2	0
Vanilla Fudge Cookie	4 oz	110	2	0
Weight Watchers				
Artic D'Lites	1 bar	130	0	5
Berries 'n Creme Mousse	2 bars	70	1	0
Caramel Nut Bars	1 bar	130	0	5
Chocolate Chip Cookie Dough Sundae	1 (5.43 oz)	180	2	5
Chocolate Dip	1 bar	100	0	5
Chocolate Mousse Bar	2 bars	70	4	5
Chocolate Treat	1 bar	100	1	10
Crispy Pralines 'n Creme Bars	1 bar	130	0	5
English Toffee Crunch Bars	1 bar	120	0	5
Light Cookie Dough Craze	½ cup	140	1	5
Oh! So Very Vanilla!	½ cup	120	1	5
Orange Vanilla Treat	2 bars	70	3	5

FOOD	PORTION	CALS.	FIB.	CHOL.
Weight Watchers (CONT.)				
Positively Praline Crunch	½ cup	140	0	5
Praline Toffee Crunch Parfait	1 (5.1 oz)	190	2	5
Reckless Rocky Road	½ cup	140	1	5
Triple Chocolate Tornado	½ cup	150	1	5
Vanilla Sandwich	1 bar	160	1	5
TAKE-OUT				
cone vanilla light soft serve	1 (4.6 oz)	164	—	28
gelato chocolate hazelnut	½ cup (5.3 oz)	370	2	92
gelato vanilla	½ cup (3 oz)	211	0	151
sundae caramel	1 (5.4 oz)	303	—	25
sundae hot fudge	1 (5.4 oz)	284	—	21
sundae strawberry	1 (5.4 oz)	269	—	21

ICE CREAM CONES AND CUPS

FOOD	PORTION	CALS.	FIB.	CHOL.
sugar cone	1	40	tr	0
wafer cone	1	17	tr	0
Comet				
Cups	1 (5 g)	20	tr	0
Sugar Cones	1 (12 g)	50	tr	0
Waffle Cone	1 (17 g)	70	1	0
Dutch Mill				
Chocolate Covered Wafer Cups	1 (0.5 oz)	80	0	0
Keebler				
Sugar Cones	1	45	—	0
Vanilla Cups	1	15	—	0
Oreo				
Chocolate Cones	1 (13 g)	50	tr	0
Teddy Grahams				
Cinnamon Cones	1 (0.5 oz)	60	tr	0

ICE CREAM TOPPINGS
(*see also* SYRUP)

FOOD	PORTION	CALS.	FIB.	CHOL.
marshmallow cream	1 jar (7 oz)	615	—	0
marshmallow cream	1 oz	88	—	0
pineapple	2 tbsp (1.5 oz)	106	—	0
pineapple	1 cup (11.5 oz)	861	—	0
strawberry	2 tbsp (1.5 oz)	107	—	0
strawberry	1 cup (11.5 oz)	863	—	0
walnuts in syrup	2 tbsp (1.4 oz)	167	—	0
Ben & Jerry's				
Hot Fudge	(1.3 oz)	140	2	10
Crumpy				
Chocolate Hazelnut Spread	1 tbsp (0.5 oz)	80	0	0

FOOD	PORTION	CALS.	FIB.	CHOL.
Hershey				
Chocolate Fudge	2 tbsp	100	—	5
Chocolate Shoppe Candy Bar Sprinkles York	2 tbsp (1.1 oz)	170	2	<5
Kraft				
Butterscotch	2 tbsp (1.4 oz)	130	0	<5
Caramel	2 tbsp (1.4 oz)	120	0	0
Chocolate	2 tbsp (1.4 oz)	110	1	0
Hot Fudge	2 tbsp (1.4 oz)	140	tr	0
Pineapple	2 tbsp (1.4 oz)	110	0	0
Strawberry	2 tbsp (1.4 oz)	110	0	0
Marzetti				
Caramel Apple	2 tbsp	60	0	5
Caramel Apple Reduced Fat	2 tbsp	30	0	5
Peanut Butter Caramel	2 tbsp	60	1	0
Planters				
Nut	2 tbsp (0.5 oz)	100	1	0
Smucker's				
Chocolate	2 tbsp	130	—	0
Magic Shell Chocolate Fudge	2 tbsp	190	—	0
Pineapple	2 tbsp	130	—	0
Strawberry	2 tbsp	120	—	0

ICED TEA
(see also TEA/HERBAL TEA)
MIX

FOOD	PORTION	CALS.	FIB.	CHOL.
instant artificially sweetened lemon flavored as prep w/ water	8 oz	5	—	0
instant sweetened lemon flavor as prep w/ water	9 oz	87	—	0
instant unsweetened lemon flavor as prep w/ water	8 oz	4	—	0
Bigelow				
Nice Over Ice	5 fl oz	1	—	0
Celestial Seasonings				
Iced Delight	8 fl oz	4	—	0
Crystal Light				
Decaffeinated Sugar Free	8 oz	2	—	0
Sugar Free	8 oz	3	—	0
Lipton				
Calorie Free Decaf as prep	1 serv	0	0	0
Calorie Free as prep	1 serv	0	0	0
Citrus as prep	1 serv	90	0	0

FOOD	PORTION	CALS.	FIB.	CHOL.
Lipton (CONT.)				
Decaf Lemon as prep	1 serv	90	0	0
Family Size Bags Lemon as prep	1 qt	0	0	0
Family Size Bags Lemon Lime as prep	1 qt	0	0	0
Family Size Bags Peach as prep	1 qt	0	0	0
Lemon as prep	1 serv	90	0	0
Lemon Lime as prep	1 serv	90	0	0
No Lemon as prep	1 serv	80	0	0
Sugar Free Decaf as prep	1 serv	5	0	0
Sugar Free Lemon as prep	1 serv	5	0	0
Sugar Free No Lemon as prep	1 serv	0	0	0
Sugar Free Peach as prep	1 serv	5	0	0
Sugar Free Raspberry as prep	1 serv	5	0	0
Sugar Free Tropical as prep	1 serv	5	0	0
Tea & Lemonade as prep	1 serv	90	0	0
Tea Bag Herbal Iced Refresher as prep	1 serv	0	0	0
Tropical as prep	1 serv	90	0	0
Nestea				
100% Instant Tea as prep	8 oz	2	—	0
Ice Teasers Citrus as prep	8 oz	6	—	0
Ice Teasers Lemon as prep	8 oz	6	—	0
Ice Teasers Orange as prep	8 oz	6	—	0
Ice Teasers Tropical as prep	8 oz	6	—	0
Ice Teasers Wild Cherry as prep	8 oz	6	—	0
Lemon as prep	8 oz	6	—	0
Peach as prep	8 oz	88	—	0
Raspberry as prep	8 oz	88	—	0
Sugarfree as prep	8 oz	4	—	0
READY-TO-DRINK				
Arizona				
Lemon	1 bottle (16 oz)	180	—	0
Raspberry	8 fl oz	95	—	0
Lipton				
Chilled Diet Lemon	8 fl oz	0	0	0
Chilled Lemon	8 fl oz	80	0	0
Chilled No Lemon	8 fl oz	90	0	0
Chilled Peach	8 fl oz	80	0	0
Chilled Raspberry	8 fl oz	80	0	0
Royal Mistic				
Diet	12 fl oz	8	—	0
Lemon	12 fl oz	144	—	0

FOOD	PORTION	CALS.	FIB.	CHOL.
Royal Mistic (CONT.)				
Orange	12 fl oz	144	—	0
Wild Berry	12 fl oz	144	—	0
Schweppes				
Ice Tea	8 fl oz	90	0	0
Shasta				
Ice Tea	12 oz	124	—	0
Sipps				
Ice Tea	8.45 oz	100	—	0
Snapple				
Cranberry	8 fl oz	110	—	0
Diet	8 fl oz	0	—	0
Diet Peach	8 fl oz	0	—	0
Diet Raspberry	8 fl oz	0	—	0
Lemon	8 fl oz	110	—	0
Mango	8 fl oz	110	—	0
Mint	8 fl oz	120	—	0
Old Fashioned	8 fl oz	80	—	0
Orange	8 fl oz	110	—	0
Peach	8 fl oz	110	—	0
Raspberry	8 fl oz	120	—	0
Strawberry	8 fl oz	100	—	0
Tropicana				
Diet Lemon Fruit	8 fl oz	15	—	0
Lemon Fruit	8 fl oz	100	—	0
Peach Fruit	1 bottle (10 fl oz)	140	—	0
Peach Fruit	8 fl oz	120	—	0
Peach Fruit	1 can (11.5 fl oz)	160	—	0
Raspberry Fruit	8 fl oz	120	—	0
Raspberry Fruit	1 bottle (10 fl oz)	140	—	0
Raspberry Fruit	1 can (11.5 fl oz)	160	—	0
Tangerine Fruit	1 can (11.5 fl oz)	170	—	0
Tangerine Fruit	1 bottle (10 fl oz)	140	—	0
Tangerine Fruit	8 fl oz	110	—	0
Twister Apple Berry	8 fl oz	100	—	0
Twister Lemon Citrus	8 fl oz	110	—	0
Turkey Hill				
Diet Decaffeinated	1 cup (8 oz)	0	—	0
Raspberry Cooler	1 cup (8 oz)	110	—	0
Regular	1 cup (8 oz)	90	—	0
Veryfine				
With Lemon	8 oz	80	—	0

ICES AND ICE POPS

(*see also* ICE CREAM AND FROZEN DESSERTS, PUDDING POPS, SHERBET, YOGURT FROZEN)

FOOD	PORTION	CALS.	FIB.	CHOL.
fruit & juice bar	1 (3 fl oz)	75	—	0
gelatin pop	1 (1.5 oz)	31	—	0
ice coconut pineapple	½ cup (4 fl oz)	109	—	0
ice fruit w/ Equal	1 bar (1.7 oz)	12	—	0
ice lime	½ cup (4 fl oz)	75	—	0
ice pop	1 (2 fl oz)	42	—	0
Ben & Jerry's				
Cherry Pop	1	330	—	55
Bresler's				
All Flavors Ice	3.5 oz	120	—	0
Chiquita				
Fruit & Juice Bar Cherry	1 bar (2 oz)	50	—	0
Fruit & Juice Bar Raspberry	1 bar (2 oz)	50	—	0
Fruit & Juice Bar Raspberry Banana	1 bar (2 oz)	50	—	0
Fruit & Juice Bar Strawberry	1 bar (2 oz)	50	—	0
Fruit & Juice Bar Strawberry Banana	1 bar (2 oz)	50	—	0
Cool Creations				
10 Pack	1 pop (2 oz)	60	0	0
Lion King Cone	1 (4 oz)	280	1	15
Mickey Mouse Bar	1 (4 oz)	170	0	15
Mickey Mouse Bar	1 (2.5 oz)	110	0	10
Surprise Pops	1 (2 oz)	60	0	0
Crystal Light				
Berry Blend	1 bar	13	—	0
Cherry	1 bar	13	—	0
Fruit Punch	1 bar	14	—	0
Orange	1 bar	13	—	0
Pina Colada	1 bar	14	—	0
Pineapple	1 bar	14	—	0
Pink Lemonade	1 bar	14	—	0
Raspberry	1 bar	13	—	0
Strawberry	1 bar	13	—	0
Strawberry Daiquiri	1 bar	14	—	0
Dole				
Fruit 'N Juice Coconut	1 bar (4 oz)	210	0	10
Fruit 'N Juice Lemonade	1 bar (4 oz)	120	0	0
Fruit 'N Juice Lime	1 bar (4 oz)	110	0	0
Fruit 'N Juice Peach Passion	1 bar (2.5 oz)	70	0	0
Fruit 'N Juice Pineapple Coconut	1 bar (4 oz)	140	0	0
Fruit 'N Juice Pineapple Orange Banana	1 bar (2.5 oz)	70	0	0

FOOD	PORTION	CALS.	FIB.	CHOL.
Dole (CONT.)				
Fruit 'N Juice Pineapple Orange Banana	1 bar (4 oz)	110	0	0
Fruit 'N Juice Raspberry	1 bar (2.5 oz)	70	0	0
Fruit 'N Juice Strawberry	1 bar (4 oz)	110	0	0
Fruit 'N Juice Strawberry	1 bar (2.5 oz)	70	0	0
Fruit Juice Grape	1 bar (1.75 oz)	45	0	0
Fruit Juice No Sugar Added Grape	1 bar (1.75 oz)	25	0	0
Fruit Juice No Sugar Added Strawberry	1 bar (1.75 oz)	25	0	0
Fruit Juice Raspberry	1 bar (1.75 oz)	45	0	0
Fruit Juice Strawberry	1 bar (1.75 oz)	45	0	0
Flintstones				
Rock Pops	1 (3.5 oz)	80	0	0
Frozfruit				
Strawberry	1 (4 oz)	80	1	0
Good Humor				
Big Stick Cherry Pineapple	1 (3.6 fl oz)	50	0	0
Big Stick Popsicle	1 (3.6 fl oz)	50	—	0
Calippo Cherry	1 (3.8 fl oz)	100	—	0
Calippo Grape Lemon	1 (3.9 fl oz)	90	—	0
Calippo Orange	1 (3.9 fl oz)	90	—	0
Citrus Bites	1 (1.8 oz)	35	—	0
Creamsicle Orange	1 (1.8 fl oz)	70	0	5
Creamsicle Orange	1 (2.8 fl oz)	110	0	10
Creamsicle Orange Raspberry	1 (2.6 fl oz)	100	0	10
Creamsicle Sugar Free	1 (1.8 fl oz)	25	—	0
Fudgsicle Bar	1 (2.8 fl oz)	90	1	5
Fudgsicle Pop	1 (1.8 fl oz)	60	0	5
Fudgsicle Sugar Free	1 (1.8 fl oz)	40	1	<5
Fun Box Fudge Bar	1 (2.3 fl oz)	80	0	5
Fun Box Pops	1 (2 fl oz)	35	—	0
Fun Box Twin Box Cherry	1 (2.6 fl oz)	50	—	0
Fun Box Twin Pop Banana	1 (2.6 fl oz)	50	—	0
Fun Box Twin Pop Blue Raspberry	1 (2.6 fl oz)	50	—	0
Fun Box Twin Pop Cherry Lemon	1 (2.6 fl oz)	50	—	0
Fun Box Twin Pop Orange Cherry Grape	1 (2.6 fl oz)	50	—	0
Fun Box Twin Pop Root Beer	1 (2.6 fl oz)	50	—	0
Garfield Bar	1 (3.9 fl oz)	90	—	0
Hyperstripe	1 (2.8 fl oz)	80	—	0

FOOD	PORTION	CALS.	FIB.	CHOL.

Good Humor (CONT.)

FOOD	PORTION	CALS.	FIB.	CHOL.
Ice Stripe Cherry Orange	1 (1.5 fl oz)	35	0	0
Jumbo Jet Star	1 (4.7 fl oz)	80	—	0
Laser Blazer	1 (2.6 oz)	70	—	0
Popsicle All Natural	1 (1.8 fl oz)	45	—	0
Popsicle Orange Cherry Grape	1 (1.8 fl oz)	45	—	0
Popsicle Rainbow Pops	1 (1.8 fl oz)	45	—	0
Popsicle Rootbeer Banana Lime	1 (1.8 fl oz)	45	—	0
Popsicle Strawberry Raspberry Wildberry	1 (1.8 fl oz)	45	—	0
Popsicle Supersicle Traffic Signal	1	80	—	0
Popsicle Twin Pop Cherry	1 (2.6 fl oz)	70	—	0
Popsicle Twin Pop Orange Cherry Grape Lime	1 (2.6 fl oz)	70	—	0
Snow Cone	1	60	—	5
Snowfruit Coconut Bar	1 (3.75 fl oz)	150	1	10
Snowfruit Orange Bar	1	140	tr	0
Snowfruit Strawberry Bar	1	120	tr	0
Snowfruit Tropical Fruit Bar	1	110	—	0
Sugar Free Pop Orange Cherry Grape	1 (1.8 fl oz)	15	—	0
Supersicle Cherry Banana	1 (4.7 fl oz)	80	—	0
Supersicle Cherry Cola	1 (4.7 fl oz)	80	—	0
Supersicle Double Fudge	1 (4.7 fl oz)	150	1	10
Supersicle Firecracker	1 (4.7 fl oz)	90	—	0
Supersicle Firecracker Jr.	1	72	—	0
Supersicle Sour Tower	1	80	—	0
Swirl Bubble Gum	1 (2.7 fl oz)	55	—	0
Swirl Cherry Banana	1 (2.7 fl oz)	55	—	0
Torpedo Cherry	1 (1.8 fl oz)	35	0	0
Twister Blue Raspberry Cherry Cherry Cola Cherry	1 (1.8 fl oz)	45	—	0
Twister Cherry Lemon Orange Lemon	1 (1.8 fl oz)	45	—	0
Vampire's Deadly Secret	1 (2.8 fl oz)	100	—	0
Watermelon Bar	1 (3.6 fl oz)	80	—	0

Haagen-Dazs

FOOD	PORTION	CALS.	FIB.	CHOL.
Sorbet Banana Strawberry	½ cup (4 oz)	140	tr	0
Sorbet Chocolate	½ cup (4 oz)	130	2	0
Sorbet Mango	½ cup (4 oz)	120	tr	0
Sorbet Orchard Peach	½ cup (4 oz)	140	tr	0
Sorbet Raspberry	½ cup (4 oz)	120	1	0

FOOD	PORTION	CALS.	FIB.	CHOL.
Haagen-Dazs (CONT.)				
Sorbet Strawberry	½ cup (4 oz)	130	1	0
Sorbet Zesty Lemon	½ cup (4 oz)	130	tr	0
Sorbet & Cream Orange	½ cup (3.7 oz)	200	0	60
Sorbet & Cream Raspberry	½ cup (3.7 oz)	190	tr	60
Sorbet Bar Chocolate	1 (2.7 oz)	80	1	0
Sorbet Bar Wild Berry	1 (2.7 oz)	90	tr	0
Hood				
Hendrie's Sizzle'N Sour Stix	1 bar (2 oz)	80	0	5
Hoodsie Pop	1 (3.3 oz)	60	—	0
Natural Blenders Pineappple	1 bar (1 oz)	60	—	0
Natural Blenders Raspberry	1 bar (1 oz)	60	—	0
Natural Blenders Strawberry	1 bar (1 oz)	60	—	0
Pop Banana	1 (3.3 oz)	60	—	0
Pop Blue Raspberry	1 (3.3 oz)	60	—	0
Pop Cherry	1 (3.3 oz)	60	—	0
Pop Grape	1 (3.3 oz)	60	—	0
Pop Orange	1 (3.3 oz)	60	—	0
Pop Root Beer	1 (3.3 oz)	60	—	0
Super Sortment Juice Bars	1 bar (1.9 oz)	40	—	0
Jell-O				
Mixed Berry	1 bar	31	—	0
Orange	1 bar	31	—	0
Orange Pineapple	1 bar	31	—	0
Raspberry	1 bar	29	—	0
Raspberry Peach	1 bar	29	—	0
Strawberry	1 bar	31	—	0
Strawberry Banana	1 bar	31	—	0
Kool-Aid				
Berry Punch	1 bar	31	—	0
Cherry	1 bar	42	—	0
Grape	1 bar	42	—	0
Mountain Berry Punch	1 bar	42	—	0
Lifesavers				
Ice Pops	1	35	0	0
Ice Pops	1 (1.75 oz)	35	0	0
Tofutti				
Frutti Apricot Mango	4 fl oz	100	—	0
Frutti Three Berry	4 fl oz	100	—	0
Vitari				
Passion-Fruit	4 oz	80	—	0

FOOD	PORTION	CALS.	FIB.	CHOL.
Vitari (CONT.)				
Peach	4 oz	80	—	0
ICING				
(*see* CAKE)				
INSTANT BREAKFAST				
(*see* BREAKFAST DRINKS)				
JACKFRUIT				
fresh	3½ oz	70	—	0
JALAPENO				
(*see* PEPPERS)				
JAM/JELLY/PRESERVES				
all flavors jam	1 pkg (0.5 oz)	34	tr	0
all flavors jam	1 tbsp (0.7 oz)	48	tr	0
all flavors jelly	1 pkg (0.5 oz)	38	tr	0
all flavors jelly	1 tbsp (0.7 oz)	52	tr	0
all flavors preserve	1 pkg (0.5 oz)	34	tr	0
ail flavors preserve	1 tbsp (0.7 oz)	48	tr	0
apple butter	1 tbsp (0.6 oz)	33	—	0
apple butter	1 cup (9.9 oz)	519	—	0
apple jelly	1 pkg (0.5 oz)	38	tr	0
apple jelly	1 tbsp (0.7 oz)	52	tr	0
apricot jam	3½ oz	250	—	0
blackberry jam	3½ oz	237	—	0
cherry jam	3½ oz	250	—	0
orange jam	3½ oz	243	—	0
orange marmalade	1 tbsp (0.7 oz)	49	—	0
orange marmalade	1 pkg (0.5 oz)	34	—	0
plum jam	3½ oz	241	—	0
quince jam	3½ oz	236	—	0
raspberry jam	3½ oz	248	—	0
raspberry jelly	3½ oz	259	—	0
red currant jam	3½ oz	237	—	0
red currant jelly	3½ oz	265	—	0
rose hip jam	3½ oz	250	—	0
strawberry jam	1 tbsp (0.7 oz)	48	tr	0
strawberry jam	1 pkg (0.5 oz)	34	tr	0
strawberry preserve	1 tbsp (0.7 oz)	48	tr	0
strawberry preserve	1 pkg (0.5 oz)	34	tr	0
BAMA				
Apple Butter	2 tsp	25	—	0
Apple Jelly	2 tsp	30	—	0

FOOD	PORTION	CALS.	FIB.	CHOL.
BAMA (CONT.)				
Grape Jelly	2 tsp	30	—	0
Peach Preserves	2 tsp	30	—	0
Red Plum Jam	2 tsp	30	—	0
Strawberry Preserves	2 tsp	30	—	0
Eden				
Apple Butter	1 tbsp (0.5 fl oz)	25	0	0
Estee				
Apple Reduced Calorie	1 pkg (0.5 oz)	10	—	0
Apple Slice	1 tbsp (0.5 oz)	10	—	0
Apricot	1 tbsp (0.5 oz)	5	—	0
Blackberry	1 tbsp (0.5 oz)	5	—	0
Cherry	1 tbsp (0.5 oz)	5	—	0
Grape	1 tbsp (0.5 oz)	10	—	0
Orange	1 tbsp (0.5 oz)	10	—	0
Peach	1 tbsp (0.5 oz)	5	—	0
Red Raspberry	1 tbsp (0.5 oz)	5	—	0
Strawberry	1 tbsp (0.5 oz)	10	—	0
Harvest Moon				
Apricot Fruit Spread	1 tbsp (0.6 oz)	35	—	0
Blueberry Fruit Spread	1 tbsp (0.6 oz)	35	—	0
Cherry Fruit Spread	1 tbsp (0.6 oz)	35	—	0
Grape Fruit Spread	1 tbsp (0.6 oz)	35	—	0
Peach Fruit Spread	1 tbsp (0.6 oz)	35	—	0
Raspberry Fruit Spread	1 tbsp (0.6 oz)	35	—	0
Strawberry Fruit Spread	1 tbsp (0.6 oz)	35	—	0
Home Brands				
All Flavors Jelly	2 tsp	35	—	0
All Flavors Preserves	2 tsp	35	—	0
Kraft				
Apple Jelly	1 tbsp (0.7 oz)	60	0	0
Apple Strawberry Jelly	1 tbsp (0.7 oz)	50	0	0
Apricot Preserves	1 tbsp (0.7 oz)	50	0	0
Blackberry Jelly	1 tbsp (0.7 oz)	50	0	0
Blackberry Preserves	1 tbsp (0.7 oz)	50	tr	0
Grape Jam	1 tbsp (0.7 oz)	60	0	0
Grape Jelly	1 tbsp (0.7 oz)	50	0	0
Grape Reduced Calorie	1 tbsp (0.6 oz)	20	0	0
Guava Jelly	1 tbsp (0.7 oz)	50	0	0
Orange Marmalade	1 tbsp (0.7 oz)	50	0	0
Peach Preserves	1 tbsp (0.7 oz)	50	0	0
Pineapple Preserves	1 tbsp (0.7 oz)	50	0	0
Red Currant Jelly	1 tbsp (0.7 oz)	50	0	0
Red Plum Jam	1 tbsp (0.7 oz)	60	0	0

FOOD	PORTION	CALS.	FIB.	CHOL.
Kraft (CONT.)				
Red Raspberry Preserves	1 tbsp (0.7 oz)	50	0	0
Strawberry Jam	1 tbsp (0.7 oz)	50	0	0
Strawberry Jelly	1 tbsp (0.7 oz)	60	0	0
Strawberry Preserves	1 tbsp (0.7 oz)	50	0	0
Strawberry Reduced Calorie	1 tbsp	20	0	0
Red Wing				
Apple Jelly	1 tbsp (0.7 oz)	50	0	0
Apple Blackberry Jelly	1 tbsp (0.7 oz)	50	0	0
Apple Cherry Jelly	1 tbsp (0.7 oz)	50	0	0
Apple Currant Jelly	1 tbsp (0.7 oz)	50	0	0
Apple Grape Jelly	1 tbsp (0.7 oz)	50	0	0
Apple Raspberry Jelly	1 tbsp (0.7 oz)	50	0	0
Apple Strawberry Jelly	1 tbsp (0.7 oz)	50	0	0
Black Raspberry Jelly	1 tbsp (0.7 oz)	50	0	0
Blackberry Jelly	1 tbsp (0.7 oz)	50	0	0
Cherry Jelly	1 tbsp (0.7 oz)	50	0	0
Concord Grape Jelly	1 tbsp (0.7 oz)	50	0	0
Crabapple Jelly	1 tbsp (0.7 oz)	50	0	0
Cranberry Jelly	1 tbsp (0.7 oz)	50	0	0
Cranberry Grape Jelly	1 tbsp (0.7 oz)	50	0	0
Currant Jelly	1 tbsp (0.7 oz)	50	0	0
Damson Plum Jelly	1 tbsp (0.7 oz)	50	0	0
Elderberry Jelly	1 tbsp (0.7 oz)	50	0	0
Grape Jelly	1 tbsp (0.7 oz)	50	0	0
Mint Jelly	1 tbsp (0.7 oz)	50	0	0
Mint Apple Jelly	1 tbsp (0.7 oz)	50	0	0
Mixed Fruit Jelly	1 tbsp (0.7 oz)	50	0	0
Red Plum Jelly	1 tbsp (0.7 oz)	50	0	0
Red Raspberry Jelly	1 tbsp (0.7 oz)	50	0	0
Strawberry Jelly	1 tbsp (0.7 oz)	50	0	0
Strawberry Apple Jelly	1 tbsp (0.7 oz)	50	0	0
S&W				
Apricot Pineapple Reduced Calorie Preserves	1 tsp	4	—	0
Blueberry Reduced Calorie Jam	1 tsp	4	—	0
Concord Grape Reduced Calorie Jelly	1 tsp	4	—	0
Orange Marmalade Reduced Calorie	1 tsp	4	—	0
Red Raspberry Reduced Calorie Jam	1 tsp	4	—	0
Red Tart Cherry Reduced Calorie Preserves	1 tsp	4	—	0

FOOD	PORTION	CALS.	FIB.	CHOL.
S&W (CONT.)				
Strawberry Reduced Calorie Jam	1 tsp	4	—	0
Smucker's				
All Flavors Jam	1 tsp	18	—	0
All Flavors Jelly	1 tsp	18	—	0
All Flavors Low Sugar Spread	1 tsp	8	—	0
All Flavors Preserves	1 tsp	18	—	0
All Flavors Simply Fruit	1 tsp	16	—	0
All Flavors Single Serving Jelly	½ oz	38	—	0
All Flavors Single Serving Preserves	½ oz	38	—	0
All Flavors Slenderella	1 tsp	7	—	0
Apple Butter Autumn Harvest	1 tsp	12	—	0
Apple Butter Simply Fruit	1 tsp	12	—	0
Apple Butter Natural	1 tsp	12	—	0
Apple Cider Butter	1 tsp	12	—	0
Blackberry Single Serving Imitation Jelly	1 pkg (0.4 oz)	4	—	0
Cherry Single Serving Imitation Jelly	1 pkg (0.4 oz)	4	—	0
Grape Single Serving Imitation Jelly	1 pkg (0.4 oz)	4	—	0
Orange Marmalade	1 tsp	18	—	0
Peach Butter	1 tsp	15	—	0
Pumpkin Butter Autumn Harvest	1 tsp	12	—	0
Tree Of Life				
Apricot Fruit Spread	1 tbsp (0.6 oz)	45	—	0
Blueberry Fruit Spread	1 tbsp (0.6 oz)	35	—	0
Cherry Fruit Spread	1 tbsp (0.6 oz)	40	—	0
Grape Fruit Spread	1 tbsp (0.6 oz)	35	—	0
Peach Fruit Spread	1 tbsp (0.6 oz)	45	—	0
Raspberry Fruit Spread	1 tbsp (0.6 oz)	30	—	0
Strawberry Fruit Spread	1 tbsp (0.6 oz)	35	—	0
White House				
Apple Butter	1 oz	50	1	0

JAPANESE FOOD
(*see* ORIENTAL FOOD, SUSHI)

JAVA PLUM

fresh	1 cup	82	—	0
fresh	3	5	—	0

FOOD	PORTION	CALS.	FIB.	CHOL.

JELLY
(see JAM/JELLY/PRESERVES)

JERUSALEM ARTICHOKE
(see ARTICHOKE)

JEW'S EAR
pepeao dried	½ cup	36	—	0
pepeao raw sliced	1 cup	25	—	0

JUJUBE
fresh	3½ oz	105	—	0

KALE
FRESH
chopped cooked	½ cup	21	—	0
raw chopped	½ cup	21	—	0
scotch chopped cooked	½ cup	18	—	0
Dole				
Chopped	½ cup	17	—	0
FROZEN				
chopped cooked	½ cup	20	—	0

KETCHUP
ketchup	1 tbsp	16	tr	0
ketchup	1 pkg (0.2 oz)	6	tr	0
low sodium	1 tbsp	16	tr	0
Del Monte				
Ketchup	1 tbsp (0.5 oz)	15	0	0
Hain				
Natural	1 tbsp	16	—	0
Natural No Salt Added	1 tbsp	16	—	0
Healthy Choice				
Ketchup	1 tbsp (0.5 oz)	9	tr	0
Heinz				
Hot	1 tbsp	14	—	0
Lite	1 tbsp	8	—	0
Hunt's				
Ketchup	1 tbsp (0.6 oz)	16	0	0
No Salt Added	1 tbsp (0.6 oz)	16	0	0
McIlhenny				
Ketchup	1 tbsp (0.6 oz)	23	tr	0
Spicy	1 tbsp (0.6 oz)	23	tr	tr
Muir Glen				
Organic	1 tbsp (0.6 oz)	15	0	0
Red Wing				
Extra Fancy	1 tbsp (0.6 oz)	20	0	0

FOOD	PORTION	CALS.	FIB.	CHOL.
Smucker's				
Ketchup	1 tsp	8	—	0
Tree Of Life				
Ketchup	1 tbsp (0.5 oz)	10	—	0
Salsa Ketchup	1 tbsp (0.5 oz)	10	—	0
KIDNEY				
beef simmered	3 oz	122	—	329
lamb braised	3 oz	117	—	481
pork braised	3 oz	128	—	408
veal braised	3 oz	139	—	672
KIDNEY BEANS				
CANNED				
kidney beans	1 cup	208	—	0
red	1 cup	216	—	0
B&M				
Red Baked Beans	½ cup (4.6 oz)	170	6	<5
Eden				
Organic	½ cup (4.4 oz)	100	10	0
Friend's				
Red Baked Beans	½ cup (4.6 oz)	160	6	<5
Goya				
Spanish Style	7.5 oz	140	10	0
Green Giant				
Dark Red	½ cup	90	5	0
Light Red	½ cup	90	5	0
Hanover				
Dark Red	½ cup	110	—	0
Light Red In Sauce	½ cup	120	—	0
Hunt's				
Red	½ cup (4.5 oz)	94	5	0
Progresso				
Red	½ cup (4.6 oz)	110	8	0
S&W				
Dark Red Lite 50% Less Salt	½ cup	120	—	0
Dark Red Premium	½ cup	120	—	0
Water Pack	½ cup	90	—	0
Trappey				
Dark Red	½ cup (4.5 oz)	130	8	0
Light Red	½ cup (4.5 oz)	120	8	0
Light Red New Orleans Style With Bacon	½ cup (4.5 oz)	110	6	0
Light Red With Jalapeno	½ cup (4.5 oz)	110	6	0
With Chili Gravy	½ cup (4.5 oz)	110	7	0

FOOD	PORTION	CALS.	FIB.	CHOL.
Van Camp's				
Dark Red	½ cup (4.6 oz)	90	6	0
Light Red	½ cup (4.6 oz)	90	6	0
DRIED				
california red cooked	1 cup	219	—	0
cooked	1 cup	225	—	0
red cooked	1 cup	225	—	0
royal red cooked	1 cup	218	—	0
Arrowhead				
Red	¼ cup (1.6 oz)	160	10	0
Hurst				
Kidney Beans	1.2 oz	120	10	0
SPROUTS				
cooked	1 lb	152	—	0
raw	½ cup	27	—	0

KIWI JUICE
After The Fall

Kiwi Bear	1 cup (8 oz)	100	0	0

KIWIS

fresh	1 med	46	3	0
Dole				
Kiwis	2	90	4	0
Sonoma				
Dried	7-8 pieces (1 oz)	90	2	0

KNISH
Joshua's

Coney Island Potato	1 (4.6 oz)	280	1	0
TAKE-OUT				
cheese & blueberry	1 (7 oz)	378	—	40
cheese & cherry	1 (7 oz)	378	—	40
everything	1 (7 oz)	221	—	0
kashe	1 (7 oz)	270	—	0
potato	1 lg (7 oz)	332	1	72
potato	1 med (3.5 oz)	166	tr	36
potato w/ broccoli & cheese	1 (7 oz)	312	—	24
potato w/ spinach & mushroom	1 (7 oz)	214	—	0

KOHLRABI

raw sliced	½ cup	19	—	0
sliced cooked	½ cup	24	—	0

KUMQUATS

fresh	1	12	—	*

FOOD	PORTION	CALS.	FIB.	CHOL.

LAMB
(see also LAMB DISHES)
FRESH

FOOD	PORTION	CALS.	FIB.	CHOL.
cubed lean only braised	3 oz	190	—	92
cubed lean only broiled	3 oz	158	—	77
ground broiled	3 oz	240	—	82
leg lean & fat Choice roasted	3 oz	219	—	79
loin chop w/ bone lean & fat Choice broiled	1 chop (2.3 oz)	201	—	64
loin chop w/ bone lean only Choice broiled	1 chop (1.6 oz)	100	—	44
rib chop lean & fat Choice broiled	3 oz	307	—	84
rib chop lean only Choice broiled	3 oz	200	—	78
shank lean & fat Choice braised	3 oz	206	—	90
shank lean & fat Choice roasted	3 oz	191	—	77
shoulder chop w/ bone lean & fat Choice braised	1 chop (2.5 oz)	244	—	84
shoulder chop w/ bone lean only Choice braised	1 chop (1.9 oz)	152	—	66
sirloin lean & fat Choice roasted	3 oz	248	—	82

FROZEN

FOOD	PORTION	CALS.	FIB.	CHOL.
New Zealand lean & fat cooked	3 oz	259	—	93
New Zealand lean only cooked	3 oz	175	—	93

LAMB DISHES
TAKE-OUT

FOOD	PORTION	CALS.	FIB.	CHOL.
curry	¾ cup	345	—	89
stew	¾ cup	124	2	29

LAMBSQUARTERS

FOOD	PORTION	CALS.	FIB.	CHOL.
chopped cooked	½ cup	29	—	0

LECITHIN
(see SOY)

LEEKS

FOOD	PORTION	CALS.	FIB.	CHOL.
chopped cooked	¼ cup	8	—	0
cooked	1 (4.4 oz)	38	—	0
freeze dried	1 tbsp	1	—	0
raw	1 (4.4 oz)	76	—	0
raw chopped	¼ cup	16	—	0

LEMON
FRESH

FOOD	PORTION	CALS.	FIB.	CHOL.
lemon	1 med	22	—	0
peel	1 tbsp	0	—	0

FOOD	PORTION	CALS.	FIB.	CHOL.
wedge	1	5	—	0
Dole				
Lemon	1	18	0	0

LEMON EXTRACT
Virginia Dare

Extract	1 tsp	22	—	0

LEMON JUICE

bottled	1 tbsp	3	—	0
fresh	1 tbsp	4	—	0
frzn	1 tbsp	3	—	0
After The Fall				
Spicy Lemon	1 can (12 oz)	150	0	0
Realemon				
Juice	1 fl oz	6	—	0

LEMONADE
FROZEN

as prep w/ water	1 cup	100	—	0
not prep	1 can (6 oz)	397	—	0
Bright & Early				
Lemonade	8 fl oz	120	—	0
Minute Maid				
Country Style	8 fl oz	120	—	0
Cranberry Lemonade	8 fl oz	80	—	0
Lemonade	8 fl oz	110	—	0
Pink	8 fl oz	120	—	0
Raspberry	8 fl oz	120	—	0
Seneca				
as prep	8 fl oz	110	1	0
MIX				
powder as prep w/ water	9 fl oz	113	—	0
powder w/ Equal	1 pitcher (67 oz)	40	—	0
Country Time				
Mix	8 fl oz	82	—	0
Pink	8 fl oz	82	—	0
Pink Sugar Free	8 fl oz	4	—	0
Sugar Free	8 fl oz	4	—	0
Crystal Light				
Mix	8 fl oz	5	—	0
Kool-Aid				
Mix	8 fl oz	99	—	0
Pink	8 fl oz	99	—	0
Sugar Free	8 fl oz	4	—	0

FOOD	PORTION	CALS.	FIB.	CHOL.
Kool-Aid (cont.)				
Sugar Sweetened Pink	8 fl oz	82	—	0
READY-TO-DRINK				
After The Fall				
Apple Raspberry	1 bottle (10 oz)	120	—	0
Crystal Geyser				
Juice Squeeze Pink	1 bottle (12 fl oz)	140	—	0
Diet Rite				
Salt/Sodium Free	8 fl oz	2	—	0
Fruitopia				
Lemonade	8 fl oz	120	—	0
Minute Maid				
Chilled	8 fl oz	110	—	0
Cranberry Chilled	8 fl oz	120	—	0
Juices To Go	1 bottle (16 fl oz)	110	—	0
Juices To Go	1 can (11.5 fl oz)	160	—	0
Juices To Go Cranberry Lemonade	1 bottle (16 fl oz)	110	—	0
Juices To Go Raspberry Lemonade	1 bottle (16 fl oz)	120	—	0
Pink Chilled	8 fl oz	110	—	0
Raspberry Chilled	8 fl oz	120	—	0
Mott's				
Lemonade	10 fl oz	160	0	0
Nehi				
Lemonade	8 fl oz	130	—	0
Newman's Own				
Roadside Virginia	8 fl oz	100	—	0
Ocean Spray				
Lemonade	8 fl oz	110	0	0
With Cranberry Juice	8 fl oz	110	0	0
With Raspberry Juice	8 fl oz	110	0	0
Odwalla				
Honey	8 fl oz	70	0	0
Strawberry	8 fl oz	150	2	0
Royal Mistic				
Lemonade Limeade	16 fl oz	230	—	0
Tropical Pink	16 fl oz	230	—	0
Santa Cruz				
Organic	8 oz	100	—	0
Shasta				
Lemonade	12 fl oz	146	—	0
Sipps				
Lemonade	8.45 fl oz	85	—	0

FOOD	PORTION	CALS.	FIB.	CHOL.
Snapple				
Diet Pink	8 fl oz	13	—	0
Lemonade	8 fl oz	110	—	0
Pink	8 fl oz	110	—	0
Strawberry	8 fl oz	110	—	0
Tropicana				
Lemonade	1 can (11.5 oz)	160	—	0
Lemonade	8 fl oz	110	—	0
Twister Wild Berry	8 fl oz	120	—	0
Turkey Hill				
Lemonade	8 fl oz	110	—	0
Veryfine				
Lemonade	8 fl oz	120	—	0

LENTILS
CANNED
Health Valley

Fast Menu Hearty Lentils Garden Vegetables	7½ oz	150	16	0
Fast Menu Organic Lentils With Tofu Weiner	7½ oz	170	15	0

DRIED

cooked	1 cup	231	—	0
Hurst				
Lentils	1.2 oz	120	11	0

MIX
Casbah

Pilaf as prep	1 cup	200	2	0

SPROUTS

raw	½ cup	40	—	0

TAKE-OUT

indian sambar	1 serv	236	9	10

LETTUCE
(*see also* SALAD)

bibb	1 head (6 oz)	21	2	0
boston	1 head (6 oz)	21	2	0
boston	2 leaves	2	tr	0
iceberg	1 leaf	3	tr	0
iceberg	1 head (19 oz)	70	5	0
looseleaf shredded	½ cup	5	—	0
romaine shredded	½ cup	4	tr	0
Dole				
Butter	1 head	21	2	0
Iceberg	⅙ med head	20	1	0

FOOD	PORTION	CALS.	FIB.	CHOL.
Dole (CONT.)				
Leaf shredded	1½ cups	12	1	0
Romaine shredded	1½ cups	18	1	0
Western Express				
Hearts Of Romaine	6 leaves (3 oz)	20	1	0

LIMA BEANS
CANNED
large	1 cup	191	—	0
lima beans	½ cup	93	—	0
Allen				
Green	½ cup (4.5 oz)	120	8	0
Green & White	½ cup (4.5 oz)	110	9	0
Del Monte				
Green	½ cup (4.4 oz)	80	4	0
East Texas Fair				
Green	½ cup (4.5 oz)	120	8	0
S&W				
Small Fancy	½ cup	80	—	0
Seneca				
Limas	½ cup	80	5	0
Trappey				
Baby Green With Bacon	½ cup (4.5 oz)	120	6	0

DRIED
baby cooked	1 cup	229	17	0
cooked	½ cup	104	—	0
large cooked	1 cup	217	14	0

FROZEN
cooked	½ cup	94	—	0
fordhook cooked	½ cup	85	—	0
Birds Eye				
Baby	½ cup	130	—	0
Fordhook	½ cup	100	—	0
Green Giant				
Harvest Fresh	½ cup	80	4	0
In Butter Sauce	½ cup	100	5	5
Hanover				
Baby	½ cup	110	—	0
Fordhook	½ cup	100	—	0

LIME
fresh	1	20	—	0

LIME JUICE
bottled	1 tbsp	3	—	0

FOOD	PORTION	CALS.	FIB.	CHOL.
fresh	1 tbsp	4	—	0
After The Fall				
Caribbean Lime	1 can (12 oz)	170	0	0
Key West	1 cup (8 oz)	100	0	0
Odwalla				
Summertime Lime	8 fl oz	90	0	0
Realime				
Juice	1 oz	6	—	0

LINGCOD

FOOD	PORTION	CALS.	FIB.	CHOL.
baked	3 oz	93	—	57
fillet baked	5.3 oz	164	—	101

LIQUOR/LIQUEUR

(*see also* BEER AND ALE, CHAMPAGNE, DRINK MIXERS, MALT, WINE, WINE COOLERS)

FOOD	PORTION	CALS.	FIB.	CHOL.
anisette	⅔ oz	74	0	0
apricot brandy	⅔ oz	64	0	0
benedictine	⅔ oz	69	0	0
bloody mary	5 oz	116	—	0
bourbon & soda	4 oz	105	—	0
coffee liqueur	1½ oz	174	—	0
cognac	3.5 oz	233	0	0
creme de menthe	1½ oz	186	—	0
curacao liqueur	⅔ oz	54	0	0
daiquiri	2 oz	111	—	0
gin	1½ oz	110	—	0
gin & tonic	7.5 oz	171	—	0
gin rickey	4 oz	150	—	0
manhattan	2 oz	128	—	0
martini	2½ oz	156	—	0
mint julep	10 oz	210	0	0
old-fashioned	2½ oz	127	0	0
pina colada	4½ oz	262	—	0
planter's punch	3½ oz	175	—	0
rum	1½ oz	97	—	0
screwdriver	7 oz	174	—	0
sloe gin fizz	2½ oz	132	0	0
tequila sunrise	5½ oz	189	—	0
tom collins	7½ oz	121	—	0
vodka	1½ oz	97	—	0
whiskey	1½ oz	105	—	0
whiskey sour	3 oz	123	—	0
whiskey sour mix not prep	1 pkg (0.6 oz)	64	—	0

FOOD	PORTION	CALS.	FIB.	CHOL.

LIVER
(see also PATE)

FOOD	PORTION	CALS.	FIB.	CHOL.
beef braised	3 oz	137	—	331
beef pan-fried	3 oz	184	—	410
chicken stewed	1 cup (5 oz)	219	—	883
duck raw	1 (1.5 oz)	60	—	227
lamb braised	3 oz	187	—	426
lamb fried	3 oz	202	—	419
pork braised	3 oz	141	—	302
turkey simmered	1 cup (5 oz)	237	—	876
veal braised	3 oz	140	—	477
veal fried	3 oz	208	—	280
Dakota Lean				
Beef raw	3 oz	100	—	150

LOBSTER
(see also CRAYFISH)
CANNED
Progresso

FOOD	PORTION	CALS.	FIB.	CHOL.
Rock Lobster Sauce	½ cup (4.3 oz)	100	2	5
FRESH				
northern cooked	1 cup	142	—	104
northern cooked	3 oz	83	—	61
northern raw	1 lobster (5.3 oz)	136	—	143
northern raw	3 oz	77	—	81
spiny steamed	3 oz	122	—	76
spiny steamed	1 (5.7 oz)	233	—	146
TAKE-OUT				
newburg	1 cup	485	—	455

LOGANBERRIES

FOOD	PORTION	CALS.	FIB.	CHOL.
frzn	1 cup	80	—	0

LONGANS

FOOD	PORTION	CALS.	FIB.	CHOL.
fresh	1	2	—	0

LOQUATS

FOOD	PORTION	CALS.	FIB.	CHOL.
fresh	1	5	—	0

LOTUS

FOOD	PORTION	CALS.	FIB.	CHOL.
root raw sliced	10 slices	45	—	0
root sliced cooked	10 slices	59	—	0
seeds dried	1 oz	94	—	0

LOX
(see SALMON)

LUPINES

FOOD	PORTION	CALS.	FIB.	CHOL.
dried cooked	1 cup	197	—	0

FOOD	PORTION	CALS.	FIB.	CHOL.
LYCHEES				
fresh	1	6	—	0
Ka-Me				
Whole Pitted In Syrup	15 pieces (5 oz)	130	0	0
MACADAMIA NUTS				
dried	1 oz	199	—	0
oil roasted	1 oz	204	—	0
Mauna Loa				
Candy Glazed	1 oz	170	—	5
Chocolate Covered	1 oz	170	—	0
Honey Roasted	1 oz	200	—	0
Macadamia Nut Brittle	1 oz	150	—	6
Roasted & Salted	1 oz	210	—	0
MACARONI				
(*see* PASTA)				
MACE				
ground	1 tsp	8	—	0
MACKEREL				
CANNED				
jack	1 cup	296	—	150
jack	1 can (12.7 oz)	563	—	285
FRESH				
atlantic cooked	3 oz	223	—	64
atlantic raw	3 oz	174	—	60
jack baked	3 oz	171	—	51
jack fillet baked	6.2 oz	354	—	106
king baked	3 oz	114	—	58
king fillet baked	5.4 oz	207	—	105
pacific baked	3 oz	171	—	51
pacific fillet baked	6.2 oz	354	—	106
spanish cooked	3 oz	134	—	62
spanish cooked	1 fillet (5.1 oz)	230	—	107
spanish raw	3 oz	118	—	65
MALT				
nonalcoholic	12 fl oz	32	—	0
Bartles & Jaymes				
Malt Cooler Berry	12 fl oz	210	—	0
Malt Cooler Black Cherry	12 fl oz	190	—	0
Malt Cooler Light Berry	12 fl oz	140	—	0
Malt Cooler Mandarin Lemon	12 fl oz	210	—	0
Malt Cooler Margarita	12 fl oz	250	—	0

FOOD	PORTION	CALS.	FIB.	CHOL.
Bartles & Jaymes (CONT.)				
Malt Cooler Original	12 fl oz	180	—	0
Malt Cooler Peach	12 fl oz	200	—	0
Malt Cooler Pina Colada	12 fl oz	270	—	0
Malt Cooler Planter's Punch	12 fl oz	220	—	0
Malt Cooler Red Sangria	12 fl oz	190	—	0
Malt Cooler Strawberry	12 fl oz	200	—	0
Malt Cooler Strawberry Daiquiri	12 fl oz	220	—	0
Malt Cooler Tropical	12 fl oz	220	—	0
Olde English				
Malt	12 oz	163	—	0
Schaefer				
Malt	12 oz	165	—	0
Schlitz				
Malt	12 oz	177	—	0

MALTED MILK

chocolate as prep w/ milk	1 cup	229	—	34
chocolate flavor powder	3 heaping tsp (¾ oz)	79	—	1
natural flavor as prep w/ milk	1 cup	237	—	37
natural flavor powder	3 heaping tsp (¾ oz)	87	—	4
Carnation				
Chocolate	3 heaping tsp (21 g)	79	—	1
Original	3 heaping tsp (21 g)	90	—	4
Kraft				
Instant Chocolate	3 tsp (0.7 oz)	80	tr	0
Instant Chocolate as prep w/ 2% milk	1 serv (9.5 oz)	200	tr	20
Instant Natural	3 tsp (0.7 oz)	90	0	5
Instant Natural as prep w/ 2% milk	1 serv (9.5 oz)	210	0	25

MAMMY-APPLE

| fresh | 1 | 431 | — | 0 |

MANGO

fresh	1	135	—	0
CANNED				
Ka-Me				
Mango	4 pieces (5 oz)	102	0	0

FOOD	PORTION	CALS.	FIB.	CHOL.
DRIED				
Sonoma				
Pieces	8 pieces (2 oz)	180	0	0
MANGO JUICE				
After The Fall				
Hawaiian Mango	1 can (12 oz)	180	0	0
Mango Ginger	1 can (12 oz)	150	0	0
Fresh Samantha				
Mango Mama	1 cup (8 oz)	125	2	0
Kern's				
Nectar	6 fl oz	100	—	0
Libby				
Nectar	1 can (11.5 fl oz)	210	—	0
Snapple				
Diet Mango Madness	8 fl oz	13	—	0
Mango Madness Cocktail	8 fl oz	110	—	0
MARGARINE				
(*see also* BUTTER BLENDS, BUTTER SUBSTITUTES)				
squeeze soybean & cottonseed	1 tsp	34	—	0
stick corn	1 tsp	34	—	0
stick corn	1 stick (4 oz)	815	—	0
stick salted	1 tsp	39	—	0
stick salted	1 stick (4 oz)	815	—	0
stick unsalted	1 stick (4 oz)	809	—	0
stick unsalted	1 tsp	34	—	0
tub corn	1 tsp	34	—	0
tub corn	1 cup	1626	—	0
tub diet	1 tsp	17	—	0
tub diet	1 cup	800	—	0
tub safflower	1 tsp	34	—	0
tub safflower	1 cup	1626	—	0
tub salted	1 tsp	34	—	0
tub salted	1 cup	1626	—	0
tub soybean salted	1 cup	1626	—	0
tub soybean salted	1 tsp	34	—	0
tub soybean unsalted	1 cup	1626	—	0
tub soybean unsalted	1 tsp	34	—	0
tub unsalted	1 cup	1626	—	0
tub unsalted	1 tsp	34	—	0
Blue Bonnet				
Stick	1 tbsp	100	—	0
Tub	1 tbsp	100	—	0
Whipped	1 tbsp	80	—	0

FOOD	PORTION	CALS.	FIB.	CHOL.
Chiffon				
Stick	1 tbsp	100	—	0
Tub	1 tbsp (0.5 oz)	100	0	0
Whipped	1 tbsp (0.3 oz)	70	0	0
Fleischmann's				
Stick	1 tbsp	100	—	0
Stick Light Corn Oil	1 tbsp	80	—	0
Stick Sweet Unsalted	1 tbsp	100	—	0
Hain				
Stick Safflower	1 tbsp	100	—	0
Stick Safflower Unsalted	1 tbsp	100	—	0
Tub Safflower	1 tbsp	100	—	0
Hollywood				
Safflower	1 tbsp	100	—	0
Safflower Unsalted Sweet	1 tbsp	100	—	0
Soft Spread	1 tbsp	90	0	0
I Can't Believe It's Not Butter				
Tub	1 tbsp	90	—	0
Krona				
Stick	1 tbsp	100	—	15
Land O'Lakes				
Stick	1 tbsp (0.5 oz)	90	—	0
Stick With Sweet Cream	1 tbsp (0.5 oz)	90	—	0
Stick With Sweet Cream Unsalted	1 tbsp (0.5 oz)	90	—	0
Tub	1 tbsp (0.5 oz)	80	—	0
Tub With Sweet Cream	1 tbsp (0.5 oz)	80	—	0
Mazola				
Stick	1 tbsp (14 g)	100	—	0
Stick	1 cup (229 g)	1650	—	0
Stick Unsalted	1 tbsp (14 g)	100	—	0
Stick Unsalted	1 cup (229 g)	1635	—	0
Tub Diet	1 cup (235 g)	815	—	0
Tub Diet	1 tbsp (14 g)	50	—	0
Tub Light Corn Oil Spread	1 tbsp (14 g)	50	—	0
Mother's				
Stick	1 tbsp	100	—	0
Stick Unsalted	1 tbsp	100	—	0
Tub Salted	1 tbsp	100	—	0
Tub Unsalted	1 tbsp	100	—	0
Nucanola				
Stick	1 tbsp	90	—	0
Parkay				
Squeeze	1 tbsp (0.5 oz)	80	0	0

FOOD	PORTION	CALS.	FIB.	CHOL.
Parkay (CONT.)				
Stick	1 tbsp (0.5 oz)	90	0	0
Stick ⅓ Less Fat	1 tbsp (0.5 oz)	70	0	0
Tub	1 tbsp (0.5 oz)	60	0	0
Tub Light	1 tbsp (0.5 oz)	50	0	0
Tub Soft	1 tbsp (0.5 oz)	100	0	0
Tub Soft Diet	1 tbsp (0.5 oz)	50	0	0
Whipped	1 tbsp (0.3 oz)	70	0	0
Promise				
Spread Soft	1 tbsp	80	—	0
Spread Stick	1 tbsp	90	—	0
Spread Light Soft	1 tbsp	50	—	0
Spread Light Stick	1 tbsp	50	—	0
Ultra Soft	1 tbsp	30	—	0
Ultra Spread Fat Free	1 tbsp	5	—	0
Smart Balance				
No Trans Fat	1 tbsp (0.5 oz)	120	—	0
No Trans Fat Light	1 tbsp (0.5 oz)	45	—	0
No Trans Fat Spread	1 tbsp (0.5 oz)	80	—	0
Smart Beat				
Light Unsalted	1 tbsp (0.5 oz)	25	—	0
Squeeze Fat Free	1 tbsp (0.5 oz)	5	—	0
Super Light Trans Fat Free	1 tbsp (0.5 oz)	20	—	0
Tub	1 tbsp	25	—	0
Tub Unsalted	1 tbsp	25	—	0
Touch Of Butter				
Squeeze	1 tbsp (0.5 oz)	80	0	0
Stick	1 tbsp (0.5 oz)	90	0	0
Tree Of Life				
Canola Soft	1 tbsp (0.5 oz)	100	—	0
Stick 100% Soy	1 tbsp (0.5 oz)	100	—	0
Stick 100% Soy Salt Free	1 tbsp (0.5 oz)	100	—	0
Stick Canola Soy	1 tbsp (0.5 oz)	100	—	0
Stick Canola Soy Salt Free	1 tbsp (0.5 oz)	100	—	0
Weight Watchers				
Light	1 tbsp	45	0	0
Light Sodium Free	1 tbsp	45	0	0
Reduced Fat Stick	1 tbsp	60	0	0

MARINADE
(*see* SAUCE)

MARJORAM

dried	1 tsp	2	—	0

FOOD	PORTION	CALS.	FIB.	CHOL.
MARSHMALLOW				
marshmallow	1 reg (0.3 oz)	23	—	0
marshmallow	1 cup (1.6 oz)	146	—	0
Campfire				
Large	2	40	—	0
Miniature	24	40	—	0
Joyva				
Twists Chocolate Covered	2 (1.5 oz)	190	0	0
Kraft				
Funmallows	4 (1.1 oz)	110	0	0
Funmallows Miniature	½ cup (1.1 oz)	100	0	0
Jet-Puffed	5 (1.2 oz)	110	0	0
Marshmallow Creme	2 tbsp (0.4 oz)	40	0	0
Miniature	½ cup (1.1 oz)	100	0	0
Teddy Bear Cocoa-Flavored	½ cup (1.1 oz)	100	0	0
MATZO				
plain	1 (1 oz)	112	1	0
whole wheat	1 (1 oz)	99	3	0
Goodman's				
Matzo Ball Mix 50% Less Salt	2 tbsp (0.5 oz)	50	0	0
Matzo Ball Mix as prep	2 tbsp (0.5 oz)	60	1	0
Horowitz Margareten				
Egg Milk Chocolate Coated	1 oz	97	1	8
Manischewitz				
Daily Thin Tea	1	103	tr	0
Dietetic Thins	1	91	tr	0
Egg Dark Chocolate Coated	½ matzo (1 oz)	97	1	8
Egg n' Onion	1	112	—	15
Matzo Cracker Miniatures	10	90	—	0
Matzo Farfel	1 cup	180	—	0
Matzo Meal	1 cup	514	tr	0
Passover	1	129	—	0
Passover Egg	1	132	—	25
Passover Egg Matzo Crackers	10	108	—	20
Salted Thin	1	100	tr	0
Unsalted	1	110	tr	0
Wheat Matzo Crackers	10	90	—	0
Whole Wheat w/ Bran	1	110	1	0
Streit's				
Dietetic	1 (1 oz)	100	1	0
Lightly Salted	1 (1 oz)	110	1	0
Matzoh Meal	¼ cup (1 oz)	110	1	0
Passover	1 (1 oz)	110	1	0

FOOD	PORTION	CALS.	FIB.	CHOL.
Streit's (CONT.)				
Unsalted	1 (0.9 oz)	100	1	0
Whole Wheat	1 (1 oz)	110	4	0

MAYONNAISE

(*see also* MAYONNAISE TYPE SALAD DRESSING, RELISH)

FOOD	PORTION	CALS.	FIB.	CHOL.
mayonnaise	1 cup	1577	—	130
mayonnaise	1 tbsp	99	—	8
reduced calorie	1 tbsp	34	—	4
reduced calorie	1 cup	556	—	58
sandwich spread	1 tbsp	60	—	12
Best Foods				
Cholesterol Free Reduced Calorie	1 tbsp (15 g)	50	—	0
Cholesterol Free Reduced Calorie	1 cup (233 g)	760	—	0
Light	1 cup (233 g)	760	—	90
Light	1 tbsp (15 g)	50	—	5
Real	1 tbsp	100	—	5
Real	1 cup	1570	—	95
Hain				
Canola	1 tbsp	60	—	0
Canola	1 tbsp	100	—	5
Cold Processed	1 tbsp	110	—	5
Eggless No Salt Added	1 tbsp	110	—	0
Light Low Sodium	1 tbsp	60	—	10
Real No Salt Added	1 tbsp	110	—	5
Safflower	1 tbsp	110	—	5
Hellmann's				
Cholesterol Free Reduced Calorie	1 tbsp (15 g)	50	—	0
Cholesterol Free Reduced Calorie	1 cup (233 g)	760	—	0
Light Reduced Calorie	1 tbsp (15 g)	50	—	5
Light Reduced Calorie	1 cup (233 g)	760	—	90
Mayonnaise	1 tbsp	100	—	5
Mayonnaise	1 cup (220 g)	1570	—	95
Hollywood				
Canola	1 tbsp	100	—	5
Mayonnaise	1 tbsp	110	—	5
Safflower	1 tbsp	100	—	5
Kraft				
Free	1 tbsp (0.6 oz)	10	0	0
Light	1 tbsp (0.5 oz)	50	0	0

FOOD	PORTION	CALS.	FIB.	CHOL.
Kraft (CONT.)				
Real	1 tbsp (0.5 oz)	100	0	10
McIlhenny				
Spicy	1 tbsp (0.5 oz)	108	tr	8
Mother's				
Mayonnaise	1 tbsp	100	—	10
Red Wing				
"H" Style	1 tbsp (0.5 oz)	110	0	10
Smart Beat				
Canola Oil	1 tbsp	40	—	0
Corn Beat	1 tbsp	40	—	0
Fat Free	1 tbsp	10	—	0
Weight Watchers				
Fat Free	1 tbsp	10	0	0
Light	1 tbsp	25	0	5
Light Low Sodium	1 tbsp	25	0	5

MAYONNAISE TYPE SALAD DRESSING
(*see also* MAYONNAISE, RELISH)

mayonnaise type salad dressing	1 cup	916	—	60
mayonnaise type salad dressing	1 tbsp	57	—	4
reduced calorie w/o cholesterol	1 tbsp	68	—	0
reduced calorie w/o cholesterol	1 cup	1084	—	0
Bright Day				
Salad Dressing	1 tbsp	60	—	0
Miracle Whip				
Free	1 tbsp (0.6 oz)	15	0	0
Light	1 tbsp (0.5 oz)	40	0	0
Salad Dressing	1 tbsp (0.5 oz)	70	0	5
Nayonaise				
Cholesterol Free	1 tbsp (0.5 oz)	35	tr	0
Fat Free	1 tbsp (0.5 oz)	11	tr	0
Spin Blend				
Cholesterol Free	1 tbsp	40	—	0
Dressing	1 tbsp	60	—	10
Weight Watchers				
Fat Free Whipped Dressing	1 tbsp	15	0	0

MEAT STICKS

jerky beef	1 oz	96	—	32
jerky beef	1 lg piece (0.7 oz)	67	—	22
smoked	1 (0.7 oz)	109	—	26
smoked	1 oz	156	—	38
Tombstone				
Beef Jerky	1 stick (0.5 oz)	35	0	15

FOOD	PORTION	CALS.	FIB.	CHOL.
Tombstone (CONT.)				
Beef Sticks	1 (0.8 oz)	110	0	20
Snappy Sticks	1 (0.8 oz)	110	0	20

MEAT SUBSTITUTES

(*see also* BACON SUBSTITUTES, CHICKEN SUBSTITUTES, SAUSAGE
SUBSTITUTES, TURKEY SUBSTITUTES)

FOOD	PORTION	CALS.	FIB.	CHOL.
simulated sausage	1 link (25 g)	64	—	0
simulated sausage	1 patty (38 g)	97	—	0
simulated meat product	1 oz	88	—	0
Boca Burgers				
Original	1 patty (2.5 oz)	110	4	3
Green Giant				
Harvest Burgers Original	1 (3 oz)	140	5	0
Harvest Direct				
TVP Beef Chunks	3.5 oz	280	18	0
TVP Beef Chunks Flavored	3.5 oz	250	17	0
TVP Beef Strips	3.5 oz	280	18	0
TVP Ground Beef	3.5 oz	280	18	0
TVP Ground Beef Flavored	3.5 oz	250	17	0
Jaclyn's				
Salisbury Steak Style Dinner	11 oz	260	—	0
Sirloin Strips Style Dinner	12 oz	290	—	0
Ken & Robert's				
Veggie Burger	1 (62 g)	110	—	0
LaLoma				
Big Franks	1 (51 g)	110	—	0
Corn Dogs	1 (71 g)	190	—	0
Dinner Cuts	2 pieces (99 g)	110	—	0
Griddle Steaks	1 piece (54 g)	140	—	0
Nuteena	½ in slice (65 g)	160	—	0
Patty Mix	¼ cup (16 g)	50	—	0
Redi-Burger	½ in slice (68 g)	130	—	0
Savory Dinner Loaf Mix not prep	¼ cup (16 g)	50	—	0
Savory Meatballs	7 (70 g)	190	—	0
Sizzle Burger	1 patty (71 g)	220	—	0
Sizzle Franks	2 (68 g)	170	—	0
Swiss Steak	1 piece (92 g)	170	—	0
Tender Bits	4 pieces (57 g)	80	—	0
Tender Rounds	6 pieces (73 g)	120	—	0
Vege-Burger	½ cup (108 g)	110	—	0
Vita-Burger Chunk	¼ cup (21 g)	70	—	0
Vita-Burger Granules	3 tbsp (21 g)	70	—	0

FOOD	PORTION	CALS.	FIB.	CHOL.
Lightlife				
American Grill	2.75 oz	110	—	0
Barbecue Grill	2.75 oz	130	—	0
Smart Deli Slices	2 slices (1.5 oz)	44	—	0
Smart Dogs	1 (1.5 oz)	40	—	0
Smart Dogs To Go	1 (5 oz)	115	—	0
Tofu Pups	1 (1.5 oz)	92	—	0
Vegetarian Sloppy Joe	4.3 oz	130	—	0
Midland Harvest				
Burger n' Loaf Chili w/o Beans	0.8 oz	90	2	0
Burger n' Loaf Herbs & Spice	3.2 oz	140	4	0
Burger n' Loaf Italian	3.2 oz	140	4	0
Burger n' Loaf Original	3.2 oz	140	4	0
Burger n' Loaf Sloppy Joe w/o Sauce	0.8 oz	80	1	0
Burger n' Loaf Taco	2.7 oz	90	1	0
Morningstar Farms				
Garden Grain Patties	1 patty (2.5 oz)	120	4	5
NewMenu				
VegiBurger	1 patty (3 oz)	110	1	0
VegiDogs	1 (1.5 oz)	45	0	0
Quorn				
Burger	1 patty (3 oz)	100	4	0
Sovex				
Better Than Burger?	½ cup (1.9 oz)	165	9	0
Soy Is Us				
Beef Not!	½ cup (1.75 oz)	140	9	0
Spring Creek				
Soysage	1 patty (1.6 oz)	63	—	0
Trader Joe's				
French Village Burger Champignon No Soy No Preservatives	1 patty (3.4 oz)	190	6	10
White Wave				
Meatless Healthy Franks	1 (1.5 oz)	90	0	0
Meatless Jumbo Franks	1 (3 oz)	170	0	0
Meatless Sandwich Slices Beef	2 slices (1.6 oz)	90	1	0
Meatless Sandwich Slices Bologna	2 slices (1.6 oz)	120	1	0
Meatless Sandwich Slices Pastrami	2 slices (1.6 oz)	90	1	0
Meatless Healthy Franks	1 (1.5 oz)	90	—	0
Veggie Burger	1 patty (2.5 oz)	110	2	0

FOOD	PORTION	CALS.	FIB.	CHOL.
Zoglo's				
Crispy Vegetarian Cutlets	1 (3.5 oz)	200	2	0
Savory Vegetarian Kebabs	1 serv (2.8 oz)	135	2	0
Tender Vegetarian Burgers	1 (2.6 oz)	150	2	0
Vegetable Patties	1 (2.6 oz)	130	2	0
Vegetarian Franks	1 (2.6 oz)	125	2	0

MELON
(see also individual names)
FRESH
Chiquita
Cantalene	1 cup	60	—	0
Honey Mist	1 cup	80	—	0

FROZEN
melon balls	1 cup	55	—	0
Big Valley				
Mixed	¾ cup (4.9 oz)	40	1	0

MEXICAN FOOD
(see also SALSA, SAUCE, SPANISH FOOD, TORTILLA)

MILK
(see also CHOCOLATE, COCOA, MILK DRINKS, MILKSHAKE)
CANNED
condensed sweetened	1 oz	123	—	13
condensed sweetened	1 cup	982	—	104
evaporated	½ cup	169	—	37
evaporated skim	½ cup	99	—	5
Carnation				
Evaporated	2 tbsp	40	—	10
Evaporated Lowfat	2 tbsp	25	—	5
Lite Evaporated Skimmed	½ cup (4 fl oz)	100	—	5
Sweetened Condensed	2 tbsp	130	—	10
Pet				
Evaporated	½ cup	170	—	36
Evaporated Filled	½ cup	150	—	5
Evaporated Light Skimmed	½ cup	100	—	10

DRIED
buttermilk	1 tbsp	25	—	5
nonfat instantized	1 pkg (3.2 oz)	244	—	12
Carnation				
Nonfat	⅓ cup dry	80	—	<5
Sanalac				
as prep	8 oz	80	0	4

REFRIGERATED
1%	1 cup	102	—	10

FOOD	PORTION	CALS.	FIB.	CHOL.
1%	1 qt	409	—	39
1% protein fortified	1 qt	477	—	39
1% protein fortified	1 cup	119	—	10
2%	1 cup	121	—	18
2%	1 qt	485	—	73
buttermilk	1 cup	99	—	9
buttermilk	1 qt	396	—	34
goat	1 cup	168	—	28
goat	1 qt	672	—	111
human	1 cup	171	—	34
indian buffalo	1 cup	236	—	46
low sodium	1 cup	149	—	33
skim	1 cup	86	—	4
skim	1 qt	342	—	18
skim protein fortified	1 qt	400	—	20
skim protein fortified	1 cup	100	—	5
whole	1 cup	150	—	33
BodyWise				
Nonfat	8 fl oz	100	0	5
CalciMilk				
CalciMilk	8 fl oz	102	0	10
Farmland				
1%	8 fl oz	100	0	10
2%	8 fl oz	130	0	20
Cholesterol Reduced	8 fl oz	150	—	10
Easylac 1%	8 fl oz	100	—	10
Easylac Nonfat	8 fl oz	90	—	5
Skim	8 fl oz	80	0	<5
Skim Plus	8 fl oz	100	—	5
Friendship				
Buttermilk	8 fl oz	120	0	15
Hood				
1%	1 cup (8 oz)	110	0	15
Better Taste 2%	1 cup (8 oz)	130	0	20
Buttermilk	1 cup (8 oz)	90	0	<5
Whole	1 cup (8 oz)	150	0	35
Lactaid				
1%	8 fl oz	102	0	10
Nonfat	8 fl oz	86	0	4
Nuform				
1%	1 cup (8 oz)	120	0	15
Skim	1 cup (8 oz)	100	0	<5
Silovet				
Skim	1 cup (8 oz)	90	0	<5

FOOD	PORTION	CALS.	FIB.	CHOL.
Weight Watchers				
Skim	1 cup	90	0	5
SHELF-STABLE				
Parmalat				
1%	1 cup (8 oz)	110	0	15
2%	1 cup (8 oz)	130	0	20
Skim	1 cup (8 oz)	90	0	5
Whole	1 cup (8 oz)	160	0	35

MILK DRINKS
(*see also* BREAKFAST DRINKS, CHOCOLATE, COCOA, MILKSHAKE)

FOOD	PORTION	CALS.	FIB.	CHOL.
chocolate milk	1 cup	208	—	30
chocolate milk	1 qt	833	—	122
chocolate milk 1%	1 cup	158	—	7
chocolate milk 1%	1 qt	630	—	29
chocolate milk 2%	1 cup	179	—	17
strawberry flavor mix as prep w/ whole milk	9 oz	234	—	33
Body Wise				
Chocolate Nonfat Milk	1 cup (8 fl oz)	180	1	5
Hershey				
Chocolate Milk 2%	1 cup	190	—	20
Hood				
Chocolate Lowfat	1 cup (8 oz)	150	0	10
Lactaid				
Chocolate Milk 1%	8 fl oz	158	tr	7
Parmalat				
Chocolate 2%	1 box (8 oz)	180	1	20

MILK SUBSTITUTES
(*see also* COFFEE WHITENERS)

FOOD	PORTION	CALS.	FIB.	CHOL.
imitation milk	1 cup	150	—	tr
imitation milk	1 qt	600	—	2
Better Than Milk				
Carob	8 fl oz	130	—	0
Chocolate	8 fl oz	125	—	0
Light	8 fl oz	80	—	0
Natural	8 fl oz	90	—	0
Eden				
Original	8 fl oz	130	0	0
Original	1 pkg (8.8 oz)	135	0	0
EdenBlend				
Original	8 fl oz	120	0	0
EdenRice				
Milk	8 fl oz	110	0	0

FOOD	PORTION	CALS.	FIB.	CHOL.
Edensoy				
Carob	8 fl oz	150	0	0
Extra Original	8 fl oz	130	0	0
Extra Original	1 pkg (8.8 oz)	140	0	0
Extra Vanilla	1 pkg (8.8 fl oz)	150	0	0
Extra Vanilla	8 fl oz	140	0	0
Vanilla	8 fl oz	150	0	0
Vanilla	1 pkg (8.8 fl oz)	150	0	0
Health Valley				
Soo Moo	1 cup	120	0	0
Rice Dream				
Carob Lite	8 fl oz	150	—	0
Chocolate	8 fl oz	190	—	0
Chocolate	8 fl oz	190	—	0
Lite Organic Original	8 fl oz	130	—	0
Lite Vanilla	8 fl oz	130	—	0
Spring Creek				
!Honey Vanilla	1 oz	23	—	0
Original	1 oz	21	—	0
Plain	1 oz	15	—	0
Vegelicious				
Milk	8 fl oz	100	—	0
Vitamite				
Non-Dairy 2% Fat	1 cup (8 oz)	110	0	0
Non-Dairy Nonfat	1 cup (8 oz)	90	0	0
Vitasoy				
Carob Supreme	8 fl oz	210	1	0
Cocoa Light	8 fl oz	130	1	0
Original Creamy	8 fl oz	160	1	0
Original Light	8 fl oz	90	1	0
Rich Cocoa	8 fl oz	210	1	0
Vanilla Light	8 fl oz	110	1	0
Vanilla Delite	8 fl oz	190	1	0
Westsoy				
Cocoa Lite	8 fl oz	140	—	0
Plain Lite	8 fl oz	100	—	0
Vanilla Lite	8 fl oz	110	—	0
MILKFISH				
baked	3 oz	162	—	57
MILKSHAKE				
chocolate	10 oz	360	—	37
strawberry	10 oz	319	—	31
thick shake chocolate	10.6 oz	356	—	32

FOOD	PORTION	CALS.	FIB.	CHOL.
thick shake vanilla	11 oz	350	—	37
vanilla	10 oz	314	—	32
Hood				
Shake Up Chocolate	1 cup (8 oz)	240	0	20
Shake Up Strawberry	1 cup (8 oz)	220	0	20
Shake Up Vanilla	1 cup (8 oz)	220	0	20
MicroMagic				
Chocolate	1 (10.5 oz)	290	—	40
Milky Way				
Shake	1 (10 fl oz)	390	0	60
Parmalat				
Shake A Shake Chocolate	1 box (6 oz)	180	1	15
Shake A Shake Orange Vanilla	1 box (6 oz)	110	0	10
Shake A Shake Vanilla	1 box (6 oz)	170	0	15
Weight Watchers				
Chocolate Fudge Shake Mix as prep	1 pkg	80	2	0

MILLET

cooked	½ cup	143	—	0

MINERAL/BOTTLED WATER

FOOD	PORTION	CALS.	FIB.	CHOL.
Artesia				
Almund	7 oz	0	—	0
Cranberi	7 oz	0	—	0
Lemin	7 oz	0	—	0
Orange	7 oz	0	—	0
Plain	7 oz	0	—	0
Canada Dry				
Sparkling Water	8 fl oz	0	0	0
Crystal Geyser				
Sparking Natural Wild Cherry	1 bottle (12 fl oz)	0	—	0
Sparkling Lemon	1 bottle (12 fl oz)	0	—	0
Sparkling Mineral	1 bottle (12 fl oz)	0	—	0
Sparkling Natural Cola Berry	1 bottle (12 fl oz)	0	—	0
Sparkling Orange	1 bottle (12 fl oz)	0	—	0
Diamond Spring				
Water	1 qt	0	—	0
Evian				
Water	1 liter	0	0	0
Glennpatrick				
Irish Spring Pure	8 oz	0	—	0
LaCroix				
Sparkling Berry	12 fl oz	0	—	0
Sparkling Lemon	12 fl oz	0	—	0

FOOD	PORTION	CALS.	FIB.	CHOL.
LaCroix (CONT.)				
Sparkling Lime	12 fl oz	0	—	0
Sparkling Orange	12 fl oz	0	—	0
Sparkling Regular	12 fl oz	0	—	0
Mountain Valley				
Mineral Water	1 qt	0	—	0
San Pellegrino				
Mineral Water	1 liter (33.8 oz)	0	—	0
Saratoga				
Sparkling	1 liter	0	—	0
Water Joe				
Caffeine Enhanced	8 fl oz	0	—	0
MISO				
miso	½ cup	284	7	0
Eden				
Genmai Miso Organic	1 tbsp (0.5 oz)	25	tr	0
Hacho Miso Organic	1 tbsp (0.5 oz)	35	1	0
Kome Miso Organic	1 tbsp (0.6 oz)	25	tr	0
Mugi Miso Organic	1 tbsp (0.6 oz)	25	1	0
Shiro Miso Organic	1 tbsp (0.6 oz)	35	1	0
MOLASSES				
blackstrap	1 tbsp (0.7 oz)	47	—	0
blackstrap	1 cup (11.5 oz)	771	—	0
molasses	1 tbsp (0.7 oz)	53	—	0
molasses	1 cup (11.5 oz)	873	—	0
Brer Rabbit				
Dark	2 tbsp	110	—	0
Light	2 tbsp	110	—	0
McIlhenny				
Molasses	1 tbsp (0.7 oz)	66	tr	0
Tree Of Life				
Blackstrap	1 tbsp (0.5 oz)	45	—	0
MONKFISH				
baked	3 oz	82	—	27
MOOSE				
roasted	3 oz	114	—	66
MOTH BEANS				
dried cooked	1 cup	207	—	0
MOUSSE				
FROZEN				
Pepperidge Farm				
San Francisco Chocolate Mousse	1	490	—	150

FOOD	PORTION	CALS.	FIB.	CHOL.
Sara Lee				
Chocolate	1 slice (2.7 oz)	260	—	20
Chocolate Light	1 (3 oz)	170	—	10
Weight Watchers				
Chocolate Mousse	1 (2.75 oz)	190	3	5
Praline Pecan	1 (2.71 oz)	170	0	0
Triple Chocolate Caramel Mousse	1 (2.75 oz)	200	2	5
HOME RECIPE				
chocolate	½ cup (7.1 oz)	447	—	299
crab	¼ cup	364	—	136
orange	½ cup	87	—	1
MIX				
Jell-O				
Rich & Luscious Chocolate	½ cup	145	—	9
Rich & Luscious Chocolate Fudge	½ cup	143	—	9
Knorr				
Dark Chocolate as prep	½ cup	90	—	5
Milk Chocolate as prep	½ cup	90	—	5
White Chocolate as prep	½ cup	80	—	5
Royal				
Chocolate Mousse No-Bake	⅛ pie	130	—	0
TAKE-OUT				
chocolate	½ cup (7.1 oz)	447	—	299

MUFFIN
FROZEN

Health Valley

FOOD	PORTION	CALS.	FIB.	CHOL.
Almond & Date Oat Bran Fancy Fruit	1	180	8	0
Fat Free Apple Spice	1	140	5	0
Fat Free Banana	1	130	5	0
Fat Free Raisin Spice	1	140	5	0
Oat Bran Fancy Fruit Blueberry	1	140	8	0
Oat Bran Fancy Fruit Raisin	1	180	8	0
Rice Bran Fancy Fruit Raisin	1	210	6	0
Pepperidge Farm				
Banana Nut	1	170	—	30
Blueberry	1	170	1	25
Cholesterol Free Multi Grain Muesli	1	200	—	0
Cholesterol Free Oatbran With Apple	1	190	—	0

FOOD	PORTION	CALS.	FIB.	CHOL.
Pepperidge Farm (CONT.)				
Cholesterol Free Raisin Bran	1	170	—	0
Cinnamon Swirl	1	190	1	35
Corn	1	180	—	30
Sara Lee				
Apple Oat Bran	1	190	—	0
Apple Spice	1	220	—	0
Blueberry	1	200	—	0
Blueberry Free & Light	1	120	—	0
Golden Corn	1	240	—	0
Oat Bran	1	210	—	0
Raisin Bran	1	220	—	0
Weight Watchers				
Banana Nut	1 (2.5 oz)	190	3	5
Blueberry	1 (2.5 oz)	250	4	45
Chocolate Chocolate Chip	1 (2.5 oz)	200	1	5
Harvest Honey Bran	1 (2.5 oz)	220	10	0
HOME RECIPE				
blueberry as prep w/ 2% milk	1 (2 oz)	163	—	21
blueberry as prep w/ whole milk	1 (2 oz)	165	—	23
corn as prep w/ 2% milk	1 (2 oz)	180	—	24
corn as prep w/ whole milk	1 (2 oz)	183	—	25
plain as prep w/ 2% milk	1 (2 oz)	169	—	22
plain as prep w/ whole milk	1 (2 oz)	172	—	24
wheat bran as prep w/ 2% milk	1 (2 oz)	161	—	19
wheat bran as prep w/ whole milk	1 (2 oz)	164	—	20
MIX				
blueberry	1 (1¾ oz)	149	—	23
corn	1 (1.75 oz)	160	—	31
wheat bran as prep	1 (1¾ oz)	138	—	34
Arrowhead				
Bran	⅓ cup (1.4 oz)	150	7	0
Oat Bran Wheat Free	⅓ cup (1.5 oz)	160	7	0
Betty Crocker				
Apple Cinnamon	1	120	—	25
Apple Cinnamon No Cholesterol Recipe	1	110	—	0
Banana Nut	1	120	—	25
Banana Nut No Cholesterol Recipe	1	110	—	0
Cinnamon Streusel	1	200	—	30
Oat Bran	1	190	—	35
Oat Bran No Cholesterol Recipe	1	180	—	0
Twice The Blueberries	1	120	—	20

FOOD	PORTION	CALS.	FIB.	CHOL.
Betty Crocker (CONT.)				
Twice The Blueberries No Cholesterol Recipe	1	110	—	0
Wild Blueberry	1	120	—	25
Wild Blueberry Light	1	70	—	20
Wild Blueberry Light No Cholesterol Recipe	1	70	—	0
Wild Blueberry No Cholesterol Recipe	1	110	—	0
Flako				
Corn	⅓ cup (1.4 oz)	160	1	0
Hain				
Oat Bran Apple Cinnamon	1	140	5	0
Oat Bran Banana Nut	1	140	4	0
Oat Bran Raspberry Spice	1	140	4	0
Jiffy				
Apple Cinnamon as prep	1	190	1	33
Banana Nut as prep	1	180	1	27
Blueberry as prep	1	190	1	36
Bran Date	1	110	—	10
Bran With Dates as prep	1	170	3	36
Corn as prep	1	180	1	0
Honey Date as prep	1	170	1	30
Oatmeal as prep	1	180	2	27
Wanda's				
Blue Corn	¼ cup mix per serv (1.2 oz)	130	1	0
READY-TO-EAT				
blueberry	1 (2 oz)	158	2	17
oat bran wheat free	1 (2 oz)	154	4	0
Arnold				
Bran'nola	1 (2.3 oz)	160	2	0
Raisin	1 (2.3 oz)	160	2	0
Dutch Mill				
Apple Oat Bran	1 (2 oz)	180	1	0
Banana Walnut	1 (2 oz)	220	1	5
Carrot	1 (2 oz)	190	1	30
Corn	1 (2 oz)	190	1	40
Cranberry Orange	1 (2 oz)	170	1	55
Raisin Bran	1 (2 oz)	230	3	30
Freihofer's				
Corn Toasters	1 (1.3 oz)	130	0	15
Hostess				
Mini Apple Cinnamon	5 (2 oz)	260	3	45

FOOD	PORTION	CALS.	FIB.	CHOL.
Hostess (CONT.)				
Mini Banana Nut	5 (2 oz)	260	tr	40
Mini Blueberry	5 (2 oz)	240	tr	40
Mini Chocolate Chip	5 (2 oz)	260	1	35
Muffin Loaf Blueberry	1 (3.8 oz)	440	2	80
Oat Bran	1 (1.5 oz)	160	tr	0
Oat Bran Banana Nut	1 (1.5 oz)	150	1	0

MULBERRIES
fresh	1 cup	61	—	0

MULLET
striped cooked	3 oz	127	—	54
striped raw	3 oz	99	—	42

MUNG BEANS
DRIED
cooked	1 cup	213	—	0

SPROUTS
canned	½ cup	8	—	0
cooked	½ cup	13	—	0
raw	½ cup	16	—	0
stir fried	½ cup	31	—	0

MUNGO BEANS
dried cooked	1 cup	190	—	1

MUSHROOMS
CANNED
chanterelle	3½ oz	12	6	0
pieces	½ cup	19	—	0
whole	1 (0.4 oz)	3	—	0
B In B				
Mushrooms	¼ cup	12	1	0
With Garlic	¼ cup	12	1	0
Empress				
Button	2 oz	14	—	0
Button Sliced	2 oz	14	—	0
Pieces & Stems	2 oz	14	—	0
Straw Broken	2 oz	10	—	0
Green Giant				
Oriental Straw	¼ cup	12	1	0
Pieces And Stems	¼ cup	12	1	0
Sliced	¼ cup	12	1	0
Whole	¼ cup	12	1	0
Ka-Me				
Stir Fry	½ cup (4.5 oz)	20	2	0

FOOD	PORTION	CALS.	FIB.	CHOL.
Ka-Me (CONT.)				
Straw Whole Peeled	½ cup (4.5 oz)	20	2	0
Seneca				
Mushrooms	½ cup	25	2	0
DRIED				
chanterelle	3½ oz	89	60	0
shitake	4 (½ oz)	44	—	0
FRESH				
chanterelle	3½ oz	11	6	0
enoki raw	1 (4 in)	2	—	0
morel	3½ oz	9	7	0
raw	1 (½ oz)	5	tr	0
raw sliced	½ cup	9	tr	0
shitake cooked	4 (2.5 oz)	40	—	0
sliced cooked	½ cup	21	1	0
whole cooked	1 (0.4 oz)	3	—	0
Mother Earth				
Organic	4 oz	35	tr	0
FROZEN				
Empire				
Breaded	7 (2.8 oz)	90	1	0

MUSSELS

FOOD	PORTION	CALS.	FIB.	CHOL.
blue raw	3 oz	73	—	24
blue raw	1 cup	129	—	42
fresh blue cooked	3 oz	147	—	48

MUSTARD

FOOD	PORTION	CALS.	FIB.	CHOL.
dry mustard seed yellow	1 tsp	15	—	0
yellow ready-to-use	1 tsp	5	—	0
Blanchard & Blanchard				
Mustard	1 tsp (5 g)	0	0	0
Eden				
Hot Organic	1 tsp (5 g)	0	0	0
Grey Poupon				
Country Dijon	1 tsp	6	0	0
Dijon	1 tsp	6	0	0
Parisian	1 tsp	6	0	0
Hain				
Stone Ground	1 tbsp	14	—	0
Stone Ground No Salt Added	1 tbsp	14	—	0
Heinz				
Mild Yellow	1 tbsp	8	—	0
Spicy Brown	1 tbsp	14	—	0

FOOD	PORTION	CALS.	FIB.	CHOL.
Ka-Me				
Hot Mustard Powder Chinese Style	¼ tsp (1 g)	5	1	0
Kosciuszko				
Spicy Brown	1 tsp	5	—	0
Kraft				
Mustard	1 tsp (0.2 oz)	0	0	0
McIlhenny				
Coarse Ground	1 tsp (0.2 oz)	4	tr	0
Spicy	1 tsp (0.2 oz)	6	1	0
Plochman				
Dijon	1 tsp (5 g)	7	—	0
Spoonable Salad	1 tsp (5 g)	4	—	0
Squeeze Salad	1 tsp (5 g)	4	—	0
Stone Ground	1 tsp (5 g)	6	—	0
Tree Of Life				
Dijon	1 tsp (5 g)	0	—	0
Dijon Imported	1 tsp (5 g)	5	—	0
Low Sodium	1 tsp (5 g)	3	—	0
Stone Ground	1 tsp (5 g)	0	—	0
Yellow	1 tsp (5 g)	0	—	0
MUSTARD GREENS				
CANNED				
Allen				
Mustard Greens	½ cup (4.1 oz)	30	3	0
Sunshine				
Mustard Greens	½ cup (4.1 oz)	30	3	0
FRESH				
chopped cooked	½ cup	11	—	0
raw chopped	½ cup	7	—	0
FROZEN				
chopped cooked	½ cup	14	—	0
NATTO				
natto	½ cup	187	—	0
NAVY BEANS				
CANNED				
navy	1 cup	296	—	0
Allen				
Navy Beans	½ cup (4.5 oz)	110	6	0
Eden				
Organic	½ cup (4.3 oz)	100	7	0
Hanover				
Navy	½ cup	100	—	0

FOOD	PORTION	CALS.	FIB.	CHOL.
Trappey				
With Bacon	½ cup (4.5 oz)	110	7	0
With Bacon & Jalapeno	½ cup (4.5 oz)	110	7	0
DRIED				
cooked	1 cup	259	—	0
SPROUTS				
cooked	3½ oz	78	—	0
raw	½ cup	35	—	0

NECTARINE

FOOD	PORTION	CALS.	FIB.	CHOL.
fresh	1	67	2	0
Dole				
Nectarine	1	70	3	0

NEUFCHATEL

FOOD	PORTION	CALS.	FIB.	CHOL.
neufchatel	1 oz	74	—	22
neufchatel	1 pkg (3 oz)	221	—	65
Philadelphia				
Neufchatel	1 oz	70	0	20
Spreadery				
Classic Ranch	2 tbsp (1 oz)	60	0	20
Garden Vegetable	2 tbsp (1 oz)	70	0	20
Garlic & Herb	2 tbsp (1 oz)	80	0	20
With Strawberry	1 oz	70	—	15
WisPride				
Garden Vegetable Cup	2 tbsp (1.1 oz)	60	0	15
Garlic & Herb Cup	2 tbsp (1.1 oz)	60	0	15

NONDAIRY CREAMERS
(*see* COFFEE WHITENERS)

NONDAIRY WHIPPED TOPPINGS
(*see* WHIPPED TOPPINGS)

NOODLE DISHES
(*see also* NOODLES, PASTA DINNERS)

FOOD	PORTION	CALS.	FIB.	CHOL.
CANNED				
Micro Cup Meals				
Noodles & Chicken	1 cup (10.4 oz)	250	2	45
Van Camp's				
Noodlee Weenee	1 can (8 oz)	230	1	20
FROZEN				
Luigino's				
Stroganoff	1 pkg (8 oz)	310	2	55
MIX				
Kraft				
Chicken Egg Noodle	1 cup	330	1	60

FOOD	PORTION	CALS.	FIB.	CHOL.
La Choy				
Ramen Noodles Beef as prep	1 cup	200	4	0
Ramen Noodles Chicken as prep	1 cup	200	4	0
Lipton				
Noodles & Sauce Alfredo	⅔ cup (2.2 oz)	250	1	75
Noodles & Sauce Alfredo Broccoli as prep	⅔ cup (2.2 oz)	260	2	75
Noodles & Sauce Alfredo Carbonara	⅔ cup (2.2 oz)	260	2	85
Noodles & Sauce Beef	⅔ cup (2.1 oz)	220	2	60
Noodles & Sauce Butter	⅔ cup (2.2 oz)	260	2	65
Noodles & Sauce Butter & Herb	⅔ cup (2.2 oz)	250	2	65
Noodles & Sauce Cheddar & Bacon	⅔ cup (2.1 oz)	230	2	65
Noodles & Sauce Cheese	⅔ cup (2.3 oz)	250	1	65
Noodles & Sauce Chicken	⅔ cup (2.1 oz)	230	2	60
Noodles & Sauce Chicken Broccoli	⅔ cup (2.1 oz)	220	2	60
Noodles & Sauce Chicken Tetrazzini	⅔ cup (2 oz)	220	2	65
Noodles & Sauce Creamy Chicken	⅔ cup (2.1 oz)	230	2	65
Noodles & Sauce Parmesan	⅔ cup (2.1 oz)	250	2	70
Noodles & Sauce Romanoff	⅔ cup (2.3 oz)	260	2	70
Noodles & Sauce Sour Cream & Chive	⅔ cup (2.2 oz)	260	2	70
Noodles & Sauce Stroganoff	⅔ cup (2 oz)	210	2	65
Minute				
Microwave Chicken Flavored	½ cup	157	—	36
Microwave Parmesan	½ cup	178	—	47
Noodles By Leonardo				
Macaroni & Cheese as prep	1 cup (2.5 oz)	250	2	0
SHELF-STABLE				
Micro Cup Meals				
Noodles & Chicken	1 cup (7.5 oz)	180	1	30
TAKE-OUT				
noodle pudding	½ cup	132	—	27
NOODLES				
cellophane	1 cup	492	—	0
chow mein	1 cup	237	—	0
egg	1 cup (38 g)	145	—	36
egg cooked	1 cup	212	—	53

FOOD	PORTION	CALS.	FIB.	CHOL.
japanese soba cooked	½ cup	56	—	0
japanese soba not prep	2 oz	192	—	0
japanese somen cooked	½ cup	115	—	0
japanese somen not prep	2 oz	203	—	0
spinach/egg cooked	1 cup	211	—	52
spinach/egg not prep	1 cup	145	—	36
Creamette				
Egg	2 oz	221	—	70
Golden Grain				
Egg	2 oz	210	2	65
Herb's				
Egg Fine	2 oz	220	2	60
Egg Medium	2 oz	220	2	60
Kluski Medium	2 oz	220	2	60
Kluski Wide	2 oz	220	2	60
Hodgson Mill				
Veggie Egg	2 oz	200	2	35
Whole Wheat Egg	2 oz	190	4	30
Whole Wheat Spinach Egg	2 oz	190	5	30
Ka-Me				
Chinese Egg	½ cup (2 oz)	210	2	53
Chinese Plain	½ cup (2 oz)	200	1	0
Chuka Soba Curly Noodles	2 oz	200	1	0
Lo Mein Wide Chinese	½ cup (2 oz)	200	1	0
Py Mai Fun Rice Sticks	2 oz	193	0	0
Sai Fun Bean Thread	1 cup (2 oz)	190	1	0
Soba Shin Shu Japanese Buckwheat	2 oz	200	2	0
Tomoshiraga Somen Noodles	2 oz	190	1	0
Udon Japanese Thick	2 oz	190	1	0
La Choy				
Chow Mein Narrow	½ cup	150	tr	0
Chow Mein Wide	½ cup	150	tr	0
Rice	½ cup	130	tr	0
Mueller's				
Egg	2 oz (57 g)	220	—	55
Noodle Trio	2 oz (57 g)	220	—	55
Noodles By Leonardo				
Egg Fine	2 oz	210	2	80
Egg Medium	2 oz	210	2	80
Egg Wide	2 oz	210	2	80
San Giorgio				
Egg	2 oz	210	—	70

FOOD	PORTION	CALS.	FIB.	CHOL.
Shofar				
No Yolks	2 oz	210	3	0
NOPALES				
cooked	1 cup (5.2 oz)	23	—	0
raw sliced	1 cup (3 oz)	14	—	0
raw sliced	½ cup (1.5 oz)	7	—	0
NUTMEG				
ground	1 tsp	12	—	0
Watkins				
Ground	¼ tsp (0.5 g)	0	0	0

NUTRITIONAL SUPPLEMENTS

(*see also* BREAKFAST BAR, BREAKFAST DRINKS, SPORTS DRINKS)

FOOD	PORTION	CALS.	FIB.	CHOL.
BeneFit				
Nutrition Bar	1 (2 oz)	240	tr	0
Boost				
Chocolate	1 can (8 oz)	240	0	5
Vanilla	8 oz	240	0	5
Calorie Shed				
Shake Fat Free No Sugar Caramel Ripple	½ cup (4 fl oz)	70	2	5
Shake Fat Free No Sugar Chocolate	½ cup (4 fl oz)	70	2	5
Shake Fat Free No Sugar Marshmellow Nougat	½ cup (4 fl oz)	70	2	5
Fi-Bar				
Apple	1 (1 oz)	90	5	0
Cocoa Almond	1	130	4	0
Cocoa Peanut	1	130	4	0
Cranberry & Wild Berries	1 (1 oz)	100	4	0
Lemon	1 (1 oz)	90	5	0
Mandarin Orange	1 (1 oz)	99	5	0
Nuggets Almond Cappuccino Crunch	1 pkg	136	—	0
Nuggets Almond Butter Crunch	1 pkg	163	—	0
Nuggets Coconut Almond Crunch	1 pkg	136	—	0
Nuggets Peanut Butter Crunch	1 pkg	160	—	0
Raspberry	1 (1 oz)	100	4	0
Strawberry	1 (1 oz)	100	4	0
Treat Yourself Right Almond	1	152	5	0
Treat Yourself Right Peanutty Butter	1	152	5	0

FOOD	PORTION	CALS.	FIB.	CHOL.
Fi-Bar (CONT.)				
Vanilla Almond	1	130	4	0
Vanilla Peanut	1	130	4	0
Gatorade				
GatorBar	1 (1.17 oz)	110	1	0
GatorLode	1 can (11.6 fl oz)	280	—	0
GatorPro	1 can (11 fl oz)	360	0	0
ReLode	1 pkt (0.75 oz)	80	—	0
GeniSoy				
Soy Protein Bar Chocolate	1 bar (2.2 oz)	210	1	0
Soy Protein Bar Chocolate Coated	1 bar (2.2 oz)	220	1	0
Gookinaid				
Lemonade	1 cup (8 fl oz)	45	—	0
Malsovit				
Mealwafers	2	152	—	0
Meal On The Go				
Apple	1 bar (3 oz)	294	5	0
Banana w/ Pecans	1 bar (3 oz)	289	8	0
Original	1 bar (3 oz)	286	7	0
Nancy Grey's				
Shake Hi-Protein Black Raspberry	1 cup (8 fl oz)	340	0	65
Shake Hi-Protein Chocolate	1 cup (8 fl oz)	340	0	65
Shake Hi-Protein Vanilla	1 cup (8 fl oz)	340	0	65
NiteBite				
Chocolate Fudge	1 bar (0.9 oz)	100	0	5
Peanut Butter	1 bar (0.9 oz)	100	0	5
Nutra/Balance				
EggPro	4 oz	200	—	18
Frozen Pudding Butterscotch	4 oz	225	—	0
Frozen Pudding Chocolate	4 oz	225	—	0
Frozen Pudding Tapioca	4 oz	225	—	0
Frozen Pudding Vanilla	4 oz	225	—	0
NutraShake				
Chocolate	4 oz	200	—	18
Strawberry	4 oz	200	—	18
Vanilla	4 oz	200	—	18
With Fiber Strawberry	6 oz	300	—	0
With Fiber Vanilla	6 oz	300	—	0
Power Bar				
Malt-Nut	1 bar (2.3 oz)	230	3	0
Sego				
Lite Chocolate	10 fl oz	150	—	5

FOOD	PORTION	CALS.	FIB.	CHOL.
Sego (CONT.)				
Lite Dutch Chocolate	10 fl oz	150	—	5
Lite French Vanilla	10 fl oz	150	—	5
Lite Strawberry	10 fl oz	150	—	5
Lite Vanilla	10 fl oz	150	—	5
Very Chocolate	10 fl oz	225	—	5
Very Chocolate Malt	10 fl oz	225	—	5
Very Strawberry	10 fl oz	225	—	5
Very Vanilla	10 fl oz	225	—	5
Slim-Fast				
Powder Chocolate as prep w/ skim milk	8 oz	190	2	9
Powder Chocolate Malt as prep w/ skim milk	8 oz	190	2	9
Powder Strawberry as prep w/ skim milk	8 oz	190	2	9
Powder Vanilla as prep w/ skim milk	8 oz	190	2	6
Sustacal				
Vanilla	8 oz	240	tr	<5
Sweet Success				
Chewy Bar Chocolate Brownie	1 (1.6 oz)	120	3	<5
Chewy Bar Chocolate Peanut Butter	1 (1.6 oz)	120	3	<5
Chewy Bar Chocolate Raspberry	1 (1.6 oz)	120	3	<5
Chewy Bar Chocolate Chip	1 (1.6 oz)	120	3	<5
Chewy Bar Oatmeal Raisin	1 (1.6 oz)	120	3	<5
Chocolate Raspberry Truffle	1 can (10 fl oz)	200	6	5
Chocolate Raspberry as prep w/ skim milk	9 fl oz	180	6	6
Chocolate Mocha Supreme	1 can (10 fl oz)	200	6	5
Chocolate Mocha Supreme as prep w/ skim milk	9 fl oz	180	6	6
Classic Chocolate Chip as prep w/ skim milk	9 fl oz	180	6	6
Creamy Milk Chocolate	1 can (10 fl oz)	200	6	5
Creamy Milk Chocolate	1 carton (12 fl oz)	220	6	<5
Creamy Milk Chocolate as prep w/ skim milk	9 fl oz	180	6	6
Creamy Vanilla Delight as prep w/ skim milk	9 fl oz	180	6	6
Dark Chocolate Fudge	1 can (10 fl oz)	200	6	5
Dark Chocolate Fudge	1 carton (12 fl oz)	220	6	<5

FOOD	PORTION	CALS.	FIB.	CHOL.
Sweet Success (CONT.)				
Dark Chocolate Fudge as prep w/ skim milk	9 fl oz	180	6	6
Rich Chocolate Almond	1 can (10 fl oz)	200	6	5
Rich Chocolate Almond	1 carton (12 fl oz)	220	6	<5
Rich Chocolate Almond as prep w/ skim milk	9 fl oz	180	6	6
Smooth Vanilla Creme	1 can (10 fl oz)	200	6	5
The Pumper				
Body Building MilkShake Chocolate & Banana	1 serv (13.5 oz)	390	3	10
Ultra Slim-Fast				
Cafe Mocha as prep w/ skim milk	8 oz	200	4	8
Chocolate Royale as prep w/ skim milk	8 oz	200	5	8
Crunch Bar Cocoa Almond	1	110	3	0
Crunch Bar Cocoa Raspberry	1	100	3	0
Crunch Bar Vanilla Almond	1	110	3	0
Dutch Chocolate as prep w/ water	8 oz	220	5	0
French Vanilla as prep w/ skim milk	8 oz	190	4	8
French Vanilla as prep w/ water	8 oz	220	4	8
Fruit Juice Mix as prep w/ fruit juice	8 oz	200	6	12
Nutrition Bar Dutch Chocolate	1	130	6	5
Nutrition Bar Peanut Butter	1	140	7	5
Pina Colada as prep w/ skim milk	8 oz	180	6	8
Ready-To-Drink Chocolate Royale	11 oz	230	5	5
Ready-To-Drink Chocolate Royale	12 oz	250	5	5
Ready-To-Drink French Vanilla	11 oz	230	5	5
Ready-To-Drink French Vanilla	12 oz	220	5	5
Ready-To-Drink Strawberry Supreme	12 oz	220	5	5
Strawberry as prep w/ skim milk	8 oz	190	4	8
Strawberry Supreme as prep w/ water	8 oz	220	4	8
Vita-J				
Apple Juice	11.5 fl oz	8	—	0

FOOD	PORTION	CALS.	FIB.	CHOL.
Vita-J (CONT.)				
Fruit Punch	11.5 fl oz	8	—	0
Grapefruit Cocktail w/ Raspberry	11.5 fl oz	8	—	0
Orange Juice	11.5 fl oz	8	—	0
NUTS MIXED				
(see also individual names)				
dry roasted w/ peanuts	1 oz	169	—	0
dry roasted w/ peanuts salted	1 oz	169	—	0
oil roasted w/ peanuts	1 oz	175	—	0
oil roasted w/ peanuts salted	1 oz	175	—	0
oil roasted w/o peanuts	1 oz	175	—	0
oil roasted w/o peanuts salted	1 oz	175	—	0
Fisher				
Mixed Deluxe Lightly Salted	1 oz	180	—	0
Mixed Deluxe Salted	1 oz	180	—	0
Mixed Oil Roasted 25% More Cashews Lightly Salted	1 oz	180	—	0
Mixed Oil Roasted 25% More Cashews Salted	1 oz	180	—	0
Nut & Fruit Pina Colada	1 oz	150	—	0
Nut & Fruit Raisin Cranberry	1 oz	150	—	0
Nut & Fruit Tropical Fruit	1 oz	140	—	0
Nut Toppings Oil Roasted With Peanuts	1 oz	190	—	0
Peanuts Cashews	1 oz	170	—	0
Guy's				
Mixed With Peanuts	1 oz	180	—	0
Tasty Mix	1 oz	130	—	0
Planters				
Cashews & Peanuts Honey Roasted	1 oz	150	2	0
Deluxe Oil Roasted	1 oz	170	2	0
Dry Roasted	1 oz	170	2	0
Honey Roasted	1 oz	140	2	0
Lightly Salted Oil Roasted	1 oz	170	2	0
No Brazils Lightly Salted Oil Roasted	1 oz	170	2	0
No Brazils Oil Roasted	1 oz	170	2	0
Oil Roasted	1 oz	170	2	0
Select Mix Cashews Almonds & Macadamias Oil Roasted	1 oz	170	2	0
Select Mix Cashews Almonds & Pecans Oil Roasted	1 oz	170	2	0

FOOD	PORTION	CALS.	FIB.	CHOL.
Planters (CONT.)				
Unsalted Oil Roasted	1 oz	170	3	0
OCTOPUS				
fresh steamed	3 oz	140	—	82
OHELOBERRIES				
fresh	1 cup	39	—	0
OIL				
(*see also* FAT)				
almond	1 cup	1927	—	0
almond	1 tbsp	120	—	0
apricot kernel	1 cup	1927	—	0
apricot kernel	1 tbsp	120	—	0
avocado	1 tbsp	124	—	0
avocado	1 cup	1927	—	0
babassu palm	1 tbsp	120	—	0
butter oil	1 cup	1795	—	524
butter oil	1 tbsp	112	—	33
canola	1 cup	1927	—	0
canola	1 tbsp	124	—	0
coconut	1 tbsp	117	—	0
corn	1 cup	1927	—	0
corn	1 tbsp	120	—	0
cottonseed	1 cup	1927	—	0
cottonseed	1 tbsp	120	—	0
cupu assu	1 tbsp	120	—	0
grapeseed	1 tbsp	120	—	0
hazelnut	1 cup	1927	—	0
hazelnut	1 tbsp	120	—	0
mustard	1 cup	1927	—	0
mustard	1 tbsp	124	—	0
oat	1 tbsp	120	—	0
olive	1 tbsp	119	—	0
olive	1 cup	1909	—	0
palm	1 tbsp	120	—	0
palm	1 cup	1927	—	0
palm kernel	1 tbsp	117	—	0
palm kernel	1 cup	1879	—	0
peanut	1 cup	1909	—	0
peanut	1 tbsp	119	—	0
poppyseed	1 tbsp	120	—	0
poppyseed	3.5 fl oz	900	—	0
rice bran	1 tbsp	120	—	0

FOOD	PORTION	CALS.	FIB.	CHOL.
safflower	1 cup	1927	—	0
safflower	1 tbsp	120	—	0
sesame	1 tbsp	120	—	0
sheanut	1 tbsp	120	—	0
soybean	1 tbsp	120	—	0
soybean	1 cup	1927	—	0
sunflower	1 tbsp	120	—	0
sunflower	1 cup	1927	—	0
teaseed	1 tbsp	120	—	0
tomatoseed	1 tbsp	120	—	0
vegetable soybean & cottonseed	1 tbsp	120	—	0
vegetable soybean & cottonseed	1 cup	1927	—	0
walnut	1 tbsp	120	—	0
walnut	1 cup	1927	1	0
wheat germ	1 tbsp	120	—	0
Arrowhead				
Hazelnut	1 tbsp (0.5 fl oz)	120	0	0
Bertolli				
Classico	1 tbsp	120	—	0
Extra Light	1 tbsp	120	—	0
Extra Virgin	1 tbsp	120	—	0
Crisco				
Corn Canola	1 tbsp (0.5 fl oz)	120	—	0
Oil	1 tbsp (0.5 fl oz)	120	—	0
Puritan Canola	1 tbsp (0.5 fl oz)	120	0	0
Eden				
Hot Pepper Sesame	1 tbsp (0.5 oz)	130	0	0
Toasted Sesame	1 tbsp (0.5 oz)	130	0	0
Hain				
All Blend	1 tbsp	120	—	0
Almond	1 tbsp	120	—	0
Apricot Kernel	1 tbsp	120	—	0
Avocado	1 tbsp	120	—	0
Canola	1 tbsp	120	—	0
Canola Organic	1 tbsp	120	—	0
Coconut	1 tbsp	120	—	0
Corn	1 tbsp	120	—	0
Garlic & Oil	1 tbsp	120	—	0
Olive	1 tbsp	120	—	0
Peanut	1 tbsp	120	—	0
Rice Bran	1 tbsp	120	—	0
Safflower	1 tbsp	120	—	0
Safflower Hi-Oleic	1 tbsp	120	—	0
Safflower Organic	1 tbsp	120	—	0

FOOD	PORTION	CALS.	FIB.	CHOL.
Hain (CONT.)				
Sesame	1 tbsp	120	—	0
Soy	1 tbsp	120	—	0
Sunflower	1 tbsp	120	—	0
Sunflower Organic	1 tbsp	120	—	0
Walnut	1 tbsp	120	—	0
Hollywood				
Canola	1 tbsp	120	—	0
Peanut	1 tbsp	120	—	0
Safflower	1 tbsp	120	—	0
Soy	1 tbsp	120	—	0
Sunflower	1 tbsp	120	—	0
House Of Tsang				
Hot Chili Sesame	1 tsp (5 g)	45	0	0
Mongolian Fire	1 tsp (5 g)	45	0	0
Pure Sesame	1 tsp (5 g)	45	0	0
Singapore Curry	1 tsp (5 g)	45	0	0
Wok Oil	1 tbsp (0.5 oz)	130	0	0
Italica				
Olive Oil	1 tbsp	120	—	0
Ka-Me				
Chili Hot	1 tbsp (0.5 fl oz)	130	0	0
Sesame	1 tbsp (0.5 fl oz)	130	0	0
Sesame Tempura	1 tbsp (0.5 fl oz)	130	0	0
Mazola				
No Stick	2.5 second spray (0.2 g)	2	—	0
Oil	1 cup (221 g)	1955	—	0
Oil	1 tbsp (14 g)	120	—	0
Orville Redenbacher's				
Oil	1 tbsp	120	0	0
Pam				
Butter	1 sec spray (0.266 g)	2	—	0
Cooking Spray	1 sec spray (0.266 g)	2	—	0
Olive Oil	1 sec spray (0.266 g)	2	—	0
Pump	1 spray (0.43 g)	4	—	0
Planters				
Peanut	1 tbsp (0.5 oz)	120	—	0
Popcorn	1 tbsp (0.5 oz)	120	—	0
Pompeian				
Olive	1 tbsp	130	—	0

FOOD	PORTION	CALS.	FIB.	CHOL.
Progresso				
Olive Extra Light	1 tbsp	119	0	0
Olive Extra Mild	1 tbsp (0.5 oz)	120	0	0
Olive Extra Virgin	1 tbsp (0.5 oz)	120	0	0
Olive Riviera Blend	1 tbsp (0.5 oz)	120	0	0
Smart Beat				
Canola	1 tbsp	120	—	0
Oil	1 tbsp	120	—	0
Tree Of Life				
Almond	1 tbsp (0.5 g)	130	—	0
Apricot Kernel	1 tbsp (0.5 g)	130	—	0
Avocado	1 tbsp (0.5 g)	130	—	0
Macadamia Nut	1 tbsp (0.5 g)	130	—	0
Olive Extra Virgin Organic	1 tbsp (0.5 g)	130	—	0
Sesame	1 tbsp (0.5 g)	130	—	0
Toasted Sesame	1 tbsp (0.5 oz)	130	0	0
Weight Watchers				
Butter Spray	⅓ second spray	0	0	0
Cooking Spray	⅓ second spray	0	0	0
Wesson				
Canola	1 tbsp	120	0	0
Cooking Spray Lite	0.5 sec spray	0	0	0
Corn	1 tbsp	120	0	0
Olive	1 tbsp	120	0	0
Sunflower	1 tbsp	120	0	0
Vegetable	1 tbsp	120	0	0
FISH OIL				
cod liver	1 tbsp	123	—	78
herring	1 tbsp	123	—	104
menhaden	1 tbsp	123	—	71
salmon	1 tbsp	123	—	66
sardine	1 tbsp	123	—	97
Hain				
Cod Liver	1 tbsp	120	—	85
Cod Liver Cherry	1 tbsp	120	—	75
Cod Liver Mint	1 tbsp	120	—	85
OKRA				
CANNED				
Allen				
Cut	½ cup (4.4 oz)	25	3	0
McIlhenny				
Pickled	2 pieces (1 oz)	7	1	0
Trappey				
Cocktail Hot	2 pieces (1 oz)	8	1	0

FOOD	PORTION	CALS.	FIB.	CHOL.
Trappey (CONT.)				
Cocktail Mild	1 piece (1 oz)	9	1	0
Creole Gumbo	½ cup (4.2 oz)	35	3	0
Cut	½ cup (4.4 oz)	25	3	0
FRESH				
raw	8 pods	36	—	0
raw sliced	½ cup	19	—	0
sliced cooked	½ cup	25	—	0
sliced cooked	8 pods	27	—	0
FROZEN				
sliced cooked	1 pkg (10 oz)	94	—	0
sliced cooked	½ cup	34	—	0
Hanover				
Cut	½ cup	25	—	0
Whole	½ cup	35	—	0
OLIVES				
green	3 extra lg	15	tr	0
green	4 med	15	tr	0
ripe	1 sm	4	tr	0
ripe	1 lg	5	tr	0
ripe	1 colossal	12	—	0
ripe	1 jumbo	7	—	0
Progresso				
Oil Cured	6 (0.5 oz)	80	1	0
Olive Salad (drained)	2 tbsp (0.8 oz)	25	1	0
S&W				
Ripe Extra Large	3.5 oz	163	—	0
Ripe Pitted Large	3.5 oz	163	—	0
Tee Pee				
Spanish Green	2 oz	98	—	0
ONION				
CANNED				
chopped	½ cup	21	—	0
whole	1 (2.2 oz)	12	—	0
S&W				
Whole Small	½ cup	35	—	0
Vlasic				
Lightly Spiced Cocktail Onions	1 oz	4	—	0
Watkins				
Liquid Spice	1 tbsp (0.5 oz)	120	0	0
DRIED				
flakes	1 tbsp	16	—	0
powder	1 tsp	7	—	0

FOOD	PORTION	CALS.	FIB.	CHOL.
Watkins				
Flakes	¼ tsp (1 g)	0	0	0
FRESH				
chopped cooked	½ cup	47	—	0
raw chopped	1 tbsp	4	tr	0
raw chopped	½ cup	30	—	0
scallions raw chopped	1 tbsp	2	tr	0
scallions raw sliced	½ cup	16	1	0
welsh raw	3½ oz	34	—	0
Antioch Farms				
Vidalia	1 med	60	3	0
Dole				
Green Chopped	1 tbsp	2	tr	0
Medium	1	60	3	0
FROZEN				
chopped cooked	½ cup	30	—	0
chopped cooked	1 tbsp	4	—	0
rings	7 (2.5 oz)	285	—	0
rings cooked	2 (0.7 oz)	81	—	0
whole cooked	3½ oz	28	—	0
Birds Eye				
Polybag Whole Small	½ cup	30	2	0
Small With Cream Sauce	½ cup	100	1	10
Kineret				
Rings	6 (3 oz)	200	0	0
Ore Ida				
Chopped	¾ cup (3 oz)	25	1	0
Onion Ringers	6 pieces (3 oz)	240	2	0
Southland				
Chopped	2 oz	15	—	0
TAKE-OUT				
rings breaded & fried	8 to 9	275	—	14

ORANGE

CANNED

FOOD	PORTION	CALS.	FIB.	CHOL.
Del Monte				
Mandarin In Heavy Syrup	½ cup (4.4 oz)	80	tr	0
Dole				
Mandarin Segments	½ cup	70	—	0
Pineapple Mandarin Segments	½ cup	80	—	0
Empress				
Mandarin	5.5 oz	100	—	0
Mandarin From Japan	5.5 oz	35	—	0
S&W				
Mandarin Natural Style	½ cup	60	—	0

FOOD	PORTION	CALS.	FIB.	CHOL.
S&W (CONT.)				
Mandarin Selected Sections in Heavy Syrup	½ cup	76	—	0
Mandarin Unsweetened	½ cup	28	—	0
FRESH				
california navel	1	65	3	0
california valencia	1	59	3	0
florida	1	69	4	0
peel	1 tbsp	6	—	0
sections	1 cup	85	4	0
Dole				
Orange	1	50	6	0

ORANGE EXTRACT

FOOD	PORTION	CALS.	FIB.	CHOL.
Virginia Dare	1 tsp	22	—	0

ORANGE JUICE

FOOD	PORTION	CALS.	FIB.	CHOL.
canned	1 cup	104	—	0
chilled	1 cup	110	—	0
fresh	1 cup	111	—	0
frzn as prep	1 cup	112	1	0
frzn not prep	6 oz	339	2	0
orange drink	6 oz	94	—	0
After The Fall				
Juice	1 bottle (10 oz)	110	—	0
Bright & Early				
Chilled	8 fl oz	120	—	0
Frozen	8 fl oz	120	—	0
Del Monte				
Juice	8 fl oz	110	tr	0
Fresh Samantha				
Juice	1 cup (8 oz)	109	1	0
Hawaiian Punch				
Drink	6 oz	100	—	0
Hi-C				
Box	8.45 fl oz	130	—	0
Drink	8 fl oz	130	—	0
Drink	1 can (11.5 fl oz)	180	—	0
Hood				
From Concentrate	1 cup (8 oz)	120	—	0
Select	1 cup (8 oz)	120	—	0
With Calcium	1 cup (8 oz)	120	—	0
Juice Works				
Drink	6 oz	90	—	0

FOOD	PORTION	CALS.	FIB.	CHOL.
Kool-Aid				
Drink	8 oz	98	—	0
Sugar Sweetened	8 oz	79	—	0
Libby				
Juice	6 fl oz	80	—	0
Minute Maid				
Box	8.45 fl oz	120	—	0
Calcium Rich Chilled	8 fl oz	120	—	0
Calcium Rich frzn	8 fl oz	120	—	0
Chilled	8 fl oz	110	—	0
Country Style Chilled	8 fl oz	110	—	0
Country Style frzn	8 fl oz	110	—	0
Juices To Go	1 can (11.5 fl oz)	160	—	0
Juices To Go	1 bottle (16 fl oz)	110	—	0
Juices To Go	1 bottle (10 fl oz)	140	—	0
Orange Punch Box	8.45 fl oz	130	—	0
Premium Choice Chilled	8 fl oz	110	—	0
Pulp Free Chilled	8 fl oz	110	—	0
Pulp Free frzn	8 fl oz	110	—	0
Reduced Acid frzn	8 fl oz	110	—	0
Mott's				
From Concentrate	10 fl oz	130	0	0
Ocean Spray				
Juice	8 fl oz	120	0	0
S&W				
100% Unsweetened	6 oz	83	—	0
Sippin' Pak				
100% Pure	8.45 fl oz	110	—	0
Snapple				
Juice	10 fl oz	130	—	0
Orangeade	8 oz	120	—	0
Tang				
Breakfast Crystals Sugar Free as prep	6 oz	5	—	0
Breakfast Crystals as prep	6 oz	86	—	0
Fruit Box	8.45 oz	127	—	0
Tropical Orange	8.45 fl oz	146	—	0
Tree Of Life				
Juice	8 fl oz	110	0	0
Tree Top				
Juice	6 oz	90	—	0
Tropicana				
Double Vitamin C with Vitamin E	8 fl oz	110	—	0

FOOD	PORTION	CALS.	FIB.	CHOL.
Tropicana (CONT.)				
Frozen as prep	6 fl oz	110	—	0
Juice	8 fl oz	110	—	0
Juice	1 container (6 fl oz)	80	—	0
Juice	1 container (10 fl oz)	130	—	0
Juice	1 container (8 fl oz)	110	—	0
Pure Premium Calcium & Extra Vitamin C	8 fl oz	110	—	0
Pure Premium Vitamins C&E	8 fl oz	110	—	0
Season's Best	1 can (11.5 fl oz)	140	—	0
Season's Best	1 bottle (10 fl oz)	130	—	0
Season's Best	1 bottle (7 fl oz)	90	—	0
Season's Best Homestyle	8 fl oz	110	—	0
Veryfine				
100%	8 oz	121	—	0
Orange Drink	8 oz	140	—	0

OREGANO
ground	1 tsp	5	—	0
Watkins				
Liquid Spice	1 tbsp (0.5 oz)	120	0	0

ORGAN MEATS
(*see* BRAINS, GIBLETS, GIZZARDS, HEART, KIDNEY, LIVER, SWEETBREADS)

ORIENTAL FOOD
(*see also* DINNER, EGG ROLLS, NOODLES, RICE, SUSHI)
CANNED
chow mein chicken	1 cup	95	—	8
La Choy				
Bi-Pack Beef Pepper	¾ cup	80	2	17
Bi-Pack Chow Mein Chicken	¾ cup	80	1	18
Bi-Pack Chow Mein Pork	¾ cup	80	2	14
Bi-Pack Chow Mein Shrimp	¾ cup	70	1	19
Bi-Pack Sweet & Sour Chicken	¾ cup	120	2	13
Bi-Pack Teriyaki Chicken	¾ cup	85	1	20
Dinner Chow Mein Chicken	¾ pkg	300	2	16
Entree Beef Pepper Oriental	¾ cup	100	2	36
Entree Chow Mein Beef	¾ cup	40	2	16
Entree Chow Mein Chicken	¾ cup	70	4	16
Entree Chow Mein Meatless	¾ cup	25	2	0
Entree Chow Mein Shrimp	¾ cup	35	2	50
Entree Sweet & Sour Chicken	¾ cup	240	1	19

FOOD	PORTION	CALS.	FIB.	CHOL.
La Choy (CONT.)				
Entree Sweet & Sour Pork	¾ cup	250	1	18
FRESH				
wonton wrappers	1	23	—	1
FROZEN				
Banquet				
Chow Mein Chicken	1 pkg (9 oz)	400	3	30
Birds Eye				
Easy Recipe Chicken Teriyaki not prep	½ pkg	160	4	0
Easy Recipe Oriental Beef not prep	½ pkg	100	8	0
Internationals Chinese Stir Fry not prep	3.3 oz	35	2	0
Japanese Stir Fry International not prep	3.3 oz	30	2	0
Chun King				
Beef Pepper Steak	1 pkg (13 oz)	300	5	10
Chow Mein Chicken	1 pkg (13 oz)	370	4	45
Imperial Chicken	1 pkg (13 oz)	460	5	25
Sweet & Sour Pork	1 pkg (13 oz)	450	4	20
Walnut Chicken	1 pkg (13 oz)	460	5	35
Lean Cuisine				
Chicken Chow Mein With Rice	1 meal (9 oz)	210	2	35
Luigino's				
Chicken & Almonds With Rice	1 pkg (8 oz)	250	3	20
Chop Suey Pork With Rice	1 pkg (8.5 oz)	210	2	15
Lo Mein Chicken	1 pkg (8 oz)	320	3	15
Lo Mein Shrimp	1 pkg (8 oz)	190	4	15
Oriental Beef & Peppers With Rice	1 pkg (8 oz)	230	2	10
Pasta Favorites				
Chicken Lo Mein	1 pkg (10.5 oz)	270	5	20
Rice Gourmet				
Chicken Teriyaki Rice Bowl	1 bowl (10.9 oz)	430	1	25
Stouffer's				
Chicken Chow Mein With Rice	1 pkg (10.6 oz)	260	3	30
Chicken Oriental	1 pkg (9.75 oz)	320	2	40
Stir-Fry Teriyaki	1 pkg (9 oz)	260	4	30
Tyson				
Stir Fry Kit With Yoshida Oriental Sauce	10.6 oz	330	—	80

FOOD	PORTION	CALS.	FIB.	CHOL.
Weight Watchers				
Chicken Chow Mein	1 pkg (9 oz)	200	3	25
MIX				
Kikkoman				
Chow Mein Seasoning	1⅛ oz pkg	98	—	tr
Teriyaki Baste & Glaze	1 tbsp	24	—	tr
La Choy				
Dinner Classics Egg Foo Young	2 patties + 3 oz sauce	170	1	275
Dinner Classics Pepper Steak	¾ cup	180	1	60
Dinner Classics Sweet & Sour	¾ cup	310	tr	50
TAKE-OUT				
chicken teriyaki	¾ cup	399	—	92
chicken teriyaki w/ rice	1 serv (11 oz)	430	1	25
chop suey w/ beef & pork	1 cup	300	—	68
chop suey w/ pork	1 cup	375	2	62
chow mein chicken	1 cup	255	—	75
chow mein pork	1 cup	425	3	89
chow mein shrimp	1 cup	221	3	55
chow mein vegetable	1 serv (8 oz)	90	4	0
sweet & sour pork	1 serv (8 oz)	250	2	30
szechuan chicken w/ lo mein	1 cup (5.3 oz)	190	0	5
wonton fried	½ cup (1 oz)	111	1	31
wonton soup	1 cup	205	1	89

OSTRICH
ostrich	3 oz	127	—	54

OYSTERS
CANNED

eastern	3 oz	58	—	46
eastern	1 cup	170	—	136
Bumble Bee				
Whole	½ cup (3.5 oz)	100	0	55
FRESH				
eastern cooked	3 oz	117	—	93
eastern cooked	6 med	58	—	46
eastern raw	1 cup	170	—	136
eastern raw	6 med	58	—	46
TAKE-OUT				
battered & fried	6 (4.9 oz)	368	—	109
breaded & fried	6 (4.9 oz)	368	—	109
eastern breaded & fried	6 med (88 g)	173	—	72
eastern breaded & fried	3 oz	167	—	69
oysters rockefeller	3 oysters	66	—	38
stew	1 cup	278	tr	100

FOOD	PORTION	CALS.	FIB.	CHOL.

PANCAKE/WAFFLE SYRUP
(see also SYRUP)

FOOD	PORTION	CALS.	FIB.	CHOL.
low calorie	1 tbsp	12	0	0
maple	1 cup (11.1 oz)	824	—	0
maple	1 tbsp (0.8 oz)	52	—	0
pancake syrup	1 tbsp (0.7 oz)	57	—	0
pancake syrup	1 cup (11 oz)	903	—	0
pancake syrup light	1 oz	46	—	0
pancake syrup w/ butter	1 tbsp (0.7 oz)	59	—	1
pancake syrup w/ butter	1 cup (11 oz)	933	—	14
Alaga				
Breakfast	2 tbsp	108	—	0
Butter Lite	2 tbsp	54	—	0
Honey Flavored	2 tbsp	124	—	0
Lite	2 tbsp	54	—	0
Aunt Jemima				
Butter Rich	¼ cup (2.8 oz)	210	—	0
Butterlite	¼ cup (2.5 oz)	100	—	0
Lite	¼ cup (2.5 oz)	100	—	0
Syrup	¼ cup (2.8 oz)	210	—	0
Brer Rabbit				
Dark	2 tbsp	120	—	0
Light	2 tbsp	120	—	0
Estee				
Lite Maple	¼ cup (2.4 oz)	80	—	0
Golden Griddle				
Syrup	1 tbsp (20 g)	50	—	0
Syrup	1 cup (321 g)	885	—	0
Karo				
Syrup	1 tbsp (21 g)	60	—	0
Log Cabin				
Country Kitchen	1 oz	103	—	0
Lite	1 oz	49	—	0
Mrs.Richardson's				
Lite	¼ cup (2.5 oz)	100	—	0
Original Recipe	¼ cup (2.8 oz)	210	—	0
Red Wing				
Lite	¼ cup (2 oz)	100	0	0
Syrup	¼ cup (2 oz)	210	0	0
Tastee				
Maple	2 tbsp	113	—	0
Syrup	2 tbsp	121	—	0
Tree Of Life				
Maple	¼ cup (2.1 oz)	200	—	0

FOOD	PORTION	CALS.	FIB.	CHOL.
Whitfield				
White Label	2 tbsp	121	—	0
Yellow Label	2 tbsp	125	—	0
Yellow Label Butter Flavor	2 tbsp	117	—	0
Yellow Label Maple Flavor	2 tbsp	117	—	0

PANCAKES
FROZEN

FOOD	PORTION	CALS.	FIB.	CHOL.
buttermilk	1 (1.3 oz) 4 in diam	83	—	3
plain	1 (1.3 oz) 4 in diam	83	—	3
Aunt Jemima				
Blueberry	3 (3.4 oz)	210	2	15
Buttermilk	3 (3 oz)	180	2	15
Lowfat	3 (3.4 oz)	130	8	0
Original	3 (3.4 oz)	200	2	15
Healthy Starts				
Pancakes w/ LeanLinks	6 oz	360	—	0
Jimmy Dean				
Flapstick	1 (2.5 oz)	240	1	20
Flapstick Blueberry	1 (2.5 oz)	260	1	15
Quaker				
Lite Pancakes & Lite Links	1 pkg (6 oz)	310	—	48
Lite Pancakes & Lite Syrup	1 pkg (6 oz)	260	—	32
Pancakes & Sausages	1 pkg (6 oz)	420	—	62
Weight Watchers				
Buttermilk	2 (2.5 oz)	140	—	10
HOME RECIPE				
blueberry	1 (4 in diam)	84	—	21
plain	1 (4 in diam)	86	—	23
MIX				
buckwheat	1 (4 in diam)	62	—	20
sugar free low sodium	1 (3 in diam)	44	—	0
whole wheat	1 (4 in diam)	92	—	27
Arrowhead				
Multigrain Pancake & Waffle Mix	¼ cup (1.2 oz)	120	3	0
Aunt Jemima				
Buckwheat Pancake & Waffle Mix	¼ cup (1.4 oz)	120	4	0
Buttermilk Pancake & Waffle Mix	⅓ cup (1.9 oz)	190	2	10
Original Pancake & Waffle Mix	⅓ cup (1.6 oz)	150	1	0
Pancake & Waffle Mix Regular	⅓ cup (1.9 oz)	190	1	15
Pancake & Waffle Mix Whole Wheat	¼ cup (1.4 oz)	130	3	0

FOOD	PORTION	CALS.	FIB.	CHOL.
Bisquick				
Apple Cinnamon Shake 'N Pour	3 (4 in diam)	240	—	0
Blueberry Shake 'N Pour	3 (4 in diam)	270	—	0
Buttermilk Shake 'N Pour	3 (4 in diam)	250	—	0
Original Shake 'N Pour	3 (4 in diam)	250	—	0
Estee				
Pancake Mix Fat Free as prep	4 (4 in diam)	180	1	0
Fast Shake				
Blueberry	1 serv (2.5 oz)	251	—	2
Buttermilk	1 serv (2.5 oz)	258	—	2
Original	1 serv (2.5 oz)	266	—	tr
Health Valley				
Pancake Mix not prep	1 oz	100	3	0
Hodgson Mill				
Buckwheat	⅓ cup (1.8 oz)	160	1	0
Stone-Buhr				
Buckwheat	¼ cup (1.4 oz)	130	3	0
Oat Bran	¼ cup (1.4 oz)	130	2	0
Whole Wheat	¼ cup (1.4 oz)	120	3	0
Wanda's				
Blue Corn	⅓ cup mix per serv (1.7 oz)	170	2	0
TAKE-OUT				
buckwheat	1 (4 in diam)	55	—	20
potato	1 (4 in diam)	78	tr	60
w/ butter & syrup	3	519	—	57

PANCREAS
(*see* SWEETBREADS)

PAPAYA
CANNED
Ka-Me

Papaya	¾ cup	120	1	0

DRIED
Sonoma

Pieces	2 pieces (2 oz)	200	6	0

FRESH

cubed	1 cup	54	—	0
papaya	1	117	—	0

PAPAYA JUICE

nectar	1 cup	142	—	0
Goya				
Nectar	6 oz	110	—	0

FOOD	PORTION	CALS.	FIB.	CHOL.
Kern's				
Nectar	6 fl oz	110	—	0
Libby				
Nectar	1 can (11.5 fl oz)	210	—	0
PAPRIKA				
paprika	1 tsp	6	—	0
Watkins				
Ground	¼ tsp (0.5 oz)	0	0	0
PARSLEY				
dry	1 tsp	1	—	0
dry	1 tbsp	1	—	0
fresh chopped	½ cup	11	—	0
Dole				
Chopped	1 tbsp	10	tr	0
PARSNIPS				
fresh cooked	1 (5.6 oz)	130	—	0
fresh sliced cooked	½ cup	63	—	0
raw sliced	½ cup	50	—	0
PASSION FRUIT				
purple fresh	1	18	—	0
PASSION FRUIT JUICE				
purple	1 cup	126	—	0
yellow	1 cup	149	—	0
Snapple				
Passion Supreme	10 fl oz	160	—	0
PASTA				
(*see also* NOODLES, PASTA DINNERS, PASTA SALAD)				
DRY				
corn cooked	1 cup	176	—	0
elbows	1 cup	389	—	0
elbows cooked	1 cup	197	—	0
protein fortified cooked	1 cup	188	—	0
shells	1 cup	389	—	0
shells cooked	1 cup	197	—	0
spaghetti	2 oz	211	—	0
spaghetti cooked	1 cup	197	—	0
spaghetti protein fortified cooked	1 cup	229	—	0
spinach spaghetti	2 oz	212	—	0
spinach spaghetti cooked	1 cup	183	—	0
spirals	1 cup	389	—	0
spirals cooked	1 cup	197	—	0

FOOD	PORTION	CALS.	FIB.	CHOL.
vegetable	1 cup	308	—	0
vegetable cooked	1 cup	171	—	0
whole wheat	1 cup	365	—	0
whole wheat cooked	1 cup (4.9 oz)	174	—	0
whole wheat spaghetti	2 oz	198	—	0
whole wheat spaghetti cooked	1 cup	174	—	0
Anthony				
Pasta	2 oz	210	tr	0
Barilla				
Pennette Rigate	1⅓ cups (2 oz)	200	2	0
Bella Via				
Angel Hair	2 oz	200	—	0
Artichoke Angel Hair as prep	⅝ cup	200	—	0
Artichoke Spaghetti as prep	⅝ cup	200	—	0
Elbows	2 oz	200	—	0
Fettucini as prep	⅝ cup	200	—	0
Linguini	2 oz	200	—	0
Penne as prep	⅝ cup	200	—	0
Rotelli	2 oz	200	—	0
Shells	2 oz	200	—	0
Spaghetti	2 oz	200	—	0
Ziti	2 oz	200	—	0
Classico				
Gnocchi Di Toscana	1 cup (2 oz)	210	2	0
Creamette				
Linguini Egg	2 oz	221	—	70
Rotelle	2 oz	210	—	0
Rotini Rainbow	2 oz	210	—	0
Spaghetti Egg	2 oz	221	—	70
Spaghetti Thin	2 oz	210	—	0
Ziti	2 oz	210	—	0
De Bole's				
Whole Wheat Organic Elbows	2 oz	210	5	0
DeFino				
Lasagna No Boil	1 oz	102	—	0
Ribbons No Boil	2 oz	204	—	0
Delverde				
Spaghetti Whole Wheat	2 oz	206	5	0
Eden				
Elbows Whole Wheat Organic	2 oz	210	6	0
Elbows Whole Wheat Vegetable Organic	2 oz	210	6	0
Kudzu And Sweet Potato Pasta	2 oz	190	0	0
Kudzu Kiri Pasta	2 oz	190	0	0

FOOD	PORTION	CALS.	FIB.	CHOL.
Eden (CONT.)				
Mung Bean Pasta Harusame	2 oz	190	0	0
Ribbons Durum Wheat Curry Organic	2 oz	220	3	0
Ribbons Durum Wheat Organic	2 oz	220	3	0
Ribbons Durum Wheat Paella Organic	2 oz	220	3	0
Ribbons Durum Wheat Parsley Garlic Organic	2 oz	220	3	0
Ribbons Durum Wheat Pesto Organic	2 oz	220	3	0
Ribbons Whole Wheat Spinach Organic	2 oz	200	7	0
Rice Pasta Bifun	2 oz	200	0	0
Shells Durum Wheat Vegetable Organic	2 oz	210	2	0
Soba 100% Buckwheat	2 oz	200	3	0
Soba 40% Buckwheat	2 oz	190	3	0
Soba Lotus Root	2 oz	190	4	0
Soba Mugwort	2 oz	190	2	0
Soba Wild Yam Jinenjo	2 oz	190	2	0
Spaghetti Durum Wheat Organic	2 oz	210	2	0
Spaghetti Kamut Organic	2 oz	210	6	0
Spaghetti Parsley Garlic Organic	2 oz	210	2	0
Spaghetti Whole Wheat Organic	2 oz	210	6	0
Spirals Durum Wheat Vegetable Organic	2 oz	210	2	0
Spirals Kamut Organic	2 oz	210	6	0
Spirals Sesame Rice Organic	2 oz	200	6	0
Spirals Whole Wheat Vegetable Organic	2 oz	210	6	0
Udon	2 oz	190	3	0
Udon Brown Rice	2 oz	190	2	0
Gioia				
Pasta	2 oz	210	tr	0
Golden Grain				
Pasta	2 oz	203	0	0
Hanover				
Spaghetti Wheels	½ cup	90	—	0
Health Valley				
Lasagna Whole Wheat	2 oz	170	7	0
Lasagna Spinach Whole Wheat	2 oz	170	7	0

FOOD	PORTION	CALS.	FIB.	CHOL.
Health Valley (CONT.)				
Spaghetti Amaranth	2 oz	170	9	0
Spaghetti Oat Bran	2 oz	120	4	0
Spaghetti Spinach Whole Wheat	2 oz	170	7	0
Spaghetti Whole Wheat	2 oz	170	7	0
Hodgson Mill				
Spaghetti Whole Wheat Spinach not prep	2 oz	190	5	0
Veggie Bows not prep	2 oz	200	1	0
Veggie Rotini not prep	2 oz	200	1	0
Veggie Wagon Wheels not prep	2 oz	200	1	0
Whole Wheat Spirals not prep	2 oz	190	6	0
La Molisana				
Radiatori	2 oz	230	—	0
Luplni				
Elbow uncooked	½ cup (2 oz)	190	5	0
Spaghetti Light uncooked	½ cup (2 oz)	190	5	0
Spaghetti With Triticale	½ pkg (2 oz)	190	6	0
Luxury				
Pasta	2 oz	210	tr	0
Merlino's				
Pasta	2 oz	210	tr	0
Mueller's				
Dinosaurs	2 oz (57 g)	210	—	0
Jungle Animals	2 oz (57 g)	210	—	0
Lasagne	2 oz (57 g)	210	—	0
Monsters	2 oz (57 g)	210	—	0
Outer Space	2 oz	210	—	0
Spaghetti	2 oz (57 g)	210	—	0
Teddy Bears	2 oz (57 g)	210	—	0
Twists Tri Color	2 oz (57 g)	210	—	0
Noodles By Leonardo				
Capellini	2 oz	200	2	0
Elbows not prep	½ cup (2 oz)	200	2	0
Fettucini	2 oz	200	2	0
Linguine not prep	½ cup (2 oz)	200	2	0
Rigatoni	2 oz	200	2	0
Rotini	2 oz	200	2	0
Shells not prep	½ cup (2 oz)	200	2	0
Spaghetti not prep	½ cup (2 oz)	200	2	0
Spaghettini	2 oz	200	2	0
Vermicelli not prep	½ cup (2 oz)	200	2	0

FOOD	PORTION	CALS.	FIB.	CHOL.
Penn Dutch				
Pasta	2 oz	210	tr	0
Pomi				
Capellini	2 oz	210	—	0
Prince				
Egg	2 oz	221	1	70
Pasta	2 oz	210	tr	0
Rainbow	2 oz	210	1	0
Spinach Egg	2 oz	220	1	70
Pritikin				
Spaghetti Whole Wheat	⅛ box (2 oz)	190	—	0
Spiral	⅔ cup (2 oz)	190	—	0
Red Cross				
Pasta	2 oz	210	tr	0
Ronco				
Pasta	2 oz	210	tr	0
Ronzoni				
Elbows	¾ cup (2 oz)	210	—	0
Fettucini	¾ cup (2 oz)	210	—	0
Fusilli	¾ cup (2 oz)	210	—	0
Lasagne	¾ cup (2 oz)	210	—	0
Manicotti	¾ cup (2 oz)	210	—	0
Mostaccioli	¾ cup (2 oz)	210	—	0
Rigatoni	¾ cup (2 oz)	210	—	0
Rotelle uncooked	¾ cup (2 oz)	210	—	0
Rotini uncooked	¾ cup (2 oz)	210	—	0
Shells uncooked	¾ cup (2 oz)	210	—	0
Shells Jumbo	¾ cup (2 oz)	210	—	0
Spaghetti not prep	¾ cup (2 oz)	210	—	0
Tubettini	¾ cup (2 oz)	210	—	0
San Giorgio				
Bowties Egg	2 oz	210	—	70
Capellini	2 oz	210	2	0
Elbow Macaroni	2 oz	210	2	0
Fettuccine Egg	2 oz	210	—	70
Fettuccini Florentine	2 oz	210	—	70
Lasagne	2 oz	210	2	0
Linguini	2 oz	210	2	0
Manicotti	2 oz	210	2	0
Mostaccioli Rigati	2 oz	210	—	0
Rigatoni	2 oz	210	2	0
Rotini	2 oz	210	2	0
Shells	2 oz	210	2	0
Spaghetti	2 oz	210	2	0

FOOD	PORTION	CALS.	FIB.	CHOL.
San Giorgio (CONT.)				
Spaghetti Thin	2 oz	210	2	0
Vermicelli	2 oz	210	2	0
Ziti Cut	2 oz	210	2	0
Tree Of Life				
Cajun as prep	⅝ cup (4.9 oz)	200	1	0
Confetti as prep	⅝ cup (4.9 oz)	200	1	0
Garlic & Parsley as prep	⅝ cup (4.9 oz)	200	1	0
Jamaican Spice as prep	⅝ cup (4.9 oz)	200	1	0
Lemon Pepper as prep	⅝ cup (4.9 oz)	200	1	0
Spinach as prep	⅝ cup (4.9 oz)	200	1	0
Tex Mex as prep	⅝ cup (4.9 oz)	200	1	0
Thai as prep	⅝ cup (4.9 oz)	200	1	0
Tomato Basil as prep	⅝ cup (4.9 oz)	200	1	0
Vimco				
Pasta	2 oz	210	tr	0
FRESH				
plain made w/ egg cooked	2 oz	75	—	19
spinach made w/ egg cooked	2 oz	74	—	19
Contadina				
Angel's Hair	1¼ cup (2.8 oz)	240	2	90
Fettuccine	1¼ cup (2.9 oz)	250	2	85
Fettuccine Cholesterol Free	1 cup (2.9 oz)	240	2	0
Light Ravioli Cheese	1 cup (3.1 oz)	240	2	60
Light Ravioli Garden Vegetable	1¼ cup (3.8 oz)	290	3	65
Light Tortellini Garlic & Cheese	1 cup (3.6 oz)	280	3	55
Linguine	1¼ cup (3 oz)	260	2	95
Linguine Cholesterol Free	1¼ cup (3.1 oz)	250	2	0
Ravioli Beef And Garlic	1¼ cup (4 oz)	350	3	110
Ravioli Cheese	1 cup (3.1 oz)	280	2	85
Ravioli Chicken And Rosemary	1¼ cup (4 oz)	330	3	85
Tagliatelli Spinach	1¼ cup (3.1 oz)	270	4	105
Tortellini Spinach Three Cheese	¾ cup (3.1 oz)	280	3	55
Tortelloni Cheese	¾ cup (3 oz)	260	3	45
Tortelloni Cheese And Basil	1 cup (4 oz)	360	3	65
Tortelloni Chicken And Prosciutto	1 cup (3.8 oz)	360	3	75
Tortelloni Chicken And Vegetable	¾ cup (2.9 oz)	260	2	45
Tortelloni Spicy Italian Sausage And Bell Pepper	1 cup (3.6 oz)	330	3	90
Di Giorno				
Angel's Hair	2 oz	160	1	0
Fettuccine	2.5 oz	190	2	0

FOOD	PORTION	CALS.	FIB.	CHOL.
Di Giorno (CONT.)				
Fettuccine Spinach	2.5 oz	190	2	0
Linguine	2.5 oz	190	2	0
Linguine Herb	2.5 oz	190	2	0
Ravioli Italian Herb Cheese	1 cup (3.8 oz)	350	2	45
Ravioli Light Cheese & Garlic	1 cup (3.7 oz)	270	1	5
Ravioli Light Tomato & Cheese	1 cup (3.7 oz)	280	2	10
Ravioli With Italian Sausage	¾ cup (3.6 oz)	340	2	50
Tortellini Cheese	¾ cup (2.8 oz)	260	1	30
Tortellini Mozzarella Garlic	1 cup (3.5 oz)	300	1	45
Tortellini Mushroom	1 cup (3.4 oz)	290	2	30
Tortellini Red Hot Pepper Cheese	1 cup (3.4 oz)	310	3	40
Tortellini With Chicken And Herbs	1 cup (3.2 oz)	260	1	35
Tortellini With Meat	¾ cup (3.1 oz)	290	1	40
Herb's				
Fettucine Bell Pepper Basil	2 oz	220	2	60
Fettucine Parsley Garlic	2 oz	220	2	60
Fettucine Spinach	2 oz	220	2	60
Ribbons Vegetable	2 oz	220	2	60
Ribbons Whole Wheat	2 oz	200	7	0
Rotini Mixed Vegetable	2 oz	210	2	0
Shells Mixed Vegetable	2 oz	210	2	0
Trios				
Ravioli Cracked Pepper Garlic Cheese	1 cup (4.3 oz)	340	0	50
HOME RECIPE				
made w/ egg cooked	2 oz	74	—	23
made w/o egg cooked	2 oz	71	—	0

PASTA DINNERS

(*see also* DINNER, PASTA SALAD)

CANNED

Chef Boyardee

FOOD	PORTION	CALS.	FIB.	CHOL.
ABC's & 1,2,3's In Cheese Flavor Sauce	7.5 oz	180	—	3
ABC's & 1,2,3's w/ Mini Meatballs	7.5 oz	260	2	17
Beef Ravioli	7.5 oz	190	2	11
Beefaroni	7.5 oz	220	2	18
Cheese Ravioli In Meat Sauce	7.5 oz	200	—	10
Dinosaurs In Cheese Flavor Sauce	7.5 oz	180	—	3

FOOD	PORTION	CALS.	FIB.	CHOL.
Chef Boyardee (CONT.)				
Dinosaurs w/ Meatballs	7.5 oz	240	4	17
Elbows In Beef Sauce	7.5 oz	210	—	15
Lasagna	7.5 oz	230	—	18
Lasagna In Garden Vegetable Sauce	7.5 oz	170	—	3
Macaroni & Cheese	7.5 oz	180	1	20
Pasta Rings & Meatballs	7.5 oz	220	4	25
Rigatoni	7.5 oz	210	—	17
Rings & Franks	7.5 oz	190	3	20
Shells In Meat Sauce	7.5 oz	210	—	15
Shells In Mushroom Sauce	7.5 oz	170	—	2
Spaghetti & Meat Balls	7.5 oz	230	—	20
Tic Tac Toes In Cheese Flavor Sauce	7.5 oz	170	3	2
Tic Tac Toes w/ Mini Meatballs	7.5 oz	250	3	16
Turtles In Sauce	7.5 oz	160	2	3
Turtles w/ Meatballs	7.5 oz	210	2	20
Hormel				
Lasagna	1 can (7.5 oz)	250	1	25
Spaghetti & Meatballs	1 can (7.5 oz)	210	2	20
Kid's Kitchen				
Cheezy Mac & Beef	1 cup (7.5 oz)	250	0	30
Noodle Rings & Chicken	1 cup (7.5 oz)	150	1	20
Spaghetti Rings & Franks	1 cup (7.5 oz)	230	3	15
Progresso				
Beef Ravioli	1 cup (9.1 oz)	260	4	5
Cheese Ravioli	1 cup (9.1 oz)	220	4	<5
Van Camp's				
Spaghetti Weenee	1 can (8 oz)	230	1	20
FROZEN				
Armour				
Classics Chicken Fettucini	1 meal (10 oz)	230	6	25
Banquet				
Family Entree Lasagna w/ Meat Sauce	1 serv (8 oz)	240	5	15
Family Entree Macaroni & Beef	1 serv (8 oz)	230	3	25
Family Entree Macaroni & Cheese	1 serv (8 oz)	300	2	25
Family Entree Noodles & Chicken	1 serv (8 oz)	210	2	40
Family Entree Noodles & Beef	1 serv (7.47 oz)	140	2	35
Birds Eye				
Easy Recipe Chicken Alfredo not prep	½ pkg	160	3	0

FOOD	PORTION	CALS.	FIB.	CHOL.
Birds Eye (CONT.)				
Easy Recipe Chicken Primavera not prep	½ pkg	80	7	0
Budget Gourmet				
Cheese Ravioli	1 meal (9.5 oz)	290	—	30
Lasagna Italian Sausage	1 meal (10 oz)	430	—	45
Lasagna Vegetable	1 meal (10.5 oz)	390	—	15
Lasagne Three Cheese	1 meal (10 oz)	390	—	70
Lasagne With Meat Sauce	1 meal (9.4 oz)	290	—	30
Linguini With Shrimp & Clams	1 meal (9.5 oz)	280	—	45
Linguini With Shrimp And Clams	1 meal (10 oz)	270	—	50
Macaroni & Cheese	1 meal (5.75 oz)	230	—	35
Macaroni & Cheese With Cheddar & Parmesan	1 meal (10.5 oz)	330	—	30
Manicotti Cheese	1 meal (10 oz)	440	—	75
Pasta Alfredo With Broccoli	1 meal (5.5 oz)	210	—	30
Penne Pasta With Chunky Tomato Sauce & Italian Sausage	1 meal (10 oz)	320	—	5
Rigatoni In Cream Sauce With Broccoli & Chicken	1 meal (10.8 oz)	290	—	30
Spaghetti With Chunky Tomato & Meat Sauce	1 meal (10 oz)	300	—	35
Tortellini Cheese	1 meal (5.5 oz)	200	—	20
Ziti In Marinara Sauce	1 meal (6.25 oz)	200	—	10
Dining Light				
Cheese Cannelloni	9 oz	310	—	70
Formagg				
Penne Pasta Alfredo	⅔ cup (5 oz)	190	0	0
Penne Pasta Primavera	⅔ cup (5 oz)	190	0	0
Vegetable Pasta & Caesar Italian Garden	⅔ cup (5 oz)	190	0	0
Green Giant				
Garden Gourmet Creamy Mushroom	1 pkg	220	3	25
Garden Gourmet Pasta Dijon	1 pkg	260	4	55
Garden Gourmet Pasta Florentine	1 pkg	230	4	25
Garden Gourmet Rotini Cheddar	1 pkg	230	5	20
One Serve Cheese Tortellini	1 pkg	260	—	25
One Serve Macaroni & Cheese	1 pkg	230	—	25

FOOD	PORTION	CALS.	FIB.	CHOL.
Green Giant (CONT.)				
One Serve Pasta Marinara	1 pkg	180	—	0
One Serve Pasta Parmesan With Green Peas	1 pkg	170	—	10
Pasta Accents Creamy Cheddar	½ cup	100	—	5
Pasta Accents Garden Herb	½ cup	80	—	5
Pasta Accents Garlic Seasoning	½ cup	110	—	5
Pasta Accents Pasta Primavera	½ cup	110	—	5
Healthy Choice				
Beef Macaroni Casserole	1 meal (8.5 oz)	200	5	15
Cheese Ravioli Parmigiana	1 meal (9 oz)	250	6	20
Chicken Broccoli Alfredo	1 meal (12.1 oz)	370	6	45
Chicken Fettucini Alfredo	1 meal (8.5 oz)	250	3	30
Classics Pasta Shells Marinara	1 meal (12 oz)	360	5	25
Classics Turkey Fettuccine Alla Crema	1 meal (12.5 oz)	350	5	30
Fettucini Alfredo	1 meal (8 oz)	240	3	10
Lasagna Roma	1 meal (13.5 oz)	390	9	15
Macaroni & Cheese	1 meal (9 oz)	290	4	15
Spaghetti Bolognese	1 meal (10 oz)	260	5	15
Three Cheese Manicotti	1 meal (11 oz)	310	7	20
Vegetable Pasta Italiano	1 meal (10 oz)	220	6	0
Zucchini Lasagna	1 meal (14 oz)	330	11	10
Kid Cuisine				
Macaroni & Cheese	1 pkg (10.6 oz)	420	3	25
Mini Cheese Ravioli	1 pkg (9.82 oz)	320	6	10
Le Menu				
Entree LightStyle Garden Vegetables Lasagna	10½ oz	260	—	25
Entree LightStyle Lasagna With Meat Sauce	10 oz	290	—	30
Entree LightStyle Meat Sauce & Cheese Tortellini	8 oz	250	—	15
Entree LightStyle Spaghetti With Beef Sauce And Mushrooms	9 oz	280	—	15
LightStyle 3-Cheese Stuffed Shells	10 oz	280	—	25
LightStyle Cheese Tortellini	10 oz	230	—	15
Lean Cuisine				
Cannelloni Cheese	1 meal (9.1 oz)	270	3	30
Cheddar Bake With Pasta	1 meal (9 oz)	220	3	20
Chicken Fettucini	1 pkg (9 oz)	270	2	45
Fettucini Alfredo	1 meal (9 oz)	270	2	15

FOOD	PORTION	CALS.	FIB.	CHOL.
Lean Cuisine (CONT.)				
Fettucini Primavera	1 meal (10 oz)	260	4	35
Lasagna Classic Cheese	1 meal (11.5 oz)	290	5	30
Lasagna Tuna	1 meal (9.75 oz)	230	3	20
Lasagna Zucchini	1 meal (11 oz)	240	4	15
Lasagne With Meat Sauce	1 pkg (10.25 oz)	270	5	25
Macaroni & Beef	1 pkg (10 oz)	280	3	25
Macaroni & Cheese	1 pkg (9 oz)	270	2	20
Marinara Twist	1 pkg (10 oz)	240	4	5
Ravioli Cheese	1 meal (8.5 oz)	250	4	55
Rigatoni	1 pkg (9 oz)	180	4	20
Spaghetti & Meatballs	1 pkg (9.5 oz)	290	4	30
Spaghetti With Meat Sauce	1 meal (11.5 oz)	290	4	20
Life Choice				
Linguini Roma	1 meal (13.2 oz)	230	6	0
Sun Dried Tomato Manicotti	1 meal (11.65 oz)	220	7	5
Vegetable Lasagna Primavera	1 meal (11.2 oz)	170	8	5
Luigino's				
& Pomodoro Sauce With Meatballs	1 pkg (9 oz)	320	2	15
& Pomodoro Sauce With Meatballs	1 cup (6.3 oz)	270	2	10
Cheese Ravioli & Alfredo With Broccoli Sauce	1 pkg (8.5 oz)	420	2	70
Cheese Tortellini & Alfredo Sauce With Broccoli	1 pkg (8 oz)	390	2	65
Fettuccine Alfredo	1 pkg (9.4 oz)	390	4	30
Fettuccine Alfredo	1 cup (7.5 oz)	330	3	20
Fettuccine Alfredo With Broccoli	1 pkg (9.2 oz)	360	4	25
Fettuccine Carbonara	1 pkg (9 oz)	360	3	35
Lasagna Alfredo	1 cup (6.3 oz)	300	2	25
Lasagna Alfredo	1 pkg (9 oz)	360	2	30
Lasagna Pollo	1 pkg (9 oz)	320	3	30
Lasagna With Meat Sauce	1 pkg (9 oz)	290	2	20
Lasagna With Meat Sauce	1 cup (7.2 oz)	240	2	15
Lasagna With Vegetables	1 pkg (9 oz)	290	2	20
Linguini With Clams & Sauce	1 pkg (9 oz)	270	2	10
Linguini With Red Sauce	1 pkg (9 oz)	260	3	0
Linguini With Seafood	1 pkg (9 oz)	290	4	0
Macaroni & Cheese	1 cup (7.2 oz)	310	2	15
Macaroni & Cheese	1 pkg (9 oz)	370	3	20
Marinara Sauce Penne Pasta Italian Sausage & Peppers	1 pkg (9 oz)	350	2	35

FOOD	PORTION	CALS.	FIB.	CHOL.
Luigino's (CONT.)				
Marinara Sauce Penne Pasta Italian Sausage & Peppers	1 cup (7.4 oz)	290	2	30
Meat Ravioli & Pomodoro Sauce	1 pkg (8.5 oz)	320	3	50
Minestrone With Penne Pasta	1 cup (6.3 oz)	180	1	5
Penne Pollo	1 pkg (9 oz)	330	3	20
Penne Primavera	1 pkg (9 oz)	350	3	25
Rigatoni Pomodoro Italiano	1 pkg (9 oz)	290	4	0
Shells & Cheese With Jalapenos	1 pkg (8.5 oz)	360	2	30
Spaghetti Bolognese	1 pkg (9 oz)	270	4	20
Spaghetti Marinara	1 pkg (10 oz)	250	3	0
Spinach Ravioli & Primavera Sauce	1 pkg (8.5 oz)	360	2	45
Morton				
Macaroni & Cheese	1 serv (8 oz)	220	2	15
Mrs. Paul's				
Entrees Light Seafood Lasagne	9½ oz	290	—	57
Entrees Light Seafood Rotini	9 oz	240	—	25
Seafood Rotini	9 oz	240	—	25
Palmazone				
Macaroni 'n Cheese	½ pkg (6 oz)	260	—	20
Pasta Favorites				
Chicken Pasta Primavera	1 pkg (10.5 oz)	330	6	25
Fettuccini Alfredo	1 pkg (10.5 oz)	370	4	30
Italian Sausage & Peppers	1 pkg (10.5 oz)	340	7	10
Lasagna	1 pkg (10.5 oz)	290	6	10
Macaroni & Cheese	1 pkg (10.5 oz)	350	5	20
Pasta Primavera	1 pkg (10.5 oz)	320	7	20
Spaghetti w/ Meatballs	1 pkg (10.5 oz)	370	6	35
Vegetable Lasagna	1 pkg (10.5 oz)	260	7	10
White Cheddar & Rotini	1 pkg (10.5 oz)	350	6	15
Senor Felix's				
Lasagna Southwestern	1 serv (6 oz)	160	2	15
Stouffer's				
Beef Ravioli	1 pkg (9.5 oz)	370	5	80
Cheese Manicotti	1 pkg (9 oz)	340	7	50
Cheese Ravioli With Tomato Sauce	1 pkg (9.5 oz)	360	4	85
Cheese Shells With Tomato Sauce	1 pkg (9.25 oz)	340	5	50
Cheese Tortellini With Alfredo Sauce	1 pkg (8.9 oz)	550	5	160

FOOD	PORTION	CALS.	FIB.	CHOL.
Stouffer's (CONT.)				
Cheese Tortellini With Tomato Sauce	1 pkg (9.25 oz)	290	4	105
Fettucini Alfredo	1 pkg (10 oz)	480	3	100
Four Cheese Lasagna	1 pkg (10.75 oz)	410	3	55
Homestyle Chicken Fettucini	1 pkg (10.5 oz)	380	3	65
Lasagna With Meat Sauce	1 cup (7 oz)	260	4	35
Lasagna With Meat Sauce	1 pkg (10.5 oz)	360	5	50
Lunch Express Cheese Lasagna Casserole	1 pkg (9.5 oz)	270	5	15
Lunch Express Cheese Ravioli	1 pkg (8.5 oz)	310	2	60
Lunch Express Chicken Fettucini	1 pkg (10.25 oz)	250	4	35
Lunch Express Chicken Alfredo	1 pkg (9.6 oz)	360	3	60
Lunch Express Fettucini Primavera	1 pkg (10.25 oz)	420	4	95
Lunch Express Lasagna With Meat Sauce	1 pkg (10 oz)	350	4	40
Lunch Express Macaroni & Cheese & Broccoli	1 pkg (9.5 oz)	240	5	20
Lunch Express Macaroni & Cheese With Broccoli	1 pkg (10.4 oz)	360	3	30
Lunch Express Pasta & Chicken Marinara	1 pkg (9.1 oz)	270	4	20
Lunch Express Pasta & Tuna Casserole	1 pkg (9.6 oz)	280	4	20
Lunch Express Pasta & Turkey Dijon	1 pkg (9.9 oz)	270	6	30
Lunch Express Rigatoni With Meat Sauce	1 pkg (10.75 oz)	340	3	30
Lunch Express Spaghetti With Meat Sauce	1 pkg (9.6 oz)	320	5	30
Lunch Express Swedish Meatballs With Pasta	1 pkg (10.25 oz)	530	3	65
Macaroni & Cheese	1 cup (6 oz)	330	2	30
Macaroni & Beef	1 pkg (11.5 oz)	340	4	50
Noodles Romanoff	1 pkg (12 oz)	460	4	60
Spaghetti With Meat Sauce	1 pkg (12.9 oz)	430	6	40
Spaghetti With Meatballs	1 pkg (12.6 oz)	420	5	45
Tuna Noodle Casserole	1 pkg (10 oz)	330	3	40
Turkey Tettrazini	1 pkg (10 oz)	360	2	40
Vegetable Lasagna	1 cup (8 oz)	280	2	25
Vegetable Lasagna	1 pkg (10.5 oz)	370	3	35
Tabatchnick				
Macaroni & Cheese	7.5 oz	280	2	26

FOOD	PORTION	CALS.	FIB.	CHOL.
Tyson				
Parmigiana	1 pkg (11.25 oz)	380	—	36
Ultra Slim-Fast				
Pasta Primavera	12 oz	340	5	25
Spaghetti With Beef & Mushroom Sauce	12 oz	370	0	25
Weight Watchers				
Angel Hair Pasta	1 pkg (9 oz)	180	7	0
Cheese Manicotti	1 pkg (9.25 oz)	290	4	20
Chicken Fettucini	1 pkg (8.25 oz)	280	2	40
Fettucini Alfredo With Broccoli	1 pkg (8.5 oz)	220	6	15
Garden Lasagne	1 pkg (11 oz)	230	6	5
Italian Cheese Lasagna	1 pkg (11 oz)	300	7	25
Lasagna Florentine	1 pkg (10 oz)	210	5	10
Lasagna Curls With Italian Vegetables	1 pkg (9.5 oz)	170	2	5
Lasagna With Meat Sauce	1 pkg (10.25 oz)	290	7	15
Macaroni & Cheese	1 pkg (9 oz)	260	7	20
Macaroni & Beef	1 pkg (8.5 oz)	220	4	10
Penne Pasta With Sun-Dried Tomatoes	1 pkg (10 oz)	290	8	15
Ravioli Florentine	1 pkg (8.5 oz)	200	4	5
Spaghetti With Meat Sauce	1 pkg (10 oz)	250	6	10
Tuna Noodle Casserole	1 pkg (9.5 oz)	240	5	15
HOME RECIPE				
macaroni & cheese	1 cup	430	—	44
spaghetti w/ meatballs & tomato sauce	1 cup	330	—	89
MIX				
Casbah				
Pasta Fasul	1 pkg (1.6 oz)	150	2	0
Hain				
Pasta & Sauce Creamy Parmesan	¼ pkg	150	—	10
Pasta & Sauce Primavera	¼ pkg	140	—	10
Pasta & Sauce Tangy Cheddar	¼ pkg	180	—	3
Kraft				
Cheddar Cheese Egg Noodle	1 cup (8 oz)	430	1	70
Macaroni & Cheese Deluxe Original	1 cup (6.1 oz)	320	1	25
Macaroni & Cheese Dinosaurs	1 cup (6.8 oz)	390	1	10
Macaroni & Cheese Flintstones	1 cup (6.8 oz)	390	1	10
Macaroni & Cheese Milk White Cheddar	1 cup (6.8 oz)	390	1	10

FOOD	PORTION	CALS.	FIB.	CHOL.
Kraft (CONT.)				
Macaroni & Cheese Original	1 cup (6.9 oz)	390	1	10
Macaroni & Cheese Santa Mac	1 cup	390	1	10
Macaroni & Cheese Spirals	1 cup (6.8 oz)	390	1	10
Macaroni & Cheese Super Mario Bros	1 cup (6.8 oz)	390	1	10
Macaroni & Cheese Teddy Bears	1 cup (6.8 oz)	390	1	10
Macaroni & Cheese Thick 'N Creamy	1 cup (6.1 oz)	320	2	25
Spaghetti Mild American	1 cup (8.1 oz)	270	3	<5
Spaghetti Tangy Italian	1 cup (7.9 oz)	270	3	<5
Spaghetti With Meat Sauce	1 cup (8.2 oz)	330	3	15
Lipton				
Golden Saute Angel Hair Chicken	⅓ cup (2.1 oz)	210	2	0
Golden Saute Angel Hair Parmesan	⅓ cup (2.2 oz)	240	2	10
Golden Saute Chicken Herb Parmesan	½ cup (2.2 oz)	230	3	<5
Golden Saute Chicken Stir Fry	½ cup (2.2 oz)	220	2	0
Golden Saute Garlic Butter	½ cup (2.1 oz)	230	2	<5
Golden Saute Penne Herb & Garlic	⅓ cup (2.1 oz)	230	2	5
Pasta & Sauce Cheddar Broccoli as prep	½ cup (2.4 oz)	260	1	10
Pasta & Sauce Cheese Bow Ties	½ cup (2 oz)	230	1	10
Pasta & Sauce Chicken Primavera as prep	½ cup (2 oz)	220	1	5
Pasta & Sauce Creamy Garlic as prep	½ cup (2.4 oz)	260	1	10
Pasta & Sauce Herb Tomato as prep	½ cup (2.3 oz)	240	3	0
Pasta & Sauce Primavera as prep	½ cup (2.2 oz)	240	2	10
Pasta & Sauce Three Cheese as prep	½ cup (2.2 oz)	240	1	10
Minute				
Microwave Cheddar Cheese Broccoli And Pasta as prep	½ cup	160	—	11
Nile Spice				
Pasta'n Sauce Mediterranean	1 pkg	210	2	10
Pasta'n Sauce Parmesan	1 pkg	200	1	10
Pasta'n Sauce Primavera	1 pkg	200	2	10

FOOD	PORTION	CALS.	FIB.	CHOL.
Uncle Ben				
Country Inn Pasta & Sauce Angel Hair Parmesan	1 serv (2.2 oz)	245	3	13
Country Inn Pasta & Sauce Broccoli & White Cheddar	1 serv (2.2 oz)	240	2	8
Country Inn Pasta & Sauce Butter & Herb	1 serv (2 oz)	230	1	10
Country Inn Pasta & Sauce Creamy Garlic	1 serv (2.4 oz)	261	2	8
Country Inn Pasta & Sauce Fettuccine Alfredo	1 serv (2.2 oz)	310	2	12
Country Inn Pasta & Sauce Herb Linguine	1 serv (2.2 oz)	240	2	5
Country Inn Pasta & Sauce Mushroom Fettuccine	1 serv (2.2 oz)	250	2	12
Country Inn Pasta & Sauce Vegetable Alfredo	1 serv (2.2 oz)	240	2	11
Velveeta				
Rotini & Cheese Broccoli	1 cup (7.2 oz)	400	2	45
Shells & Cheese Bacon	1 cup (6.8 oz)	360	1	40
Shells & Cheese Original	1 cup (6.6 oz)	360	1	40
Shells & Cheese Salsa	1 cup (7.5 oz)	380	2	40
SHELF-STABLE				
Chef Boyardee				
Microwave Main Meal Beans & Pasta	10.5 oz	200	10	10
Microwave Main Meal Beef Ravioli Suprema	10.5 oz	290	5	10
Microwave Main Meal Cheese Ravioli Suprema	10.5 oz	290	5	10
Microwave Main Meal Fettuccine	10.5 oz	290	6	25
Microwave Main Meal Lasagna	10.5 oz	290	5	20
Microwave Main Meal Meat Tortellini	10.5 oz	220	6	30
Microwave Main Meal Noodles w/ Chicken	10.5 oz	170	3	20
Microwave Main Meal Peas & Pasta	10.5 oz	190	6	0
Microwave Main Meal Spaghetti Suprema	10.5 oz	200	7	20
Microwave Main Meal Zesty Macaroni	10.5 oz	290	5	25
Microwave Main Meal Ziti In Sauce	10.5 oz	210	7	0

FOOD	PORTION	CALS.	FIB.	CHOL.
Kid's Kitchen				
Microwave Meals Beefy Macaroni	1 cup (7.5 oz)	190	2	30
Microwave Meals Macaroni & Cheese	1 cup (7.5 oz)	260	1	35
Microwave Meals Mini Ravioli	1 cup (7.5 oz)	240	3	20
Microwave Meals Spaghetti Ring & Meatballs	1 cup (7.5 oz)	250	3	20
Lunch Bucket				
Lasagna With Meatsauce	1 pkg (7.5 oz)	220	—	30
Light'n Healthy Italian Style Pasta	1 pkg (7.5 oz)	130	—	10
Light'n Healthy Pasta In Wine Sauce	1 pkg (7.5 oz)	130	—	10
Light'n Healthy Pasta'n Garden Vegetables	1 pkg (7.5 oz)	150	—	0
Pasta'n Chicken	1 pkg (7.5 oz)	180	—	45
Spaghetti'n Meatsauce	1 pkg (7.5 oz)	240	—	30
Micro Cup Meals				
Lasagna	1 cup (7.5 oz)	230	2	35
Lasagna & Beef Tomato Sauce	1 cup	359	3	34
Macaroni & Beef With Vegetables	1 cup	285	6	26
Macaroni & Cheese	1 cup (7.5 oz)	260	1	35
Ravioli Tomato Sauce	1 cup (7.5 oz)	260	3	20
Spaghetti & Meat Sauce	1 cup (7.5 oz)	220	4	30
My Own Meal				
Cheese Tortellini	1 pkg (10 oz)	340	6	15
Top Shelf				
Italian Lasagna	1 bowl (10 oz)	350	3	50
Spaghetti With Meat Sauce	1 bowl (10 oz)	240	3	20
TAKE-OUT				
lasagna	1 piece (2.5 in x 2.5 in)	374	2	107
macaroni & cheese	1 cup	230	—	24
manicotti	¾ cup (6.4 oz)	273	2	77
rigatoni w/ sausage sauce	¾ cup	260	3	59
spaghetti w/ meatballs & cheese	1 cup	407	—	104

PASTA MACHINE MIX

FOOD	PORTION	CALS.	FIB.	CHOL.
Wanda's				
Dried Tomato	⅓ cup mix per serv (1.9 oz)	202	1	0
Durum & Semolina	⅓ cup mix per serv (1.9 oz)	199	1	0

FOOD	PORTION	CALS.	FIB.	CHOL.
Wanda's (CONT.)				
Semolina Blend	⅓ cup mix per serv (1.9 oz)	202	1	0
Spinach	⅓ cup mix per serv (1.9 oz)	202	1	0
Whole Wheat & Semolina	⅓ cup mix per serv (1.9 oz)	198	4	0

PASTA SALAD
MIX
Kraft

Pasta Salad Classic Ranch With Bacon	¾ cup (4.7 oz)	360	2	15
Pasta Salad Creamy Caesar	¾ cup (4.8 oz)	350	2	15
Pasta Salad Garden Primavera	¾ cup (5 oz)	280	2	<5
Pasta Salad Light Italian	¾ cup (5 oz)	190	2	<5
Pasta Salad Parmesan Peppercorn	¾ cup (4.9 oz)	360	2	20

TAKE-OUT

elbow macaroni salad	3.5 oz	160	—	0
italian style pasta salad	3.5 oz	140	—	0
mustard macaroni salad	3.5 oz	190	—	0
pasta salad w/ vegetables	3.5 oz	140	—	0

PASTRY
(*see* BROWNIE, CAKE, DANISH PASTRY)

PATE
CANNED

goose liver smoked	1 tbsp (13 g)	60	—	20
goose liver smoked	1 oz	131	—	43
Sells				
Liver	2.08 oz	190	—	90

PEACH
CANNED

halves in heavy syrup	1 half	60	—	0
halves in light syrup	1 half	44	—	0
halves juice pack	1 half	34	—	0
halves water pack	1 half	18	—	0
spiced in heavy syrup	1 fruit	66	—	0
spiced in heavy syrup	1 cup	180	—	0
Del Monte				
Halves Cling In Heavy Syrup	½ cup (4.5 oz)	100	1	0
Halves Cling Lite	½ cup (4.4 oz)	60	1	0
Halves Cling Melba In Heavy Syrup	½ cup (4.5 oz)	100	1	0

FOOD	PORTION	CALS.	FIB.	CHOL.
Del Monte (CONT.)				
Halves Freestone In Heavy Syrup	½ cup (4.5 oz)	100	1	0
Sliced Cling Fruit Naturals	½ cup (4.4 oz)	60	1	0
Sliced Cling In Heavy Syrup	½ cup (4.5 oz)	100	1	0
Sliced Cling Lite	½ cup (4.4 oz)	60	1	0
Sliced Freestone In Heavy Syrup	½ cup (4.5 oz)	100	1	0
Sliced Freestone Lite	½ cup (4.4 oz)	60	1	0
Snack Cups Diced Fruit Naturals	1 serv (4.5 oz)	60	1	0
Snack Cups Diced Fruit Naturals EZ-Open Lid	1 serv (4.2 oz)	60	1	0
Snack Cups Diced In Heavy Syrup	1 serv (4.5 oz)	100	1	0
Snack Cups Diced In Heavy Syrup EZ-Open Lid	1 serv (4.2 oz)	90	1	0
Snack Cups Diced Lite	1 serv (4.5 oz)	60	1	0
Snack Cups Diced Lite EZ-Open Lid	1 serv (4.2 oz)	60	1	0
Whole Cling In Heavy Syrup	½ cup (4.2 oz)	100	tr	0
Hunt's				
Halves	½ cup (4.5 oz)	100	1	0
Slices	½ cup (4.5 oz)	100	1	0
Libby				
Halves Yellow Cling Lite	½ cup (4.4 oz)	60	1	0
Sliced Yellow Cling Lite	½ cup (4.4 oz)	60	1	0
S&W				
Halves Clingstone	½ cup	100	—	0
Halves Clingstone Diet	½ cup	30	—	0
Halves Clingstone Unsweetened	½ cup	30	—	0
Halves Freestone Diet	½ cup	30	—	0
Halves Freestone In Heavy Syrup	½ cup	100	—	0
Sliced Clingstone Diet	½ cup	30	—	0
Sliced Clingstone Unsweetened	½ cup	30	—	0
Sliced Freestone Diet	½ cup	30	—	0
Sliced Freestone In Heavy Syrup	½ cup	100	—	0
Sliced Yellow Cling Natural Style	½ cup	90	—	0
Sliced Yellow Cling Premium In Heavy Syrup	½ cup	100	—	0

FOOD	PORTION	CALS.	FIB.	CHOL.
S&W (CONT.)				
Whole Yellow Cling Spiced In Heavy Syrup	½ cup	90	—	0
Yellow Cling Natural Lite	½ cup	50	—	0
DRIED				
halves	10	311	11	0
halves	1 cup	383	13	0
halves cooked w/ sugar	½ cup	139	—	0
halves cooked w/o sugar	½ cup	99	—	0
Del Monte				
Sun Dried	⅓ cup (1.4 oz)	90	5	0
Mariani				
Peaches	¼ cup	140	—	0
Sonoma				
Pieces	3-5 pieces (1.4 oz)	120	1	0
FRESH				
peach	1	37	1	0
sliced	1 cup	73	—	0
Dole				
Peach	2	70	1	0
FROZEN				
slices sweetened	1 cup	235	—	0
Big Valley				
Freestone	⅔ cup (4.9 oz)	50	1	0
PEACH JUICE				
nectar	1 cup	134	—	0
Goya				
Nectar	6 oz	110	—	0
Kern's				
Nectar	6 fl oz	110	—	0
Libby				
Nectar	1 can (11.5 fl oz)	210	—	0
Mott's				
Fruit Basket Orchard Peach Juice Cocktail as prep	8 fl oz	130	0	0
Smucker's				
Juice	8 oz	120	—	0
Snapple				
Dixie Peach	10 fl oz	140	—	0
PEANUT BUTTER				
chunky	1 cup	1520	17	0
chunky	2 tbsp	188	2	0
chunky w/o salt	2 tbsp	188	2	0

FOOD	PORTION	CALS.	FIB.	CHOL.
chunky w/o salt	1 cup	1520	17	0
smooth	1 cup	1517	15	0
smooth	2 tbsp	188	2	0
smooth w/o salt	1 cup	1517	15	0
smooth w/o salt	2 tbsp	188	2	0
Arrowhead				
Creamy	2 tbsp (1.1 oz)	200	1	0
Crunchy	2 tbsp (1.1 oz)	200	1	0
BAMA				
Creamy	2 tbsp	200	—	0
Crunchy	2 tbsp	200	—	0
Jelly & Peanut Butter	2 tbsp	150	—	0
Crazy Richard's				
Natural Creamy	2 tbsp (1.1 oz)	190	2	0
Erewhon				
Chunky	2 tbsp (32 g)	190	—	0
Chunky Unsalted	2 tbsp (32 g)	190	—	0
Creamy	2 tbsp (32 g)	190	—	0
Creamy Unsalted	2 tbsp (32 g)	190	—	0
Estee				
Chunky Sodium Free	2 tbsp (1 oz)	190	2	0
Chunky Sodium Free Sorbitol Sweetened	2 tbsp (1 oz)	190	2	0
Creamy Sodium Free	2 tbsp (1 oz)	190	2	0
Creamy Sodium Free Sorbitol Sweetened	2 tbsp (1 oz)	190	2	0
Health Valley				
Chunky No Salt	2 tbsp	170	2	0
Creamy No Salt	2 tbsp	170	3	0
Hollywood				
Creamy	1 tbsp	35	1	0
Crunchy	1 tbsp	35	1	0
Unsalted	1 tbsp	35	1	0
Home Brand				
Natural Lightly Salted	2 tbsp	210	—	0
Natural Unsalted	2 tbsp	210	—	0
No-Sugar Added	2 tbsp	180	—	0
Peanut Butter	2 tbsp	210	—	0
Jif				
Creamy	2 tbsp (1.1 oz)	190	2	0
Extra Crunchy	2 tbsp (1.1 oz)	190	2	0
Reduced Fat	2 tbsp (1.3 oz)	190	2	0
Simply Creamy	2 tbsp (1.1 oz)	190	2	0
Simply Extra Crunchy	2 tbsp (1.1 oz)	190	2	0

FOOD	PORTION	CALS.	FIB.	CHOL.
Peter Pan				
Creamy	2 tbsp	190	2	0
Creamy Salt Free	2 tbsp	190	2	0
Crunchy	2 tbsp	190	2	0
Crunchy Salt Free	2 tbsp	190	2	0
Red Wing				
Creamy	2 tbsp (1.1 oz)	200	2	0
Crunchy	2 tbsp (1.1 oz)	200	2	0
Reese's				
Peanut Butter Chips	¼ cup (1.5 oz)	230	—	5
Skippy				
Creamy	1 cup (263 g)	1540	—	0
Creamy w/ 2 slices white bread	1 sandwich	340	—	0
Reduced Fat Creamy	2 tbsp	190	1	0
Super Chunk	1 cup (260 g)	1540	—	0
Super Chunk	2 tbsp (32 g)	190	—	0
Super Chunk w/ 2 slices white bread	1 sandwich	340	—	0
Smucker's				
Goober Grape	2 tbsp	180	—	0
Honey Sweetened	2 tbsp	200	—	0
Natural	2 tbsp	200	—	0
Natural No-Salt Added	2 tbsp	200	—	0
Tree Of Life				
Creamy	2 tbsp (1 oz)	190	1	0
Creamy No Salt	2 tbsp (1 oz)	190	1	0
Creamy Organic	2 tbsp (1 oz)	190	1	0
Creamy Organic No Salt	2 tbsp (1 oz)	190	1	0
Crunchy	2 tbsp (1 oz)	190	1	0
Crunchy No Salt	2 tbsp (1 oz)	190	1	0
Crunchy Organic	2 tbsp (1 oz)	190	1	0
Crunchy Organic No Salt	2 tbsp (1 oz)	190	1	0
Peanut Wonder 78% Less Fat	2 tbsp (1 oz)	100	1	0
PEANUTS				
chocolate coated	10 (1.4 oz)	208	—	4
chocolate coated	1 cup (5.2 oz)	773	—	13
cooked	½ cup	102	—	0
dry roasted	1 oz	164	2	0
dry roasted	1 cup	855	12	0
oil roasted	1 oz	163	2	0
oil roasted	1 cup	837	13	0
oil roasted w/o salt	1 cup	837	13	0
oil roasted w/o salt	1 oz	163	2	0

FOOD	PORTION	CALS.	FIB.	CHOL.
spanish oil roasted	1 oz	162	2	0
spanish oil roasted w/o salt	1 oz	162	2	0
unroasted	1 oz	159	—	0
valencia oil roasted	1 oz	165	2	0
valencia oil roasted	1 cup	848	9	0
valencia oil roasted w/o salt	1 oz	165	2	0
valencia oil roasted w/o salt	1 cup	848	9	0
virginia oil roasted	1 cup	826	—	0
virginia oil roasted	1 oz	161	—	0
Beer Nuts				
Peanuts	1 pkg (1 oz)	180	—	0
Fisher				
Party Peanuts	1 oz	160	—	0
Salted-In-Shell shelled	1 oz	170	—	0
Spanish Roasted	1 oz	180	—	0
Frito Lay				
Dry Roasted	1.2 oz	190	—	0
Salted	1 oz	170	—	0
Guy's				
Dry Roasted	1 oz	170	—	0
Spanish Salted	1 oz	170	—	0
Lance				
Honey Toasted	1 pkg (39 g)	230	—	0
Roasted w/ Shell	1 pkg (50 g)	190	—	0
Salted	1 pkg (32 g)	190	—	0
Salted Tube	1 pkg (42 g)	240	—	0
Little Debbie				
Salted	1 pkg (1.2 oz)	230	2	0
Pennant				
Oil Roasted	1 oz	170	3	0
Planters				
Cocktail Lightly Salted Oil Roasted	1 oz	170	2	0
Cocktail Oil Roasted	1 oz	170	3	0
Cocktail Unsalted Oil Roasted	1 oz	170	2	0
Dry Roasted	1 oz	160	3	0
Fun Size! Oil Roasted	2 pkg (1 oz)	170	2	0
Heat Hot Spicy Oil Roasted	1 pkg (1.7 oz)	290	4	0
Heat Hot Spicy Oil Roasted	1 oz	160	2	0
Heat Hot Spicy Oil Roasted	1 pkg (2 oz)	330	5	0
Heat Mild Spicy Oil Roasted	1 oz	160	2	0
Honey Roasted	1 oz	160	2	0
Honey Roasted Dry Roasted	1 pkg (1.7 oz)	260	3	0
Lightly Salted Dry Roasted	1 oz	160	3	0

FOOD	PORTION	CALS.	FIB.	CHOL.
Planters (CONT.)				
Lightly Salted Dry Roasted	1 pkg (1.75 oz)	290	4	0
Lightly Salted Oil Roasted	1 pkg (1.8 oz)	300	4	0
Munch'N Go Singles Heat Hot Spicy Oil Roasted	1 pkg (2.5 oz)	410	6	0
Reduced Fat Honey Roasted	⅓ cup (1 oz)	130	2	0
Salted Oil Roasted	1 pkg (1 oz)	170	2	0
Spanish Oil Roasted	1 oz	170	2	0
Spanish Raw	1 oz	150	3	0
Sweet N Crunchy	1 oz	140	2	0
Unsalted Dry Roasted	1 oz	160	3	0
Weight Watchers				
Honey Roasted	1 pkg (0.7 oz)	100	2	0
PEAR				
CANNED				
halves in heavy syrup	1 cup	188	—	0
halves in heavy syrup	1 half	68	—	0
halves in light syrup	1 half	45	—	0
halves juice pack	1 cup	123	—	0
halves water pack	1 half	22	—	0
Del Monte				
Halves Fruit Naturals	½ cup (4.4 oz)	60	1	0
Halves In Heavy Syrup	½ cup (4.5 oz)	100	1	0
Halves Lite	½ cup (4.4 oz)	60	1	0
Sliced In Heavy Syrup	½ cup (4.5 oz)	100	1	0
Sliced Lite	½ cup (4.4 oz)	60	1	0
Snack Cups Diced In Heavy Syrup	1 serv (4.5 oz)	100	1	0
Snack Cups Diced In Heavy Syrup EZ-Open Lid	1 serv (4.2 oz)	90	1	0
Snack Cups Diced Lite	1 serv (4.5 oz)	60	1	0
Snack Cups Diced Lite EZ-Open Lid	1 serv (4.2 oz)	60	1	0
Libby				
Halves Lite	½ cup (4.3 oz)	60	1	0
Sliced Lite	½ cup (4.3 oz)	60	1	0
S&W				
Halves Bartlett In Heavy Syrup	½ cup	100	—	0
Halves Bartlett Peeled Unsweetened	½ cup	35	—	0
Halves Peeled Diet	½ cup	35	—	0
Quartered Peeled Diet	½ cup	35	—	0
Sliced Natural Light Bartlett	½ cup	60	—	0

FOOD	PORTION	CALS.	FIB.	CHOL.
S&W (CONT.)				
Sliced Natural Style	½ cup	80	—	0
DRIED				
halves	10	459	—	0
halves	1 cup	472	—	0
halves cooked w/ sugar	½ cup	196	—	0
halves cooked w/o sugar	½ cup	163	—	0
Mariani				
Pears	¼ cup	150	—	0
Sonoma				
Pieces	3-4 pieces (1.4 oz)	120	3	0
FRESH				
asian	1 (4.3 oz)	51	—	0
pear	1	98	4	0
sliced w/ skin	1 cup	97	4	0
Dole				
Pear	1	100	4	0

PEAR JUICE

nectar	1 cup	149	—	0
Goya				
Nectar	6 oz	120	—	0
Kern's				
Nectar	6 fl oz	120	—	0
Libby				
Nectar	1 can (11.5 fl oz)	220	3	0

PEAS
CANNED

green	½ cup	59	—	0
green low sodium	½ cup	59	—	0
Allen				
Crowder	½ cup (4.5 oz)	110	8	0
Purple Hull	½ cup (4.4 oz)	120	6	0
Crest Top				
Early June	½ cup (4.5 oz)	100	6	0
Del Monte				
Sweet	½ cup (4.4 oz)	60	4	0
Sweet 50% Less Salt	½ cup (4.4 oz)	60	4	0
Sweet No Salt Added	½ cup (4.4 oz)	60	4	0
Sweet Very Young	½ cup (4.4 oz)	60	4	0
East Texas Fair				
Cream Peas	½ cup (4.4 oz)	120	5	0
Crowder	½ cup (4.5 oz)	110	8	0
Lady Peas With Snaps	½ cup (4.3 oz)	100	4	0

FOOD	PORTION	CALS.	FIB.	CHOL.
East Texas Fair (CONT.)				
Peas 'n Pork	½ cup (4.5 oz)	110	5	0
Pepper Peas	½ cup (4.5 oz)	120	6	0
Purple Hull	½ cup (4.4 oz)	120	6	0
White Acre	½ cup (4.3 oz)	100	5	0
Green Giant				
Sweet	½ cup	50	4	0
Homefolks				
Crowder	½ cup (4.5 oz)	110	8	0
Purple Hull	½ cup (4.4 oz)	120	6	0
Owatonna				
Early June or Sweet	½ cup	70	—	0
S&W				
Petit Pois	½ cup	70	—	0
Sweet	½ cup	70	—	0
Sweet Water Pack	½ cup	40	—	0
Veri-Green Sweet	½ cup	70	—	0
Seneca				
Natural Pack	½ cup	60	4	0
Peas	½ cup	50	5	0
Sunshine				
Field Peas	½ cup (4.4 oz)	120	6	0
Lady Peas	½ cup (4.3 oz)	100	5	0
Trappey				
Field Peas With Bacon	½ cup (4.5 oz)	90	5	0
Field Peas With Snaps And Bacon	½ cup (4.5 oz)	110	4	0
DRIED				
split cooked	1 cup	231	—	0
Bascom's				
Yellow Split as prep	½ cup	110	—	0
FRESH				
green cooked	½ cup	67	—	0
green raw	½ cup	58	—	0
snap peas cooked	½ cup	34	2	0
snap peas raw	½ cup	30	2	0
Dole				
Sugar Peas	½ cup	30	2	0
FROZEN				
green cooked	½ cup	63	—	0
snap peas cooked	1 pkg (10 oz)	132	—	0
snap peas cooked	½ cup	42	—	0
Birds Eye				
Green	½ cup	80	4	0

FOOD	PORTION	CALS.	FIB.	CHOL.
Birds Eye (CONT.)				
In Butter Sauce	½ cup	80	3	5
Polybag Deluxe Tender Tiny	½ cup	60	4	0
Polybag Green	½ cup	70	2	0
Sugar Snap Deluxe	½ cup	45	4	0
Tender Tiny Deluxe	½ cup	60	4	0
Chun King				
Snow Pea Pods	½ pkg (3 oz)	35	2	0
Green Giant				
Harvest Fresh Early June	½ cup	60	3	0
Harvest Fresh Sugar Snap	½ cup	30	2	0
Harvest Fresh Sweet	½ cup	50	3	0
In Butter Sauce	½ cup	80	4	5
One Serve In Butter Sauce	1 pkg	90	5	5
Sugar Snap Sweet Select	½ cup	30	2	0
Sweet	½ cup	50	4	0
Hanover				
Petite	½ cup	70	—	0
Snow Peas	½ cup	35	—	0
Sweet	½ cup	70	—	0
Le Seur				
Early In Butter Sauce	½ cup	80	3	5
Early Select	½ cup	60	4	0
Tree Of Life				
Peas	⅔ cup (3.1 oz)	70	4	0
SHELF-STABLE				
Green Giant				
Mini Sweet	½ cup	60	4	0
SPROUTS				
raw	½ cup	77	—	0
PECANS				
dried	1 oz	190	2	0
dry roasted	1 oz	187	—	0
dry roasted salted	1 oz	187	—	0
halves dried	1 cup	721	7	0
oil roasted	1 oz	195	—	0
oil roasted salted	1 oz	195	—	0
Planters				
Chips	1 pkg (2 oz)	390	7	0
Gold Measure Halves	1 pkg (2 oz)	390	3	0
Halves	1 oz	190	2	0
Honey Roasted	1 oz	180	2	0
Pieces	1 oz	190	2	0

FOOD	PORTION	CALS.	FIB.	CHOL.
Planters (CONT.)				
Pieces	1 pkg (2 oz)	390	3	0
PECTIN				
powder	¼ pkg (0.4 oz)	39	—	0
powder	1 pkg (1.75 oz)	163	—	0
Certo				
Liquid	1 tbsp	2	—	0
Slim Set				
Packet	1 pkg	208	14	0
Powder	1 tbsp	3	tr	0
Sure-Jell				
Light	¼ pkg	33	—	0
Powder	¼ pkg	38	—	0
PEPPER				
black	1 tsp	5	—	0
cayenne	1 tsp	6	—	0
red	1 tsp	6	—	0
white	1 tsp	7	—	0
Ac'cent				
Lemon	½ tsp	0	0	0
Seasoned	½ tsp	0	0	0
Lawry's				
Lemon	1 tsp	6	tr	0
Watkins				
Black	¼ tbsp (0.5 g)	0	0	0
Cajun	¼ tbsp (0.5 g)	0	0	0
Cracked Black	¼ tbsp (0.5 g)	0	0	0
Dijon	¼ tbsp (0.5 g)	0	0	0
Garlic Peppercorn Blend	¼ tbsp (1 g)	0	0	0
Herb	¼ tbsp (0.5 g)	0	0	0
Italian	¼ tbsp (0.5 g)	0	0	0
Lemon	¼ tbsp (1 g)	0	0	0
Mexican	¼ tbsp (0.5 g)	0	0	0
Red Pepper Flakes	¼ tsp (0.5 oz)	0	0	0
Royal Pepper Blend	¼ tbsp (0.5 g)	0	0	0
PEPPERS				
CANNED				
chili green hot	1 (2.6 oz)	18	—	0
chili green hot chopped	½ cup	17	—	0
chili red hot	1 (2.6 oz)	18	—	0
chili red hot chopped	½ cup	17	—	0
green halves	½ cup	13	—	0

FOOD	PORTION	CALS.	FIB.	CHOL.
jalapeno chopped	½ cup	17	—	0
red halves	½ cup	13	—	0
Chi-Chi's				
Chilies Diced Green	2 tbsp (1.2 oz)	10	0	0
Chilies Green Whole	¾ pepper (1 oz)	10	0	0
Jalapenos Green Wheels	1 oz	10	0	0
Jalapenos Green Whole	1 oz	10	0	0
Jalapenos Red Wheels	1 oz	10	0	0
Jalapenos Red Whole	1 oz	15	0	0
Del Monte				
Chilpotle In Spice Sauce	2 tbsp (1.1 oz)	20	1	0
Hot Chili	4 (1 oz)	10	tr	0
Jalapeno Nacho Pickled Sliced	2 tbsp (1 oz)	5	tr	0
Jalapeno Pickled Sliced	2 tbsp (1.1 oz)	5	tr	0
Jalapeno Pickled Whole	2 tbsp (1.1 oz)	5	tr	0
Jalapeno Whole	1 (0.7 oz)	3	tr	0
Hebrew National				
Filet	¼ pepper (1 oz)	9	—	0
Hot Cherry	⅓ pepper (1 oz)	11	—	0
Red Filet	¼ pepper (1 oz)	9	—	0
McIlhenny				
Jalapeno Nacho Slices	12 slices (1.1 oz)	7	1	0
Old El Paso				
Green Chilies Chopped	2 tbsp (1 oz)	5	1	0
Green Chilies Whole	1 (1.2 oz)	10	1	0
Jalapenos Peeled	3 (1 oz)	10	1	0
Jalapenos Pickled	2 (0.9 oz)	5	0	0
Jalapenos Slices	2 tbsp (1.1 oz)	15	1	0
Progresso				
Cherry (drained)	2 tbsp (0.9 oz)	30	1	0
Fried (drained)	2 tbsp (0.9 oz)	60	1	0
Hot Cherry	1 (1 oz)	15	0	0
Pepper Salad (drained)	2 tbsp (0.9 oz)	25	1	0
Roasted	½ piece (1 oz)	10	0	0
Tuscan (drained)	3 (1 oz)	10	1	0
Rosoff's				
Sweet	¼ pepper (1 oz)	9	—	0
Schorr's				
Filet Peppers	1 oz	9	—	0
Trappey				
Banana Mild	3 peppers (1 oz)	6	1	0
Banana Sliced Rings	21 slices (1 oz)	6	1	0
Cherry Hot	2 peppers (1 oz)	7	1	0
Cherry Mild	2 peppers (1 oz)	10	1	0

FOOD	PORTION	CALS.	FIB.	CHOL.
Trappey (CONT.)				
Dulcito Italian Pepperoncini	4 peppers (1 oz)	8	1	0
In Vinegar Hot	15 peppers (1 oz)	9	tr	0
Jalapeno Hot Sliced	21 slices (1 oz)	4	1	tr
Jalapeno Whole	2 peppers (1 oz)	11	1	tr
Serano	7 peppers (1 oz)	7	tr	0
Tempero Golden Greek Pepperoncini	4 peppers (1 oz)	7	1	0
Torrido Santa Fe Grande	3 peppers (1 oz)	10	tr	0
Vlasic				
Hot Banana Pepper Rings	1 oz	4	—	0
Hot Cherry	1 oz	10	—	0
Jalapeno Mexican Hot	1 oz	8	—	0
Mexican Tiny Hot	1 oz	6	—	0
Mild Cherry	1 oz	8	—	0
Mild Greek Pepperoncini Salad Peppers	1 oz	4	—	0
DRIED				
green	1 tbsp	1	—	0
red	1 tbsp	1	—	0
FRESH				
chili green hot raw	1	18	—	0
chili green hot raw chopped	½ cup	30	—	0
chili red hot raw	1 (1.6 oz)	18	—	0
chili red raw chopped	½ cup	30	—	0
green chopped cooked	½ cup	19	—	0
green cooked	1 (2.6 oz)	20	—	0
green raw	1 (2.6 oz)	20	1	0
green raw chopped	½ cup	13	1	0
red chopped cooked	½ cup	19	—	0
red cooked	1 (2.6 oz)	20	—	0
red raw	1 (2.6 oz)	20	1	0
red raw chopped	½ cup	13	1	0
yellow raw	1 (6.5 oz)	50	—	0
yellow raw	10 strips	14	—	0
Dole				
Medium	1	25	2	0
FROZEN				
green chopped not prep	1 oz	6	—	0
red chopped	1 oz	6	—	0
Southland				
Green Diced	2 oz	10	—	0

FOOD	PORTION	CALS.	FIB.	CHOL.
Southland (CONT.)				
Sweet Red & Green Cut	2 oz	15	—	0
PERCH				
FRESH				
cooked	1 fillet (1.6 oz)	54	—	53
cooked	3 oz	99	—	98
ocean perch atlantic cooked	1 fillet (1.8 oz)	60	—	27
ocean perch atlantic cooked	3 oz	103	—	46
ocean perch atlantic raw	3 oz	80	—	36
raw	3 oz	77	—	76
FROZEN				
Van De Kamp's				
Battered Fillets	2 (4 oz)	300	0	25
PERSIMMONS				
dried japanese	1	93	—	0
fresh	1	32	—	0
fresh japanese	1	118	—	0
Sonoma				
Dried	6-8 pieces (1.4 oz)	140	3	0
PHYLLO DOUGH				
phyllo dough	1 oz	85	—	0
sheet	1	57	—	0
Ekizian				
Sheets	½ lb	865	—	123
PICANTE				
(*see* SALSA)				
PICKLES				
dill	1 (2.3 oz)	12	—	0
dill low sodium	1 (2.3 oz)	12	1	0
dill low sodium sliced	1 slice	1	tr	0
dill sliced	1 slice	1	tr	0
gherkins	3½ oz	21	—	0
kosher dill	1 (2.3 oz)	12	1	0
polish dill	1 (2.3 oz)	12	1	0
quick sour	1 (1.2 oz)	4	—	0
quick sour low sodium	1 (1.2 oz)	4	—	0
quick sour sliced	1 slice	1	—	0
sweet	1 (1.2 oz)	41	tr	0
sweet gherkin	1 sm (½ oz)	20	—	0
sweet low sodium	1 (1.2 oz)	41	tr	0
sweet sliced	1 slice	7	tr	0

FOOD	PORTION	CALS.	FIB.	CHOL.
Claussen				
Bread 'N Butter Slices	1 slice	7	—	0
Dill Spears	1 spear	4	—	0
Kosher Halves	1 half	9	—	0
Kosher Slices	1 slice	1	—	0
Kosher Whole	1	9	—	0
No Garlic Dills	1	17	—	0
Del Monte				
Dill Halves	¼ pickle (1 oz)	5	tr	0
Dill Hamburger Chips	5 pieces (1 oz)	5	0	0
Dill Sweet Chips	5 pieces (1 oz)	40	tr	0
Dill Sweet Gherkin	2 pickles (1 oz)	40	tr	0
Dill Sweet Midgets	3 pickles (1 oz)	40	tr	0
Dill Sweet Whole	2 pickles (1 oz)	40	tr	0
Dill Tiny Kosher	1½ pickle (1 oz)	5	tr	0
Dill Whole Pickles	1½ pickle (1 oz)	5	tr	0
Hebrew National				
Half Sour	½ pickle (1 oz)	4	—	0
Kosher	⅓ pickle (1 oz)	4	—	0
Kosher Barrel Cured Dill	1 pkg	23	—	0
Kosher Barrel Cured Hot Dill	1 pkg	23	—	0
Kosher Chips	3 slices (1 oz)	4	—	0
Kosher Halves	⅓ pickle (1 oz)	4	—	0
Kosher Large	⅕ pickle (1 oz)	4	—	0
Kosher Spears	½ spear (1 oz)	4	—	0
Sour Garlic	⅓ pickle (1 oz)	3	—	0
McIlhenny				
Hot N' Sweet	4 (1 oz)	42	tr	0
Rosoff's				
Half Sour	⅓ pickle (1 oz)	4	—	0
Half Sour Spears	½ spear (1 oz)	4	—	0
Kosher	⅓ pickle (1 oz)	4	—	0
Kosher Halves	⅓ pickle (1 oz)	4	—	0
Schorr's				
Garlic	⅓ pickle (1 oz)	3	—	0
Half Sour	½ spear (1 oz)	4	—	0
Half Sour	⅓ pickle (1 oz)	4	—	0
Kosher Deli	½ pickle (1 oz)	4	—	0
Kosher Halves	⅓ pickle (1 oz)	4	—	0
Kosher Spears	½ spear (1 oz)	4	—	0
Kosher Whole	⅓ pickle (1 oz)	4	—	0
Vlasic				
Bread & Butter Chips	1 oz	30	—	0
Bread & Butter Chunks	1 oz	25	—	0

FOOD	PORTION	CALS.	FIB.	CHOL.
Vlasic (CONT.)				
Bread & Butter Stixs	1 oz	18	—	0
Deli Bread & Butter	1 oz	25	—	0
Deli Dill Halves	1 oz	4	—	0
Half-The-Salt Hamburger Dill Chips	1 oz	2	—	0
Half-The-Salt Kosher Crunchy Dills	1 oz	4	—	0
Half-The-Salt Kosher Dill Spears	1 oz	4	—	0
Half-The-Salt Sweet Butter Chips	1 oz	30	—	0
Hot & Spicy Garden Mix	1 oz	4	—	0
Kosher Baby Dills	1 oz	4	—	0
Kosher Crunchy Dills	1 oz	4	—	0
Kosher Dill Gherkins	1 oz	4	—	0
Kosher Dill Spears	1 oz	4	—	0
Kosher Snack Chunks	1 oz	4	—	0
No Garlic Dill Spears	1 oz	4	—	0
Original Dills	1 oz	2	—	0
Polish Snack Chunk Dills	1 oz	4	—	0
Zesty Crunchy Dills	1 oz	4	—	0
Zesty Dill Snack Chunks	1 oz	4	—	0
Zesty Dill Spears	1 oz	4	—	0
PIE (*see also* PIE CRUST)				
CANNED FILLING				
apple	1 can (21 oz)	599	6	0
apple	⅛ can (2.6 oz)	74	1	0
cherry	1 can (21 oz)	683	—	0
cherry	⅛ can (2.6 oz)	85	—	0
pumpkin pie mix	1 cup	282	—	0
Libby				
Pumpkin Pie Mix	½ cup	100	2	0
FROZEN				
apple	⅛ of 9 in pie (4.4 oz)	297	2	0
blueberry	⅛ of 9 in pie (4.4 oz)	289	—	0
cherry	⅛ of 9 in pie (4.4 oz)	325	1	0
chocolate creme	⅙ of 8 in pie (4 oz)	344	—	6
coconut creme	⅙ of 7 in pie (2.2 oz)	191	1	0

FOOD	PORTION	CALS.	FIB.	CHOL.
lemon meringue	1/6 of 8 in pie (4.5 oz)	303	1	51
peach	1/6 of 8 in pie (4.1 oz)	261	—	0
Banquet				
Apple	1/5 pie (4 oz)	300	2	5
Banana Cream	1/3 pie (4.7 oz)	350	1	<5
Cherry	1/5 pie (4 oz)	290	2	5
Chocolate Cream	1/3 pie (4.7 oz)	360	3	<5
Coconut Cream	1/3 pie (4.7 oz)	350	2	<5
Lemon Cream	1/3 pie (4.7 oz)	360	2	<5
Mincemeat	1/5 pie (4 oz)	310	2	10
Peach	1/5 pie (4 oz)	260	2	5
Pumpkin	1/6 pie (4 oz)	250	3	20
Kineret				
Apple Homestyle	1/6 pie (4 oz)	313	1	0
Mrs. Smith's				
Apple	1/10 of 10 in pie (4.6 oz)	280	1	0
Apple	1/8 of 9 in pie (4.6 oz)	370	2	0
Apple	1/6 of 8 in pie (4.3 oz)	270	1	0
Apple Cranberry	1/6 of 8 in pie (4.3 oz)	280	1	0
Apple Lattice Ready To Serve	1/5 of 8 in pie (4.6 oz)	310	2	0
Banana Cream	1/4 of 8 in pie (3.4 oz)	250	1	0
Berry	1/6 of 8 in pie (4.3 oz)	280	0	0
Blackberry	1/6 of 8 in pie (4.3 oz)	280	1	0
Blueberry	1/6 of 8 in pie	260	1	0
Boston Cream	1/8 of 8 in pie (2.4 oz)	170	0	25
Cherry	1/6 of 8 in pie	270	1	0
Cherry	1/10 of 10 in pie (4.6 oz)	410	—	10
Cherry	1/8 of 9 in pie (4.6 oz)	320	1	0
Cherry Lattice Ready To Serve	1/5 of 8 in pie (4.6 oz)	320	1	0
Chocolate Cream	1/4 of 8 in pie (3.4 oz)	290	1	0

FOOD	PORTION	CALS.	FIB.	CHOL.
Mrs. Smith's (CONT.)				
Coconut Cream	¼ of 8 in pie (3.4 oz)	280	0	0
Coconut Custard	⅕ of 8 in pie (5 oz)	280	0	75
Dutch Apple	⅙ of 8 in pie	310	1	0
Dutch Apple	⅒ of 10 in pie (4.6 oz)	320	1	0
Dutch Apple	⅑ of 9 in pie (4.5 oz)	300	2	0
French Silk Cream	⅕ of 8 in pie (4.8 oz)	410	1	5
Hearty Pumpkin	⅕ of 8 in pie (5.2 oz)	280	2	60
Lemon Cream	¼ of 8 in pie (3.4 oz)	270	0	0
Lemon Meringue	⅕ of 8 in pie (4.8 oz)	300	0	65
Mince	⅙ of 8 in pie (4.3 oz)	300	2	0
Peach	⅙ of 8 in pie	260	1	0
Peach	⅛ of 9 in pie (4.6 oz)	310	1	0
Pecan	⅛ of 10 in pie (4.5 oz)	500	1	60
Pumpkin	⅑ of 10 in pie (5.1 oz)	250	1	50
Pumpkin	⅕ of 8 in pie (5.2 oz)	270	1	45
Red Raspberry	⅙ of 8 in pie (4.3 oz)	280	0	0
Strawberry Rhubarb	⅕ of 8 in pie (4.8 oz)	520	1	70
Strawberry Rhubarb	⅙ of 8 in pie (4.3 oz)	280	0	0
Pepperidge Farm				
Hyannis Boston Cream Pie	1	230	2	70
Mississippi Mud	1	310	—	60
Sara Lee				
Apple Homestyle	1 slice (4 oz)	280	—	0
Apple Homestyle High	1 slice (4.9 oz)	400	—	0
Apple Streusel Free & Light	1 slice (2.9 oz)	170	—	0
Blueberry Homestyle	1 slice (4 oz)	300	—	0
Cherry Homestyle	1 slice (4 oz)	270	—	0
Cherry Streusel Free & Light	1 slice (3.6 oz)	160	—	0

FOOD	PORTION	CALS.	FIB.	CHOL.
Sara Lee (CONT.)				
Dutch Apple Homestyle	1 slice (4 oz)	300	—	0
Mince Homestyle	1 slice (4 oz)	300	—	0
Peach Homestyle	1 slice (3.4 oz)	280	—	0
Pecan Homestyle	1 slice (3.4 oz)	400	—	55
Pumpkin Homestyle	1 slice (4 oz)	240	—	40
Raspberry Homestyle	1 slice (4 oz)	280	—	0
Weight Watchers				
Chocolate Mocha	1 (2.75 oz)	170	2	5
Mississippi Mud	1 (5.04 oz)	180	2	5
HOME RECIPE				
apple	⅛ of 9 in pie (5.4 oz)	411	3	0
banana cream	⅛ of 9 in pie (5.2 oz)	398	—	75
blueberry	⅛ of 9 in pie (5.2 oz)	360	—	0
butterscotch	⅛ of 9 in pie (4.5 oz)	355	—	78
cherry	⅛ of 9 in pie (6.3 oz)	486	—	0
coconut creme	⅛ of 9 in pie (4.7 oz)	396	—	77
custard	⅛ of 9 in pie (4.5 oz)	262	2	87
lemon meringue	⅛ of 9 in pie (4.5 oz)	362	2	68
mince	⅛ of 9 in pie (5.8 oz)	477	—	0
pecan	⅛ of 9 in pie (4.3 oz)	502	4	106
pumpkin	⅛ of 9 in pie (5.4 oz)	316	4	65
vanilla cream	⅛ of 9 in pie (4.4 oz)	350	—	78
MIX				
chocolate mousse no-bake	⅛ of 9 in pie (3.3 oz)	247	—	0
Jell-O				
Banana Cream as prep w/ whole milk	⅙ of 8 in pie	103	—	11
Chocolate Cream Pie No Bake Dessert	⅛ pie	260	—	29
Chocolate Mousse	⅛ pie	259	—	29

FOOD	PORTION	CALS.	FIB.	CHOL.
Jell-O (CONT.)				
Coconut Cream	⅛ pie	258	—	29
Coconut Cream as prep w/ whole milk	⅙ of 8 in pie	111	—	11
Lemon	⅙ of 8 in pie	175	—	92
Pumpkin	⅛ pie	253	—	31
Royal				
Key Lime Pie Filling	mix for 1 serv	50	—	0
Lemon Pie Filling	mix for 1 serv	50	0	0
SNACK				
apple	1 (3 oz)	266	—	13
cherry	1 (3 oz)	266	—	13
lemon	1 (3 oz)	266	—	13
Drake's				
Apple	1 (2 oz)	210	—	0
Blueberry	1 (2 oz)	210	—	0
Cherry	1 (2 oz)	220	—	0
Lemon	1 (2 oz)	210	—	0
Lance				
Pecan	1 (38 g)	350	—	40
Little Debbie				
Marshmallow Banana	1 pkg (1.4 oz)	160	0	0
Marshmallow Banana	1 pkg (2 oz)	240	0	0
Marshmallow Banana	1 pkg (2.7 oz)	320	0	0
Marshmallow Chocolate	1 pkg (1.4 oz)	160	1	0
Marshmallow Chocolate	1 pkg (2.7 oz)	320	1	0
Marshmallow Chocolate	1 pkg (2 oz)	240	1	0
Oatmeal Creme	1 pkg (1.3 oz)	170	1	0
Oatmeal Creme	1 pkg (2.5 oz)	300	1	0
Oatmeal Creme	1 pkg (3 oz)	360	2	0
Raisin Creme	1 pkg (1.2 oz)	140	1	0
Raisin Creme	1 pkg (2.5 oz)	290	0	0
Tastykake				
Apple	1 pkg (113 g)	300	2	0
Banana Creme	1 pkg (120 g)	380	2	25
Blueberry	1 pkg (113 g)	310	2	0
Cherry	1 pkg (113 g)	300	2	0
Coconut Creme	1 pkg (113 g)	380	2	65
French Apple	1 pkg (120 g)	350	2	0
Lemon	1 pkg (113 g)	320	2	40
Lemon Lime	1 pkg (113 g)	320	1	45
Peach	1 pkg (113 g)	300	—	0
Pineapple Cheese	1 pkg (120 g)	340	2	20
Pumpkin	1 pkg (4 oz)	320	2	30

FOOD	PORTION	CALS.	FIB.	CHOL.
Tastykake (CONT.)				
Strawberry	1 pkg (113 g)	340	1	0
Tasty Klair	1 pkg (113 g)	400	2	55
TAKE-OUT				
coconut custard	⅙ of 8 in pie (3.6 oz)	271	—	36
custard	⅙ of 9 in pie	330	—	169
pecan	⅙ of 8 in pie (4 oz)	452	4	36
pumpkin	⅙ of 8 in pie (3.8 oz)	229	3	22

PIE CRUST

(*see also* PIE)

FOOD	PORTION	CALS.	FIB.	CHOL.
FROZEN				
puff pastry baked	1 shell (1.4 oz)	223	—	0
Pet-Ritz				
Deep Dish	⅙ pie (1 oz)	130	—	7
Graham Cracker	⅙ pie (0.83 oz)	110	—	7
Regular	⅙ pie (0.83 oz)	110	—	7
Tart Shells	1	150	—	7
HOME RECIPE				
9-inch crust	1	900	—	0
baked	⅛ of 9 in crust (0.8 oz)	119	—	0
baked	9 in shell (6.3 oz)	949	—	0
MIX				
as prep	9 in crust (5.6 oz)	801	—	0
as prep	⅛ of 9 in pie (0.7 oz)	100	—	0
Betty Crocker				
Pie Crust	1/16 pkg	120	—	0
Sticks	1/16 pkg	120	—	0
Flako				
Mix	¼ cup (0.9 oz)	130	1	5
Jiffy				
as prep	1/7 crust	180	tr	5
READY-TO-EAT				
chocolate cookie crumb baked	9 in crust (7.7 oz)	1130	—	3
chocolate cookie crumb baked	⅛ of 9 in pie (1 oz)	139	—	0
chocolate cookie crumb chilled	⅛ of 9 in pie (1 oz)	142	—	0
chocolate cookie crumb chilled	9 in crust (7.8 oz)	1127	—	3
graham cracker baked	9 in crust (8.4 oz)	1181	—	0
graham cracker baked	⅛ of 9 in pie (1 oz)	148	—	0
graham cracker chilled	⅛ of 9 in pie (1 oz)	150	—	0

FOOD	PORTION	CALS.	FIB.	CHOL.
graham cracker chilled	9 in crust (8.6 oz)	1182	—	0
vanilla wafer cracker crumbs baked	⅛ of 9 in pie (0.8 oz)	119	—	9
vanilla wafer cracker crumbs baked	9 in crust (6.1 oz)	937	—	69
vanilla wafer cracker crumbs chilled	⅛ of 9 in pie (0.8 oz)	117	—	9
vanilla wafer cracker crumbs chilled	9 in crust (6.2 oz)	934	—	69
Generic Label				
Graham	⅛ pie (0.7 oz)	110	1	0
Honey Maid				
Graham	⅙ crust (1 oz)	140	tr	0
Nabisco				
Nilla	⅙ crust (1 oz)	140	0	<5
Oreo				
Crumb Crust	⅙ crust (1 oz)	140	tr	0
Ready Crust				
Chocolate	⅛ of 9 in pie	100	—	0
Chocolate	1 (3 in diam)	110	—	0
Graham	1 (3 in diam)	110	—	0
Graham	⅛ of 9 in pie	100	—	0
REFRIGERATED				
Pillsbury				
All Ready	⅛ of 2 crust pie	240	—	15

PIEROGI
FROZEN

FOOD	PORTION	CALS.	FIB.	CHOL.
Empire				
Potato Cheese	3 (4.6 oz)	260	5	5
Potato Onion	3 (4.6 oz)	250	4	0
Golden				
Potato Cheese	3 (4 oz)	250	—	35
Mrs. T's				
Potato And Cheddar Cheese	1 (1.3 oz)	60	—	<2
Potato And Onion	1 (1.3 oz)	50	—	<2
Sauerkraut	1	60	—	2
TAKE-OUT				
pierogi	¾ cup (4.4 oz)	307	—	49

PIG'S EARS AND FEET

FOOD	PORTION	CALS.	FIB.	CHOL.
ears frzn simmered	1 ear (3.7 oz)	183	—	99
feet pickled	1 lb	923	—	419
feet pickled	1 oz	58	—	26
feet simmered	2.5 oz	138	—	71

FOOD	PORTION	CALS.	FIB.	CHOL.
Hormel				
Pickled Feet	2 oz	80	0	45
Pickled Hocks	2 oz	110	0	45
PIGEON				
w/ skin & bone	3.5 oz	169	—	110
PIGEON PEAS				
dried cooked	½ cup	102	—	0
dried cooked	1 cup	204	—	0
PIGNOLIA				
(*see* PINE NUTS)				
PIKE				
northern cooked	½ fillet (5.4 oz)	176	—	78
northern cooked	3 oz	96	—	43
northern raw	3 oz	75	—	33
roe raw	3½ oz	130	—	360
walleye baked	3 oz	101	—	94
walleye fillet baked	4.4 oz	147	—	137
PILLNUTS				
canarytree dried	1 oz	204	—	0
PIMIENTOS				
canned	1 slice	0	—	0
canned	1 tbsp	3	—	0
Dromedary				
Pimientos	1 oz	10	—	0
PINE NUTS				
pignolia dried	1 tbsp	51	—	0
pignolia dried	1 oz	146	—	0
pinyon dried	1 oz	161	—	0
Progresso				
Pignoli	1 jar (1 oz)	170	0	0
PINEAPPLE				
CANNED				
chunks in heavy syrup	1 cup	199	—	0
chunks juice pack	1 cup	150	—	0
crushed in heavy syrup	1 cup	199	—	0
slices in heavy syrup	1 slice	45	—	0
slices in light syrup	1 slice	30	—	0
slices juice pack	1 slice	35	—	0
slices water pack	1 slice	19	—	0
tidbits in heavy syrup	1 cup	199	—	0

FOOD	PORTION	CALS.	FIB.	CHOL.
tidbits in juice	1 cup	150	—	0
tidbits in water	1 cup	79	—	0
Del Monte				
Chunks In Heavy Syrup	½ cup (4.3 oz)	90	1	0
Chunks In Its Own Juice	½ cup (4.4 oz)	70	1	0
Crushed In Heavy Syrup	½ cup (4.4 oz)	90	1	0
Crushed In Its Own Juice	½ cup (4.3 oz)	70	1	0
Sliced In Heavy Syrup	½ cup (4.1 oz)	90	1	0
Sliced In Its Own Juice	½ cup (4 oz)	60	1	0
Snack Cups Tidbits In Juice	1 serv (4.5 oz)	70	1	0
Snack Cups Tidbits In Juice EZ-Open Lid	1 serv (4.2 oz)	60	1	0
Spears In Its Own Juice	½ cup (4.3 oz)	70	1	0
Tidbits In Its Own Juice	½ cup (4.3 oz)	70	1	0
Wedges In Its Own Juice	½ cup (4.3 oz)	70	1	0
Dole				
All Cuts Juice Pack	½ cup	70	—	0
All Cuts Syrup Pack	½ cup	90	—	0
Empress				
Chunk	4 oz	70	—	0
Crushed	4 oz	70	—	0
Sliced	4 oz	70	—	0
Libby				
Crushed	1 cup with juice	140	—	0
Sliced In Unsweetened Juice	1 cup with juice	140	—	0
S&W				
Hawaiian Slice In Heavy Syrup	½ cup	90	—	0
Hawaiian Slice Juice Pack	½ cup	70	—	0
Sliced Unsweetened	½ cup	60	—	0
DRIED				
Sonoma				
Pieces	2 pieces (1.4 oz)	140	2	0
FRESH				
diced	1 cup	77	2	0
slice	1 slice	42	1	0
Chiquita				
Fresh	1 cup	90	—	0
Dole				
Pineapple	2 slices	90	2	0
FROZEN				
chunks sweetened	½ cup	104	—	0

PINEAPPLE JUICE

FOOD	PORTION	CALS.	FIB.	CHOL.
canned	1 cup	139	—	0

FOOD	PORTION	CALS.	FIB.	CHOL.
frzn as prep	1 cup	129	—	0
frzn not prep	6 oz	387	—	0
After The Fall				
Mandarin Pineapple	1 can (12 oz)	150	0	0
Bright & Early				
Frozen	8 fl oz	120	—	0
Del Monte				
Juice	8 fl oz	110	0	0
Juice	6 fl oz	80	0	0
Juice	1 serv (11.5 oz)	190	1	0
Dole				
100% frzn as prep	8 fl oz	130	0	0
Chilled	6 fl oz	90	—	0
Minute Maid				
Box	8.45 fl oz	130	—	0
Frozen	8 fl oz	110	—	0
S&W				
Unsweetened	6 oz	100	—	0
Tree Top				
Juice	6 oz	100	—	0
Veryfine				
100%	8 oz	125	—	0

PINK BEANS
CANNED
Goya

Spanish Style	7.5 oz	140	10	0

DRIED

cooked	1 cup	252	—	0

PINTO BEANS
CANNED

pinto	1 cup	186	—	0
Allen				
Pinto Beans	½ cup (4.5 oz)	110	7	0
Brown Beauty				
Pinto Beans	½ cup (4.5 oz)	110	7	0
East Texas Fair				
Pinto Beans	½ cup (4.5 oz)	110	7	0
Eden				
Organic	½ cup (4.4 oz)	90	6	0
Gebhardt				
Pinto Beans	4 oz	100	5	0
Goya				
Spanish Style	7.5 oz	140	10	0

FOOD	PORTION	CALS.	FIB.	CHOL.
Green Giant				
Picante	½ cup	100	6	0
Pinto Beans	½ cup	90	5	0
Old El Paso				
Pinto Beans	½ cup (4.6 oz)	110	7	0
Progresso				
Pinto Beans	½ cup (4.6 oz)	110	7	0
Trappey				
Jalapinto With Bacon	½ cup (4.5 oz)	120	8	0
With Bacon	½ cup (4.5 oz)	120	7	0
DRIED				
cooked	1 cup	235	—	0
Arrowhead				
Dried	¼ cup (1.5 oz)	150	8	0
Bean Cuisine				
Dried	½ cup	115	5	0
Hurst				
Pinto Beans	1.2 oz	120	10	0
With Spanish Seasoning	1.3 oz	120	6	0
FROZEN				
cooked	3 oz	152	—	0
SPROUTS				
cooked	3½ oz	22	—	0
raw	3½ oz	62	—	0

PINYON
(*see* PINE NUTS)

PISTACHIOS
dried	1 oz	164	3	0
dried	1 cup	739	14	0
dry roasted	1 oz	172	—	0
dry roasted salted	1 oz	172	—	0
dry roasted salted	1 cup	776	—	0
Dole				
Shelled	1 oz	163	—	0
Shells On	1 oz	90	—	0
Fisher				
Red Tint	1 oz	170	—	0
Lance				
Pistachios	1 pkg (32 g)	100	—	0
Planters				
Munch'N Go Singles Shelled Dry Roasted	1 pkg (2 oz)	330	6	0
Red Salted Dry Roasted	1 pkg	160	3	0

FOOD	PORTION	CALS.	FIB.	CHOL.
Planters (CONT.)				
Uncolored Dry Roasted	½ cup	160	3	0
Sonoma				
Salted Shelled	¼ cup (1 oz)	190	3	0
PITANGA				
fresh	1 cup	57	—	0
fresh	1	2	—	0
PIZZA				
DOUGH				
Boboli				
Shell + Sauce	⅛ lg shell (2.6 oz)	170	1	5
Shell + Sauce	⅙ sm shell (2.6 oz)	170	1	5
House of Pasta				
Frozen	⅛ of 14 in pie (1.9 oz)	140	1	0
Jiffy				
as prep	¼ crust	180	2	0
Sassafras				
Cornmeal Pizza Crust	1 slice (1.4 oz)	140	1	0
Italian Pizza Crust Mix	1 slice (1.4 oz)	140	1	0
Wanda's				
Crust Mix Oregano & Basil	⅒ pie (1.4 oz)	149	1	0
Crust Mix Oregano & Basil Whole Wheat	⅒ pie (1.4 oz)	141	5	0
Watkins				
Crust Mix	⅛ pkg (1.8 oz)	180	2	0
FROZEN				
Celeste				
Italian Bread Deluxe	1 (5.1 oz)	290	3	15
Italian Bread Garlic & Herb Zesty Chicken	1 (5 oz)	260	3	20
Italian Bread Pepperoni	1 (5 oz)	320	3	20
Italian Bread Zesty Four Cheese	1 (4.6 oz)	300	3	25
Large Cheese	¼ pie (4.4 oz)	320	3	25
Large Deluxe	¼ pie (5.5 oz)	350	4	20
Large Pepperoni	¼ pie (4.7 oz)	350	3	20
Large Suprema With Meat	⅕ pie (4.6 oz)	290	3	15
Large Zesty Four Cheese	¼ pie (4.4 oz)	330	3	30
Small Cheese	1 (7.5 oz)	540	4	45
Small Deluxe	1 (8.2 oz)	540	6	25
Small Hot & Zesty Four Cheese	1 (7 oz)	530	4	50
Small Original Four Cheese	1 (7 oz)	540	4	50
Small Pepperoni	1 (6.7 oz)	520	4	25

FOOD	PORTION	CALS.	FIB.	CHOL.
Celeste (CONT.)				
Small Sausage	1 (7.5 oz)	530	5	25
Small Suprema Vegetable	1 (7.5 oz)	480	5	5
Small Suprema With Meat	1 (9 oz)	580	7	30
Small Zesty Four Cheese	1 (7 oz)	530	4	50
Croissant Pocket				
Stuffed Sandwich Pepperoni Pizza	1 piece (4.5 oz)	350	3	30
Empire				
3 Pack	1 (3 oz)	210	7	20
Bagel	1 (2 oz)	150	0	15
English Muffin	1 (2 oz)	130	1	15
Pizza	½ pie (5 oz)	340	2	30
Healthy Choice				
French Bread Cheese	1 (5.6 oz)	310	6	10
French Bread Pepperoni	1 (6 oz)	360	5	25
French Bread Sausage	1 (6 oz)	330	6	20
French Bread Supreme	1 (6.35 oz)	340	5	25
Hot Pocket				
Stuffed Sandwich Pepperoni & Sausage Pizza	1 (4.5 oz)	340	3	30
Stuffed Sandwich Pepperoni Pizza	1 (4.5 oz)	350	2	30
Kid Cuisine				
Cheese	1 (8 oz)	430	5	20
Hamburger	1 (8.3 oz)	400	6	25
Kineret				
Bagel Pizza	2 (4 oz)	300	1	30
Slice	1 (4.9 oz)	490	2	20
Lean Cuisine				
French Bread Cheese	1 pkg (6 oz)	350	4	20
French Bread Deluxe	1 pkg (6.1 oz)	350	5	30
French Bread Pepperoni	1 pkg (5.25 oz)	330	4	25
Lean Pockets				
Stuffed Sandwich Pizza Deluxe	1 (4.5 oz)	270	2	25
MicroMagic				
Deep Dish Combination	1 (6.5 oz)	605	—	28
Deep Dish Pepperoni	1 (6.5 oz)	615	—	42
Deep Dish Sausage	1 (6.5 oz)	590	—	18
Old El Paso				
Pizza Burrito Pepperoni	1 (3.5 oz)	260	0	20
Pizza Burrito Sausage	1 (3.5 oz)	260	0	15
Small World				
Four Cheese	1 (4 oz)	240	1	13

FOOD	PORTION	CALS.	FIB.	CHOL.
Special Delivery				
Organic	1/3 pizza (5.3 oz)	320	1	20
Organic Soy Kaas	1/3 pizza (5.3 oz)	320	1	0
Stouffer's				
French Bread Bacon Cheddar	1 piece (5.8 oz)	440	4	30
French Bread Cheese	1 piece (5.2 oz)	350	3	15
French Bread Cheeseburger	1 piece (6 oz)	440	5	55
French Bread Deluxe	1 piece (6.2 oz)	440	5	35
French Bread Double Cheese	1 piece (5.9 oz)	420	3	30
French Bread Garden Vegetable	1 piece (5.8 oz)	340	4	15
French Bread Pepperoni	1 piece (5.6 oz)	420	3	35
French Bread Pepperoni & Mushroom	1 piece (6.1 oz)	430	3	30
French Bread Sausage	1 piece (6 oz)	420	4	35
French Bread Sausage & Pepperoni	1 piece (6.25 oz)	460	4	40
French Bread Vegetable Deluxe	1 piece (6.4 oz)	380	5	25
French Bread White Pizza	1 piece (5.1 oz)	460	5	25
Lunch Express Deluxe	1 pkg (6.6 oz)	460	4	45
Lunch Express Double Cheese	1 pkg (5.9 oz)	420	3	35
Lunch Express Pepperoni	1 pkg (5.75 oz)	440	4	40
Lunch Express Sausage	1 pkg (6.5 oz)	460	3	40
Lunch Express Sausage & Pepperoni	1 pkg (6.4 oz)	500	4	60
Tombstone				
12 in Canadian Bacon	1/5 pie (5.5 oz)	360	2	40
12 in Cheese & Hamburger	1/5 pie (4.4 oz)	320	2	30
12 in Cheese & Pepperoni	1/5 pie (4.4 oz)	340	2	35
12 in Cheese & Sausage	1/5 pie (4.4 oz)	320	2	30
12 in Cheese Sausage & Mushroom	1/5 pie (4.5 oz)	320	2	30
12 in Deluxe	1/5 pie (4.7 oz)	320	2	30
12 in Extra Cheese	1/5 pie (5.1 oz)	370	2	30
12 in Sausage & Pepperoni	1/5 pie (4.4 oz)	340	2	35
12 in Special Order Four Cheese	1/5 pie (5.2 oz)	400	2	40
12 in Special Order Four Meat	1/6 pie (4.7 oz)	350	2	40
12 in Special Order Pepperoni	1/6 pie (4.5 oz)	360	2	40
12 in Special Order Super Supreme	1/6 pie (4.8 oz)	350	2	40
12 in Special Order Three Sausage	1/6 pie (4.6 oz)	340	2	35
12 in Supreme	1/5 pie (4.6 oz)	330	2	35
12 in ThinCrust Italian Style Three Cheese	1/4 pie (4.8 oz)	380	2	45

FOOD	PORTION	CALS.	FIB.	CHOL.
Tombstone (CONT.)				
9 in Cheese & Hamburger	⅓ pie (4.1 oz)	310	2	30
9 in Cheese & Pepperoni	⅓ pie (4.1 oz)	340	2	30
9 in Cheese & Sausage	⅓ pie (4.1 oz)	310	2	30
9 in Deluxe	⅓ pie (4.5 oz)	320	2	30
9 in Extra Cheese	⅓ pie (5.6 oz)	420	3	30
9 in Pepperoni & Sausage	⅓ pie (4.4 oz)	360	2	35
9 in Special Order Four Meat	⅓ pie (5.3 oz)	400	2	45
9 in Special Order Pepperoni	⅓ pie (5.1 oz)	400	2	45
9 in Special Order Super Supreme	⅓ pie (5.5 oz)	400	2	45
9 in Special Order Three Sausage	⅓ pie (5.2 oz)	390	2	40
Double Top Pepperoni With Double Cheese	⅙ pie (4.5 oz)	350	2	45
Double Top Sausage & Pepperoni With Double Cheese	⅙ pie (4.7 oz)	360	2	45
Double Top Sausage With Double Cheese	⅙ pie (4.7 oz)	350	2	40
For One ½ Less Fat Cheese	1 pie (6.5 oz)	360	3	15
For One ½ Less Fat Pepperoni	1 pie (6.7 oz)	400	4	35
For One ½ Less Fat Supreme	1 pie (7.7 oz)	400	4	35
For One ½ Less Fat Vegetable	1 pie (7.2 oz)	360	5	15
For One Cheese & Pepperoni	1 pie (7 oz)	580	3	50
For One Extra Cheese	1 pie (7 oz)	540	3	45
For One Italian Sausage	1 pie (7 oz)	560	2	55
For One Sausage & Pepperoni	1 pie (7 oz)	590	3	55
For One Supreme	1 pie (7.5 oz)	570	3	50
Light Supreme	⅕ pie (4.8 oz)	270	3	20
Light Vegetable	⅕ pie (4.6 oz)	240	3	10
ThinCrust Italian Style Four Meat Combo	¼ pie (5.1 oz)	410	2	50
ThinCrust Italian Style Pepperoni	¼ pie (5 oz)	420	2	55
ThinCrust Italian Style Sausage	¼ pie (5.1 oz)	400	2	50
ThinCrust Italian Style Supreme	¼ pie (5.3 oz)	400	2	45
ThinCrust Mexican Style Supreme Taco	¼ pie (5.1 oz)	380	2	50
Weight Watchers				
Deluxe Combo	1 (6.57 oz)	380	6	40
Deluxe Pocket Pizza Sandwich	1 (5 oz)	300	4	15
Extra Cheese	1 (5.74 oz)	390	6	35
Pepperoni	1 (5.56 oz)	390	4	45

FOOD	PORTION	CALS.	FIB.	CHOL.
SAUCE				
Boboli				
Sauce	1 pkg (1.2 oz)	20	1	0
Sauce	¼ cup (2.5 oz)	40	1	0
Eden				
Pizza Pasta Sauce	½ cup (4.4 oz)	80	3	0
Muir Glen				
Organic	¼ cup (2.2 oz)	40	2	0
Progresso				
Pizza Sauce	¼ cup (2.2 oz)	35	1	0
Ragu				
Quick Traditional	3 tbsp (1.7 oz)	35	—	0
Tree Of Life				
Sauce	¼ cup (1.9 oz)	30	—	0
TAKE-OUT				
cheese	12 in pie	1121	—	74
cheese	⅛ of 12 in pie	140	—	9
cheese deep dish individual	1 (5.5 oz)	460	2	20
cheese meat & vegetables	12 in pie	1472	—	165
cheese meat & vegetables	⅛ of 12 in pie	184	—	21
pepperoni	⅛ of 12 in pie	181	—	14
pepperoni	12 in pie	1445	—	115
PLANTAINS				
fresh uncooked	1 (6.3 oz)	218	—	0
sliced cooked	½ cup	89	—	0
Chifles				
Plantain Chips	1 pkg (2 oz)	170	2	0
PLUMS				
CANNED				
purple in heavy syrup	3	119	—	0
purple in heavy syrup	1 cup	320	—	0
purple in light syrup	3	83	—	0
purple in light syrup	1 cup	158	—	0
purple juice pack	3	55	—	0
purple juice pack	1 cup	146	—	0
purple water pack	1 cup	102	—	0
purple water pack	3	39	—	0
S&W				
Halves Purple Fancy Unpeeled In Extra Heavy Syrup	½ cup	135	—	0
Whole Purple Fancy Unpeeled In Extra Heavy Syrup	½ cup	135	—	0
Whole Unpeeled Diet	½ cup	52	—	0

FOOD	PORTION	CALS.	FIB.	CHOL.
FRESH				
plum	1	36	—	0
sliced	1 cup	91	—	0
Dole				
Plums	2	70	1	0
POI				
poi	½ cup	134	—	0
POKEBERRY SHOOTS				
cooked	½ cup	16	—	0
raw	½ cup	18	—	0
Allen				
Pokeberry Shoots	½ cup (4.1 oz)	35	3	0
POLENTA				
(*see* CORNMEAL)				
POLLACK				
atlantic fillet baked	5.3 oz	178	—	137
atlantic baked	3 oz	100	—	77
POMEGRANATES				
pomegranate	1	104	—	0
POMPANO				
florida cooked	3 oz	179	—	54
florida raw	3 oz	140	—	43
POPCORN				
(*see also* CHIPS, POPCORN CAKES, PRETZELS, SNACKS)				
air-popped	1 cup (0.3 oz)	31	2	0
air-popped	1 oz	108	4	0
caramel coated w/ peanuts	⅔ cup (1 oz)	114	1	0
cheese	1 oz	149	3	3
cheese	1 cup (0.4 oz)	58	1	1
oil popped	1 oz	142	3	0
oil popped	1 cup (0.4 oz)	55	1	0
Barrel O' Fun				
Baked Curl	1 oz	150	0	0
Caramel Corn	1 oz	115	1	0
Corn Pop	1 oz	190	0	0
Popcorn	1 oz	160	1	0
White Cheddar Pops	1 oz	170	0	0
Cheetos				
Cheddar Cheese	0.5 oz	80	—	0
Chesters				
Cheddar Cheese	0.5 oz	80	—	0
Microwave	3 cups	110	—	0
Microwave Butter	3 cups	120	—	0

FOOD	PORTION	CALS.	FIB.	CHOL.
Chesters (CONT.)				
Microwave Cheese	3 cups	110	—	0
Popcorn	0.5 oz	70	—	0
Estee				
No Sugar Added Caramel	1 cup (1 oz)	120	1	0
Greenfield				
Caramel	1 cup (1 oz)	120	—	0
Jiffy Pop				
Bag Butter	3 cups	90	2	0
Bag Lite	3 cups	70	2	0
Bag Regular	3 cups	100	2	0
Glazed Popcorn Clusters	1 oz	120	1	5
Microwave Butter	4 cups	140	3	0
Microwave Regular	4 cups	140	3	0
Pan Butter	4 cups	130	2	0
Pan Regular	4 cups	130	2	0
Lance				
Cheese	1 pkg (25 g)	130	—	5
Plain	1 pkg (25 g)	140	—	0
White Cheddar Cheese	1 pkg (25 g)	140	—	5
Louise's				
Fat-Free Apple Cinnamon	1 oz	100	1	0
Fat-Free Buttery Toffee	1 oz	100	1	0
Fat-Free Caramel	1 oz	100	1	0
Newman's Own				
Oldstyle Picture Show	3⅓ cups	80	—	0
Oldstyle Picture Show Microwave Natural Butter	3 cups	150	4	0
Oldstyle Picture Show Microwave No Salt	3 cups	150	4	0
Oldstyle Picture Show Microwave Light Butter	3 cups	90	4	0
Oldstyle Picture Show Microwave Light Natural	3 cups	90	4	0
Orville Redenbacher's				
Gourmet Hot Air	3 cups	40	3	0
Gourmet Original	3 cups	80	3	0
Gourmet White	3 cups	80	3	0
Microwave Gourmet	3 cups	100	3	0
Microwave Gourmet Butter	3 cups	100	3	0
Microwave Gourmet Butter Toffee	2½ cups	210	2	tr
Microwave Gourmet Caramel	2½ cups	240	2	tr
Microwave Gourmet Cheddar Cheese	3 cups	130	3	2

FOOD	PORTION	CALS.	FIB.	CHOL.
Orville Redenbacher's (CONT.)				
Microwave Gourmet Frozen	3 cups	100	3	0
Microwave Gourmet Frozen Butter	3 cups	100	3	0
Microwave Gourmet Light	3 cups	70	3	0
Microwave Gourmet Light Butter	3 cups	70	3	0
Microwave Gourmet Salt Free	3 cups	100	3	0
Microwave Gourmet Salt Free Butter	3 cups	100	3	0
Microwave Gourmet Sour Cream 'n Onion	3 cups	160	3	0
Pop Secret				
Butter Flavor	3 cups	100	2	1
Butter Flavor Singles	6 cups	250	4	0
Light Butter Flavor	3 cups	70	2	0
Light Butter Flavor Singles	6 cups	140	4	0
Light Natural Flavor	3 cups	70	2	0
Light Natural Flavor Singles	6 cups	150	4	0
Natural Flavor	3 cups	100	2	0
Natural Flavor Salt Free	3 cups	100	2	0
Pop Chips	1½ cups (1 oz)	130	1	0
Pop Qwiz Butter Flavor	3 cups	100	2	0
Pop Qwiz Natural Flavor	3 cups	100	2	0
Smartfood				
Cheddar Cheese	0.5 oz	80	—	6
Light Butter	0.5 oz	70	—	8
Snyder's				
Butter	1 oz	140	3	0
Ultra Slim-Fast				
Lite N' Tasty	½ oz	60	2	0
Weight Watchers				
Butter	1 pkg (0.66 oz)	90	3	0
Butter Toffee	1 pkg (0.9 oz)	110	1	0
Caramel	1 pkg (0.9 oz)	100	1	0
Microwave	1 pkg (1 oz)	90	8	0
White Cheddar Cheese	1 pkg (0.66 oz)	90	2	0

POPCORN CAKES

FOOD	PORTION	CALS.	FIB.	CHOL.
popcorn cake	1 (0.3 oz)	38	—	u
General Mills				
Popcorn Bars Caramel	1 (0.6 oz)	70	0	u
Mother's				
Butter Flavor	1 (0.3 oz)	35	0	0

FOOD	PORTION	CALS.	FIB.	CHOL.
Mother's (CONT.)				
Unsalted	1 (0.3 oz)	35	0	0
Quaker				
Blueberry Crunch	1 (0.5 oz)	50	—	0
Butter Mini	6 (0.5 oz)	50	2	0
Butter Popped	1 (0.3 oz)	35	—	0
Caramel	1 (0.5 oz)	50	—	0
Caramel Mini	5 (0.5 oz)	50	1	0
Cheddar Cheese Mini	6 (0.5 oz)	50	1	0
Lightly Salted Mini	7 (0.5 oz)	50	2	0
Monterey Jack	1 (0.4 oz)	40	—	0
Strawberry Crunch	1 (0.5 oz)	50	—	0
White Cheddar	1 (0.4 oz)	40	—	0

POPOVER

home recipe as prep w/ 2% milk	1 (1.4 oz)	87	—	46
home recipe as prep w/ whole milk	1 (1.4 oz)	90	—	47

POPPY SEEDS

poppy seeds	1 tsp	15	—	0

PORK

(*see also* BACON, BACON SUBSTITUTES, CANADIAN BACON, DELI MEATS/ COLD CUTS, HAM, SAUSAGE)

CANNED				
Hormel				
Pickled Tidbits	2 oz	100	0	45
FRESH				
blade chop roasted	1 (3.1 oz)	321	—	79
center loin chop broiled	1 (3.1 oz)	275	—	84
center loin roasted	3 oz	259	—	78
center loin chop lean & fat braised	1 chop (2.6 oz)	266	—	81
center loin chop lean & fat broiled	1 chop (3.1 oz)	275	—	84
center loin chop lean & fat panfried	1 chop (3.1 oz)	333	—	92
center loin chop lean & fat roasted	1 chop (3.1 oz)	268	—	80
center loin chop lean only braised	1 chop (2.1 oz)	166	—	68
center loin chop lean only broiled	1 chop (2.5 oz)	166	—	71
center loin chop lean only panfried	1 chop (2.4 oz)	178	—	71
center loin chop lean only roasted	1 chop (2.4 oz)	180	—	68
center loin lean & fat braised	3 oz	301	—	91
center loin lean & fat panfried	3 oz	318	—	87
center loin lean only broiled	3 oz	196	—	83
center loin lean only panfried	3 oz	226	—	91

FOOD	PORTION	CALS.	FIB.	CHOL.
center loin lean only roasted	3 oz	204	—	78
chop loin bone-in lean & fat roasted	3 oz	199	—	68
chop rib bone-in lean & fat roasted	3 oz	217	—	62
ham fresh rump half lean & fat roasted	3 oz	233	—	81
ham fresh rump half lean only roasted	3 oz	187	—	81
ham fresh shank half lean & fat roasted	3 oz	258	—	78
ham fresh shank half lean only roasted	3 oz	183	—	78
ham fresh whole lean & fat roasted	3 oz	250	—	79
ham fresh whole lean only roasted	3 oz	187	—	80
leg loin & shoulder lean only roasted	3 oz	198	—	79
loin blade chop lean & fat braised	1 chop (3.1 oz)	321	—	79
loin blade chop lean & fat braised	1 chop (2.4 oz)	275	—	72
loin blade chop lean & fat panfried	1 chop (3.1 oz)	368	—	85
loin blade chop lean only braised	1 chop (1.8 oz)	156	—	57
loin blade chop lean only broiled	1 chop (2.1 oz)	177	—	59
loin blade chop lean only panfried	1 chop (2.2 oz)	175	—	60
loin blade chop lean only roasted	1 chop (2.5 oz)	198	—	63
loin blade lean & fat braised	3 oz	348	—	92
loin blade lean & fat broiled	3 oz	334	—	83
loin blade lean & fat panfried	3 oz	352	—	81
loin blade lean & fat roasted	3 oz	310	—	76
loin blade lean only broiled	3 oz	255	—	85
loin blade lean only panfried	3 oz	240	—	82
loin blade lean only roasted	3 oz	238	—	76
loin chop lean & fat braised	1 chop (2.5 oz)	261	—	73
loin chop lean & fat roasted	1 chop (2.9 oz)	262	—	74
loin chop lean & fat braised	1 chop (2.3 oz)	267	—	67
loin chop lean & fat broiled	1 chop (2.7 oz)	295	—	76
loin chop lean & fat panfried	1 chop (2.9 oz)	337	—	72
loin chop lean & fat roasted	1 chop (2.8 oz)	274	—	68
loin chop lean only braised	1 chop (1.8 oz)	147	—	51
loin chop lean only broiled	1 chop (2.1 oz)	165	—	60
loin chop lean only panfried	1 chop (2 oz)	157	—	49
loin chop lean only roasted	1 chop (2.3 oz)	167	—	54
loin lean & fat braised	3 oz	312	—	87
loin lean & fat broiled	3 oz	294	—	80

FOOD	PORTION	CALS.	FIB.	CHOL.
loin lean only braised	3 oz	232	—	90
loin lean only broiled	3 oz	218	—	81
loin lean only roasted	3 oz	204	—	77
loin w/ fat roasted	3 oz	271	—	77
lungs braised	3 oz	84	—	329
pancreas braised	3 oz	186	—	268
rib chop lean only braised	1 chop (1.8 oz)	147	—	51
rib chop lean only panfried	1 chop (2 oz)	160	—	60
rib chop lean only roasted	1 chop (2.2 oz)	162	—	52
rib chop lean & fat braised	1 chop (2.2 oz)	246	—	64
rib chop lean & fat broiled	1 chop (2.6 oz)	264	—	72
rib chop lean & fat roasted	1 chop (2.6 oz)	252	—	64
shoulder arm picnic cured lean & fat roasted	3 oz	238	—	49
shoulder arm picnic cured lean only roasted	3 oz	145	—	41
shoulder arm picnic lean only braised	3 oz	211	—	97
shoulder arm picnic lean only roasted	3 oz	194	—	81
shoulder arm picnic lean & fat braised	3 oz	293	—	93
shoulder arm picnic lean & fat roasted	3 oz	281	—	80
shoulder blade boston steak lean & fat braised	1 steak (5.6 oz)	594	—	178
shoulder blade boston steak lean & fat broiled	1 steak (6.5 oz)	647	—	190
shoulder blade boston steak lean & fat roasted	1 steak (6.5 oz)	594	—	179
shoulder blade boston steak lean only braised	1 steak (4.6 oz)	382	—	151
shoulder blade boston steak lean only broiled	1 steak (5.3 oz)	413	—	159
shoulder blade boston steak lean only roasted	1 steak (5.5 oz)	404	—	155
shoulder blade roll cured lean & fat	3 oz	304	—	60
shoulder boston blade lean & fat braised	3 oz	316	—	95
shoulder boston blade lean & fat broiled	3 oz	297	—	87
shoulder boston blade lean & fat roasted	3 oz	273	—	82

FOOD	PORTION	CALS.	FIB.	CHOL.
shoulder boston blade lean only braised	3 oz	250	—	99
shoulder boston blade lean only broiled	3 oz	233	—	89
shoulder boston blade lean only roasted	3 oz	218	—	83
shoulder whole lean only roasted	3 oz	207	—	82
shoulder whole roasted	3 oz	277	—	81
sirloin chop lean & fat braised	1 chop (2.4 oz)	250	—	75
sirloin chop lean & fat broiled	1 chop (2.8 oz)	278	—	81
sirloin chop lean & fat roasted	1 chop (2.8 oz)	244	—	76
sirloin chop lean only braised	1 chop (1.9 oz)	149	—	63
sirloin chop lean only broiled	1 chop (2.3 oz)	165	—	67
sirloin chop lean only roasted	1 chop (2.5 oz)	175	—	67
spareribs braised	3 oz	338	—	103
spleen braised	3 oz	127	—	428
tail simmered	3 oz	336	—	110
tenderloin lean only roasted	3 oz	141	—	79
Oscar Mayer				
Sweet Morsel Smoked Boneless Pork Shoulder	3 oz	180	0	50

PORK DISHES
FROZEN
Jimmy Dean

BBQ Pork Rib Sandwich	1 (5.4 oz)	440	1	55

TAKE-OUT

pork roast	2 oz	70	—	40

POSOLE
(*see* HOMINY)

POT PIE
FROZEN
Award Brand

Beef	1 (7 oz)	350	3	20
Chicken	1 (7 oz)	350	3	30
Banquet				
Family Entree Chicken Pie	1 serv (8 oz)	450	6	35
Macaroni & Cheese	1 pkg (6.5 oz)	200	2	10
Vegetable & Cheese	1 (7 oz)	390	3	15
Vegetable Pie w/ Beef	1 (7 oz)	330	3	25
Vegetable Pie w/ Chicken	1 (7 oz)	350	3	40
Vegetable Pie w/ Turkey	1 (7 oz)	370	3	45
Empire				
Chicken	1 (8.1 oz)	440	11	30

FOOD	PORTION	CALS.	FIB.	CHOL.
Empire (CONT.)				
Turkey	1 (8.1 oz)	470	11	25
Great Value				
Beef	1 (7 oz)	390	3	35
Chicken	1 (7 oz)	380	2	35
Turkey	1 (7 oz)	400	3	35
Morton				
Beef	1 (7 oz)	310	2	15
Chicken	1 (7 oz)	320	3	25
Macaroni & Cheese	1 (6 oz)	160	3	10
Turkey	1 (7 oz)	300	2	25
Ozark Valley				
Chicken	1 (7 oz)	330	2	35
Macaroni & Cheese	1 (6.5 oz)	160	0	<5
Turkey	1 (7 oz)	280	2	30
Stouffer's				
Beef Pie	1 pkg (10 oz)	450	3	65
Chicken Pie	1 pkg (10 oz)	520	3	70
Chicken Pie	½ pkg (8 oz)	460	3	65
Turkey	1 cup (8 oz)	500	3	55
Turkey	1 pkg (10 oz)	530	3	65
TAKE-OUT				
beef	⅓ of 9 in pie (7.4 oz)	515	—	42
chicken	⅓ of 9 in pie (8.1 oz)	545	—	56

POTATO
(*see also* CHIPS, KNISH)

FOOD	PORTION	CALS.	FIB.	CHOL.
CANNED				
potatoes	½ cup	54	—	0
Allen				
Refried Potatoes	½ cup (4.5 oz)	150	11	0
Butterfield				
Diced	⅔ cup (5.7 oz)	100	3	0
Sliced	½ cup (5.7 oz)	100	4	0
Whole	2½ pieces (5.6 oz)	90	2	0
Del Monte				
New Sliced	⅔ cup (5.4 oz)	60	2	0
New Whole	⅔ cup (5.5 oz)	60	2	0
Hormel				
Au Gratin & Bacon	1 can (7.5 oz)	250	2	25
Scalloped & Ham	1 can (7.5 oz)	260	1	35
S&W				
New Potatoes Extra Small	½ cup	45	—	0

FOOD	PORTION	CALS.	FIB.	CHOL.
Seneca				
Potatoes	½ cup	80	2	0
Sunshine				
Whole	2½ pieces (5.6 oz)	90	2	0
FRESH				
baked skin only	1 skin (2 oz)	115	2	0
baked w/ skin	1 (6½ oz)	220	—	0
baked w/o skin	1 (5 oz)	145	2	0
baked w/o skin	½ cup	57	1	0
boiled	½ cup	68	1	0
microwaved	1 (7 oz)	212	—	0
microwaved w/o skin	½ cup	78	—	0
raw w/o skin	1 (3.9 oz)	88	—	0
Yukon Gold				
Fresh	1 (5.3 oz)	110	—	0
FROZEN				
french fries	10 strips	111	2	0
french fries thick cut	10 strips	109	—	0
potato puffs	½ cup	138	—	0
potato puffs as prep	1	16	—	0
Budget Gourmet				
Baked With Broccoli And Cheese	1 pkg (10.5 oz)	300	—	30
Cheddared Potatoes	1 pkg (5.5 oz)	260	—	35
Cheddared Potatoes With Broccoli	1 pkg (5 oz)	150	—	20
Three Cheese Potatoes	1 pkg (5.75 oz)	220	—	30
Empire				
Crinkle Cut French Fries	½ cup (3 oz)	90	7	0
Latkes Potato Pancakes	1 (2 oz)	80	8	0
Latkes Mini Potato Pancakes	2 (2 oz)	90	6	0
Golden				
Potato Pancakes	1 (1.33 oz)	71	—	4
Green Giant				
One Serve Au Gratin	1 pkg	200	—	20
One Serve Potatoes & Broccoli In Cheese Sauce	1 pkg	130	—	5
Healthy Choice				
Cheddar Broccoli Potatoes	1 meal (10.5 oz)	310	8	10
Garden Potato Casserole	1 meal (9.25 oz)	200	6	10
Kineret				
Crinkle Cut	18 pieces (3 oz)	120	2	0
Kugel	1 piece (2.5 oz)	150	1	30
Latkes	1 (1.5 oz)	90	2	0

FOOD	PORTION	CALS.	FIB.	CHOL.
Kineret (CONT.)				
Latkes Mini	10 (3 oz)	160	2	0
Lean Cuisine				
Deluxe Cheddar	1 pkg (10.4 oz)	270	3	30
MicroMagic				
French Fries Low Fat	1 pkg (3 oz)	130	3	0
Oh Boy!				
Stuffed With Cheddar Cheese	1 (6 oz)	130	4	0
Stuffed With Real Bacon	1 (6 oz)	120	4	5
Ore Ida				
Cheddar Browns	1 patty (3 oz)	90	1	<5
Cottage Fries	14 pieces (3 oz)	130	1	0
Crispers!	17 pieces (3 oz)	220	2	0
Crispers! Nacho	10 pieces (3 oz)	170	2	0
Crispers! Texas	3 oz	170	2	0
Crispy Crowns!	12 pieces (3 oz)	100	2	0
Crispy Crunchies	12 pieces (3 oz)	160	2	0
Deep Fries Crinkle Cuts	18 pieces (3 oz)	160	2	0
Deep Fries French Fries	22 pieces (3 oz)	160	2	0
Dinner Fries Country Style	8 pieces (3 oz)	110	1	0
Fast Fries	23 pieces (3 oz)	140	2	0
Fast Fries Ranch	22 pieces (3 oz)	150	1	0
Golden Crinkles	16 pieces (3 oz)	120	2	0
Golden Fries	16 pieces (3 oz)	120	1	0
Golden Patties	1 (2.5 oz)	140	1	0
Golden Twirls	28 pieces (3 oz)	160	2	0
Hash Browns Country Style	1 cup (2.6 oz)	60	1	0
Hash Browns Shredded	1 patty (3 oz)	70	1	0
Hash Browns Southern Style	¾ cup (3 oz)	70	2	0
Hot Tots	9 pieces (3 oz)	150	2	0
Mashed Natural Butter	½ cup (2.1 oz)	80	tr	<5
Microwave Crinkle Cuts	1 pkg (3.5 oz)	180	2	0
Microwave Hash Browns	1 patty (2 oz)	110	tr	0
Microwave Tater Tots	1 pkg (3.75 oz)	190	2	0
O'Brien Potatoes	¾ cup (3 oz)	60	2	0
Pixie Crinkles	33 pieces (3 oz)	140	3	0
Shoestrings	38 pieces (3 oz)	150	2	0
Snackin' Fries	1 pkg (5 oz)	180	3	0
Snackin' Fries Extra Zesty	1 pkg (5 oz)	180	4	0
Tater ABC's	10 pieces (3 oz)	190	2	0
Tater Tots	9 pieces (3 oz)	160	2	0
Tater Tots Bacon	9 pieces (3 oz)	150	1	0
Tater Tots Onion	9 pieces (3 oz)	150	2	0
Toaster Hash Browns	2 patties (3.5 oz)	190	1	0

FOOD	PORTION	CALS.	FIB.	CHOL.
Ore Ida (CONT.)				
Topped Broccoli & Cheese	½ (6 oz)	150	4	10
Topped Salsa & Cheese	½ (5.5 oz)	160	3	10
Topped Vegetable Primavera	1 (6.13 oz)	160	—	<5
Twice Baked Butter	1 (5 oz)	200	4	0
Twice Baked Cheddar Cheese	1 (5 oz)	190	3	0
Twice Baked Ranch	1 (5 oz)	180	3	0
Twice Baked Sour Cream & Chives	1 (5 oz)	180	3	0
Waffle Fries	15 pieces (3 oz)	140	2	0
Wedges With Skin	9 pieces (3 oz)	110	2	0
Zesties!	12 pieces (3 oz)	160	1	0
Stouffer's				
Au Gratin	½ cup (2.25 oz)	130	1	15
Baked Broccoli & Cheese	1 pkg (10.1 oz)	320	4	25
Baked Cheddar Cheese & Bacon	1 pkg (9.4 oz)	380	5	40
Lunch Express Baked Broccoli & Cheese	1 pkg (10.25 oz)	250	6	25
Scalloped	½ cup (2.25 oz)	130	2	5
Weight Watchers				
Baked Broccoli & Cheese	1 pkg (10 oz)	230	6	10
HOME RECIPE				
au gratin	½ cup	160	—	29
mashed	½ cup	111	—	2
scalloped	½ cup	105	—	14
MIX				
instant mashed flakes as prep w/ whole milk & butter	½ cup	118	—	15
instant mashed flakes not prep	½ cup	78	—	0
instant mashed granules as prep w/ whole milk & butter	½ cup	114	—	15
instant mashed granules not prep	½ cup	372	—	0
Country Store				
Mashed not prep	⅓ cup	70	—	0
Kraft				
Potatoes & Cheese Au Gratin	½ cup	130	—	40
Potatoes & Cheese Broccoli Au Gratin	½ cup	120	—	40
Potatoes & Cheese Scalloped	½ cup	140	—	25
Potatoes & Cheese Scalloped With Ham	½ cup	150	—	15
REFRIGERATED				
Simply Potatoes				
Au Gratin	¼ pkg (3 oz)	130	—	21

FOOD	PORTION	CALS.	FIB.	CHOL.
Simply Potatoes (CONT.)				
Hash Browns	⅓ pkg (4 oz)	100	—	0
Hash Browns Onion	⅓ pkg (4 oz)	120	—	0
Hash Browns Southwest Style	⅓ pkg (4 oz)	100	—	0
Mashed	⅓ pkg (4 oz)	90	—	0
Scalloped	¼ pkg (3 oz)	100	—	17
SHELF-STABLE				
Lunch Bucket				
Scalloped	1 pkg (7.5 oz)	160	—	35
Micro Cup Meals				
Scalloped Potatoes & Ham	1 cup (10.4 oz)	360	3	40
Scalloped Potatoes With Ham	1 cup (7.5 oz)	260	2	35
Pantry Express				
Augratin	½ cup	120	2	5
TAKE-OUT				
au gratin w/ cheese	½ cup	178	—	18
baked topped w/ cheese sauce	1	475	—	19
baked topped w/ cheese sauce & bacon	1	451	—	30
baked topped w/ cheese sauce & broccoli	1	402	—	20
baked topped w/ cheese sauce & chili	1	481	—	31
baked topped w/ sour cream & chives	1	394	—	23
french fried in beef tallow	1 lg	358	—	20
french fried in beef tallow	1 reg	237	—	13
french fried in vegetable oil	1 reg	235	—	0
french fried in vegetable oil	1 lg	355	—	0
indian yogurt potatoes	1 serv	315	0	18
mashed w/ whole milk & margarine	⅓ cup	66	—	2
mustard potato salad	3.5 oz	120	—	0
o'brien	1 cup	157	—	7
potato pancakes	1 (1.3 oz)	101	—	35
potato salad	½ cup	179	—	86
potato salad	⅓ cup	108	—	57
potato salad w/ vegetables	3.5 oz	120	—	0
scalloped	½ cup	127	—	7
POTATO STARCH				
potato starch	3½ oz	335	—	0
Manischewitz				
Potato Starch	1 cup	570	—	0

FOOD	PORTION	CALS.	FIB.	CHOL.

POUT
ocean baked	3 oz	86	—	57
ocean fillet baked	4.8 oz	139	—	91

PRESERVE
(*see* JAM/JELLY/PRESERVES)

PRETZELS
(*see also* CHIPS, POPCORN, SNACKS)

dutch twist	4 (2.1 oz)	229	2	0
pretzels	1 oz	108	1	0
rods	4 (2 oz)	229	2	0
sticks	10	10	—	tr
sticks	120 (2 oz)	229	2	0
twist	1 (½ oz)	65	—	tr
twists	10 (2.1 oz)	229	2	0
whole wheat	2 sm (1 oz)	103	—	0
whole wheat	2 med (2 oz)	205	—	0
Barrel O' Fun				
Mini	1 oz	110	1	0
Sticks	1 oz	110	1	0
Twists	1 oz	110	1	0
Estee				
Dutch Unsalted	2 (1.1 oz)	130	1	0
Nuggets Ranch Reduced Sodium	23 (1 oz)	130	tr	0
Nuggets Reduced Sodium	30 (1 oz)	120	1	0
Unsalted	23 (1 oz)	120	1	0
Formagg				
Pretzel Nuts	1 oz	120	tr	0
J&J				
Soft	1 (2.25 oz)	170	—	0
Soft Bites	5 bites	110	—	0
Lance				
Twist	1 pkg (42 g)	150	—	0
Manischewitz				
Bagel Pretzels Original	4 (1 oz)	110	1	0
Mister Salty				
Chips	16 (1 oz)	110	tr	0
Dutch	2 (1.1 oz)	120	1	0
Fat Free Chips	16 (1 oz)	100	1	0
Mini	22 (1 oz)	110	1	0
Sticks Fat Free	47 (1 oz)	110	1	0
Twist Fat Free	9 (1 oz)	110	1	0

FOOD	PORTION	CALS.	FIB.	CHOL.
Mr. Phipps				
Chips Lower Sodium	16 (1 oz)	120	tr	0
Chips Original	16 (1 oz)	120	tr	0
Chips Original Fat Free	16 (1 oz)	100	tr	0
Planters				
Twists	1 oz	100	1	0
Twists	1 pkg (1.5 oz)	160	1	0
Quinlan				
Beers	1 oz	110	1	0
Hard Sourdough	1 oz	110	1	0
Logs	1 oz	110	1	0
Nuggets	1 oz	110	1	0
Rods	1 oz	110	1	0
Sticks	1 oz	110	1	0
Thins	1 oz	110	1	0
Rold Gold				
Bavarian	3 pieces (1 oz)	120	—	0
Pretzel Chips	1 oz	110	—	0
Pretzel Chips Cheese	1 oz	120	—	0
Rods	3 pieces (1 oz)	110	—	0
Snack Mix	½ cup (1 oz)	140	—	0
Sour Dough	1½ pieces (1 oz)	110	—	0
Sticks	50 pieces (1 oz)	110	—	0
Thin Twist	10 pieces (1 oz)	110	—	0
Tiny Twist	15 pieces (1 oz)	110	—	0
Snyder's				
Logs	1 oz	310	—	0
Minis	1 oz	310	—	0
Minis Unsalted	1 oz	310	—	0
Nibblers	1 oz	310	—	0
Oat Bran	1 oz	120	—	0
Old Fashioned Hard	1 oz	111	—	0
Old Fashioned Hard Unsalted	1 oz	100	—	0
Old Tyme	1 oz	310	—	0
Old Tyme Unsalted	1 oz	110	—	0
Rods	1 oz	310	—	0
Sourdough Hard Buttermilk Ranch	1 oz	130	0	0
Sourdough Hard Cheddar Cheese	1 oz	160	0	0
Sourdough Hard Honey Mustard & Onion	1 oz	130	0	0
Stix	1 oz	310	—	0
Very Thins	1 oz	310	—	0

FOOD	PORTION	CALS.	FIB.	CHOL.
Sunshine				
California Pretzels	1 oz	110	1	0
Ultra Slim-Fast				
Lite N' Tasty	1 oz	100	4	0
Wege				
Sourdough	1 oz	102	—	0
Unsalted	1 oz	102	—	0
Whole Wheat	1 oz	109	—	0
Weight Watchers				
Oat Bran Nuggets	1 pkg (1.5 oz)	170	3	0

PRICKLYPEAR

fresh	1	42	—	0

PRUNE JUICE

canned	1 cup	181	3	0
Del Monte				
Juice	8 fl oz	170	1	0
S&W				
Unsweetened	6 oz	120	—	0

PRUNES
CANNED

in heavy syrup	5	90	—	0
in heavy syrup	1 cup	245	—	0
DRIED				
cooked w/ sugar	½ cup	147	7	0
cooked w/o sugar	½ cup	113	6	0
dried	10	201	6	0
dried	1 cup	385	12	0
Del Monte				
Pitted	¼ cup (1.4 oz)	120	3	0
Unpitted	⅓ cup (1.4 oz)	110	1	0
Mariani				
Pitted	¼ cup	140	—	0
Whole	¼ cup	140	—	0
Sonoma				
Pitted	¼ cup (1.4 oz)	120	3	0
Sunsweet				
Orange Essence Pitted Prunes	6 (1.4 oz)	100	3	0

PUDDING
(*see also* CUSTARD, PUDDING POPS)
HOME RECIPE

bread pudding	½ cup (4.4 oz)	212	—	83
bread pudding	1 recipe 6 serv (26.4 oz)	1266	—	434

FOOD	PORTION	CALS.	FIB.	CHOL.
chocolate as prep w/ whole milk	½ cup (5.5 oz)	221	—	17
corn	⅔ cup	181	—	122
rice	½ cup (5.3 oz)	217	—	17
MIX				
lemon	½ cup (5.1 oz)	163	—	77
Knorr				
Creme Caramel Flan & Sauce as prep	½ cup + 1 tbsp sauce	190	—	20
*My*T*Fine*				
Butterscotch	mix for 1 serv	90	—	0
Chocolate	mix for 1 serv	100	0	0
Chocolate Almond	mix for 1 serv	100	—	0
Chocolate Fudge	mix for 1 serv	100	1	0
Lemon	mix for 1 serv	90	—	0
Vanilla	mix for 1 serv	90	0	0
Vanilla Tapioca	mix for 1 serv	80	—	0
Royal				
Banana Cream	mix for 1 serv	80	0	0
Banana Cream Instant	mix for 1 serv	90	—	0
Butterscotch	mix for 1 serv	90	0	0
Butterscotch Instant	mix for 1 serv	90	—	0
Cherry Vanilla Instant	mix for 1 serv	90	0	0
Chocolate	mix for 1 serv	90	0	0
Chocolate Chocolate Chip Instant	mix for 1 serv	110	0	0
Chocolate Instant	mix for 1 serv	110	0	0
Chocolate Peanut Butter Instant	mix for 1 serv	110	0	0
Dark 'n Sweet Chocolate	mix for 1 serv	90	1	0
Dark 'n Sweet Instant	mix for 1 serv	110	0	0
Lemon Instant	mix for 1 serv	90	—	0
Pistachio Instant	mix for 1 serv	90	0	0
Strawberry Instant	mix for 1 serv	100	—	0
Vanilla	mix for 1 serv	80	0	0
Vanilla Chocolate Chip Instant	mix for 1 serv	90	0	0
Vanilla Instant	mix for 1 serv	90	—	0
MIX WITH 2% MILK				
banana	½ cup (4.9 oz)	142	—	9
banana instant	½ cup (5.2 oz)	152	—	9
chocolate	½ cup (5 oz)	150	—	9
chocolate instant	½ cup (5.2 oz)	149	—	9
coconut cream	½ cup (4.9 oz)	148	—	9
coconut cream instant	½ cup (5.2 oz)	157	—	0
lemon instant	½ cup (5.2 oz)	155	—	9
rice	½ cup (5.1 oz)	161	—	9

FOOD	PORTION	CALS.	FIB.	CHOL.
tapioca	½ cup (5 oz)	147	—	9
vanilla	½ cup (4.9 oz)	141	—	9
vanilla instant	½ cup (5 oz)	147	—	9
Jell-O				
Banana Instant Sugar Free	½ cup	84	—	9
Chocolate Instant Sugar Free	½ cup	92	—	9
Chocolate Sugar Free	½ cup	91	—	9
Pistachio Instant Sugar Free	½ cup	94	—	9
Vanilla Instant Sugar Free	½ cup	82	—	9
MIX WITH SKIM MILK				
D-Zerta				
Butterscotch	½ cup	68	—	2
Chocolate	½ cup	65	—	2
Vanilla	½ cup	69	—	2
Emes				
Dietetic	½ cup (4 fl oz)	71	—	0
MIX WITH WHOLE MILK				
banana	½ cup (4.9 oz)	157	—	17
banana instant	½ cup (5.2 oz)	167	—	17
chocolate	½ cup (5 oz)	158	—	17
chocolate instant	½ cup (5.2 oz)	164	—	17
coconut cream	½ cup (4.9 oz)	160	—	17
coconut cream instant	½ cup (5.2 oz)	172	—	17
lemon instant	½ cup (5.2 oz)	169	—	17
rice	½ cup (5.1 oz)	175	—	17
tapioca	½ cup (5 oz)	161	—	17
vanilla	½ cup (4.9 oz)	155	—	17
vanilla instant	½ cup (5 oz)	181	—	16
Jell-O				
Banana Cream Instant	½ cup	165	—	17
Butter Pecan Instant	½ cup	170	—	17
Butterscotch	½ cup	169	—	17
Butterscotch Instant	½ cup	164	—	17
Chocolate Fudge Instant	½ cup	175	—	17
Chocolate Instant	½ cup	176	—	17
Chocolate Tapioca Americana	½ cup	169	—	17
Coconut Cream Instant	½ cup	178	—	17
French Vanilla	½ cup	169	—	17
French Vanilla Instant	½ cup	165	—	17
Golden Egg Custard Americana	½ cup	167	—	85
Lemon Instant	½ cup	168	—	17
Milk Chocolate Instant	½ cup	179	—	17
Pineapple Cream Instant	½ cup	165	—	17
Pistachio Instant	½ cup	170	—	17

FOOD	PORTION	CALS.	FIB.	CHOL.
Jell-O (CONT.)				
Rice Americana	½ cup	175	—	17
Vanilla	½ cup	156	—	17
Vanilla Instant	½ cup	168	—	17
Vanilla Tapioca Americana	½ cup	160	—	17
READY-TO-EAT				
chocolate	1 pkg (5 oz)	189	—	5
lemon	1 pkg (5 oz)	177	—	0
vanilla	1 pkg (4 oz)	146	—	8
Del Monte				
Snack Cups Banana	1 serv (4 oz)	140	0	0
Snack Cups Butterscotch	1 serv (4 oz)	140	0	0
Snack Cups Chocolate	1 serv (4 oz)	160	0	0
Snack Cups Chocolate Fudge	1 serv (4 oz)	150	0	0
Snack Cups Chocolate Peanut Butter	1 serv (4 oz)	160	0	0
Snack Cups Lite Chocolate	1 serv (4 oz)	100	0	0
Snack Cups Lite Vanilla	1 serv (4 oz)	90	0	0
Snack Cups Tapioca	1 serv (4 oz)	140	0	0
Snack Cups Vanilla	1 serv (4 oz)	150	0	0
Hunt's				
Snack Pack Banana	1 (4 oz)	158	0	tr
Snack Pack Butterscotch	1 (4 oz)	153	0	1
Snack Pack Chocolate	1 (4 oz)	167	0	1
Snack Pack Chocolate Fudge	1 (4 oz)	167	0	1
Snack Pack Chocolate Marshmallow	1 (4 oz)	155	0	tr
Snack Pack Fat Free Chocolate	1 (4 oz)	96	0	tr
Snack Pack Fat Free Tapioca	1 (4 oz)	95	0	tr
Snack Pack Fat Free Vanilla	1 (4 oz)	93	0	1
Snack Pack Lemon	1 (4 oz)	162	0	0
Snack Pack Swirl Chocolate Caramel	1 (4 oz)	168	0	1
Snack Pack Swirl Chocolate Peanut Butter	1 (4 oz)	166	0	1
Snack Pack Swirl Milk Chocolate	1 (4 oz)	164	0	1
Snack Pack Swirl Smores	1 (4 oz)	154	0	1
Snack Pack Tapioca	1 (4 oz)	151	0	1
Snack Pack Vanilla	1 (4 oz)	163	0	1
Imagine Foods				
Lemon Dream	1 (4 oz)	120	—	0
Jell-O				
Chocolate	1 (4 oz)	171	—	1

FOOD	PORTION	CALS.	FIB.	CHOL.
Jell-O (CONT.)				
Chocolate Caramel Swirl	1 (4 oz)	175	—	2
Chocolate Fudge	1 (4 oz)	171	—	1
Chocolate Fudge Milk Chocolate Swirl	1 (4 oz)	171	—	2
Chocolate Vanilla Swirl	1 (4 oz)	175	—	2
Chocolate Vanilla Swirl	1 (5.5 oz)	240	—	2
Light Chocolate	1 (4 oz)	104	—	5
Light Chocolate Fudge	1 (4 oz)	101	—	3
Light Chocolate Vanilla	1 (4 oz)	104	—	5
Light Vanilla	1 (4 oz)	104	—	6
Milk Chocolate	1 (4 oz)	173	—	2
Tapioca	1 (5.5 oz)	229	—	2
Tapioca	1 (4 oz)	167	—	2
Vanilla	1 (4 oz)	182	—	2
Vanilla	1 (5.5 oz)	250	—	2
Vanilla Chocolate Swirl	1 (4 oz)	178	—	2
Kozy Shack				
Banana	1 pkg (4 oz)	130	1	10
Chocolate	1 pkg (4 oz)	140	1	5
Light Chocolate	1 pkg (4 oz)	110	1	5
Light Vanilla	1 pkg (4 oz)	110	0	10
Rice	1 pkg (4 oz)	130	1	17
Tapioca	1 pkg (4 oz)	140	0	5
Vanilla	1 pkg (4 oz)	130	1	10
Snack Pack				
Banana	4.25 oz	145	0	1
Butterscotch	4.25 oz	170	0	1
Chocolate	4.25 oz	170	0	1
Chocolate Marshmallow	4.25 oz	165	0	1
Chocolate Fudge	4.25 oz	165	0	1
Lemon	4.25 oz	150	tr	0
Light Chocolate	4.25 oz	100	0	1
Light Tapioca	4.25 oz	100	0	1
Tapioca	4.25 oz	150	0	1
Vanilla	4.25 oz	170	0	1
Swiss Miss				
Butterscotch	4 oz	180	0	5
Chocolate	4 oz	180	0	5
Chocolate Fudge	4 oz	220	0	5
Chocolate Sundae	4 oz	220	0	5
Light Chocolate	4 oz	100	0	0
Light Chocolate Fudge	4 oz	100	0	0
Light Vanilla	4 oz	100	0	0

FOOD	PORTION	CALS.	FIB.	CHOL.
Swiss Miss (CONT.)				
Light Vanilla Chocolate Parfait	4 oz	100	0	0
Tapioca	4 oz	160	0	5
Vanilla	4 oz	190	0	5
Vanilla Parfait	4 oz	180	0	1
Vanilla Sundae	4 oz	200	0	5
Ultra Slim-Fast				
Butterscotch	4 oz	100	2	0
Chocolate	4 oz	100	2	0
Vanilla	4 oz	100	2	0
TAKE-OUT				
bread pudding	½ cup (4.4 oz)	212	—	83
bread w/ raisins	½ cup	180	—	77
chocolate	½ cup (5.5 oz)	206	—	9
rice w/ raisins	½ cup	246	4	136
tapioca	½ cup (5.3 oz)	189	—	124
vanilla	½ cup (4.3 oz)	130	—	17

PUDDING POPS

(*see also* ICE CREAM AND FROZEN DESSERTS, PUDDING)

chocolate	1 (1.6 oz)	72	—	1
vanilla	1 (1.6 oz)	75	—	1
Jell-O				
Chocolate	1 pop	79	—	1
Chocolate Caramel Swirl	1 pop	74	—	1
Chocolate Fudge	1 pop	79	—	1
Chocolate Peanut Butter Swirl	1 bar	78	—	1
Chocolate Swirl	1 pop	80	—	1
Chocolate Vanilla Swirl	1 pop	78	—	1
Deluxe Chocolate Covered	1 pop	201	—	2
Deluxe Peanuts And Chocolate	1 bar	185	—	2
Milk Chocolate	1 pop	80	—	1
Vanilla	1 pop	77	—	1

PUMMELO

fresh	1	228	—	0
sections	1 cup	71	—	0

PUMPKIN
CANNED

pumpkin	½ cup	41	—	0
Libby				
Solid Pack	½ cup	60	4	0
Owatonna				
Pumpkin	½ cup	40	—	0

FOOD	PORTION	CALS.	FIB.	CHOL.
FRESH				
cooked mashed	½ cup	24	—	0
flowers cooked	½ cup	10	—	0
flowers raw	1	0	—	0
leaves cooked	½ cup	7	—	0
leaves raw	½ cup	4	—	0
raw cubed	½ cup	15	—	0
SEEDS				
dried	1 oz	154	—	0
roasted	1 cup	1184	—	0
roasted	1 oz	148	—	0
salted & roasted	1 oz	148	—	0
salted & roasted	1 cup	1184	—	0
whole roasted	1 oz	127	—	0
whole roasted	1 cup	285	—	0
whole salted roasted	1 cup	285	—	0
whole salted roasted	1 oz	127	—	0
PURSLANE				
cooked	1 cup	21	—	0
raw	1 cup	7	—	0
QUAHOGS				
(see CLAMS)				
QUICHE				
HOME RECIPE				
lorraine	⅛ of 8 in pie	600	—	285
QUINCE				
fresh	1	53	—	0
QUINOA				
quinoa	½ cup	318	—	0
Arrowhead				
Quinoa	¼ cup (1.4 oz)	140	4	0
Eden				
not prep	¼ cup (1.6 oz)	170	3	0
RABBIT				
domestic w/o bone roasted	3 oz	167	—	70
wild w/o bone stewed	3 oz	147	—	104
RADICCHIO				
raw shredded	½ cup	5	—	0
RADISHES				
DRIED				
chinese	½ cup	157	—	0

FOOD	PORTION	CALS.	FIB.	CHOL.
daikon	½ cup	157	—	0
FRESH				
chinese raw	1 (12 oz)	62	—	0
chinese raw sliced	½ cup	8	—	0
chinese sliced cooked	½ cup	13	—	0
daikon raw	1 (12 oz)	62	—	0
daikon raw sliced	½ cup	8	—	0
daikon sliced cooked	½ cup	13	—	0
red raw	10	7	—	0
red sliced	½ cup	10	—	0
white icicle raw	1 (½ oz)	2	—	0
white icicle raw sliced	½ cup	7	—	0
Dole				
Radishes	7	20	0	0
SPROUTS				
raw	½ cup	8	—	0
RAISINS				
chocolate coated	10 (0.4 oz)	39	—	0
chocolate coated	1 cup (6.7 oz)	741	—	5
golden seedless	1 cup	437	8	0
seedless	1 cup	434	8	0
seedless	1 tbsp	27	—	0
sultanas	1 oz	88	2	0
Cinderella				
Seedless	½ cup	250	—	0
Del Monte				
Golden	¼ cup (1.4 oz)	130	2	0
Raisins	1 box (1.5 oz)	140	3	0
Raisins	¼ cup (1.4 oz)	130	2	0
Raisins	1 box (1 oz)	90	2	0
Raisins	1 box (0.5 oz)	45	tr	0
Yogurt Raisins Strawberry	1 pkg (0.9 oz)	110	tr	0
Yogurt Raisins Vanilla	1 pkg (0.9 oz)	110	tr	0
Yogurt Raisins Vanilla	1 pkg (1 oz)	120	tr	0
Yogurt Raisins Vanilla	3 tbsp (1 oz)	130	1	0
Dole				
Golden	½ cup	250	—	0
Seedless	½ cup	250	—	0
Sonoma				
Monukka Thompson	¼ cup (1.4 oz)	130	2	0
Tree Of Life				
Organic	¼ cup (1.4 oz)	130	2	0
RASPBERRIES				
CANNED				
in heavy syrup	½ cup	117	—	0

FOOD	PORTION	CALS.	FIB.	CHOL.
FRESH				
raspberries	1 cup	61	—	0
raspberries	1 pint	154	—	0
Dole				
Raspberries	1 cup	45	9	0
FROZEN				
sweetened	1 cup	256	—	0
sweetened	1 pkg (10 oz)	291	—	0
Big Valley				
Raspberries	⅔ cup (4.9 oz)	80	3	0
Birds Eye				
Whole In Lite Syrup	½ cup	100	4	0
RASPBERRY JUICE				
Crystal Geyser				
Juice Squeeze Mountain Raspberry	1 bottle (12 fl oz)	135	—	0
Fresh Samantha				
Raspberry Dream	1 cup (8 oz)	120	2	0
Kool-Aid				
Raspberry	8 oz	98	—	0
Sugar Free	8 oz	2	—	0
Smucker's				
Juice	8 oz	120	—	0
RED BEANS				
CANNED				
Allen				
Red Beans	½ cup (4.5 oz)	160	9	0
Green Giant				
Red Beans	½ cup	90	5	0
Hunt's				
Small	½ cup (4.5 oz)	89	6	0
Van Camp's				
Red Beans	½ cup (4.6 oz)	90	5	0
DRIED				
Bean Cuisine				
Dried	½ cup	115	5	0
MIX				
Bean Cuisine				
Pasta & Beans Barcelona Red With Radiatore	½ cup	170	—	tr
Mahatma				
Red Beans & Rice	1 cup	190	7	0

FOOD	PORTION	CALS.	FIB.	CHOL.
RELISH				
cranberry orange	½ cup	246	—	0
hamburger	1 tbsp	19	—	0
hamburger	½ cup	158	—	0
hot dog	1 tbsp	14	—	0
hot dog	½ cup	111	—	0
sweet	1 tbsp	19	—	0
sweet	½ cup	159	—	0
Claussen				
Pickle Relish	1 tbsp	14	—	0
Del Monte				
Hamburger	1 tbsp (0.5 oz)	20	tr	0
Hot Dog	1 tbsp (0.5 oz)	15	tr	0
Sweet Pickle	1 tbsp (0.5 oz)	20	0	0
Hellmann's				
Sandwich Spread	1 tbsp (15 g)	55	—	5
Old El Paso				
Jalapeno	1 tbsp (0.5 oz)	5	0	0
Vlasic				
Dill	1 oz	2	—	0
Hamburger	1 oz	40	—	0
Hot Piccalilli	1 oz	35	—	0
India	1 oz	30	—	0
Sweet	1 oz	30	—	0
RHUBARB				
fresh	½ cup	13	—	0
frzn	½ cup	60	—	0
frzn as prep w/ sugar	½ cup	139	—	0
RICE				
(*see also* BRAN, CEREAL, FLOUR, RICE CAKES, WILD RICE)				
BROWN				
long-grain cooked	½ cup	109	2	0
medium-grain cooked	½ cup	109	—	0
Arrowhead				
Basmati	¼ cup (1.5 oz)	150	2	0
Quick Regular	⅓ cup (1.5 oz)	150	2	0
Quick Spanish Style	¼ pkg (1.4 oz)	150	2	0
Quick Vegetable Herb	¼ pkg (1.4 oz)	150	3	0
Quick Wild Rice & Herb	¼ pkg (1.3 oz)	140	3	0
Minute				
Precooked as prep	½ cup	121	1	0
Near East				
Pilaf as prep	1 cup	220	2	0

FOOD	PORTION	CALS.	FIB.	CHOL.
S&W				
Quick Natural Long Grain	3.5 oz	110	—	0
Quick Natural Long Grain cooked	3.5 oz	119	—	0
Uncle Ben				
Brown Rice	1 serv (1.6 oz)	158	1	0
CANNED				
Old El Paso				
Mexican	½ cup (4 oz)	410	3	0
Spanish	1 cup (8.6 oz)	130	2	0
Van Camp's				
Spanish	1 cup (9 oz)	180	3	0
FROZEN				
Birds Eye				
Rice & Broccoli Au Gratin	½ pkg	150	1	10
Budget Gourmet				
Oriental Rice With Vegetables	1 pkg (5.75 oz)	230	—	20
Rice Pilaf With Green Beans	1 pkg (5.5 oz)	230	—	10
Chun King				
Fried Rice	1 pkg (8 oz)	290	5	25
Fried Rice With Chicken	1 pkg (8 oz)	270	4	25
Green Giant				
Garden Gourmet Asparagus Pilaf	1 pkg	190	3	10
Garden Gourmet Sherry Wild Rice	1 pkg	210	3	10
One Serve Rice 'N Broccoli In Cheese Sauce	1 pkg	180	—	5
One Serve Rice Peas & Mushrooms With Sauce	1 pkg	130	—	5
Rice Originals Italian Rice Spinach In Cheese Sauce	½ cup	140	—	10
Rice Originals Pilaf	½ cup	110	—	2
Rice Originals Rice 'N Broccoli In Cheese Sauce	½ cup	120	—	5
Rice Originals Rice Medley	½ cup	100	—	5
Rice Originals White & Wild	½ cup	130	—	0
Luigino's				
Fried Rice Chicken	1 pkg (8 oz)	250	2	55
Fried Rice Pork	1 pkg (8 oz)	250	2	60
Fried Rice Pork & Shrimp	1 pkg (8 oz)	250	2	55
Fried Rice Shrimp	1 pkg (8 oz)	220	2	60
Risotto Parmesano	1 pkg (8 oz)	360	2	50
MIX				
Casbah				
Jambalaya	1 pkg (1.4 oz)	130	1	0

FOOD	PORTION	CALS.	FIB.	CHOL.
Casbah (CONT.)				
La Fiesta	1 pkg (1.59 oz)	170	0	0
Nutted Pilaf as prep	1 cup	220	1	0
Pilaf as prep	1 cup	200	tr	0
Spanish Pilaf as prep	1 cup	200	1	0
Thai Yum	1 pkg (1.7 oz)	180	1	0
Goodman's				
Rice & Vermicelli For Beef	¾ cup	160	0	5
Rice & Vermicelli For Chicken	¾ cup	160	1	0
Hain				
Rice Almondine	½ cup	130	—	0
Kikkoman				
Fried Rice Seasoning Mix	1 oz pkg	91	—	tr
Kitchen Del Sol				
Mediterranean Paella Costa Brava as prep	½ cup (1.2 oz)	130	1	0
Mediterranean Sunny Lemon Pilaf as prep	½ cup (1.2 oz)	110	1	0
Mediterranean Tomato & Basil With Pine Nuts	½ cup (1 oz)	110	1	0
La Choy				
Chinese Fried Rice	¾ cup	190	tr	0
Lipton				
Golden Saute Beef	½ cup (2.1 oz)	230	1	0
Golden Saute Chicken	½ cup (2.2 oz)	240	1	0
Golden Saute Chicken Broccoli	½ cup (2.3 oz)	260	2	0
Golden Saute Fried Rice	½ cup (2.1 oz)	240	1	0
Golden Saute Herb & Butter	½ cup (2.1 oz)	240	1	<5
Golden Saute Onion Mushroom	½ cup (2.1 oz)	240	2	0
Golden Saute Oriental	½ cup (2.1 oz)	240	1	0
Golden Saute Savory Herb	½ cup (2.1 oz)	240	1	0
Golden Saute Spanish	½ cup (2.3 oz)	250	2	0
Rice & Beans Cajun as prep	½ cup (2.5 oz)	260	7	0
Rice & Sauce Alfredo Broccoli as prep	½ cup (2.2 oz)	250	1	10
Rice & Sauce Beef Broccoli as prep	½ cup (2.1 oz)	230	2	0
Rice & Sauce Beef Flavor as prep	½ cup (2.2 oz)	230	2	0
Rice & Sauce Cajun as prep	½ cup (2.2 oz)	230	2	0
Rice & Sauce Cheddar Broccoli as prep	½ cup (2.2 oz)	250	1	<5
Rice & Sauce Chicken Broccoli as prep	½ cup (2.2 oz)	250	2	<5

FOOD	PORTION	CALS.	FIB.	CHOL.
Lipton (CONT.)				
Rice & Sauce Chicken Flavor as prep	½ cup (2.2 oz)	240	1	<5
Rice & Sauce Chicken Risotto	½ cup (2.1 oz)	230	1	5
Rice & Sauce Creamy Chicken as prep	½ cup (2.2 oz)	260	2	0
Rice & Sauce Herb & Butter as prep	½ cup (2.1 oz)	240	1	10
Rice & Sauce Long Grain Mushroom	½ cup (2.2 oz)	250	1	0
Rice & Sauce Medley as prep	½ cup (2.1 oz)	240	2	<5
Rice & Sauce Mushroom as prep	½ cup (2.1 oz)	220	1	0
Rice & Sauce Oriental as prep	½ cup (2.1 oz)	230	1	<5
Rice & Sauce Original Long Grain as prep	½ cup (2.2 oz)	250	2	0
Rice & Sauce Pilaf as prep	½ cup (2.1 oz)	230	1	0
Rice & Sauce Spanish as prep	½ cup (2.2 oz)	230	2	0
Mahatma				
Broccoli & Cheese	1 cup	200	2	5
Jambalaya	1 cup (2 oz)	190	tr	0
Long Grain & Wild	1 cup (2 oz)	190	2	0
Pilaf	1 cup (2 oz)	190	tr	0
Spanish	1 cup (2 oz)	180	2	0
Yellow Rice Mix	1 cup	190	tr	0
Minute				
Microwave Broccoli Almondin	½ cup	143	—	8
Microwave Cheddar Cheese Broccoli	½ cup	164	—	11
Microwave French Pilaf	½ cup	133	—	8
Microwave Long Grain Brown And Wild	½ cup	140	—	8
Microwave Rice With Savory Cheese Sauce as prep	½ cup	162	—	11
Rice Drumstick With Vermicelli as prep	½ cup	153	—	10
Rice Rib Roast With Vermicelli as prep	½ cup	151	—	10
Near East				
Barley Pilaf as prep	1 cup	220	5	0
Beef Pilaf as prep	1 cup	220	1	0
Curry Rice as prep	1 cup	220	1	0
Lentil Pilaf as prep	1 cup	210	0	0
Long Grain & Wild as prep	1 cup	220	2	0

FOOD	PORTION	CALS.	FIB.	CHOL.
Near East (CONT.)				
Pilaf Chicken as prep	1 cup	220	1	0
Pilaf Kosher as prep	1 cup	220	1	0
Spanish Pilaf as prep	1 cup	230	1	0
Pritikin				
Mexican	⅓ cup (2 oz)	200	—	0
Oriental	⅓ cup (2 oz)	190	—	0
Success				
Beef Oriental	½ cup	190	2	0
Broccoli & Cheese	½ cup	200	2	10
Brown & Wild	½ cup	190	3	0
Classic Chicken	½ cup	150	1	0
Long Grain & Wild	½ cup	190	1	0
Pilaf	½ cup	200	2	0
Spanish	½ cup	190	1	0
Uncle Ben				
Brown & Wild Fast Cooking	1 serv (1.3 oz)	120	1	tr
Country Inn Broccoli Almondine	1 serv (1.2 oz)	124	1	tr
Country Inn Broccoli & White Cheddar	1 serv (1.2 oz)	131	1	3
Country Inn Broccoli Au Gratin	1 serv (1.1 oz)	116	1	2
Country Inn Chicken Stock	1 serv (1.2 oz)	123	1	3
Country Inn Chicken With Wild Rice	1 serv (1.1 oz)	108	1	1
Country Inn Creamy Chicken & Mushroom	1 serv (1.3 oz)	138	1	2
Country Inn Creamy Chicken & Wild Rice	1 serv (1.3 oz)	135	1	4
Country Inn Green Bean Almondine	1 serv (1.2 oz)	128	1	2
Country Inn Herbed Au Gratin	1 serv (1.2 oz)	119	1	3
Country Inn Homestyle Chicken & Vegetables	1 serv (1.3 oz)	139	1	7
Country Inn Rice Florentine	1 serv (1.2 oz)	212	1	3
Country Inn Vegetable Pilaf	1 serv (1.2 oz)	115	1	1
Long Grain & Wild Chicken Stock Sauce	1 serv (1.3 oz)	133	1	5
Long Grain & Wild Fast Cooking	1 serv (1 oz)	101	1	1
Long Grain & Wild Garden Vegetable Blend	1 serv (1.3 oz)	128	1	1
Long Grain & Wild Original	1 serv (1 oz)	96	1	tr
Watkins				
Brown & Wild	¼ cup (1.6 oz)	160	3	0

FOOD	PORTION	CALS.	FIB.	CHOL.
Watkins (CONT.)				
Calico Medley	¼ cup (1.6 oz)	160	4	0
East/West Medley	¼ cup (1.6 oz)	160	5	0
Heartland Medley	¼ cup (1.6 oz)	160	4	0
Minnesota Medley	¼ cup (1.6 oz)	160	2	0
White & Wild	¼ cup (1.6 oz)	160	1	0
TAKE-OUT				
pilaf	½ cup	84	3	22
spanish	¾ cup	363	—	35
WHITE				
glutinous cooked	½ cup	116	—	0
long-grain cooked	½ cup	131	tr	0
long-grain instant cooked	½ cup	80	tr	0
long-grain parboiled cooked	½ cup	100	tr	0
medium-grain cooked	½ cup	132	—	0
short-grain cooked	½ cup	133	—	0
starch	3½ oz	343	—	0
Arrowhead				
Basmati	¼ cup (1.5 oz)	150	tr	0
Minute				
Boil In Bag Long Grain as prep	½ cup	94	—	0
Long Grain as prep	⅔ cup	150	1	8
Rice as prep	⅔ cup	141	1	5
Rice Long Grain & Wild as prep	½ cup	149	—	10
S&W				
Long Grain cooked	3.5 oz	106	—	0
Superfino				
Arborio Rice	½ cup	100	—	0
Uncle Ben				
Boil-In-Bag	1 serv (0.9 oz)	94	tr	0
Converted	1 serv (1.2 oz)	123	tr	0
In An Instant	1 serv (1.1 oz)	111	tr	0

RICE CAKES
(*see also* POPCORN CAKES)

FOOD	PORTION	CALS.	FIB.	CHOL.
brown rice	1 (0.3 oz)	35	tr	0
brown rice & buckwheat	1 (0.3 oz)	34	tr	0
brown rice & buckwheat unsalted	1 (0.3 oz)	34	tr	0
brown rice & corn	1 (0.3 oz)	35	—	0
brown rice & rye	1 (0.3 oz)	35	tr	0
brown rice & sesame seed	1 (0.3 oz)	35	—	0
brown rice multigrain	1 (0.3 oz)	35	—	0
brown rice multigrain unsalted	1 (0.3 oz)	35	—	0
brown rice unsalted	1 (0.3 oz)	35	tr	0

FOOD	PORTION	CALS.	FIB.	CHOL.
Hain				
Mini Apple Cinnamon	½ oz	60	0	0
Mini Barbeque	½ oz	70	0	0
Mini Cheese	½ oz	60	0	<5
Mini Honey Nut	½ oz	60	0	0
Mini Nacho Cheese	½ oz	70	—	<5
Mini Plain	½ oz	60	0	0
Mini Plain No Salt Added	½ oz	60	0	0
Mini Ranch	½ oz	70	—	0
Mini Teriyaki	½ oz	50	0	0
Ka-Me				
Cheese	16 pieces (1 oz)	120	0	0
Onion	16 pieces (1 oz)	120	0	0
Plain	16 pieces (1 oz)	120	0	0
Seaweed	16 pieces (1 oz)	120	0	0
Sesame	16 pieces (1 oz)	120	0	0
Unsalted	16 pieces (1 oz)	120	0	0
Mother's				
Mini Apple	5 (0.5 oz)	50	0	0
Mini Caramel	5 (0.5 oz)	50	0	0
Mini Cinnamon	5 (0.5 oz)	50	0	0
Mini Plain Unsalted	7 (0.5 oz)	60	0	0
Multigrain Lightly Salted	1 (0.3 oz)	35	0	0
Rye Unsalted	1 (0.3 oz)	35	1	0
Wheat Unsalted	1 (0.3 oz)	35	1	0
Pritikin				
Mini Apple Crisp	5 (0.5 oz)	50	—	0
Multigrain	1 (0.3 oz)	35	—	0
Multigrain Unsalted	1 (0.3 oz)	35	—	0
Plain	1 (0.3 oz)	35	—	0
Plain Unsalted	1 (0.3 oz)	35	—	0
Sesame Low Sodium	1 (0.3 oz)	35	—	0
Sesame Unsalted	1 (0.3 oz)	35	—	0
Quaker				
Apple Cinnamon	1 (0.5 oz)	50	—	0
Banana Crunch	1 (0.5 oz)	50	—	0
Cinnamon Crunch	1 (0.5 oz)	50	—	0
Mini Apple Cinnamon	5 (0.5 oz)	50	—	0
Mini Banana Nut	5 (0.5 oz)	50	—	0
Mini Butter Popped Corn	6 (0.5 oz)	50	—	0
Mini Caramel Corn	5 (0.5 oz)	50	—	0
Mini Chocolate Crunch	5 (0.5 oz)	50	—	0
Mini Cinnamon Crunch	5 (0.5 oz)	50	—	0
Mini Honey Nut	5 (0.5 oz)	50	—	0

FOOD	PORTION	CALS.	FIB.	CHOL.
Quaker (CONT.)				
Mini Monterey Jack	6 (0.5 oz)	50	—	0
Mini White Cheddar	6 (0.5 oz)	50	—	0
Salt-Free	1 (0.3 oz)	35	—	0
Salted	1 (0.3 oz)	35	—	0
Tree Of Life				
Fat Free Mini Apple Cinnamon	15	60	0	0
Fat Free Mini Caramel	15	60	0	0
Fat Free Mini Honey Nut	15	60	0	0
Fat Free Mini Jalapeno	15	60	0	0
Fat Free Mini Plain	15	50	0	0

ROCKFISH

FOOD	PORTION	CALS.	FIB.	CHOL.
pacific cooked	1 fillet (5.2 oz)	180	—	66
pacific cooked	3 oz	103	—	38
pacific raw	3 oz	80	—	29

ROE

(see individual fish names)

FOOD	PORTION	CALS.	FIB.	CHOL.
fish	3.5 oz	39	—	105
fresh baked	1 oz	58	—	136
fresh baked	3 oz	173	—	408

ROLL

(see also BISCUIT, CROISSANT, ENGLISH MUFFIN, MUFFIN, POPOVER, SCONE)

FROZEN

Weight Watchers

FOOD	PORTION	CALS.	FIB.	CHOL.
Glazed Cinnamon Rolls	1 (2.1 oz)	200	1	5
HOME RECIPE				
dinner as prep w/ 2% milk	1 (2½ in)	111	—	12
dinner as prep w/ whole milk	1 (2½ in)	112	—	13
raisin & nut	1 (2 oz)	196	—	13
MIX				
Natural Ovens				
German Hard	1 (2.1 oz)	138	1	0
Gourmet Dinner	1 (1 oz)	50	2	0
Hearty Sandwich	1 (1.8 oz)	110	2	0
READY-TO-EAT				
brown & serve	1 (1 oz)	85	—	0
cinnamon raisin	1 (2¾ in)	223	1	40
dinner	1 (1 oz)	85	—	0
french	1 (1.3 oz)	105	—	0
hamburger multi-grain	1 (1½ oz)	113	2	0
hamburger reduced calorie	1 (1½ oz)	84	3	0

FOOD	PORTION	CALS.	FIB.	CHOL.
hard	1 (3½ in)	167	—	0
hotdog multi-grain	1 (1½ oz)	113	2	0
hotdog reduced calorie	1 (1½ oz)	84	3	0
kaiser	1 (3½ in)	167	—	0
oat bran	1 (1.2 oz)	78	1	0
rye	1 (1 oz)	81	—	0
submarine	1 (4.7 oz)	155	—	tr
wheat	1 (1 oz)	77	—	0
whole wheat	1 (1 oz)	75	—	0
Alvarado St. Bakery				
Burger Buns	1 (2.2 oz)	140	3	0
Hot Dog Buns	1 (2.2 oz)	140	3	0
Arnold				
Augusto Pan Cubano	1	230	2	0
Bakery Light	1 (1.5 oz)	80	4	0
Bran'nola Buns	1 (1.5 oz)	100	3	0
Dinner Plain	1 (0.7 oz)	50	1	tr
Dinner Sesame	1 (0.7 oz)	50	1	tr
Dutch Egg	1	130	2	0
Hamburger	1	120	2	0
Hot Dog	1 (1.5 oz)	110	1	0
Hot Dog Bran'nola	1 (1.5 oz)	110	1	0
Hot Dog New England Style	1	110	1	0
Italian 8-inch Savoni	1	210	3	0
Onion Premium	1 (2.6 oz)	180	2	0
Onion Soft	1	140	2	0
Potato	1	140	2	0
Sandwich Soft Sesame	1	130	2	0
August Bros.				
Kaiser	1	170	2	0
Onion	1	160	2	0
Sesame Cubano	1	170	2	0
Bread Du Jour				
Bavarian Cracked Wheat	1 (1.2 oz)	90	1	0
Crusty Italian	1 (1.2 oz)	80	tr	0
French Petite	1 (3.5 oz)	230	2	0
Rye	1 (1.2 oz)	90	1	0
Sourdough	1 (2.2 oz)	140	2	0
Country Kitchen				
Frankfurt	1	120	—	0
Dicarlo's				
Extra Sourdough	1 (1.6 oz)	100	1	0
French	1 (1 oz)	70	tr	0

FOOD	PORTION	CALS.	FIB.	CHOL.
Hollywood				
Dark Bread	1	40	—	0
Dinner Light Pan Special Formula	1	60	—	0
Sliced Light Special Formula	1	80	—	0
Home Pride				
Dinner Wheat	1 (1.9 oz)	160	2	0
Hamburger Potato Bun	1 (1.9 oz)	130	2	0
Hot Dog Potato Bun	1 (1.9 oz)	130	2	0
Sandwich Roll Wheat	1 (1.9 oz)	160	2	0
White	2 (1.6 oz)	130	1	0
Martin's				
Big Marty Poppy	1	170	3	0
Big Marty Sesame	1	170	3	0
Hoagie	1	240	3	0
Hoagie Sesame	1	240	4	0
Potato Dinner	1	100	1	0
Potato Long	1	140	2	0
Potato Party	1	50	1	0
Potato Sandwich	1	140	2	0
Sandwich Whole Wheat 100% Stoneground	1	160	5	0
Matthew's				
Salad Roll	1	110	2	0
Sandwich	1	110	2	0
Pepperidge Farm				
Brown 'N Serve Club	1	100	1	0
Brown 'N Serve French	½ roll	180	1	0
Brown 'N Serve Hearth	1	50	tr	0
Dinner	1	60	tr	<5
Dinner Country Style Classic	1	50	0	0
Finger Poppy Seed	1	50	tr	<5
Finger Sesame Seed	1	60	tr	<5
Frankfurter Dijon	1	160	2	0
Frankfurter Side Sliced	1	140	1	0
Frankfurter Top Sliced	1	140	1	0
Frankfurter w/ Poppy Seeds	1	130	1	0
French Style	1	100	1	0
Hamburger	1	130	1	0
Hamburger	1	130	1	0
Heat & Serve Butter Crescent	1	110	tr	15
Heat & Serve Golden Twist	1	110	tr	5
Hoagie Soft	1	210	1	0
Old Fashioned	1	50	tr	5

FOOD	PORTION	CALS.	FIB.	CHOL.
Pepperidge Farm (CONT.)				
Parker House	1	60	tr	5
Party	1	30	tr	0
Potato Sandwich	1	160	1	0
Sandwich Onion w/ Poppy Seeds	1	150	1	0
Sandwich Salad	1	110	—	10
Sandwich w/ Sesame Seeds	1	140	1	0
Soft Family	1	100	1	0
Sourdough French	1	100	1	0
Roman Meal				
Brown & Serve	2 (2 oz)	140	2	0
Dinner	2 (2 oz)	136	2	0
Hamburger	1 (1.6 oz)	111	2	0
Hotdog	1 (1.5 oz)	103	2	0
Sandwich	1 (2.7 oz)	181	3	0
Sandwich	1 (2.7 oz)	181	3	0
San Francisco				
Sourdough	1 (1.8 oz)	180	3	0
The Baker				
Honey Cinnamon Raisin	1 (2 oz)	150	4	0
Wonder				
Brown 'N Serve Buttermilk	1 (1 oz)	70	tr	0
Brown 'N Serve Wheat	1 (1 oz)	70	tr	0
Brown 'N Serve White	1 (1 oz)	70	tr	0
Dinner White Light	1 (1 oz)	60	4	0
Hamburger	1 (1.5 oz)	110	tr	0
Hamburger Light	1 (1.5 oz)	80	5	0
Hamburger Wheat	1 (2.2 oz)	170	1	0
Hot Dog	1 (1.5 oz)	110	tr	0
Hot Dog Light	1 (1.5 oz)	80	5	0
Tea Dinner Rolls	1 (1.5 oz)	80	5	0
REFRIGERATED				
crescent	1 (1 oz)	98	—	0
Pillsbury				
Best Quick Cinnamon Rolls w/ Icing	1	110	—	0
Butterflake	1	140	—	0
Crescent	1	100	—	0
ROSE APPLE				
fresh	3½ oz	32	—	0
ROSE HIP				
fresh	3½ oz	91	—	0

FOOD	PORTION	CALS.	FIB.	CHOL.
ROSELLE				
fresh	1 cup	28	—	0
ROSEMARY				
dried	1 tsp	4	—	0
ROUGHY				
orange baked	3 oz	75	—	22
RUTABAGA				
CANNED				
Sunshine				
Diced	½ cup (4.2 oz)	30	3	0
FRESH				
cooked mashed	½ cup	41	—	0
raw cubed	½ cup	25	—	0
SABLEFISH				
baked	3 oz	213	—	53
fillet baked	5.3 oz	378	—	95
smoked	1 oz	72	—	18
smoked	3 oz	218	—	55
SAFFLOWER				
seeds dried	1 oz	147	—	0
SAFFRON				
saffron	1 tsp	2	—	0
SAGE				
ground	1 tsp	2	—	0
Watkins				
Sage	¼ tsp (0.5 g)	0	0	0
SALAD				
(*see also* LETTUCE, PASTA SALAD)				
MIX				
Dole				
Caesar Salad	⅓ pkg (3.5 oz)	170	1	5
Classic Blend	3.5 oz	25	1	0
Coleslaw Blend	3.5 oz	30	2	0
French Blend	3.5 oz	25	1	0
Italian Blend	3.5 oz	25	1	0
Salad-In-A-Minute Oriental	3.5 oz	110	2	0
Salad-In-A-Minute Spinach	3.5 oz	180	3	0
Fresh Express				
American Salad	1½ cups (3 oz)	20	1	0
Caesar Salad	1½ cups (3 oz)	140	1	10

FOOD	PORTION	CALS.	FIB.	CHOL.
Fresh Express (CONT.)				
European Salad	1½ cups (3 oz)	20	1	0
Garden Salad	1½ cups (3 oz)	20	1	0
Italian Salad	1½ cups (3 oz)	20	1	0
Oriental Salad	1½ cups (3 oz)	120	1	0
Riviera Salad	1½ cups (3 oz)	10	1	0
Spinach Salad	1½ cups (3 oz)	130	3	0
TAKE-OUT				
caesar	2 cups (5 oz)	235	1	10
chef w/o dressing	1½ cups	386	—	244
tossed w/o dressing	¾ cup	16	—	0
tossed w/o dressing	1½ cups	32	—	0
tossed w/o dressing w/ cheese & egg	1½ cups	102	—	98
tossed w/o dressing w/ chicken	1½ cups	105	—	72
tossed w/o dressing w/ pasta & seafood	1½ cups (14.6 oz)	380	—	50
tossed w/o dressing w/ shrimp	1½ cups	107	—	180
waldorf	½ cup	79	1	8

SALAD DRESSING
HOME RECIPE

FOOD	PORTION	CALS.	FIB.	CHOL.
vinegar & oil	1 tbsp	72	—	0
MIX				
Good Seasons				
Blue Cheese & Herbs as prep	1 tbsp	72	—	tr
Buttermilk Farm as prep	1 tbsp	58	—	5
Cheese Garlic as prep	1 tbsp	72	—	tr
Cheese Italian as prep	1 tbsp	72	—	tr
Classic Dill	1 pkg	28	—	0
Italian as prep	1 tbsp	71	—	0
Italian Lite as prep	1 tbsp	27	—	0
Italian No Oil as prep	1 tbsp	7	—	0
Lemon & Herbs as prep	1 tbsp	71	—	0
Lite Cheese Italian as prep	1 tbsp	27	—	tr
Lite Ranch as prep	1 tbsp	29	—	3
Mild Italian as prep	1 tbsp	73	—	0
Ranch as prep	1 tbsp	57	—	5
Zesty Italian as prep	1 tbsp	71	—	0
Hain				
No Oil 1000 Island	1 tbsp	12	—	tr
No Oil Bleu Cheese	1 tbsp	14	—	<5
No Oil Buttermilk	1 tbsp	11	—	0
No Oil Caesar	1 tbsp	6	—	0

FOOD	PORTION	CALS.	FIB.	CHOL.
Hain (CONT.)				
No Oil French	1 tbsp	12	—	0
No Oil Garlic & Cheese	1 tbsp	6	—	0
No Oil Herb	1 tbsp	2	—	0
No Oil Italian	1 tbsp	2	—	0
READY-TO-EAT				
french reduced calorie	1 tbsp	22	—	1
italian reduced calorie	1 tbsp	16	—	1
russian reduced calorie	1 tbsp	23	—	1
sesame seed	1 tbsp	68	—	0
thousand island reduced calorie	1 tbsp	24	—	2
Estee				
Creamy French Fat Free	1 pkg (0.5 oz)	5	—	0
Creamy Garlic Fat Free	1 pkg (0.5 oz)	5	—	0
Fat Free Thousand Island	1 pkg (0.5 oz)	5	—	0
Hain				
1000 Island	1 tbsp	50	—	0
Canola Garden Tomato	1 tbsp	60	—	0
Canola Italian	1 tbsp	50	—	0
Canola Spicy French Mustard	1 tbsp	50	—	5
Canola Tangy Citrus	1 tbsp	50	—	0
Creamy Caesar	1 tbsp	60	—	<5
Creamy Caesar Low Salt	1 tbsp	60	—	<5
Creamy French	1 tbsp	60	—	0
Creamy Italian	1 tbsp	80	—	0
Creamy Italian No Salt Added	1 tbsp	80	—	0
Cucumber Dill	1 tbsp	80	—	5
Dijon Vinaigrette	1 tbsp	50	—	<5
Garlic & Sour Cream	1 tbsp	70	—	0
Honey & Sesame	1 tbsp	60	—	0
Italian Cheese Vinaigrette	1 tbsp	55	—	<5
Old Fashioned Buttermilk	1 tbsp	70	—	0
Poppyseed Rancher's	1 tbsp	60	—	<5
Savory Herb No Salt Added	1 tbsp	90	—	0
Swiss Cheese Vinaigrette	1 tbsp	60	—	<5
Traditional Italian	1 tbsp	80	—	0
Traditional Italian No Salt Added	1 tbsp	60	—	0
Hollywood				
Caesar	1 tbsp	70	0	0
Creamy French	1 tbsp	70	0	0
Creamy Italian	1 tbsp	90	0	0
Dijon Vinaigrette	1 tbsp	60	0	0
Italian	1 tbsp	90	0	0

FOOD	PORTION	CALS.	FIB.	CHOL.
Hollywood (CONT.)				
Italian Cheese	1 tbsp	80	0	0
Old Fashion Buttermilk	1 tbsp	75	0	0
Poppy Seed Rancher's	1 tbsp	75	0	0
Thousand Island	1 tbsp	60	0	5
Kraft				
Bacon & Tomato	2 tbsp (1.1 oz)	140	0	<5
Buttermilk Ranch	2 tbsp (1 oz)	150	0	<5
Caesar	2 tbsp (1.1 oz)	130	0	<5
Caesar Ranch	2 tbsp (1 oz)	140	0	10
Catalina French	2 tbsp (1.2 oz)	140	0	0
Catalina With Honey	2 tbsp (1.2 oz)	140	0	0
Chunky Blue Cheese	2 tbsp (1.2 oz)	90	0	10
Coleslaw	2 tbsp (1.2 oz)	150	0	25
Creamy Caesar	2 tbsp (1 oz)	140	0	10
Creamy Garlic	2 tbsp (1.1 oz)	110	0	0
Creamy Italian	2 tbsp (1.1 oz)	110	0	0
Cucumber Ranch	2 tbsp (1.1 oz)	150	0	0
Deliciously Right Bacon & Tomato	2 tbsp (1.1 oz)	60	0	<5
Deliciously Right Caesar	2 tbsp (1.1 oz)	50	0	<5
Deliciously Right Catalina French	2 tbsp (1.2 oz)	80	0	0
Deliciously Right Creamy Italian	2 tbsp (1.1 oz)	50	0	0
Deliciously Right Cucumber Ranch	2 tbsp (1.1 oz)	60	0	0
Deliciously Right French	2 tbsp (1.2 oz)	50	0	0
Deliciously Right Italian	2 tbsp (1.1 oz)	70	0	0
Deliciously Right Ranch	2 tbsp (1.1 oz)	110	0	10
Deliciously Right Thousand Island	2 tbsp (1.2 oz)	70	0	5
Free Blue Cheese	2 tbsp (1.2 oz)	50	1	0
Free Catalina	2 tbsp (1.2 oz)	45	tr	0
Free French	2 tbsp (1.2 oz)	50	tr	0
Free Honey Dijon	2 tbsp (1.2 oz)	50	1	0
Free Italian	2 tbsp (1.1 oz)	10	0	0
Free Peppercorn Ranch	2 tbsp (1.2 oz)	50	1	0
Free Ranch	1 tbsp (1.2 oz)	50	tr	0
Free Red Wine Vinegar	2 tbsp (1.1 oz)	15	0	0
Free Thousand Island	2 tbsp (1.2 oz)	45	1	0
French	2 tbsp (1.1 oz)	120	0	0
Honey Dijon	2 tbsp (1.1 oz)	150	0	0
House Italian	2 tbsp (1.1 oz)	120	0	<5
Oil-Free Italian	2 tbsp (1.1 oz)	5	0	0

FOOD	PORTION	CALS.	FIB.	CHOL.
Kraft (CONT.)				
Peppercorn Ranch	2 tbsp (1 oz)	170	0	10
Pesto Italian	2 tbsp (1.1 oz)	140	0	0
Ranch	2 tbsp (1 oz)	170	0	5
Roka Blue Cheese	2 tbsp (1.2 oz)	90	0	10
Russian	2 tbsp (1.2 oz)	130	0	0
Salsa Ranch	2 tbsp (1 oz)	130	0	10
Salsa Zesty Garden	2 tbsp (1.1 oz)	70	tr	0
Sour Cream & Onion Ranch	2 tbsp (1 oz)	170	0	10
Thousand Island	2 tbsp (1.1 oz)	110	0	10
Thousand Island With Bacon	2 tbsp (1 oz)	120	0	0
Zesty Italian	2 tbsp (1.1 oz)	110	0	0
Marzetti				
Bacon Spinach Salad	2 tbsp	80	15	1
Blue Cheese	2 tbsp	160	0	20
Buttermilk & Herb	2 tbsp	180	0	3
Buttermilk Bacon Ranch	2 tbsp	180	0	10
Buttermilk Blue Cheese	2 tbsp	160	0	10
Buttermilk Parmesan Pepper	2 tbsp	170	0	10
Buttermilk Parmesan Ranch	2 tbsp	160	0	10
Buttermilk Ranch	2 tbsp	180	0	4
Buttermilk Veggie Dip	2 tbsp	170	0	3
Caesar	2 tbsp	150	0	0
Caesar Ranch	2 tbsp	190	0	5
California French	2 tbsp	160	0	0
Celery Seed	2 tbsp	160	0	0
Chunky Blue Cheese	2 tbsp	150	0	25
Classic Caesar Ranch	2 tbsp	190	0	5
Country French	2 tbsp	150	0	10
Cracked Peppercorn	2 tbsp	140	0	30
Creamy Garlic Italian	2 tbsp	160	0	15
Creamy Italian	2 tbsp	150	0	15
Crispy Celery Seed	2 tbsp	160	0	0
Dijon Honey Mustard	2 tbsp	140	0	20
Dijon Ranch	2 tbsp	170	0	25
Dutch Sweet'N Sour	2 tbsp	160	0	0
Fat Free California French	2 tbsp	45	0	0
Fat Free Honey Dijon	2 tbsp	60	1	0
Fat Free Honey French	2 tbsp	45	0	0
Fat Free Italian	2 tbsp	15	0	0
Fat Free Peppercorn Ranch	2 tbsp	30	1	0
Fat Free Ranch	2 tbsp	30	1	0
Fat Free Raspberry	2 tbsp	70	0	0
Fat Free Slaw	2 tbsp	45	0	15

FOOD	PORTION	CALS.	FIB.	CHOL.
Marzetti (CONT.)				
Fat Free Sweet & Sour	2 tbsp	45	0	0
Fat Free Thousand Island	2 tbsp	35	0	0
Garden Ranch	2 tbsp	180	0	3
Gusto Italian	2 tbsp	120	0	0
Honey Dijon	2 tbsp	140	0	15
Honey Dijon Ranch	2 tbsp	150	0	25
Honey French	2 tbsp	160	0	0
Honey French Blue Cheese	2 tbsp	160	0	0
House Caesar	2 tbsp	150	0	5
Italian With Olive Oil	2 tbsp	120	0	0
Light Blue Cheese	2 tbsp	60	0	15
Light Buttermilk Ranch	2 tbsp	90	0	10
Light California French	2 tbsp	80	0	0
Light Chunky Blue Cheese	2 tbsp	80	0	15
Light French	2 tbsp	40	0	0
Light Honey French	2 tbsp	80	0	0
Light Italian	2 tbsp	60	0	0
Light Ranch	2 tbsp	90	0	5
Light Red Wine Vinegar & Oil	2 tbsp	20	0	0
Light Slaw	2 tbsp	60	0	30
Light Sweet & Sour	2 tbsp	100	0	0
Light Thousand Island	2 tbsp	70	0	20
Old Fashioned Poppyseed	2 tbsp	140	0	10
Olde Venice Italian	2 tbsp	130	0	0
Olde World Caesar	2 tbsp	150	0	5
Parmesan Pepper	2 tbsp	160	0	10
Peppercorn Ranch	2 tbsp	180	0	10
Poppyseed	2 tbsp	160	0	15
Potato Salad Dressing	2 tbsp	120	0	35
Ranch	2 tbsp	180	0	3
Red Wine Vinegar & Oil	2 tbsp	130	0	0
Romano Cheese Caesar	2 tbsp	150	0	15
Romano Italian	2 tbsp	160	0	0
Savory Italian	2 tbsp	110	0	0
Slaw	2 tbsp	170	0	30
Southern Slaw	2 tbsp	100	0	20
Sweet & Saucy	2 tbsp	140	0	0
Sweet & Sour	2 tbsp	160	0	0
Thousand Island	2 tbsp	150	0	25
Vintage Champagne	2 tbsp	150	0	0
Wilde Raspberry	2 tbsp	150	0	0
Nasoya				
Creamy Dill	2 tbsp (1 oz)	63	tr	0

FOOD	PORTION	CALS.	FIB.	CHOL.
Nasoya (CONT.)				
Creamy Italian	2 tbsp (1 oz)	60	tr	0
Garden Herb	2 tbsp (1 oz)	61	tr	0
Sesame Garlic	2 tbsp (1 oz)	63	tr	0
Thousand Island	2 tbsp (1 oz)	62	tr	0
Newman's Own				
Italian Light	1 tbsp (0.5 fl oz)	10	—	0
Olive Oil & Vinegar	1 tbsp (0.5 fl oz)	80	—	0
Ranch	1 tbsp (0.5 fl oz)	90	—	5
Pfeiffer				
1000 Island	2 tbsp	140	0	20
California French	2 tbsp	140	0	0
French	2 tbsp	150	0	10
Honey Dijon	2 tbsp	140	0	15
Lite Italian	2 tbsp	50	0	0
Ranch	2 tbsp	180	0	3
Savory Italian	2 tbsp	110	0	0
Pritikin				
Dijon Balsamic Vinaigrette	2 tbsp (1 oz)	3	—	0
French	2 tbsp (1 oz)	35	—	0
Honey Dijon	2 tbsp (1 oz)	45	—	0
Honey French	2 tbsp (1 oz)	40	—	0
Italian	2 tbsp (1 oz)	20	—	0
Raspberry Vinaigrette	2 tbsp (1 oz)	45	—	0
Red Wing				
"K" Dressing	1 tbsp (0.5 oz)	70	0	5
Chunky Blue Cheese	2 tbsp (1 oz)	130	0	0
Creamy Ranch	2 tbsp (1 oz)	150	0	15
French Traditional	2 tbsp (1 oz)	130	0	0
Italian Traditional	2 tbsp (1 oz)	100	0	0
Spicy Sweet French	2 tbsp (1 oz)	130	0	0
Thousand Island Thick & Rich	2 tbsp (1 oz)	110	0	15
S&W				
French Low Calorie	1 tbsp	18	—	0
Italian No-Oil	1 tbsp	2	—	0
Russian Low Calorie	1 tbsp	25	—	0
Seven Seas				
Creamy Italian	2 tbsp (1.1 oz)	110	0	0
Free Italian	2 tbsp (1.1 oz)	10	0	0
Free Ranch	2 tbsp (1.2 oz)	50	1	0
Free Red Wine Vinegar	2 tbsp (1.1 oz)	15	0	0
Green Goddess	2 tbsp (1 oz)	120	0	0
Herbs & Spices	2 tbsp (1.1 oz)	120	0	0
Ranch	2 tbsp (1 oz)	150	0	5

FOOD	PORTION	CALS.	FIB.	CHOL.
Seven Seas (CONT.)				
Red Wine Vinegar & Oil	2 tbsp (1.1 oz)	110	0	0
Reduced Calorie Creamy Italian	2 tbsp (1.1 oz)	60	0	0
Reduced Calorie Italian With Olive Oil	2 tbsp (1.1 oz)	50	0	0
Reduced Calorie Ranch	2 tbsp (1.1 oz)	100	0	0
Reduced Calorie Red Wine Vinegar & Oil	2 tbsp (1.1 oz)	60	0	0
Two Cheese Italian	2 tbsp (1.1 oz)	70	0	0
Viva Buttermilk	2 tbsp (1.1 oz)	150	0	0
Viva Caesar	2 tbsp (1.1 oz)	120	0	0
Viva Italian	2 tbsp (1.1 oz)	110	0	0
Viva Reduced Calorie Italian	2 tbsp (1.1 oz)	45	0	0
Tree Of Life				
Cafe Venice	2 tbsp (1 oz)	100	0	0
Fat Free Honey French	2 tbsp (1 oz)	35	—	0
Fat Free Italian Garlic	2 tbsp (1 oz)	20	—	0
Fat Free Oriental Ginger	2 tbsp (1 oz)	15	—	0
Frisco's Raspberry	2 tbsp (1 oz)	120	0	0
Maison Caesar	2 tbsp (1 oz)	70	0	5
Shanghai Palace	2 tbsp (1 oz)	80	0	0
Ultra Slim-Fast				
French	1 tbsp	20	0	0
Italian	1 tbsp	6	0	0
W.J. Clark				
Ginger Orange Vinaigrette	1 tbsp	73	0	0
Herbs & Romano	1 tbsp	67	0	0
Lemon Peppercorn	1 tbsp	72	0	0
Lime Cilantro Vinaigrette	1 tbsp	73	0	0
Poppy Seed	1 tbsp	75	0	0
Sweet Pepper Basil	1 tbsp	69	0	0
Tarragon Honey Mustard	1 tbsp	66	0	0
Walden Farms				
Fat Free Balsamic Vinaigrette	2 tbsp (1 oz)	15	0	0
Fat Free Bleu Cheese	2 tbsp (1 oz)	25	0	8
Fat Free Caesar	2 tbsp (1 oz)	25	0	0
Fat Free Creamy Italian With Parmesan	1 tbsp (1 oz)	25	0	0
Fat Free French Style	2 tbsp (1 oz)	25	0	0
Fat Free Honey Dijon	2 tbsp (1 oz)	25	0	0
Fat Free Italian	2 tbsp (1 oz)	10	0	0
Fat Free Ranch	2 tbsp (1 oz)	25	0	0
Fat Free Raspberry Vinaigrette	2 tbsp (1 oz)	20	0	0
Fat Free Russian	2 tbsp (1 oz)	30	0	5

FOOD	PORTION	CALS.	FIB.	CHOL.
Walden Farms (CONT.)				
Fat Free Sodium Free Italian	2 tbsp (1 oz)	10	0	0
Fat Free Sugar Free Italian	2 tbsp (1 oz)	0	0	0
Fat Free Thousand Island	2 tbsp (1 oz)	35	0	5
Italian With Sun Dried Tomato	2 tbsp (1 oz)	15	0	0
Ranch With Sun Dried Tomato	2 tbsp (1 oz)	25	0	0
Weight Watchers				
Fat Free Caesar	2 tbsp	10	0	0
Fat Free Caesar	1 pkg (0.75 oz)	6	0	0
Fat Free Creamy Italian	2 tbsp	30	0	0
Fat Free French Style	2 tbsp	40	0	0
Fat Free Honey Dijon	2 tbsp	45	0	0
Fat Free Italian	2 tbsp	10	0	0
Fat Free Ranch	2 tbsp	35	0	0
Fat Free Ranch	1 pkg (0.75 oz)	25	0	0
Salad Celebrations 3 Cheese Caesar	2 tbsp	40	0	10
Salad Celebrations Russian	2 tbsp	45	0	10
Salad Celebrations Thousand Island	2 tbsp	45	0	10
Wishbone				
Caesar Olive Oil	2 tbsp (1 oz)	90	0	0
Chunky Blue Cheese	2 tbsp (1 oz)	170	0	10
Classic House Italian	2 tbsp (1 oz)	140	0	<5
Classic Olive Oil Italian	2 tbsp (1 oz)	70	0	0
Creamy Italian	2 tbsp (1 oz)	100	0	0
Creamy Roasted Garlic	2 tbsp (1 oz)	140	0	0
Deluxe French	2 tbsp (1 oz)	120	0	0
Fat Free Chunky Blue Cheese	2 tbsp (1 oz)	35	0	0
Fat Free Creamy Roasted Garlic	2 tbsp (1 oz)	40	0	0
Fat Free Honey Dijon	2 tbsp (1 oz)	45	0	0
Fat Free Italian	2 tbsp (1 oz)	15	0	0
Fat Free Ranch	2 tbsp (1 oz)	40	0	0
Fat Free Sweet & Spicy French	2 tbsp (1 oz)	30	0	0
Fat Free Thousand Island	2 tbsp (1 oz)	35	0	0
Honey Dijon	2 tbsp (1 oz)	130	0	0
Italian	2 tbsp (1 oz)	80	0	0
Lite Caesar With Olive Oil	2 tbsp	60	0	<5
Lite Chunky Blue Cheese	2 tbsp (1 oz)	80	0	0
Lite Classic Dijon Vinaigrette	2 tbsp (1 oz)	60	0	0
Lite Creamy Italian	2 tbsp (1 oz)	60	0	<5
Lite French	2 tbsp	50	0	<5
Lite Italian	2 tbsp (1 oz)	24	0	0
Lite Ranch	2 tbsp (1 oz)	100	0	5

FOOD	PORTION	CALS.	FIB.	CHOL.
Wishbone (CONT.)				
Lite Thousand Island	2 tbsp (1 oz)	80	0	10
Olive Oil Vinaigrette	2 tbsp (1 oz)	60	0	0
Ranch	2 tbsp (1 oz)	160	0	10
Robusto Italian	2 tbsp (1 oz)	100	0	0
Russian	2 tbsp (1 oz)	110	0	0
Santa Fe	2 tbsp (1 oz)	150	0	5
Sierra	2 tbsp	150	0	0
Sweet 'N Spicy French	2 tbsp (1 oz)	130	0	0
Thousand Island	2 tbsp (1 oz)	130	0	10

SALMON
CANNED
chum w/ bone	1 can (13.9 oz)	521	—	144
chum w/ bone	3 oz	120	—	33
sockeye w/ bone	3 oz	130	—	37
sockeye w/ bone	1 can (12.9 oz)	568	—	161
Bumble Bee				
Keta	3.5 oz	160	—	60
Pink	3.5 oz	160	—	50
Pink Skinless & Boneless	3.25 oz	120	—	25
Red	3.5 oz	180	—	60
Red Skinless & Boneless	3.25 oz	130	—	30
Deming's				
Alaska Pink	½ cup	140	—	65
Alaska Red Sockeye	½ cup	170	—	65
Double Q				
Alaska Pink	½ cup	140	—	65
FRESH				
atlantic baked	3 oz	155	—	60
chinook baked	3 oz	196	—	72
chum baked	3 oz	131	—	81
coho cooked	3 oz	157	—	42
coho cooked	½ fillet (5.4 oz)	286	—	76
coho raw	3 oz	124	—	33
pink baked	3 oz	127	—	57
sockeye cooked	3 oz	183	—	74
sockeye cooked	½ fillet (5.4 oz)	334	—	135
sockeye raw	3 oz	143	—	53
SMOKED				
chinook	1 oz	33	—	7
chinook	3 oz	99	—	20
Nathan's				
Nova	2 oz	80	0	30

FOOD	PORTION	CALS.	FIB.	CHOL.
TAKE-OUT				
salmon cake	1 (3 oz)	241	—	104

SALSA

(see also KETCHUP, SAUCE, SPANISH FOOD)

Chi-Chi's

FOOD	PORTION	CALS.	FIB.	CHOL.
Hot	2 tbsp (1 oz)	10	0	0
Medium	1 tbsp (1 oz)	10	0	0
Mild	2 tbsp (1 oz)	10	0	0
Verde Medium	2 tbsp (1.2 oz)	15	0	0
Verde Mild	2 tbsp (1.2 oz)	15	0	0
Del Monte				
Mexicana	2 tbsp (1.1 oz)	5	1	0
Taquera	2 tbsp (1.1 oz)	5	1	0
Verde	2 tbsp (1.1 oz)	10	tr	0
Frito Lay				
Hot	1 oz	12	—	0
Medium	1 oz	12	—	0
Mild	1 oz	12	—	0
Guiltless Gourmet				
Picante Hot	1 oz	6	tr	0
Picante Medium	1 oz	6	tr	0
Hain				
Hot	¼ cup	22	—	0
Heluva Good Cheese				
Cheese & Salsa	2 tbsp (1.1 oz)	80	0	10
Thick & Chunky Hot	2 tbsp (1.2 oz)	10	0	0
Thick & Chunky Mild	2 tbsp (1.2 oz)	10	0	0
Hot Cha Cha				
Medium	2 tbsp (1 oz)	5	—	0
Hunt's				
Alfresco Medium	2 tbsp (1.1 oz)	10	tr	0
Alfresco Mild	2 tbsp (1.1 oz)	10	tr	0
Hot	2 tbsp (1.1 oz)	27	1	0
Medium	2 tbsp (1.1 oz)	27	1	0
Mild	2 tbsp (1.1 oz)	27	1	0
Picante Medium	2 tbsp (1.1 oz)	11	tr	0
Picante Mild	2 tbsp (1.1 oz)	11	tr	0
Louise's				
Fat Free BBQ Black Bean	1 oz	10	0	0
Fat Free Black Bean	1 oz	10	0	0
Fat Free Medium	1 oz	10	1	0
Fat Free Mild	1 oz	10	1	0
Fat Free Nacho Queso	1 oz	15	0	0

FOOD	PORTION	CALS.	FIB.	CHOL.
Muir Glen				
Organic Fat Free Hot	2 tbsp (1.1 oz)	10	0	0
Organic Fat Free Medium	2 tbsp (1.1 oz)	10	0	0
Organic Fat Free Mild	2 tbsp (1.1 oz)	10	0	0
Newman's Own				
Bandito Hot	1 tbsp (0.7 oz)	6	—	0
Bandito Medium	1 tbsp (0.7 oz)	6	—	0
Bandito Mild	1 tbsp (0.7 oz)	6	—	0
Old El Paso				
Green Chili Medium	2 tbsp (1 oz)	10	tr	0
Homestyle	2 tbsp (1 oz)	5	0	0
Homestyle Mild	2 tbsp (1 oz)	5	0	0
Picante Hot	2 tbsp (1 oz)	10	0	0
Picante Medium	2 tbsp (1 oz)	10	0	0
Picante Mild	2 tbsp (1 oz)	10	0	0
Picante Thick'n Chunky Hot	2 tbsp (1 oz)	10	0	0
Picante Thick'n Chunky Medium	2 tbsp (1 oz)	10	0	0
Picante Thick'n Chunky Mild	2 tbsp (1 oz)	10	0	0
Pico De Gallo Hot	2 tbsp (1 oz)	5	tr	0
Pico De Gallo Medium	1 tbsp (1 oz)	5	tr	0
Salsa Verde	2 tbsp (1 oz)	10	0	0
Thick'n Chunky Hot	2 tbsp (1 oz)	10	0	0
Thick'n Chunky Medium	2 tbsp (1 oz)	10	0	0
Thick'n Chunky Mild	2 tbsp (1 oz)	10	0	0
Ortega				
Hot Green Chili	1 tbsp	6	—	0
Medium Green Chili	1 tbsp	6	—	0
Mild Green Chili	1 tbsp	8	—	0
Pace				
Picante	2 tbsp (1 fl oz)	7	tr	0
Thick & Chunky	2 tbsp (1 fl oz)	12	1	0
Progresso				
Italian Hot	2 tbsp (1 oz)	30	tr	0
Italian Medium	2 tbsp (1 oz)	10	tr	0
Italian Mild	2 tbsp (1 oz)	10	tr	0
Roserita				
Chunky Hot	3 tbsp (1.5 oz)	25	tr	0
Chunky Medium	3 tbsp (1.5 oz)	25	tr	0
Chunky Mild	3 tbsp (1.5 oz)	25	tr	0
Taco Salsa Chunky Medium	3 tbsp (1.5 oz)	25	tr	0
Taco Salsa Chunky Mild	3 tbsp (1.5 oz)	25	tr	0
Tabasco				
Picante	2 tbsp (1.5 oz)	17	1	0

FOOD	PORTION	CALS.	FIB.	CHOL.
Tree Of Life				
Hot	2 tbsp (1 oz)	10	—	0
Medium	2 tbsp (1 oz)	10	—	0
Mild	2 tbsp (1 oz)	10	—	0
No Salt	2 tbsp (1 oz)	10	—	0
Watkins				
Salsa Seasoning Blend	⅛ tsp (0.5 g)	0	0	0
Tropical	2 tbsp (1 oz)	60	0	0
Wise				
Picante	2 tbsp	12	—	0
SALSIFY				
fresh sliced cooked	½ cup	46	—	0
raw sliced	½ cup	55	—	0
SALT/SEASONED SALT				
(*see also* SALT SUBSTITUTES)				
salt	1 tbsp (18 g)	0	—	0
salt	1 tsp (6 g)	0	—	0
Hain				
Sea Salt	1 tsp	0	—	0
Sea Salt Iodized	1 tsp	0	—	0
Morton				
Garlic	1 tsp	3	—	0
Iodized	1 tsp	tr	—	0
Kosher	1 tsp	0	—	0
Lite	1 tsp	tr	—	0
Nature's Season Seasoning Blend	1 tsp	3	—	0
Non-Iodized	1 tsp	0	—	0
Seasoned	1 tsp	4	—	0
Watkins				
Bacon Cheese Salt	¼ tbsp (1 g)	0	0	0
Butter Salt	¼ tbsp (1 g)	0	0	0
Cheese Salt	¼ tbsp (1 g)	0	0	0
Garlic Salt	¼ tsp (1 g)	0	0	0
Salt & Vinegar Seasoning	¼ tsp (1 g)	0	0	0
Seasoning Salt	¼ tsp (1 g)	0	0	0
Sour Cream & Onion Salt	¼ tbsp (1 g)	0	0	0
SALT SUBSTITUTES				
Cardia				
Salt Alternative	1 pkg (0.6 g)	0	—	0
Morton				
Salt Substitute	1 tsp	2	—	0

FOOD	PORTION	CALS.	FIB.	CHOL.
Mrs. Dash				
Onion & Herb	⅛ tsp (0.02 oz)	2	—	0
Papa Dash				
Lite Salt	½ tsp (1 g)	0	—	0
SAPODILLA				
fresh	1	140	—	0
fresh cut up	1 cup	199	—	0
SAPOTES				
fresh	1	301	—	0
SARDINES				
CANNED				
atlantic in oil w/ bone	2	50	—	34
atlantic in oil w/ bone	1 can (3.2 oz)	192	—	131
pacific in tomato sauce w/ bone	1 can (13 oz)	658	—	225
pacific in tomato sauce w/ bone	1	68	—	23
Del Monte				
In Tomato Sauce	1 fish (1.4 oz)	50	tr	25
Port Clyde				
In Louisiana Hot Sauce	1 can (3.75 oz)	170	0	105
In Mustard Sauce	1 can (3.75 oz)	150	1	110
In Soybean Oil Select Small	1 can (3.3 oz)	220	0	115
In Soybean Oil With Hot Chilies	1 can (3.3 oz)	155	0	80
In Soybean Oil drained	1 can (3.3 oz)	220	0	115
In Spring Water	1 can (3.3 oz)	170	0	140
In Tomato Sauce	1 can (3.75 oz)	150	0	100
SAUCE				
(*see also* BARBECUE SAUCE, GRAVY, PIZZA, SALSA, SPAGHETTI SAUCE, TOMATO)				
JARRED				
teriyaki	1 tbsp	15	—	0
teriyaki	1 oz	30	—	0
Armour				
Chili Hot Dog	¼ cup (2.2 oz)	120	—	20
Meatless Sloppy Joe Sauce	¼ cup (2.2 oz)	30	—	0
Best Foods				
Tartar	1 tbsp (14 g)	70	—	5
Bright Day				
Tartar	1 tbsp	50	—	0
Chi-Chi's				
Taco Thick & Chunky	1 tbsp (0.5 oz)	10	0	0

FOOD	PORTION	CALS.	FIB.	CHOL.
Del Monte				
Cocktail	¼ cup (2.7 oz)	100	0	0
Sloppy Joe Hickory Flavor	¼ cup (2.4 oz)	70	0	0
Sloppy Joe Italian Style	¼ cup (2.4 oz)	70	0	0
Sloppy Joe Original	¼ cup (2.4 oz)	70	0	0
El Molino				
Taco Red Mild	2 tbsp	10	—	0
Gebhardt				
Enchilada Sauce	3 tbsp (1.5 oz)	25	tr	tr
Hot Dog Chili Sauce	2 tbsp	30	tr	3
Hot Sauce	½ tsp	tr	tr	0
Gold's				
Rib	1 oz	60	—	0
Golden Dipt				
Cajun Style	1 oz	90	—	0
Creole	1 oz	20	—	0
Dijonaisse	1 oz	52	—	0
French White	1 oz	55	—	0
Ginger Teriyaki Marinade	1 oz	120	—	0
Lemon Butter Dill	1 oz	100	—	0
Lemon Herb Marinade	1 oz	130	—	0
Seafood Cocktail	1 tbsp	20	—	0
Seafood Cocktail Extra Hot	1 tbsp	20	—	0
Tartar	1 tbsp	70	—	10
Tartar Lite	1 tbsp	50	—	5
Heinz				
Worcestershire	1 tbsp	6	—	0
Hellmann's				
Tartar	1 tbsp (14 g)	70	—	5
Heluva Good Cheese				
Cocktail	¼ cup (1.6 oz)	40	—	0
Hormel				
Not-So-Sloppy-Joe Sauce	¼ cup (2.2 oz)	70	1	0
House Of Tsang				
Bangkok Padang	1 tbsp (0.6 oz)	45	0	0
Hoisin	1 tsp (6 g)	15	0	0
Mandarin Marinade	1 tbsp (0.6 oz)	25	0	0
Saigon Sizzle	1 tbsp (0.6 oz)	40	0	0
Spicy Brown Bean	1 tsp (6 g)	15	0	0
Stir Fry Classic	1 tbsp (0.6 oz)	25	0	0
Stir Fry Sweet & Sour	1 tbsp (0.6 oz)	35	0	0
Stir Fry Szechuan Spicy	1 tbsp (0.6 oz)	20	0	0
Sweet & Sour Concentrate	1 tsp (6 g)	10	0	0
Teriyaki Korean	1 tbsp (0.6 oz)	30	0	0

FOOD	PORTION	CALS.	FIB.	CHOL.
Hunt's				
Barbeque	¼ cup (2.2 oz)	57	1	0
Chicken Sensations Barbecue Flavor	1 tbsp (0.5 oz)	35	tr	0
Chicken Sensations Italian Garlic	1 tbsp (0.5 oz)	30	1	0
Chicken Sensations Lemon Herb	1 tbsp (0.5 oz)	31	tr	0
Chicken Sensations South Western	1 tbsp (0.5 oz)	27	tr	0
Pepper Sauce Original	1 tsp (5.2 g)	1	0	0
Steak	1 tbsp (0.6 oz)	10	tr	0
Just Rite				
Hot Dog	2 oz	60	tr	7
Ka-Me				
Black Bean Sauce	1 tbsp (0.5 oz)	10	1	0
Chili Sauce Hot Garlic	1 tbsp (0.5 oz)	15	1	0
Duck Sauce	2 tbsp (1 oz)	80	0	0
Fish Sauce	1 tbsp (0.5 fl oz)	10	0	0
Hoisin Sauce	2 tbsp (1 oz)	45	1	0
Hot Sauce	1 tsp (5 g)	0	0	0
Lemon Sauce	1 tbsp (0.5 oz)	45	0	0
Mandarin Orange Sauce	2 tbsp (1 oz)	80	0	0
Oyster Sauce	1 tbsp (0.5 fl oz)	10	0	0
Plum	2 tbsp (1 fl oz)	80	0	0
Stir Fry Sauce	1 tbsp	10	0	0
Sweet & Sour	2 tbsp (1 fl oz)	50	0	0
Szechuan	1 tbsp (0.5 oz)	20	2	0
Tamari	1 tbsp (0.5 fl oz)	10	0	0
Tempura Sauce	2 tbsp (1 fl oz)	15	0	0
Teriyaki Sauce	1 tbsp (0.5 fl oz)	10	0	0
Kikkoman				
Stir-Fry	1 tbsp	16	1	1
Sweet & Sour	1 tbsp	19	tr	tr
Teriyaki	1 tbsp	15	0	0
Kraft				
Sandwich Spread & Burger Sauce	1 tbsp (0.5 oz)	50	0	<5
Sweet'n Sour	2 tbsp (1.3 oz)	80	0	0
Tartar Sauce Nonfat	2 tbsp (1.1 oz)	25	tr	0
La Choy				
Duck Sauce Sweet & Sour	1 tbsp	25	tr	0
Sweet & Sour	1 tbsp	25	tr	0

FOOD	PORTION	CALS.	FIB.	CHOL.
Lawry's				
Teriyaki Marinade	2 tbsp	72	tr	0
Lea & Perrins				
Worcestershire	1 tsp	5	—	0
Worcestershire White Wine	1 tsp	4	—	0
Manwich				
Bold	¼ cup (2.2 oz)	62	1	0
Burrito	¼ cup (2.2 oz)	25	4	0
Mexican	¼ cup (2.2 oz)	27	1	0
Original	¼ cup (2.2 oz)	32	1	0
Taco	¼ cup (2.2 oz)	31	1	0
Thick & Chunky	¼ cup (2.3 oz)	44	1	0
Marzetti				
Teriyaki Stir-Fry	2 tbsp	80	0	0
McIlhenny				
7 Spice Chili	2 tbsp (1.1 fl oz)	16	1	tr
Sauce	2 tbsp (1.1 oz)	48	tr	tr
Tabasco	1 tsp	1	tr	tr
Mrs. Dash				
Steak	1 tbsp (0.4 oz)	17	—	0
Newman's Own				
Bandito Diavalo Spicy	4 oz	70	—	0
Old El Paso				
Enchilada Hot	¼ cup (2 oz)	30	0	0
Enchilada Mild	¼ cup (2 oz)	25	0	0
Green Chili Enchilada Sauce	¼ cup (2.1 oz)	30	0	0
Taco Hot	1 tbsp (0.5 oz)	5	0	0
Taco Medium	1 tbsp (0.5 oz)	5	0	0
Taco Mild	1 tbsp (0.5 oz)	5	0	0
Taco Sauce	1 tbsp (0.5 oz)	5	0	0
Taco Sauce Extra Chunky Medium	1 tbsp (0.5 oz)	5	0	0
Taco Sauce Extra Chunky Mild	1 tbsp (0.5 oz)	5	0	0
Ortega				
Taco Thick & Smooth Hot	1 tbsp	8	0	0
Taco Thick & Smooth Mild	1 tbsp	8	0	0
Taco Western Style	1 oz	8	—	0
Progresso				
Alfredo	½ cup (4.4 oz)	310	0	75
Red Wing				
Chili Sauce	1 tbsp (0.6 oz)	20	0	0
Seafood Cocktail	¼ cup (2 oz)	90	0	0
Sauce Arturo				
Original	¼ cup (2.2 fl oz)	50	0	0

FOOD	PORTION	CALS.	FIB.	CHOL.
Sauceworks				
Cocktail	¼ cup (2.3 oz)	60	tr	0
Sweet'n Sour	2 tbsp (1.2 oz)	60	0	0
Tartar	2 tbsp (1.1 oz)	100	0	10
Tartar Natural Lemon & Herb	2 tbsp (1 oz)	150	0	15
Simmer Chef				
Golden Honey Mustard	½ cup (4 fl oz)	150	1	0
Hearty Onion & Mushroom	½ cup (4 fl oz)	50	1	0
Trappey				
Indi-Pep West Indian Style Pepper Sauce	1 tsp (0.1 oz)	1	tr	0
Mexi Pep Louisiana Hot Sauce	1 tsp (0.1 oz)	tr	tr	0
Pepper Sauce	1 tsp (0.2 oz)	1	tr	0
Red Devil Buffalo Style Hot Sauce	1 tsp (0.1 oz)	1	tr	0
Red Devil Cayenne Pepper Sauce	1 tsp (0.1 oz)	1	tr	0
Worcestershire Chef Magic	1 tsp (0.1 oz)	3	tr	0
Watkins				
Beef Marinade	¼ tbsp (2 g)	5	0	0
Calypso Hot Pepper Sauce	1 tsp (5 g)	10	0	0
Caribbean Red Pepper Sauce	1 tsp (5 g)	10	0	0
Chicken & Pork Marinade	¼ tbsp (2 g)	5	0	0
Fish & Seafood Marinade	¼ tbsp (2 g)	10	0	0
Inferno Hot Pepper Sauce	2 tbsp (1 oz)	35	1	0
Meat Magic	1 tsp (6 g)	10	0	0
Steak Sauce	1 tbsp (0.5 oz)	20	0	0
MIX				
bearnaise as prep w/ milk & butter	1 cup	701	—	189
cheese as prep w/ milk	1 cup	307	—	53
curry as prep w/ milk	1 cup	270	—	35
mushroom as prep w/ milk	1 cup	228	—	34
sour cream as prep w/ milk	1 cup	509	—	91
stroganoff as prep	1 cup	271	—	38
sweet & sour as prep	1 cup	294	—	0
teriyaki as prep	1 cup	131	—	0
white as prep w/ milk	1 cup	241	—	34
Durkee				
A La King as prep	1 cup	60	0	0
Cheese as prep	¼ cup	25	0	2
Hollandaise as prep	2 tbsp	10	0	0
Nacho Cheese as prep	2 tbsp	25	0	0
White as prep	¼ cup	20	0	0

FOOD	PORTION	CALS.	FIB.	CHOL.
French's				
Cheese as prep	¼ cup	25	0	0
Hollandaise as prep	2 tbsp	10	0	0
Kikkoman				
Marinade For Meat	1 oz pkg	64	—	0
Sweet & Sour	2⅛ oz pkg	228	—	0
Teriyaki	1½ oz pkg	125	—	0
Weight Watchers				
Lemon Butter as prep	¼ cup	5	0	0

SAUERKRAUT
CANNED ½ cup 22 — 0

FOOD	PORTION	CALS.	FIB.	CHOL.
Claussen				
Canned	½ cup	17	—	0
Del Monte	½ cup (4.2 oz)	15	2	0
Eden				
Organic	½ cup (3.9 oz)	25	3	0
Hebrew National				
Gallon Kraut	½ cup	25	—	0
S&W				
Canned	½ cup	25	—	0
Seneca				
Canned	2 tbsp	5	1	0
SnowFloss				
Kraut	4 oz	28	1	0
Kraut Bavarian Style	4 oz	64	1	0
Vlasic				
Old Fashioned	1 oz	4	—	0

SAUERKRAUT JUICE
S&W

FOOD	PORTION	CALS.	FIB.	CHOL.
Juice	4 oz	14	—	0

SAUSAGE
(*see also* HOT DOG, SAUSAGE SUBSTITUTES)

FOOD	PORTION	CALS.	FIB.	CHOL.
bratwurst pork cooked	1 link (3 oz)	256	—	51
bratwurst pork	1 oz	92	—	18
bratwurst pork & beef	1 link (2.5 oz)	226	—	44
country-style pork cooked	1 patty (1 oz)	100	—	22
country-style pork cooked	1 link (½ oz)	48	—	11
italian pork cooked	1 (2.4 oz)	216	—	52
italian pork cooked	1 (3 oz)	268	—	65
kielbasa pork	1 oz	88	—	19
knockwurst pork & beef	1 (2.4 oz)	209	—	39
knockwurst pork & beef	1 oz	87	—	16

FOOD	PORTION	CALS.	FIB.	CHOL.
polish pork	1 (8 oz)	739	—	158
polish pork	1 oz	92	—	20
pork cooked	1 link (½ oz)	48	—	11
pork cooked	1 patty (1 oz)	100	—	22
smoked beef cooked	1 sausage (1.4 oz)	134	—	29
smoked pork	1 link (2.4 oz)	265	—	46
smoked pork	1 sm link (½ oz)	62	—	11
smoked pork & beef	1 link (2.4 oz)	229	—	48
smoked pork & beef	1 sm link (½ oz)	54	—	11
vienna canned	1 (½ oz)	45	—	8
vienna canned	7 (4 oz)	315	—	59
Aidells				
Andouille Cajun Cooked	1 (3.5 oz)	220	—	40
Burmese Curry Cooked	1 (3.5 oz)	220	—	20
Chicken & Apple Fresh	1 (1.9 oz)	110	—	20
Chicken & Apple Smoked	1 (3.5 oz)	220	0	30
Chicken & Turkey New Mexico Smoked	1 (3.5 oz)	220	—	40
Chicken & Turkey Thai Fresh	1 (3.5 oz)	200	—	35
Chicken & Turkey Thai Smoked	1 (3.5 oz)	220	—	30
Chicken & Turkey With Sun-Dried Tomatoes & Basil Fresh	1 (3.5 oz)	200	—	35
Chicken & Turkey With Sun-Dried Tomatoes & Basil Smoked	1 (3.5 oz)	200	—	30
Creole Hot Cooked	1 (3.5 oz)	220	—	30
Duck & Turkey Smoked	1 (3.5 oz)	220	—	60
Hunter's Cooked	1 (3.5 oz)	240	—	35
Italian Hot Fresh	1 (3.5 oz)	230	—	40
Italian Mild Fresh	1 (3.5 oz)	230	—	40
Lamb & Beef With Rosemary Fresh	1 (3.5 oz)	220	—	35
Lemon Chicken Cooked	1 (3.5 oz)	220	—	35
Mexican Chorizo Beef Fresh	1 (3.5 oz)	400	—	70
Whiskey Fennel Cooked	1 (3.5 oz)	230	—	65
Armour				
Vienna Sausage 25% Less Fat	3 (1.9 oz)	130	—	50
Vienna Sausage In BBQ Sauce	3 (2.1 oz)	160	—	45
Vienna Sausage In Beef Stock	3 (1.9 oz)	170	—	50
Vienna Sausage In Hot Sauce	3 (2.1 oz)	170	—	50
Vienna Sausage Smoked	3 (1.9 oz)	170	—	50
Banner				
Sausage Tripe	2 oz	90	—	85

FOOD	PORTION	CALS.	FIB.	CHOL.
Bilinski's				
Chicken & Vegetable	1 (3 oz)	80	tr	40
Chicken Italian With Peppers & Onions	1 (3 oz)	120	—	80
Golden Brown				
Beef	1	80	—	18
Mild	1	100	—	18
Spicy	1	100	—	18
Healthy Choice				
Low Fat Smoked	2 oz	70	1	25
Low Fat Smoked Polska Kielbasa	2 oz	70	1	25
Hebrew National				
Beef Knocks	1 (3 oz)	260	—	55
Polish Beef	1 link	240	—	50
Hormel				
Light & Lean 97 Dinner Smoked	2 oz	60	0	20
Pickled Hot	6 (2 oz)	140	0	40
Pickled Smoked	6 (2 oz)	140	0	40
Vienna	2 oz	140	0	45
Vienna Chicken	2 oz	90	0	55
Jimmy Dean				
Brick Sausage	2.5 oz	270	0	55
Bulk	2.5 oz	300	0	55
Hickory Smoked Dinner Sausage	2 oz	170	0	35
Pattie Pre-Cooked	1 (1.9 oz)	230	0	45
Polska Kielbaska	2 oz	170	0	35
Sage Pattie	1 (2 oz)	200	0	45
Sausage Pattie Raw	1 (2 oz)	200	0	40
Skinless Link	4 (2 oz)	200	0	45
Skinless Link	2 (2 oz)	200	0	45
Jones				
Brown & Serve Bacon	1	90	—	19
Brown & Serve Beef	1	90	—	18
Brown & Serve Light	1	60	—	16
Brown & Serve Regular	1	100	—	19
Cello Beef	1 slice (1 oz)	130	—	25
Cello Hot Country	1 slice (1 oz)	110	—	24
Cello Original	1 slice (1 oz)	100	—	24
Dinner Link	1	280	—	48
Golden Brown Light Links	1	60	—	16
Golden Brown Mild Pattie	1	150	—	29

FOOD	PORTION	CALS.	FIB.	CHOL.
Jones (CONT.)				
Italian	1	160	—	44
Light Link	1	70	—	21
Little Link	1	140	—	24
Patties	1	150	—	36
Scrapple	1 slice	90	—	24
Scrapple	1 slice (1½ oz)	90	—	24
Little Sizzlers				
Brown & Serve	2 patties (1.4 oz)	190	0	40
Brown & Serve	3 links (2.1 oz)	190	0	45
Cooked	3 links (1.4 oz)	210	0	45
Cooked	2 patties (2 oz)	250	0	50
Heat & Serve Pork cooked	3 links (1.4 oz)	210	0	45
Louis Rich				
Polska Kielbasa	2 oz	80	0	35
Smoked Sausage With Cheese cooked	1 (1 oz)	47	—	18
Turkey	2.5 oz	110	0	50
Turkey & Cheese Smoked	2 oz	90	0	35
Turkey Links	2 (2 oz)	90	0	45
Turkey Smoked	2 oz	90	0	35
Mr. Turkey				
Breakfast	2.5 oz	130	—	65
Hearty Blend Polish Kielbasa	1 oz	70	—	23
Hearty Blend Smoked	1 oz	70	—	23
Hot Smoked	1 oz	45	—	15
Italian Smoked	1 oz	45	—	15
Polish Kielbasa	1 oz	45	—	15
Smoked	1 oz	45	—	15
Old Smokehouse				
Summer Sausage	1 oz	110	0	30
Oscar Mayer				
Pork cooked	2 links (1.7 oz)	170	0	40
Smokies Beef	1 (1.5 oz)	120	0	25
Smokies Cheese	1 (1.5 oz)	130	0	30
Smokies Links	1 (1.5 oz)	130	0	25
Smokies Little	6 (2 oz)	170	0	35
Perdue				
Breakfast Links Turkey Cooked	2 links (2 oz)	100	—	45
Hot Italian Turkey Cooked	1 link (2.4 oz)	110	—	60
Sweet Italian Turkey Cooked	1 link (2.4 oz)	110	—	60
Rudy's Farm				
Italian Hot	2.5 oz	240	0	50
Italian Mild	2.5 oz	240	0	50

FOOD	PORTION	CALS.	FIB.	CHOL.
Rudy's Farm (CONT.)				
Italian Mild Natural Casing	1 (2 oz)	190	0	40
Morning Right Link	3 (2.9 oz)	150	0	40
Morning Right Pattie	2 (2.9 oz)	150	0	40
Pattie Pre-Cooked	1 (1.4 oz)	100	1	35
Smoked	4 (2.1 oz)	200	0	40
Sweet Link	1 (3.9 oz)	380	0	80
Shofar				
Knockwurst Beef	1 (3 oz)	260	0	50
Tyson				
Country Pork	3.5 oz	320	—	49
Wampler Longacre				
Breakfast Links	1 (2.8 oz)	170	—	20
Italian Links	1 (2.8 oz)	170	—	20
Tinderlings Garlic & Pepper	1 (3.5 oz)	143	—	55
Turkey	1 patty (2 oz)	120	—	60
Turkey	1 link (1 oz)	60	—	30
TAKE-OUT				
pork	1 link (0.5 oz)	48	—	11
pork	1 patty (1 oz)	100	—	22

SAUSAGE DISHES
FROZEN

Jimmy Dean				
Italian Sausage & Mozzarella Sandwich	1 (4.5 oz)	380	2	40

SAUSAGE SUBSTITUTES

LaLoma				
Linketts	2 (71 g)	140	—	0
Little Links	2 (46 g)	90	—	0
Lightlife				
Lean Links Breakfast	1.25 oz	69	—	0
Lean Links Italian	1.5 oz	83	—	0
White Wave				
Meatless Healthy Links	2 (1.6 oz)	140	3	0

SAVORY

ground	1 tsp	4	—	0

SCALLOP
FRESH

raw	3 oz	75	—	28
FROZEN				
Mrs. Paul's				
Fried	2 oz	160	—	10

FOOD	PORTION	CALS.	FIB.	CHOL.
HOME RECIPE				
breaded & fried	2 lg	67	—	19
TAKE-OUT				
breaded & fried	6 (5 oz)	386	—	107
SCONE				
apricot scone	1	232	—	34
Finnegan's				
Irish Raisin	1 (2.7 oz)	90	1	0
SCROD				
FROZEN				
Gorton's				
Microwave Entree Baked	1 pkg	320	—	80
SEA BASS				
(*see* BASS)				
SEA TROUT				
(*see* TROUT)				
SEAWEED				
agar dried	1 oz	87	—	0
agar fresh	1 oz	tr	—	0
irish moss fresh	1 oz	14	—	0
kelp fresh	1 oz	12	—	0
kombu fresh	1 oz	12	—	0
laver fresh	1 oz	10	—	0
nori fresh	1 oz	10	—	0
spirulina dried	1 oz	83	—	0
spirulina fresh	1 oz	7	—	0
tangle fresh	1 oz	12	—	0
wakame fresh	1 oz	13	—	0
Eden				
Agar Agar Bars	1 tbsp (2.5 oz)	10	2	0
Agar Agar Flakes	1 tbsp (2.5 oz)	10	2	0
Arame	½ cup (0.3 oz)	30	7	0
Hiziki	½ cup (0.3 oz)	30	6	0
Kombu	3.5 in piece (3.3 g)	10	1	0
Nori	1 sheet (2.5 g)	10	1	0
Sushi Nori	1 sheet (2.5 g)	10	1	0
Wakame	½ cup (0.3 oz)	25	4	0
Wakame Flakes	½ cup (0.3 oz)	25	4	0
Maine Coast				
Alaria	⅓ cup (7 g)	18	2	0
Dulse	⅓ cup (7 g)	18	2	0

FOOD	PORTION	CALS.	FIB.	CHOL.
Maine Coast (CONT.)				
Kelp	⅓ cup (7 g)	17	3	0
Kelp Crunch	1 bar (1 oz)	129	2	0
Kelp Crunch Peanut-Raisin	1 bar (1 oz)	129	2	0
Laver	⅓ cup (7 g)	22	3	0
Sea Seasoning Dulse	1 g	3	—	0
Sea Seasoning Dulse With Celery	1 g	3	—	0
Sea Seasoning Dulse With Garlic	1 g	3	—	0
Sea Seasoning Dulse With Sesame	1 g	3	—	0
Sea Seasoning Kelp	1 g	3	—	0
Sea Seasoning Kelp With Cayenne	1 g	3	—	0
Sea Seasoning Nori	1 g	3	—	0
Sea Seasoning Nori With Ginger	1 g	3	—	0

SEITAN
(*see* WHEAT)

SEMOLINA

dry	½ cup	303	3	0

SESAME

seeds	1 tsp	16	—	0
seeds dried	1 tbsp	52	—	0
seeds dried	1 cup	825	—	0
seeds roasted & toasted	1 oz	161	—	0
sesame butter	1 tbsp	95	1	0
sesame crunch candy	1 oz	146	—	0
sesame crunch candy	20 pieces (1.2 oz)	181	—	0
sesame sticks	1 oz	153	—	0
sesame sticks unsalted	1 oz	153	—	0
tahini from roasted & toasted kernels	1 tbsp	89	—	0
tahini from stone ground kernels	1 tbsp	86	—	0
tahini from unroasted kernels	1 tbsp	85	—	0
Arrowhead				
Sesame Tahini	1 oz	170	—	0
Casbah				
Tahini Sauce Mix as prep	¼ cup	160	tr	0
Eden				
Sesame Shake	½ tsp (1.5 g)	10	tr	0

FOOD	PORTION	CALS.	FIB.	CHOL.
Eden (CONT.)				
Sesame Shake Garlic	½ tsp (1.5 g)	10	tr	0
Sesame Shake Organic Seaweed	½ tsp (1.5 g)	10	tr	0
Erewhon				
Sesame Butter	2 tbsp (32 g)	190	—	0
Sesame Tahini	2 tbsp (32 g)	200	—	0
Joyva				
Tahini	2 tbsp (1 oz)	200	1	0
Planters				
Nut Mix	1 oz	150	2	0
Stone-Buhr				
Seeds Raw	4 tsp (1 oz)	180	1	0

SESBANIA
flower	1	1	—	0
flowers	1 cup	5	—	0
flowers cooked	1 cup	23	—	0

SHAD
roe raw	3½ oz	130	—	360

SHALLOTS
dried	1 tbsp	3	—	0
raw chopped	1 tbsp	7	—	0

SHARK
batter-dipped & fried	3 oz	194	—	50
raw	3 oz	111	—	43

SHELLFISH
(*see individual names*, SHELLFISH SUBSTITUTES)

SHELLFISH SUBSTITUTES
crab imitation	3 oz	87	—	17
scallop imitation	3 oz	84	—	18
shrimp imitation	3 oz	86	—	31
surimi	1 oz	28	—	8
surimi	3 oz	84	—	25
Louis Kemp				
Crab Delights Chunk Style	2 oz	54	—	10
Lobster Delights	2 oz	60	—	10
Maryland Style Cakes	2.5 oz	154	—	26
Ocean Magic				
Imitation King Crab	3 oz	80	—	15

SHELLIE BEANS
canned	½ cup	37	—	0

FOOD	PORTION	CALS.	FIB.	CHOL.
SHERBET				
(*see also* ICES AND ICE POPS)				
orange	½ cup (4 fl oz)	132	—	5
orange	½ gal	2158	—	113
orange	1 bar (2.75 fl oz)	91	—	3
orange home recipe	½ cup	120	—	9
Bresler's				
All Flavors	3.5 oz	140	—	6
Hood				
Lime Orange Lemon	½ cup (3.1 oz)	120	0	<5
Orange	½ cup (3.1 oz)	120	0	<5
Rainbow Swirl	½ cup (3.1 oz)	120	0	<5
Raspberry Orange Lime	½ cup (3.1 oz)	120	0	<5
Sealtest				
Lime	½ cup (3 oz)	130	0	5
Orange	½ cup (3 oz)	130	0	5
Rainbow Orange Red Raspberry Lime	½ cup (3 oz)	130	0	5
Red Raspberry	½ cup (3 oz)	130	0	5
SHRIMP				
CANNED				
canned	3 oz	102	—	147
canned	1 cup	154	—	222
FRESH				
cooked	3 oz	84	—	166
cooked	4 large	22	—	43
raw	4 large	30	—	43
raw	3 oz	90	—	130
FROZEN				
Gorton's				
Microwave Crunchy Shrimp	5 oz	380	—	65
Mrs. Paul's				
Entrees Light Seafood & Clams With Linguini	10 oz	240	—	40
Van De Kamp's				
Breaded Butterfly	7 (4 oz)	280	2	55
Breaded Popcorn	20 (4 oz)	270	1	35
Breaded Whole	7 (4 oz)	240	2	50
TAKE-OUT				
breaded & fried	3 oz	206	—	150
breaded & fried	6 to 8 (6 oz)	454	—	201
jambalaya	¾ cup	188	8	50

FOOD	PORTION	CALS.	FIB.	CHOL.
SMELT				
rainbow cooked	3 oz	106	—	76
rainbow raw	3 oz	83	—	60
SNACKS				
(*see also* CHIPS, FRUIT SNACKS, NUTS MIXED, POPCORN, PRETZELS)				
oriental mix	1 oz	155	—	0
pork skins	1 oz	154	—	27
pork skins barbecue	1 oz	152	—	33
trail mix	1 oz	131	—	0
trail mix	1 cup (5.3 oz)	693	—	0
trail mix tropical	1 oz	115	—	0
Bakem-ets				
Hot'N Spicy	21 pieces (1 oz)	150	—	25
Snacks	21 pieces (1 oz)	160	—	25
Big Dipper				
Bagel Chips Lowfat Barbeque	12 (1 oz)	110	1	0
Bagel Chips Lowfat Garlic	12 (1 oz)	120	1	0
Bagel Chips Lowfat Original	12 (1 oz)	110	1	0
Cheetos				
Cheddar Valley	26 pieces (1 oz)	160	1	0
Crunchy	26 pieces (1 oz)	150	1	0
Curls	15 pieces (1 oz)	150	1	0
Flamin' Hot	26 pieces (1 oz)	150	1	0
Light	38 pieces (1 oz)	140	1	0
Paws	16 pieces (1 oz)	160	1	0
Puffed Ball	38 pieces (1 oz)	160	1	0
Puffs	33 pieces (1 oz)	160	1	0
Chex				
Snack Mix Barbeque	½ cup (1.1 oz)	130	1	0
Snack Mix Cool Sour Cream And Onion	½ cup (1 oz)	130	2	0
Snack Mix Golden Cheddar	½ cup (1 oz)	130	1	0
Snack Mix Traditional	⅔ cup (1.2 oz)	150	2	0
Combos				
Cheddar Cheese Cracker	1 pkg (1.7 oz)	250	1	5
Cheddar Cheese Cracker	1 oz	140	0	5
Cheddar Cheese Pretzel	1 pkg (1.8 oz)	240	1	5
Cheddar Cheese Pretzel	1 oz	130	0	0
Chili Cheese w/ Corn Shell	1 oz	140	1	0
Chili Cheese w/ Corn Shell	1 pkg (1.7 oz)	230	2	5
Mustard Pretzel	1 pkg (1.8 oz)	230	1	0
Mustard Pretzel	1 oz	130	1	0
Nacho Cheese Pretzel	1 pkg (1.7 oz)	230	1	0

FOOD	PORTION	CALS.	FIB.	CHOL.
Combos (CONT.)				
Nacho Cheese Pretzel	1 oz	130	1	0
Nacho Cheese w/ Tortilla Shell	1 oz	140	1	0
Nacho Cheese w/ Tortilla Shell	1 pkg (1.7 oz)	230	1	0
Peanut Butter Cracker	1 oz	140	1	0
Pepperoni & Cheese Pizza	1 oz	140	0	5
Pepperoni & Cheese Pizza	1 pkg (1.7 oz)	240	1	5
Pizzeria Pretzel	1 pkg (1.8 oz)	230	1	0
Pizzeria Pretzel	1 oz	130	1	0
Tortilla Ranch	1 bag (1.7 oz)	240	1	5
Tortilla Ranch	1 oz	140	1	5
Cornnuts				
Barbecue	1 oz	120	2	0
Nacho Cheese	1 oz	120	2	0
Original	1 oz	120	2	0
Original	1 pkg (2 oz)	260	4	0
Picante	1 oz	120	2	0
Ranch	1 oz	120	2	0
Doo Dads				
Snacks	1 oz	130	—	0
Energy Food Factory				
Poprice Cheddar Cheese	½ oz	60	—	0
Poprice Herb & Garlic	½ oz	50	—	0
Poprice Lite	½ oz	50	—	0
Poprice Original No Salt	½ oz	45	—	0
Estee				
Snack Crisps Apple Cinnamon	1 pkg (0.66 oz)	90	tr	0
Snack Crisps Apple Cinnamon	27 crisps (1 oz)	130	1	0
Snack Crisps Chocolate	30 crisps (1 oz)	130	2	0
Snack Crisps Chocolate	1 pkg (0.66 oz)	90	1	0
Snack Crisps Lemon	1 pkg (0.66 oz)	90	tr	0
Snack Crisps Lemon	30 (1 oz)	130	tr	5
Snack Crisps Ranch	30 (1 oz)	130	tr	5
Snack Crisps Ranch	1 pkg (0.6 oz)	90	0	5
Snack Crisps White Cheddar	1 pkg (0.6 oz)	90	tr	5
Snack Crisps With Cheddar	27 crisps (1 oz)	130	tr	5
Frito Lay				
Corn Nuggets Toasted	1.38 oz	170	—	0
Funyums				
Onion Rings	11 pieces (1 oz)	140	1	0
Handi-Snacks				
Peanut Butter'n Crackers	1 pkg (1.1 oz)	180	1	0
Peanut Butter'n Grahamsticks	1 pkg (1.1 oz)	170	1	0

FOOD	PORTION	CALS.	FIB.	CHOL.
Hapi				
Chili Bits	½ cup (1 oz)	110	1	0
Health Valley				
Cheddar Lites	0.75 oz	40	tr	tr
Cheddar Lites With Green Onion	0.75 oz	40	tr	0
Innovative Foods				
Roasted Sweet Corn	1 pkg (0.8 oz)	76	2	0
Lance				
Cheese Balls	1 pkg (32 g)	190	—	5
Crunchy Cheese Twists	1 pkg (42 g)	260	—	0
Gold-N-Chees	1 pkg (39 g)	180	—	5
Pork Skins	1 pkg (14 g)	80	—	20
Pork Skins BBQ	1 pkg (14 g)	80	—	20
Mr. Peanut				
Peanut Butter Crisps Graham	12 pieces (1.1 oz)	150	2	0
Munchos				
Snack	16 pieces (1 oz)	160	—	0
Pita Puffs				
Barbeque	35 (1 oz)	120	1	0
Lowfat Garlic	35 (1 oz)	110	1	0
Lowfat Original	35 (1 oz)	110	1	0
Lowfat Salsa	35 (1 oz)	110	1	0
Pizza	35 (1 oz)	120	1	0
Ranch	35 (1 oz)	120	1	0
Planters				
Cheez Balls	1 oz	150	1	2
Cheez Balls	1 pkg (1 oz)	150	1	2
Cheez Curls	1 oz	150	1	2
Cheez Curls	1 pkg (1.2 oz)	190	1	2
Heat Snack Mix	1 oz	140	2	0
Snyder's				
Cheddar Cheese Twists	1 oz	150	—	0
Kruncheez	1 oz	160	—	0
Onion Toasters	1 oz	150	3	0
Snack Mix	1 oz	170	tr	0
Sopaipillas Apple & Cinnamon	1 oz	150	1	0
Splurge				
Snack Mix Fat Free Original	⅔ cup (1 oz)	100	tr	0
Ultra Slim-Fast				
Lite N' Tasty Cheese Curls	1 oz	110	3	0
Weight Watchers				
Cheese Curls	1 pkg (0.5 oz)	70	0	0
Pizza Curls	1 pkg (0.5 oz)	60	1	0

FOOD	PORTION	CALS.	FIB.	CHOL.
Weight Watchers (CONT.)				
Ranch Curls	1 pkg (0.5 oz)	60	1	0
SNAIL				
cooked	3 oz	233	—	110
raw	3 oz	117	—	55
SNAPPER				
cooked	3 oz	109	—	40
cooked	1 fillet (6 oz)	217	—	80
raw	3 oz	85	—	31
SODA				
(*see also* DRINK MIXERS, MINERAL/BOTTLED WATER, SPORTS DRINKS)				
club	12 oz	0	—	0
cola	12 oz	151	—	0
cream	12 oz	191	—	0
diet cola	12 oz	2	—	0
diet cola w/Equal	12 oz	2	—	0
diet cola w/ saccharin	12 oz	2	—	0
ginger ale	12 oz can	124	—	0
grape	12 oz	161	—	0
lemon lime	12 oz	149	—	0
orange	12 oz	177	—	0
pepper type	12 oz	151	—	0
quinine	12 oz	125	—	0
root beer	12 oz	152	—	0
tonic water	12 oz	125	—	0
7 Up				
Cherry	1 oz	13	—	0
Cherry Diet	1 oz	tr	—	0
Diet	1 oz	tr	—	0
Gold	1 oz	13	—	0
Gold Diet	1 oz	tr	—	0
Original	1 oz	12	—	0
After The Fall				
Raspberry Ginger Ale	1 can (12 oz)	150	0	0
Barrelhead				
Root Beer	8 fl oz	110	0	0
Burst				
Cola Strawberry	8 fl oz	117	—	0
Canada Dry				
Birch Beer Brown	8 fl oz	110	0	0
Birch Beer Clear	8 fl oz	110	0	0
Black Cherry Wishniak	8 fl oz	130	0	0

FOOD	PORTION	CALS.	FIB.	CHOL.
Canada Dry (CONT.)				
Cactus Cooler	8 fl oz	110	0	0
California Strawberry	8 fl oz	110	0	0
Club	8 fl oz	0	0	0
Club Sodium Free	8 fl oz	0	0	0
Concord Grape	8 fl oz	120	0	0
Diet Ginger Ale	8 fl oz	0	0	0
Diet Ginger Ale Cherry	8 fl oz	0	0	0
Diet Ginger Ale Cranberry	8 fl oz	0	0	0
Diet Ginger Ale Lemon	8 fl oz	5	0	0
Diet Tonic Water	8 fl oz	0	0	0
Diet Tonic Water Twist Of Lime	8 fl oz	0	0	0
Ginger Ale	8 fl oz	100	0	0
Ginger Ale Cherry	8 fl oz	110	0	0
Ginger Ale Cranberry	8 fl oz	100	0	0
Ginger Ale Golden	8 fl oz	100	0	0
Ginger Ale Lemon	8 fl oz	100	0	0
Half & Half	8 fl oz	110	0	0
Hi-Spot	8 fl oz	110	0	0
Island Lime	8 fl oz	140	0	0
Jamaica Cola	8 fl oz	110	0	0
Lemon Sour	8 fl oz	100	0	0
Peach	8 fl oz	120	0	0
Pina Pineapple	8 fl oz	110	0	0
Seltzer	8 fl oz	0	0	0
Seltzer Cherry	8 fl oz	0	0	0
Seltzer Cranberry Lime	8 fl oz	0	0	0
Seltzer Grapefruit	8 fl oz	0	0	0
Seltzer Lemon Lime	8 fl oz	0	0	0
Seltzer Mandarin Orange	8 fl oz	0	0	0
Seltzer Peach	8 fl oz	0	0	0
Seltzer Raspberry	8 fl oz	0	0	0
Seltzer Strawberry	8 fl oz	0	0	0
Seltzer Tropical	8 fl oz	0	0	0
Sunripe Orange	8 fl oz	140	0	0
Tahitian Treat	8 fl oz	150	0	0
Tonic Water	8 fl oz	100	0	0
Tonic Water Twist Of Lime	8 fl oz	100	0	0
Vanilla Cream	8 fl oz	120	0	0
Vichy Water	8 fl oz	0	0	0
Wild Cherry	8 fl oz	110	0	0
Clearly Canadian				
Soda	8 fl oz	0	—	0

FOOD	PORTION	CALS.	FIB.	CHOL.
Coca-Cola				
Cherry	8 fl oz	104	—	0
Classic	8 fl oz	97	—	0
Classic Caffeine-Free	8 fl oz	97	—	0
Coke II	8 fl oz	105	—	0
Diet	8 fl oz	1	—	0
Diet Cherry	8 fl oz	1	—	0
Diet Coke Caffeine-free	8 fl oz	1	—	0
Cott				
Cola	8 fl oz	110	0	0
Ginger Ale	8 fl oz	90	0	0
Grape	8 fl oz	130	0	0
Orange	8 fl oz	140	0	0
Pineapple	8 fl oz	130	0	0
Punch	8 fl oz	130	0	0
Seltzer	8 fl oz	0	0	0
Crush				
Cherry	8 fl oz	140	0	0
Grape	8 fl oz	110	0	0
Orange	8 fl oz	140	0	0
Orange Diet	8 fl oz	0	0	0
Pineapple	8 fl oz	140	0	0
Strawberry	8 fl oz	130	0	0
Tropical Fruit Punch	1 bottle (10 fl oz)	180	0	0
Tropical Fruit Punch	1 can (11.5 fl oz)	200	—	0
Diet Rite				
Black Cherry Salt/Sodium Free	8 fl oz	2	—	0
Cola	8 fl oz	1	—	0
Cola Caffeine/Sugar Free	8 fl oz	1	—	0
Cola Salt/Sodium Free	8 fl oz	1	—	0
Fruit Punch Salt/Sodium Free	8 fl oz	2	—	0
Golden Peach Salt/Sodium Free	8 fl oz	2	—	0
Key Lime Salt/Sodium Free	8 fl oz	7	—	0
Pink Grapefruit Salt/Sodium Free	8 fl oz	2	—	0
Red Raspberry Salt/Sodium Free	8 fl oz	3	—	0
Tangerine Salt/Sodium Free	8 fl oz	2	—	0
White Grape Salt/Sodium Free	8 fl oz	1	—	0
Dr Pepper				
Diet	1 oz	tr	—	0
Free	1 oz	12	—	0
Free Diet	1 oz	tr	—	0
Original	1 oz	13	—	0

FOOD	PORTION	CALS.	FIB.	CHOL.
Dr. Nehi				
Soda	8 fl oz	100	—	0
Fanta				
Ginger Ale	8 fl oz	86	—	0
Grape	8 fl oz	117	—	0
Orange	8 fl oz	118	—	0
Root Beer	8 fl oz	111	—	0
Fresca				
Soda	8 fl oz	3	—	0
Health Valley				
Ginger Ale	12 oz	153	0	0
Rootbeer Old Fashioned	12 oz	120	—	0
Sarsaparilla Rootbeer	12 oz	153	—	0
Wild Berry	12 oz	142	—	0
Hires				
Cream	8 fl oz	130	0	0
Cream Soda Diet	8 fl oz	0	0	0
Original Mocha	8 fl oz	100	0	0
Original Mocha Diet	8 fl oz	5	0	0
Root Beer	8 fl oz	130	0	0
Root Beer Diet	8 fl oz	0	0	0
Kick				
Soda	8 fl oz	120	—	0
Like				
Cola	1 oz	13	—	0
Cola Sugar Free	1 oz	tr	—	0
Lucozade				
Soda	7 oz	136	0	0
Manischewitz				
Seltzer No Salt Added No Calories	8 fl oz	0	—	0
Mello Yellow				
Diet	8 fl oz	4	—	0
Soda	8 fl oz	119	—	0
Minute Maid				
Berry	8 fl oz	111	—	0
Diet Orange	8 fl oz	2	—	0
Fruit Punch	8 fl oz	117	—	0
Grape	8 fl oz	121	—	0
Grapefruit	8 fl oz	108	—	0
Orange	8 fl oz	118	—	0
Peach	8 fl oz	110	—	0
Pineapple	8 fl oz	109	—	0
Raspberry	8 fl oz	111	—	0

FOOD	PORTION	CALS.	FIB.	CHOL.
Minute Maid (cont.)				
Soda	8 fl oz	110	—	0
Strawberry	8 fl oz	122	—	0
Mountain Dew				
Diet	8 fl oz	2	—	0
Soda	8 fl oz	118	—	0
Mr. PiBB				
Diet	8 fl oz	1	—	0
Soda	6 oz	97	—	0
Mug				
Cream	8 fl oz	122	—	0
Diet Cream	8 fl oz	2	—	0
Diet Root Beer	8 fl oz	1	—	0
Root Beer	8 fl oz	141	—	0
Nehi				
Cream	8 fl oz	120	—	0
Fruit Punch	8 fl oz	120	—	0
Ginger Ale	8 fl oz	90	—	0
Grape	8 fl oz	120	—	0
Orange	8 fl oz	130	—	0
Peach	8 fl oz	130	—	0
Pineapple	8 fl oz	130	—	0
Quinine Water	8 fl oz	90	—	0
Root Beer	8 fl oz	120	—	0
Strawberry	8 fl oz	120	—	0
Wild Red	8 fl oz	120	—	0
Old Colony				
Grape	8 fl oz	140	0	0
Orangina				
Sparkling Citrus	6 fl oz	80	—	0
Pepsi				
Caffeine Free	8 fl oz	105	—	0
Diet	8 fl oz	1	—	0
Diet Caffeine Free	8 fl oz	1	—	0
Regular	8 fl oz	105	—	0
Ramblin' Root Beer	8 fl oz	120	—	0
Razing Razberry				
Cola	8 fl oz	117	—	0
Royal Crown				
Caffeine Free Cola	8 fl oz	110	—	0
Cherry	8 fl oz	110	—	0
Cola	8 fl oz	100	—	0
Diet	8 fl oz	1	—	0
Diet Caffeine Free	8 fl oz	1	—	0

FOOD	PORTION	CALS.	FIB.	CHOL.
Royal Crown (CONT.)				
Diet Cranberry Apple Salt/Sodium Free	8 fl oz	2	—	0
Diet Cranberry Salt/Sodium Free	8 fl oz	2	—	0
Royal Mistic				
'N Juice Black Cherry	12 fl oz	146	—	0
'N Juice Peach Vanilla	12 fl oz	146	—	0
'N Juice Tangerine Orange	12 fl oz	146	—	0
'N Juice Tropical Supreme	12 fl oz	152	—	0
'N Juice Wild Berry	12 fl oz	156	—	0
Caribbean Fruit Punch	16 fl oz	230	—	0
Grape Strawberry	16 fl oz	230	—	0
Sparkling Diet With Lime Kiwi	11.1 fl oz	0	—	0
Sparkling Diet With Raspberry Boysenberry	11.1 fl oz	0	—	0
Sparkling Diet With Royal Peach	11.1 fl oz	0	—	0
Sparkling Diet With Wild Cherry	11.1 fl oz	0	—	0
Sparkling With Lime Kiwi	11.1 fl oz	112	—	0
Sparkling With Mandarin Orange Pineapple	11.1 fl oz	120	—	0
Sparkling With Mango Passion	11.1 fl oz	112	—	0
Sparkling With Raspberry Boysenberry	11.1 fl oz	112	—	0
Sparkling With Royal Peach	11.1 fl oz	112	—	0
Sparkling With Wild Cherry	11.1 fl oz	112	—	0
Schweppes				
Bitter Lemon	8 fl oz	110	0	0
Club	8 fl oz	0	0	0
Club Sodium Free	8 fl oz	0	0	0
Diet Ginger Ale	8 fl oz	0	0	0
Diet Ginger Ale Dry Grape	8 fl oz	2	0	0
Diet Ginger Ale Raspberry	8 fl oz	0	0	0
Ginger Ale	8 fl oz	90	0	0
Ginger Ale Dry Grape	8 fl oz	100	0	0
Ginger Ale Raspberry	8 fl oz	100	0	0
Ginger Beer	8 fl oz	100	0	0
Grape	8 fl oz	130	0	0
Grapefruit	8 fl oz	110	0	0
Lemon Sour	8 fl oz	110	0	0
Lemon-Lime	8 fl oz	100	0	0
Seltzer Black Berry	8 fl oz	0	0	0
Seltzer Lemon	8 fl oz	0	0	0

FOOD	PORTION	CALS.	FIB.	CHOL.
Schweppes (CONT.)				
Seltzer Lemon Lime	8 fl oz	0	0	0
Seltzer Lime	8 fl oz	0	0	0
Seltzer Orange	8 fl oz	0	0	0
Seltzer Peaches & Cream	8 fl oz	0	0	0
Seltzer Raspberry	8 fl oz	0	0	0
Tonic Citrus	8 fl oz	90	0	0
Tonic Cranberry	8 fl oz	90	0	0
Tonic Raspberry	8 fl oz	90	0	0
Tonic Water Diet	8 fl oz	0	0	0
Shasta				
Black Cherry	12 oz	162	—	0
Cherry Cola	12 oz	140	—	0
Citrus Mist	12 oz	170	—	0
Club	12 oz	0	—	0
Cola	8 oz	98	—	0
Cola	12 oz	147	—	0
Collins	12 oz	118	—	0
Creme	12 oz	154	—	0
Diet Birch Beer	12 oz	4	—	0
Diet Cola	8 oz	0	—	0
Diet Ginger Ale	8 oz	0	—	0
Diet Lemon Lime	8 oz	0	—	0
Dr. Diablo	12 oz	140	—	0
Free Cola	12 oz	151	—	0
Fruit Punch	12 oz	173	—	0
Ginger Ale	8 oz	80	—	0
Ginger Ale	12 oz	120	—	0
Grape	12 oz	177	—	0
Lemon Lime	12 oz	146	—	0
Lemon Lime	8 oz	97	—	0
Orange	12 oz	177	—	0
Red Berry	12 oz	158	—	0
Red Pop	12 oz	158	—	0
Root Beer	12 oz	154	—	0
Strawberry	12 oz	147	—	0
Tonic Water	12 oz	0	—	0
Slice				
Diet Lemon Lime	8 fl oz	5	—	0
Diet Mandarin	8 fl oz	5	—	0
Lemon Lime	8 fl oz	100	—	0
Mandarin Orange	8 fl oz	128	—	0
Red	8 fl oz	128	—	0

FOOD	PORTION	CALS.	FIB.	CHOL.
Snapple				
Amazin' Grape	8 fl oz	120	—	0
Cherry Lime Ricky	8 fl oz	110	—	0
Creme D'Vanilla	8 fl oz	130	—	0
French Cherry	8 fl oz	120	—	0
Kiwi Peach	8 fl oz	120	—	0
Kiwi Strawberry	8 fl oz	130	—	0
Mango Madness	8 fl oz	130	—	0
Passion Supreme	8 fl oz	120	—	0
Peach Melba	8 fl oz	120	—	0
Raspberry	8 fl oz	120	—	0
Seltzer Black Cherry	8 fl oz	0	—	0
Seltzer Lemon Lime	8 fl oz	0	—	0
Seltzer Original	8 fl oz	0	—	0
Seltzer Tangerine	8 fl oz	0	—	0
Tru Root Beer	8 fl oz	110	—	0
Sprite				
Diet	8 fl oz	3	—	0
Soda	8 fl oz	100	—	0
Sundrop				
Cherry	8 fl oz	130	0	0
Diet	8 fl oz	5	0	0
Soda	8 fl oz	140	0	0
Sunkist				
Cactus Cooler	8 fl oz	110	0	0
Cherry	8 fl oz	140	0	0
Diet Citrus	8 fl oz	0	0	0
Diet Orange	8 fl oz	5	0	0
Fruit Punch	8 fl oz	130	0	0
Orange	8 fl oz	140	0	0
Peach	8 fl oz	120	0	0
Pineapple	8 fl oz	140	0	0
Strawberry	8 fl oz	140	0	0
TAB				
Soda	8 fl oz	1	—	0
Tropical Chill				
Cola	8 fl oz	117	—	0
Diet	8 fl oz	1	—	0
Upper 10				
Diet	8 fl oz	3	—	0
Diet Salt/Sodium Free	8 fl oz	3	—	0
Salt Free	8 fl oz	100	—	0
Soda	8 fl oz	100	—	0

FOOD	PORTION	CALS.	FIB.	CHOL.
Welch's				
Sparkling Apple	12 oz	180	—	0
Sparkling Grape	12 oz	180	—	0
Sparkling Orange	12 oz	180	—	0
Sparkling Strawberry	12 oz	180	—	0
Wink				
Diet	8 fl oz	5	0	0
Soda	8 fl oz	130	0	0
Yoo-Hoo				
Original	9 fl oz	150	tr	0

SOLDIER BEANS
Bean Cuisine

Dried	½ cup	115	5	0

SOLE
FRESH

cooked	1 fillet (4.5 oz)	148	—	86
cooked	3 oz	99	—	58
raw	3½ oz	90	—	50

FROZEN
Gorton's

Microwave Entree In Lemon Butter	1 pkg	380	—	120
Microwave Entree In Wine Sauce	1 pkg	180	—	90
Mrs. Paul's				
Light Fillets	1 fillet	240	—	50
Van De Kamp's				
Lightly Breaded Fillets	1 (4 oz)	220	0	40
Natural Fillets	1 (4 oz)	110	0	50

TAKE-OUT

battered & fried	3.2 oz	211	—	31
breaded & fried	3.2 oz	211	—	31

SORBET
(*see* ICES AND ICE POPS)

SORGHUM

sorghum	½ cup	325	—	0

SOUFFLE
HOME RECIPE

grand marnier	1 cup	109	—	139
lemon chilled	1 cup	176	—	2
raspberry chilled	1 cup	173	—	3
spinach	1 cup	218	—	184

FOOD	PORTION	CALS.	FIB.	CHOL.

SOUP
CANNED

FOOD	PORTION	CALS.	FIB.	CHOL.
asparagus cream of as prep w/ milk	1 cup	161	—	22
asparagus cream of as prep w/ water	1 cup	87	—	5
beef broth ready-to-serve	1 can (14 oz)	27	—	1
beef broth ready-to-serve	1 cup	16	—	tr
beef noodle as prep w/water	1 cup	84	—	5
black bean turtle soup	1 cup	218	—	0
black bean as prep w/water	1 cup	116	—	0
celery cream of as prep w/ milk	1 cup	165	—	32
celery cream of as prep w/ water	1 cup	90	—	15
celery cream of not prep	1 can (10¾ oz)	219	—	34
cheese as prep w/ milk	1 cup	230	—	48
cheese as prep w/ water	1 cup	155	—	30
cheese not prep	1 can (11 oz)	377	—	72
chicken broth as prep w/ water	1 cup	39	—	1
chicken cream of as prep w/ milk	1 cup	191	—	27
chicken cream of as prep w/ water	1 cup	116	—	10
chicken gumbo as prep w/ water	1 cup	56	—	5
chicken noodle as prep w/ water	1 cup	75	—	7
chicken rice as prep w/ water	1 cup	251	—	7
clam chowder manhattan as prep w/ water	1 cup	77	—	3
clam chowder new england as prep w/ water	1 cup	95	—	5
clam chowder new england as prep w/ milk	1 cup	163	—	22
consomme w/ gelatin not prep	1 can (10½ oz)	71	—	0
consomme w/ gelatin as prep w/ water	1 cup	29	—	0
escarole ready-to-serve	1 cup	27	—	2
french onion as prep w/ water	1 cup	57	—	0
gazpacho ready-to-serve	1 cup	57	—	0
minestrone as prep w/water	1 cup	83	—	2
mushroom cream of as prep w/ milk	1 cup	203	—	20
mushroom cream of as prep w/ water	1 cup	129	—	2
oyster stew as prep w/ milk	1 cup	134	—	32
oyster stew as prep w/ water	1 cup	59	—	14
pepperpot as prep w/ water	1 cup	103	—	10

FOOD	PORTION	CALS.	FIB.	CHOL.
potato cream of as prep w/ milk	1 cup	148	—	22
potato cream of as prep w/ water	1 cup	73	—	5
scotch broth as prep w/ water	1 cup	80	—	5
split pea w/ ham as prep w/ water	1 cup	189	—	8
tomato as prep w/ milk	1 cup	160	—	17
tomato as prep w/ water	1 cup	86	—	0
vegetarian vegetable as prep w/ water	1 cup	72	—	0
vichyssoise	1 cup	148	—	22
American Original				
New England Chowder	4 oz	64	—	5
Campbell				
Chicken & Pasta With Garden Vegetables	1 cup (8.4 oz)	90	1	5
Healthy Request Bean With Bacon as prep	8 oz	140	—	5
Healthy Request Chicken Noodle as prep	8 oz	60	—	15
Healthy Request Chicken With Rice as prep	8 oz	60	—	10
Healthy Request Cream Of Chicken	8 oz	70	—	10
Healthy Request Cream Of Mushroom as prep	8 oz	60	—	<5
Healthy Request Hearty Chicken Vegetable	8 oz	120	—	20
Healthy Request Ready-To-Serve Chicken Broth	8 oz	10	—	0
Healthy Request Ready-To-Serve Hearty Minestrone	8 oz	90	—	<2
Healthy Request Ready-To-Serve Hearty Chicken Noodle	8 oz	80	—	25
Healthy Request Ready-To-Serve Hearty Chicken Rice	8 oz	110	—	20
Healthy Request Ready-To-Serve Hearty Vegetable	8 oz	110	—	0
Healthy Request Ready-To-Serve Hearty Vegetable Beef	8 oz	120	—	15
Healthy Request Tomato as prep	8 oz	90	—	0
Healthy Request Tomato as prep w/ skim milk	8 oz	130	—	<5
Healthy Request Vegetable as prep	8 oz	90	—	<5

FOOD	PORTION	CALS.	FIB.	CHOL.
Campbell (CONT.)				
Healthy Request Vegetable Beef as prep	8 oz	70	—	5
Ready-To-Serve Chunky Chicken Noodle	10¾ oz	200	—	25
College Inn				
Beef Broth	½ can (7 oz)	16	—	0
Chicken Broth	½ can (7 oz)	35	0	5
Chicken Broth Lower Salt	½ can (7 oz)	20	0	5
Gold's				
Borscht	8 oz	100	—	0
Borscht Lo-Cal	8 oz	20	—	0
Schav	8 oz	25	—	15
Gorton's				
New England Clam Chowder as prep w/ whole milk	¼ can	140	—	15
Goya				
Black Bean	7.5 oz	160	9	0
Hain				
Chicken Broth	8¾ fl oz	70	—	5
Chicken Broth No Salt Added	8¾ fl oz	60	—	5
Chicken Noodle	9½ oz	120	—	20
Chicken Noodle No Salt Added	9½ oz	120	—	25
Creamy Mushroom	9¼ fl oz	110	—	15
Italian Vegetable Pasta	9½ fl oz	160	—	20
Italian Vegetable Pasta Low Sodium	9½ fl oz	140	—	20
Minestrone	9½ fl oz	170	—	0
Minestrone No Salt Added	9½ fl oz	160	—	0
Mushroom Barley	9½ fl oz	100	—	10
New England Clam Chowder	9¼ fl oz	180	—	25
Split Pea	9½ fl oz	170	—	0
Split Pea No Salt Added	9½ fl oz	170	—	0
Turkey Rice	9½ fl oz	100	—	20
Turkey Rice No Salt Added	9½ fl oz	120	—	15
Vegetable Chicken	9½ fl oz	120	—	15
Vegetable Chicken No Salt Added	9½ fl oz	130	—	20
Vegetable Broth	9½ fl oz	45	—	0
Vegetable Broth Low Sodium	9½ fl oz	40	—	0
Vegetable Split Pea	9½ fl oz	170	—	0
Vegetable Split Pea No Salt Added	9½ fl oz	170	—	0
Vegetarian Lentil	9½ fl oz	160	—	5

FOOD	PORTION	CALS.	FIB.	CHOL.
Hain (cont.)				
Vegetarian Lentil No Salt Added	9½ fl oz	160	—	5
Vegetarian Vegetable	9½ fl oz	140	—	0
Vegetarian Vegetable No Salt Added	9½ fl oz	150	—	0
Health Valley				
Beef Broth	7.5 oz	10	0	1
Beef Broth No Salt Added	7.5 oz	10	0	1
Black Bean	7.5 oz	150	16	0
Black Bean No Salt Added	7.5 oz	150	16	0
Chicken Broth	7.5 oz	35	0	2
Chicken Broth No Salt Added	7.5 oz	35	0	2
Chunky Chicken Vegetable	7.5 oz	125	4	12
Chunky Five Bean Vegetable	7.5 oz	110	11	0
Chunky Five Bean Vegetable No Salt Added	7.5 oz	110	11	0
Chunky Vegetable Chicken No Salt Added	7.5 oz	125	4	12
Green Split Pea	7.5 oz	180	15	0
Green Split Pea No Salt Added	7.5 oz	180	15	0
Lentil	7.5 oz	220	10	0
Lentil No Salt Added	7.5 oz	220	10	0
Manhattan Clam Chowder	7.5 oz	110	2	15
Manhattan Clam Chowder No Salt Added	7.5 oz	110	2	15
Minestrone	7.5 oz	130	13	0
Minestrone No Salt Added	7.5 oz	130	13	0
Mushroom Barley	7.5 oz	100	9	0
Mushroom Barley No Salt Added	7.5 oz	100	9	0
Potato Leek	7.5 oz	130	7	0
Potato Leek No Salt Added	7.5 oz	130	7	0
Tomato	7.5 oz	130	1	0
Tomato No Salt Added	7.5 oz	130	1	0
Vegetable	7.5 oz	110	8	0
Vegetable No Salt Added	7.5 oz	110	8	0
Healthy Choice				
Bean & Ham	1 cup (8.7 oz)	184	10	5
Beef & Potato	1 cup (8.5 oz)	119	3	8
Chicken Corn Chowder	1 cup (8.8 oz)	176	2	8
Chicken Pasta	1 cup (8.6 oz)	118	1	6
Chicken With Rice	1 cup (8.4 oz)	108	1	6
Chili Beef	1 cup (9.1 oz)	166	5	10
Clam Chowder	1 cup (8.8 oz)	123	2	12

FOOD	PORTION	CALS.	FIB.	CHOL.
Healthy Choice (CONT.)				
Country Vegetable	1 cup (8.6 oz)	104	2	tr
Cream Of Chicken With Mushrooms	1 cup (8.9 oz)	127	1	8
Cream Of Chicken With Vegetables	1 cup (8.9 oz)	127	1	10
Cream Of Mushroom	1 cup (8.8 oz)	77	1	tr
Garden Vegetable	1 cup (8.6 oz)	118	3	tr
Hearty Chicken	1 cup (8.7 oz)	132	1	19
Lentil	1 cup (8.7 oz)	146	5	2
Minestrone	1 cup (8.6 oz)	112	3	2
Old Fashion Chicken Noodle	1 cup (8.8 oz)	137	1	9
Split Pea & Ham	1 cup (8.8 oz)	155	2	9
Tomato Garden	1 cup (8.6 oz)	106	3	1
Turkey With Wild Rice	1 cup (8.4 oz)	92	1	2
Vegetable Beef	1 cup (8.8 oz)	130	2	3
Hormel				
Bean & Ham	1 cup (7.5 oz)	190	7	25
Beef Vegetable	1 cup (7.5 oz)	90	2	10
Broccoli Cheese With Ham	1 cup (7.5 oz)	170	1	60
Chicken & Rice	1 cup (7.5 oz)	110	1	10
Chicken Noodle	1 cup (7.5 oz)	110	1	20
New England Clam Chowder	1 cup (7.5 oz)	130	1	25
Potato Cheese With Ham	1 cup (7.5 oz)	190	1	60
Manischewitz				
Borscht Low Calorie	8 fl oz	20	—	0
Borscht With Beets	8 fl oz	80	—	0
Schav	1 cup	11	—	0
Old El Paso				
Black Bean With Bacon	1 cup (8.6 oz)	160	7	5
Chicken Vegetable	1 cup (8.4 oz)	110	0	15
Chicken With Rice	1 cup (8.4 oz)	90	0	15
Garden Vegetable	1 cup (8.4 oz)	110	0	<5
Hearty Beef	1 cup (8.4 oz)	120	0	25
Hearty Chicken Noodle	1 cup (8.4 oz)	110	0	25
Pritikin				
Chicken & Rice	1 cup (8.8 oz)	80	—	5
Chicken Broth	1 cup (8.5 oz)	15	—	0
Chicken Pasta	1 cup (8.6 oz)	100	—	5
Hearty Vegetable	1 cup (8.8 oz)	90	—	0
Lentil	1 cup (8.4 oz)	130	—	0
Minestrone	1 cup (8.8 oz)	90	—	0
Split Pea	1 cup (9.2 oz)	140	—	0
Three Bean Chili	½ cup (4.5 oz)	90	—	0

FOOD	PORTION	CALS.	FIB.	CHOL.
Pritikin (CONT.)				
Vegetable Broth	1 cup (8.3 oz)	20	—	0
Vegetarian Vegetables	1 cup (9 oz)	100	—	0
Progresso				
Bean And Ham	1 cup (8.4 oz)	160	8	10
Beef	1 can (10.5 fl oz)	180	—	35
Beef Barley	1 cup (8.5 oz)	130	3	25
Beef Minestrone	1 cup (8.5 oz)	140	3	25
Beef Noodle	1 cup (8.5 oz)	140	1	30
Beef Vegetable & Rotini	1 cup (8 oz)	120	3	20
Broccoli & Shells	1 cup (8.5 oz)	70	3	<5
Chickarina	1 cup (8.3 oz)	120	1	20
Chicken & Wild Rice	1 cup (8.4 oz)	100	2	20
Chicken Barley	1 cup (8.5 oz)	110	3	15
Chicken Broth	1 cup ((8.2 oz)	20	0	5
Chicken Minestrone	1 cup (8.4 oz)	120	2	20
Chicken Noodle	1 cup (8.4 oz)	80	1	20
Chicken Noodle	1 can (10.5 oz)	110	1	25
Chicken Rice Vegetable	1 can (10.5 oz)	130	tr	20
Chicken Rice Vegetable	1 cup (8.4 oz)	110	tr	15
Chicken Vegetables & Penne	1 cup (8.4 oz)	100	3	10
Clam & Rotini Chowder	1 cup (8.8 oz)	200	0	10
Corn Chowder	1 cup (8.6 oz)	180	2	10
Cream Of Chicken	1 cup (8.4 oz)	170	0	35
Cream Of Mushroom	1 cup (8.4 oz)	140	1	20
Creamy Tortellini	1 cup (8.4 oz)	210	0	30
Escarole In Chicken Broth	1 cup (8.1 oz)	25	0	<5
Green Split Pea	1 cup (8.6 oz)	170	5	5
Healthy Classics Beef Barley	1 cup (8.5 oz)	140	3	20
Healthy Classics Beef Vegetable	1 cup (8.5 oz)	150	6	15
Healthy Classics Chicken Noodle	1 cup (8.3 oz)	80	1	20
Healthy Classics Chicken Rice With Vegetables	1 cup (8.4 oz)	90	1	10
Healthy Classics Cream Of Broccoli	1 cup (8.6 oz)	90	2	<5
Healthy Classics Garlic & Pasta	1 cup (8.5 oz)	100	3	<5
Healthy Classics Lentil	1 cup (8.5 oz)	120	1	0
Healthy Classics Minestrone	1 cup (8.5 oz)	120	1	0
Healthy Classics New England Clam Chowder	1 cup (8.6 oz)	120	1	5
Healthy Classics Split Pea	1 cup (8.9 oz)	180	5	<5
Healthy Classics Tomato Garden Vegetable	1 cup (8.6 oz)	100	4	0

FOOD	PORTION	CALS.	FIB.	CHOL.
Progresso (CONT.)				
Healthy Classics Vegetable	1 cup (8.4 oz)	80	1	5
Hearty Minestrone With Shells	1 cup (8.4 oz)	120	4	0
Hearty Black Bean	1 cup (8.5 oz)	170	10	<5
Hearty Chicken	1 can (10.5 fl oz)	120	0	25
Hearty Chicken & Rotini	1 cup (8.4 oz)	90	0	20
Hearty Penne In Chicken Broth	1 cup (8.4 oz)	70	0	<5
Hearty Tomato & Rotini	1 cup (8.4 oz)	90	3	5
Hearty Vegetable With Rotini	1 cup (8.4 oz)	110	3	0
Homestyle Chicken Vegetable	1 cup (8.4 oz)	100	1	15
Lentil	1 can (10.5 fl oz)	170	8	0
Lentil	1 cup (8.5 oz)	140	7	0
Lentil & Shells	1 cup (8.5 oz)	130	4	0
Lentil With Sausage	1 cup (8.5 oz)	170	5	15
Macaroni & Bean	1 cup (8.6 oz)	160	6	<5
Manhattan Clam Chowder	1 cup (8.4 oz)	110	3	10
Meatballs & Pasta Pearls	1 cup (8.3 oz)	140	0	15
Minestrone	1 can (10.5 fl oz)	170	6	0
Minestrone	1 cup (8.4 oz)	130	5	0
New England Clam Chowder	1 can (10.5 oz)	220	2	20
New England Clam Chowder	1 cup (8.4 oz)	180	2	15
Spicy Chicken & Penne	1 cup (8.5 oz)	120	0	20
Split Pea With Ham	1 cup (8.5 oz)	160	5	15
Tomato	1 cup (8.5 oz)	90	4	0
Tomato Beef & Rotini	1 cup (8.5 oz)	140	2	25
Tomato Tortellini	1 cup (8.4 oz)	120	2	10
Tortellini In Chicken Broth	1 cup (8.3 oz)	80	2	5
Vegetable	1 cup (8.4 oz)	90	3	<5
Zesty Minestrone	1 cup (8.3 oz)	150	4	10
Weight Watchers				
Chicken & Rice	1 can (10.5 oz)	110	4	10
Chicken Noodle	1 can (10.5 oz)	150	4	30
Minestrone	1 can (10.5 oz)	130	6	5
Vegetable	1 can (10.5 oz)	130	6	0
DRY				
asparagus cream of as prep w/ water	1 cup	59	—	tr
beef broth	1 pkg (0.2 oz)	14	—	1
beef broth as prep w/ water	1 cup	19	—	1
beef broth cube	1 cube (3.6 g)	6	—	tr
beef broth cube as prep w/water	1 cup	8	—	tr
celery cream of as prep w/ water	1 cup	63	—	1
chicken broth	1 pkg (0.2 oz)	16	—	1
chicken broth as prep w/water	1 cup	21	—	1

FOOD	PORTION	CALS.	FIB.	CHOL.
chicken broth cube	1 cube (4.8 g)	9	—	1
chicken broth cube, as prep w/ water	1 cup	13	—	1
chicken cream of as prep w/ water	1 cup	107	—	3
chicken noodle as prep w/ water	1 cup	53	—	3
french onion not prep	1 pkg (1.4 oz)	115	—	2
leek as prep w/ water	1 cup	71	—	3
onion as prep w/ water	1 cup	28	—	0
tomato as prep w/ water	1 cup	102	—	1
Armour				
Bouillon Cubes Beef	1 (4 g)	5	—	0
Bouillon Cubes Chicken	1 (4 g)	5	—	0
Arrowhead				
Bean & Barley	¼ cup (1.9 oz)	170	7	0
Bean Cuisine				
Bean Bouillabaisse	1 cup (7.5 fl oz)	174	5	0
Island Black Bean	1 cup (8.7 fl oz)	210	10	0
Lots of Lentil	1 cup (7.7 oz)	166	6	0
Mesa Maize	1 cup (9.2 fl oz)	179	6	0
Rocky Mountain Red Bean	1 cup (8.6 oz)	202	8	0
Santa Fe Corn Chowder	1 cup (9.2 oz)	179	6	0
Thick As Fog Split Pea	1 cup (8.6 fl oz)	189	1	0
Ultima Pasta E Fagioli	1 cup (8.6 fl oz)	179	4	0
White Bean Provencal	1 cup (7.7 fl oz)	166	6	0
Casbah				
Black Bean	1 pkg (1.7 oz)	170	9	0
Split Pea	1 pkg (2.3 oz)	230	10	0
Sweet Corn Chowder	1 pkg (1.2 oz)	125	2	0
Vegetarian Chili	1 pkg (1.8 oz)	170	7	0
Cup-A-Soup				
Chicken Vegetable as prep	1 pkg	50	0	10
Chicken Broth as prep	1 pkg	20	0	0
Chicken Noodle as prep	1 pkg	50	0	10
Cream Of Chicken as prep	1 pkg	70	0	0
Cream Of Mushroom as prep	1 pkg	60	0	0
Creamy Broccoli & Cheese as prep	1 pkg	70	1	<5
Green Pea as prep	1 pkg	110	3	0
Hearty Chicken Noodle as prep	1 pkg	60	0	10
Hearty Chicken Supreme as prep	1 pkg	90	tr	0
Hearty Harvest Vegetable as prep	1 pkg	90	2	0
Ring Noodle as prep	1 pkg	50	0	10

FOOD	PORTION	CALS.	FIB.	CHOL.
Cup-A-Soup (CONT.)				
Spring Vegetable as prep	1 pkg	50	1	10
Tomato as prep	1 pkg	90	1	<5
Virginia Pea as prep	1 pkg	130	3	0
Emes				
Beef Base	1 tsp	18	—	0
Chicken Base	1 tsp	18	—	0
Fantastic				
Cha-Cha Chili Low Fat	1 pkg	220	13	0
Golden Dipt				
Lobster Bisque	¼ pkg	30	—	2
Manhattan Clam Chowder	¼ pkg	80	—	3
New England Clam Chowder	¼ pkg	24	—	2
Seafood Chowder	¼ pkg	70	—	2
Shrimp Bisque	¼ pkg	30	—	2
Goodman's				
Cup Of Soup Beef	1 pkg (1½ cups)	180	2	45
Cup Of Soup Chicken Noodle	1 pkg (1½ cups)	180	2	45
Cup Of Soup Vegetable	1 pkg (1½ cups)	180	2	40
Matzo Ball & Soup	1 cup	40	1	0
Matzo Ball & Soup 50% Less Salt	1 serv	50	1	0
Noodleman	1 cup	45	0	10
Noodleman Low Sodium	1 cup	50	1	10
Onion	1 cup	30	1	0
Onion Low Sodium	1 cup	30	1	0
Herb-Ox				
Beef Bouillon	1 cube (3.5 g)	10	0	0
Beef Instant Bouillon Powder	1 tsp (4 g)	10	0	0
Beef Instant Broth & Seasoning Pack	1 pkg (4.5 g)	10	0	0
Beef Instant Broth & Seasoning Pack Low Sodium	1 pkg (4 g)	15	0	0
Chicken Bouillon	1 cube (4 g)	10	0	0
Chicken Instant Bouillon Powder	1 tsp (4 g)	10	0	0
Chicken Instant Broth & Seasoning Pack	1 pkg (5 g)	10	0	0
Chicken Instant Broth & Seasoning Pack Low Sodium	1 pkg (4 g)	15	0	0
Vegetable Bouillon	1 cube (4 g)	10	0	0
Hodgson Mill				
13 Bean not prep	1.5 oz	100	12	0

FOOD	PORTION	CALS.	FIB.	CHOL.
Hurst				
15 Bean Soup Beef	1 serv (1.7 oz)	160	1	0
15 Bean Soup Cajun	1 serv (1.7 oz)	160	9	0
15 Bean Soup Chicken	1 serv (1.7 oz)	160	1	0
15 Bean Soup Chili	1 serv (1.7 oz)	160	1	0
15 Bean Soup Ham	1 serv (1.7 oz)	160	1	0
Spanish-American Black Bean	1 serv (1.3 oz)	120	8	0
Ka-Me				
Won Ton Chicken not prep	1 pkg (1.25 oz)	180	1	0
Won Ton Pork not prep	1 pkg (1.25 oz)	180	1	0
Knorr				
Black Bean Cup-A-Soup as prep	1 pkg	200	9	0
Chicken Noodle Instant as prep	6 fl oz	25	—	5
Hearty Minestrone Cup-A-Soup as prep	1 pkg	150	1	2
Lentil Cup-A-Soup as prep	1 pkg	220	6	0
Navy Bean Cup-A-Soup as prep	1 pkg	140	5	0
Potato Leek Cup-A-Soup as prep	1 pkg	120	1	0
Vegetable Cup-A-Soup as prep	1 pkg	100	2	0
Kojel				
Hearty Potato With Vegetables Instant	1 serv (6 fl oz)	60	2	0
Noodle Soup Chicken Flavor Instant	1 serv (6 fl oz)	70	2	0
Split Pea Instant	1 serv (6 fl oz)	60	3	0
Tomato Instant	1 serv (6 fl oz)	50	1	0
Vegetable Chicken Couscous Instant	1 serv (6 fl oz)	80	2	0
Lipton				
Recipe Secrets Beefy Mushroom	2 tbsp	35	0	0
Recipe Secrets Beefy Onion	1 tbsp	25	0	0
Recipe Secrets Golden Herb With Lemon	2 tbsp	35	0	<5
Recipe Secrets Golden Onion	2 tbsp	60	0	0
Recipe Secrets Italian Herb With Tomato	2 tbsp	40	0	0
Recipe Secrets Onion	1 tbsp	20	tr	0
Recipe Secrets Onion Mushroom	2 tbsp	35	0	0
Recipe Secrets Savory Herb With Garlic	1 tbsp	35		0
Recipe Secrets Vegetable	2 tbsp	30	1	0

FOOD	PORTION	CALS.	FIB.	CHOL.
Lipton (CONT.)				
Soup Secrets Chicken Noodle	1 serv	80	0	15
Soup Secrets Extra Noodle	1 serv	90	tr	25
Soup Secrets Giggle Noodle	1 serv	80	0	15
Soup Secrets Hearty Chicken Noodle	1 serv	80	0	20
Soup Secrets Hearty Noodle With Vegetables	1 serv	70	tr	10
Soup Secrets Noodle With Chicken Broth	1 serv	60	0	15
Soup Secrets Ring-O-Noodle	1 serv	70	0	10
Soup Secrets Ruffle Pasta	1 serv	60	0	0
Manischewitz				
Minestrone as prep	6 fl oz	50	—	0
Split Pea as prep	6 fl oz	45	—	0
Vegetable as prep	6 fl oz	50	—	0
Maruchan				
Instant Lunch Oriental Noodles Beef	1 pkg (2.25 oz)	290	—	1
Instant Lunch Oriental Noodles Chicken	1 pkg (2.25 oz)	290	2	4
Instant Lunch Oriental Noodles Chicken Mushroom	1 pkg (2.25 oz)	280	—	0
Instant Lunch Oriental Noodles Mushroom	1 pkg (2.25 oz)	290	—	0
Instant Lunch Oriental Noodles Pork	1 pkg (2.25 oz)	290	—	0
Instant Lunch Oriental Noodles Shrimp	1 pkg (2.25 oz)	290	—	8
Instant Lunch Oriental Noodles Toast Onion	1 pkg (2.25 oz)	270	—	0
Instant Lunch Oriental Noodles Vegetable Beef	1 pkg (2.25 oz)	290	—	0
Instant Wonton Chicken	1 pkg (1.49 oz)	200	—	5
Instant Wonton Hot & Sour	1 pkg (1.49 oz)	200	—	0
Instant Wonton Oriental	1 pkg (1.49 oz)	190	—	0
Instant Wonton Pork	1 pkg (1.49 oz)	200	—	0
Instant Wonton Shrimp	1 pkg (1.49 oz)	200	—	10
Oriental Noodle Picante Style Beef	1 pkg (2.25 oz)	290	—	0
Oriental Noodle Picante Style Chicken	1 pkg (2.25 oz)	290	—	5
Oriental Noodle Picante Style Shrimp	1 pkg (2.25 oz)	300	—	5

FOOD	PORTION	CALS.	FIB.	CHOL.
Maruchan (CONT.)				
Ramen Beef	½ pkg (1.5 oz)	190	—	0
Ramen Chicken	½ pkg (1.5 oz)	190	—	0
Ramen Chicken Mushroom	½ pkg (1.5 oz)	190	—	0
Ramen Chili	½ pkg (1.5 oz)	190	—	0
Ramen Mushroom	½ pkg (1.5 oz)	190	—	0
Ramen Oriental	½ pkg (1.5 oz)	190	—	0
Ramen Pork	½ pkg (1.5 oz)	190	—	0
Ramen Shrimp	½ pkg (1.5 oz)	190	—	tr
Wonton Beef	⅓ pkg (0.68 oz)	90	—	0
Wonton Chicken	⅓ pkg (0.67 oz)	90	—	0
Wonton Pork	⅓ pkg (0.68 oz)	90	—	0
Wonton Vegetable	⅓ pkg (0.7 oz)	90	—	0
Morga				
Vegetable Bouillon No Salt Added	½ cube (5 g)	25	0	0
Vegetable Broth Fat Free	1 tsp (4 g)	10	0	0
Nile Spice				
Couscous Almondine	1 pkg	200	2	0
Couscous Garbanzo	1 pkg	220	2	0
Couscous Lentil Curry	1 pkg	200	4	0
Couscous Minestrone	1 pkg	180	2	0
Couscous Parmesan	1 pkg	200	2	10
Homestyle Black Bean	1 pkg	190	2	0
Homestyle Chicken Flavored Vegetable	1 pkg	120	4	5
Homestyle Lentil	1 pkg	180	3	0
Homestyle Minestrone	1 pkg	160	4	0
Homestyle Red Beans & Rice	1 pkg	190	3	0
Homestyle Split Pea	1 pkg	200	6	0
Homestyle Sweet Corn Chowder	1 pkg	120	0	0
Italian Tomato	1 pkg	140	2	10
Potato Leek	1 pkg	150	2	20
Potato Romano	1 pkg	140	3	15
Ultra Slim-Fast				
Beef Noodle	6 oz	45	2	5
Chicken Leek	6 oz	50	2	<2
Chicken Noodle	6 oz	45	2	5
Creamy Broccoli	6 oz	75	2	0
Creamy Tomato	6 oz	60	2	0
Hearty Vegetable	6 oz	50	2	0
Onion	6 oz	45	2	0
Potato Leek	6 oz	80	2	0

FOOD	PORTION	CALS.	FIB.	CHOL.
Weight Watchers				
Instant Beef Broth	1 pkg (0.16 oz)	10	0	0
Instant Chicken Broth	1 pkg (0.16 oz)	10	0	0
FROZEN				
Jaclyn's				
Barley & Mushroom	7.5 fl oz	90	—	0
Split Pea	7.5 fl oz	180	—	0
Vegetable	7.5 fl oz	90	—	0
Tabatchnick				
Barley Mushroom	1 serv (7.5 oz)	70	3	0
Barley Mushroom No Salt Added	1 serv (7.5 oz)	70	3	0
Broccoli Cream Of	1 serv (7.5 oz)	90	3	5
Cabbage	1 serv (7.5 oz)	60	2	0
Chicken With Dumplings	1 serv (7.5 oz)	70	1	20
Corn Chowder	1 serv (7.5 oz)	150	1	5
Minestrone	1 serv (7.5 oz)	150	10	0
New England Potato	1 serv (7.5 oz)	150	2	9
New York Chicken	1 serv (7.5 oz)	35	0	0
Old Fashion Potato	1 serv (7.5 oz)	70	2	0
Pea	1 serv (7.5 oz)	180	11	0
Pea No Salt Added	1 serv (7.5 oz)	180	11	0
Spinach Cream Of	1 serv (7.5 oz)	90	2	5
Vegetable	1 serv (7.5 oz)	110	4	0
Vegetable No Salt Added	1 serv (7.5 oz)	110	4	0
Wisconsin Cheddar Vegetable	1 serv (7.5 oz)	140	1	13
Yankee Bean	1 serv (7.5 oz)	160	11	0
SHELF-STABLE				
Lunch Bucket				
Chicken Noodle	1 pkg (7.25 oz)	90	—	25
Country Vegetable	1 pkg (7.25 oz)	70	—	0
TAKE-OUT				
beef stew soup	1 cup (8.8 oz)	221	—	60
black bean turtle soup	1 cup	241	—	0
brunswick stew soup	1 cup (8.5 oz)	232	—	71
corn & cheese chowder	¾ cup	215	3	66
gazpacho	1 cup	46	—	0
greek	¾ cup	63	2	83
hot & sour	1 serv (14 oz)	173	1	87
pasta e fagioll	1 cup (8.8 oz)	194	—	3
ratatouille	1 cup (7.5 oz)	266	—	0

SOUR CREAM
(*see also* SOUR CREAM SUBSTITUTES)

sour cream	1 cup (8 oz)	493	—	102

FOOD	PORTION	CALS.	FIB.	CHOL.
sour cream	1 tbsp (0.4 oz)	26	—	5
Breakstone				
Free	2 tbsp (1.1 oz)	35	0	<5
Half & Half	2 tbsp (1.1 oz)	45	0	15
Sour Cream	2 tbsp (1 oz)	60	0	25
Cabot				
Light	1 oz	33	—	7
Sour Cream	1 oz	60	—	13
Friendship				
Light	2 tbsp (1 oz)	35	0	10
Sour Cream	2 tbsp (1 oz)	60	0	20
Heluva Good Cheese				
Fat-Free	2 tbsp (1.1 oz)	20	0	0
Light	2 tbsp (1.1 oz)	40	0	10
Sour Cream	2 tbsp (1.1 oz)	60	0	20
Hood				
Fat Free	2 tbsp (1 oz)	20	0	0
Light	2 tbsp (1 oz)	40	0	10
Sour Cream	2 tbsp (1 oz)	60	0	20
Knudsen				
Free	2 tbsp (1.1 oz)	35	0	0
Hampshire	2 tbsp (1 oz)	60	0	25
Light	2 tbsp (1.1 oz)	40	0	10
Naturally Yours				
No Fat	2 tbsp (1 oz)	15	—	0
Sealtest				
Free	2 tbsp (1.1 oz)	35	0	<5
Light	2 tbsp (1.1 oz)	40	0	10
Sour Cream	2 tbsp (1 oz)	60	0	20

SOUR CREAM SUBSTITUTES

FOOD	PORTION	CALS.	FIB.	CHOL.
nondairy	1 cup	479	—	0
nondairy	1 oz	59	—	0
Pet				
Imitation	1 tbsp	25	—	tr
Tofutti				
Better Than Sour Cream Sour Supreme	1 oz	50	—	0

SOURSOP

FOOD	PORTION	CALS.	FIB.	CHOL.
fresh	1	416	—	0
fresh cut up	1 cup	150	—	0

SOY

(*see also* CHEESE SUBSTITUTES, ICE CREAM AND FROZEN DESSERTS, MILK SUBSTITUTES, MISO, SOY SAUCE, SOYBEANS, TEMPEH, TOFU, AND YOGURT FROZEN)

lecithin	1 tbsp	104	—	0

FOOD	PORTION	CALS.	FIB.	CHOL.
soy milk	1 cup	79	—	0
LaLoma				
Soyagen All Purpose	¼ cup	130	—	0
Soyagen Carob	¼ cup	140	—	0
Soyagen No Sucrose	¼ cup	130	—	0

SOY SAUCE

FOOD	PORTION	CALS.	FIB.	CHOL.
shoyu	1 tbsp	9	—	0
soy sauce	1 tbsp	7	—	0
tamari	1 tbsp	11	—	0
Eden				
Shoyu Organic	1 tbsp (0.5 oz)	15	0	0
Shoyu Traditional	1 tbsp (0.5 oz)	15	0	0
Tamari Organic Domestic	1 tbsp (0.5 oz)	15	0	0
Tamari Organic Imported	1 tbsp (0.5 oz)	15	0	0
House Of Tsang				
Dark	1 tbsp (0.6 oz)	10	0	0
Ginger Flavored	1 tbsp (0.6 oz)	20	0	0
Ginger Flavored Low Sodium	1 tbsp (0.6 oz)	10	0	0
Light	1 tbsp (0.6 oz)	5	0	0
Low Sodium	1 tbsp (0.6 oz)	5	0	0
Mushroom Flavored Low Sodium	1 tbsp (0.6 oz)	10	0	0
Ka-Me				
Chinese Dark	1 tbsp (0.5 fl oz)	10	0	0
Chinese Light	1 tbsp (0.5 fl oz)	5	0	0
Dark	1 tbsp (0.5 fl oz)	10	0	0
Japanese	1 tbsp (0.5 fl oz)	5	0	0
Light	1 tbsp (0.5 oz)	5	0	0
Mild	1 tbsp (0.5 fl oz)	5	0	0
Kikkoman				
Lite	1 tbsp	13	—	0
Soy Sauce	1 tbsp	12	0	0
La Choy				
Lite	½ tsp	1	tr	0
Soy Sauce	½ tsp	2	tr	0
Trappey				
Chef Magic	1 tbsp (0.5 oz)	23	tr	0
Tree Of Life				
Shoyu	1 tbsp (0.5 oz)	15	—	0
Tamari Reduced Sodium	1 tbsp (0.5 oz)	20	—	0
Tamari Wheat Free	1 tbsp (0.5 oz)	15	—	0

SOYBEANS

(*see also* MILK SUBSTITUTES, MISO, SOY, SOY SAUCE, TEMPEH, AND TOFU)

FOOD	PORTION	CALS.	FIB.	CHOL.
dried cooked	1 cup	298	—	0

FOOD	PORTION	CALS.	FIB.	CHOL.
dry-roasted	½ cup	387	—	0
green cooked	½ cup	127	4	0
honey toasted	¼ cup (1 oz)	130	0	0
roasted	½ cup	405	—	0
roasted & toasted	1 oz	129	—	0
roasted & toasted	1 cup	490	—	0
roasted & toasted salted	1 cup	490	—	0
roasted & toasted salted	1 oz	129	—	0
sprouts raw	½ cup	43	—	0
sprouts steamed	½ cup	38	—	0
sprouts stir fried	1 cup	125	—	0

SPAGHETTI
(see PASTA, PASTA DINNERS, PASTA SALAD, SPAGHETTI SAUCE)

SPAGHETTI SAUCE
(see also PIZZA, TOMATO)

JARRED

FOOD	PORTION	CALS.	FIB.	CHOL.
marinara sauce	1 cup	171	—	0
spaghetti sauce	1 cup	272	—	0
Classico				
Beef & Pork	4 fl oz	80	—	10
Four Cheese	4 fl oz	70	—	<5
Ripe Olives & Mushrooms	4 fl oz	50	—	0
Spicy Red Pepper	4 fl oz	50	—	0
Sweet Peppers & Onions	4 fl oz	50	—	0
Tomato & Basil	4 fl oz	60	—	0
Contadina				
Italian	¼ cup	15	1	0
Sauce	¼ cup	20	tr	0
Thick & Zesty	¼ cup	15	1	0
Del Monte				
Traditional	½ cup (4.4 oz)	80	tr	0
Traditional No Sugar Added	½ cup (4.4 oz)	60	tr	0
With Garlic & Onion	½ cup (4.4 oz)	70	tr	0
With Green Peppers & Mushrooms	½ cup (4.4 oz)	70	tr	0
With Meat	½ cup (4.4 oz)	40	tr	0
With Mushrooms	½ cup (4.4 oz)	80	tr	0
Eden				
Organic	½ cup (4.4 oz)	80	3	0
Organic No Salt Added	½ cup (4.4 oz)	80	3	0
Enrico's				
Fat Free Organic Basil	½ cup (4 oz)	50	4	0
Fat Free Organic Garlic	½ cup (4 oz)	50	5	0

FOOD	PORTION	CALS.	FIB.	CHOL.
Enrico's (CONT.)				
Fat Free Organic Hot Pepper	½ cup (4 oz)	50	5	0
Fat Free Organic Mushroom	½ cup (4 oz)	60	7	0
Fat Free Organic Traditional	½ cup (4 oz)	45	6	0
Healthy Choice				
Extra Chunky Garlic & Onion	½ cup (4.4 oz)	43	1	0
Extra Chunky Italian Vegetable	½ cup (4.4 oz)	39	1	0
Extra Chunky Mushroom	½ cup (4.4 oz)	41	1	0
Super Chunky Mushroom & Sweet Peppers	½ cup (4.4 oz)	44	1	0
Super Chunky Tomato, Mushroom & Garlic	½ cup (4.4 oz)	46	2	0
Super Chunky Vegetable Primavera	½ cup (4.4 oz)	46	1	0
Traditional	½ cup (4.4 oz)	47	2	0
With Meat	½ cup (4.4 oz)	47	2	2
Hunt's				
Chunky Marinara	½ cup (4.4 oz)	60	2	0
Chunky Tomato Garlic & Onion	½ cup (4.4 oz)	61	2	0
Chunky Vegetable	½ cup (4.4 oz)	63	2	0
Classic Garlic & Onion	½ cup (4.4 oz)	58	2	0
Classic Italian With Parmesan	½ cup (4.4 oz)	50	2	0
Classic Tomato & Basil	½ cup (4.4 oz)	48	4	0
Home Style With Meat	½ cup (4.4 oz)	56	2	2
Home Style With Mushrooms	½ cup (4.4 oz)	56	2	0
Homestyle Traditional	½ cup (4.4 oz)	56	2	0
Italian Cheese & Garlic	½ cup (4.5 oz)	65	2	1
Italian Sausage	½ cup (4.5 oz)	77	2	2
Old Country Garlic & Herbs	½ cup (4.4 oz)	63	3	0
Old Country Italian Style Vegetables	½ cup (4.4 oz)	64	3	0
Old Country Traditional	½ cup (4.4 oz)	53	3	0
Old Country With Meat	½ cup (4.4 oz)	56	3	tr
Old Country With Mushrooms	½ cup (4.4 oz)	53	3	0
Original Traditional	½ cup (4.4 oz)	65	4	0
Original With Meat	½ cup (4.4 oz)	65	2	3
Original With Mushrooms	½ cup (4.4 oz)	65	2	0
Mama Rizzo's				
Mushroom Onion	½ cup (4.3 oz)	60	1	0
Pepper Mushroom Onion	½ cup (4.3 oz)	60	1	0
Pepper Primavera Vegetable	½ cup (4.2 oz)	50	2	0
Pepper Tomato Basil Garlic	½ cup (4.7 oz)	60	1	0
Primavera Vegetable	½ cup (4.2 oz)	50	2	0
Tomato Basil Garlic	½ cup (4.6 oz)	60	2	0

FOOD	PORTION	CALS.	FIB.	CHOL.
Muir Glen				
Organic Cabernet Marinara	½ cup (4.4 oz)	45	2	0
Organic Chunky Style	½ cup (4.5 oz)	80	3	0
Organic Fat Free Tomato Basil	½ cup (4.3 oz)	50	2	0
Organic Garlic Onion	½ cup (4.3 oz)	50	3	0
Organic Garlic Roasted Garlic	½ cup (4.4 oz)	45	2	0
Organic Green Pepper & Mushroom	½ cup (4.5 oz)	70	4	0
Organic Italian Herb	½ cup (4.5 oz)	60	2	0
Organic Romano Cheese	½ cup (4.5 oz)	90	4	0
Organic Sun Dried Tomato	½ cup (4.4 oz)	40	2	0
Organic Sweet Pepper Onion	½ cup (4.4 oz)	40	1	0
Organic Tomato Basil	½ cup (4.3 oz)	50	2	0
Newman's Own				
Marinara	4 oz	70	—	0
Marinara With Mushrooms	4 oz	70	—	0
Sockarooni	4 oz	70	—	0
Pritikin				
Chunky Garden	½ cup (4 oz)	50	—	0
Marinara	½ cup (4 oz)	60	—	0
Original	½ cup (4 oz)	60	—	0
Progresso				
Marinara	½ cup (4.3 oz)	90	2	<5
Meat Flavored	½ cup (4.4 oz)	100	3	5
Mushroom	½ cup (4.4 oz)	100	4	<5
Sauce	½ cup (4.4 oz)	100	2	<5
Ragu				
Fino Italian Garden Medley	½ cup (4.5 oz)	90	2	0
Fino Italian Garlic & Basil	½ cup (4.5 oz)	90	2	0
Fino Italian Parmesan	½ cup (4.5 oz)	100	2	<5
Fino Italian Sliced Mushroom	½ cup (4.5 oz)	90	2	0
Fino Italian Tomato & Herb	½ cup (4.5 oz)	90	2	0
Fino Italian Zesty Tomato	½ cup (4.5 oz)	90	2	0
Gardenstyle Chunky Garden Combination	½ cup (4.5 oz)	120	3	0
Gardenstyle Chunky Green & Red Pepper	½ cup (4.5 oz)	120	2	0
Gardenstyle Chunky Mushroom & Green Pepper	½ cup (4.5 oz)	120	3	0
Gardenstyle Chunky Mushroom & Onion	½ cup (4.5 oz)	120	3	0
Gardenstyle Chunky Tomato Garlic & Onion	½ cup (4.5 oz)	120	3	0
Gardenstyle Super Mushroom	½ cup (4.5 oz)	120	3	0

FOOD	PORTION	CALS.	FIB.	CHOL.
Ragu (CONT.)				
Gardenstyle Super Vegetable Primavera	½ cup (4.5 oz)	110	4	0
Homestyle Mushroom	½ cup (4.5 oz)	120	3	0
Homestyle Tomato & Herb	½ cup (4.5 oz)	120	3	0
Homestyle With Meat	½ cup (4.5 oz)	130	3	<5
Light Chunky Mushroom	½ cup (4.4 oz)	50	2	0
Light Garden Harvest	½ cup (4.4 oz)	50	2	0
Light No Sugar Added	½ cup (4.4 oz)	60	3	0
Light Tomato & Herb	½ cup (4.4 oz)	50	2	0
Old World Style Marinara	½ cup (4.4 oz)	90	3	0
Old World Style Mushrooms	½ cup (4.4 oz)	80	3	0
Old World Style Traditional	½ cup (4.4 oz)	80	3	0
Old World Style With Meat	½ cup (4.4 oz)	90	3	<5
Sauce	4 fl oz	80	—	0
Thick & Hearty Mushroom	½ cup (4.5 oz)	120	3	0
Thick & Hearty Spaghetti Sauce	4 oz	100	—	0
Thick & Hearty Tomato & Herb	½ cup (4.5 oz)	120	3	0
Thick & Hearty With Meat	½ cup (4.5 oz)	130	3	<5
Tree Of Life				
Pasta Sauce	½ cup (4 oz)	50	—	0
Pasta Sauce Fat Free Classic	½ cup (3.9 oz)	40	0	0
Pasta Sauce Fat Free Mushroom & Basil	½ cup (3.9 oz)	30	0	0
Pasta Sauce Fat Free Onion & Garlic	½ cup (3.9 oz)	30	0	0
Pasta Sauce Fat Free Sweet Pepper	½ cup (3.9 oz)	30	0	0
Pasta Sauce No Salt	½ cup (3.9 oz)	50	—	0
Weight Watchers				
Pasta Sauce With Mushrooms	½ cup	60	4	0
MIX				
Durkee				
American Style as prep	½ cup	15	0	0
Family Style as prep	½ cup	20	0	0
Spaghetti Sauce as prep	½ cup	15	0	0
With Mushrooms as prep	½ cup	15	0	0
Zesty as prep	½ cup	20	0	0
French's				
All American as prep	½ cup	20	0	0
Italian as prep	½ cup	16	0	0
Mushroom as prep	½ cup	20	0	2
Thick as prep	½ cup	10	0	0

FOOD	PORTION	CALS.	FIB.	CHOL.
French's (CONT.)				
Zesty Pasta as prep	½ cup	20	0	0
REFRIGERATED				
Contadina				
Alfredo	½ cup (4.2 fl oz)	400	0	80
Four Cheese Sauce With White Wine & Shallots	½ cup (4.2 fl oz)	320	0	70
Light Alfredo	½ cup (4.2 fl oz)	190	0	40
Light Chunky Tomato	½ cup (4.4 fl oz)	45	3	0
Light Garden Vegetable	½ cup (4.4 fl oz)	45	3	0
Marinara	½ cup (4.4 fl oz)	80	2	0
Pesto With Basil	¼ cup (2 oz)	310	0	10
Pesto With Sun Dried Tomatoes	¼ cup (2 oz)	250	3	0
Plum Tomato With Basil	½ cup (4.4 fl oz)	70	3	0
Spicy Italian Sausage & Bell Pepper	½ cup (4.4 fl oz)	100	3	40
Di Giorno				
Alfredo	¼ cup (2.2 oz)	230	0	45
Four Cheese	¼ cup (2.2 oz)	200	0	45
Light Chunky Tomato With Basil	½ cup (4.5 oz)	70	2	0
Light Reduced Fat Alfredo	¼ cup (2.4 oz)	170	0	30
Marinara	½ cup (4.5 oz)	100	3	<5
Olive Oil & Garlic With Grated Cheese	¼ cup (2.1 oz)	370	0	20
Pesto	¼ cup (2.2 oz)	320	0	15
Plum Tomato & Mushroom	½ cup (4.4 oz)	70	2	0
Traditional Meat	½ cup (4.5 oz)	120	3	15

SPANISH FOOD

(*see also* BEANS, CHIPS, DINNER, PEPPERS, SALSA, SAUCE, SNACKS, TORTILLA)

CANNED

FOOD	PORTION	CALS.	FIB.	CHOL.
Chi-Chi's				
Picante Hot	2 tbsp (1 oz)	10	0	0
Picante Medium	2 tbsp (1 oz)	10	0	0
Picante Mild	2 tbsp (1 oz)	10	0	0
Pico De Gallo	2 tbsp (1.2 oz)	10	0	0
Derby				
Tamales	2	160	1	24
El Molino				
Green Chili Sauce Mild	2 tbsp	10	—	0
Gebhardt				
Enchiladas	2	310	2	58

FOOD	PORTION	CALS.	FIB.	CHOL.
Gebhardt (CONT.)				
Tamales	2	290	2	54
Tamales Jumbo	2	400	3	75
Guiltless Gourmet				
Picante Mild	1 oz	6	tr	0
Queso Mild Cheddar	1 oz	22	tr	tr
Hormel				
Tamales Beef	3 (7.5 oz)	280	3	35
Tamales Chicken	3 (7.5 oz)	210	2	50
Tamales Hot Spicy Beef	3 (7.5 oz)	280	3	35
Tamales Jumbo Beef	2 (6.9 oz)	270	3	35
Old El Paso				
Tamales	3 (7.2 oz)	330	5	30
Rosarita				
Enchilada Sauce Mild	2.5 oz	25	tr	0
Picante Chunky Hot	3 tbsp (2 fl oz)	18	tr	0
Picante Chunky Medium	3 tbsp (2 fl oz)	16	tr	0
Picante Chunky Mild	3 tbsp (2 oz)	25	tr	0
Van Camp's				
Tamales	2 (5.1 oz)	210	3	20
FROZEN				
Amy's Organic				
Enchilada Cheese	1 (4.7 oz)	210	2	20
Banquet				
Beef Enchilada	1 pkg (11 oz)	320	10	15
Chimichanga Meal	1 pkg (9.5 oz)	470	9	15
Enchilada Cheese	1 pkg (11 oz)	350	9	15
Enchilada Chicken	1 pkg (11 oz)	360	9	20
Family Entree Beef Enchilada w/ Cheese	1 serv (4.67 oz)	130	3	5
El Charrito				
Enchiladas 4 Grande Beef	1 pkg (16.5 oz)	890	—	65
Healthy Choice				
Beef Burrito Ranchero Medium	1 (5.4 oz)	290	6	15
Beef Burrito Ranchero Mild	1 (5.4 oz)	300	7	15
Beef Enchilada Rio Grande	1 meal (13.4 oz)	410	9	15
Burrito Chicken Con Queso	1 (5.4 oz)	280	5	10
Chicken Enchilada Supreme	1 meal (13.4 oz)	390	8	30
Enchiladas Suiza Chicken	1 meal (10 oz)	270	5	25
Fiesta Chicken Fajitas	1 meal (7 oz)	260	5	30
Jimmy Dean				
Burrito Breakfast Bacon	1 (4 oz)	260	1	70
Burrito Breakfast Sausage	1 (4 oz)	250	2	45

FOOD	PORTION	CALS.	FIB.	CHOL.
Le Menu				
Entree LightStyle Enchiladas Chicken	8 oz	280	—	35
Lean Cuisine				
Enchanadas Chicken	1 meal (9.9 oz)	220	4	30
Enchilada Suiza Chicken	1 meal (9 oz)	290	5	25
Life Choice				
Burrito Black Bean	1 meal (13.2 oz)	410	13	0
Vegetable Enchilada Sonora	1 meal (14 oz)	420	11	0
Lightlife				
Vegetarian Taco	2 oz	51	—	0
Old El Paso				
Burrito Bean & Cheese	1 (4.9 oz)	290	3	15
Burrito Beef & Bean Hot	1 (5 oz)	320	3	15
Burrito Beef & Bean Medium	1 (5 oz)	320	3	15
Burrito Beef & Bean Mild	1 (5 oz)	330	4	15
Chimichanga Beef	1 (4.5 oz)	370	3	10
Chimichanga Chicken	1 (4.5 oz)	350	2	20
Patio				
Burrito Bean & Cheese	1 (5 oz)	270	7	5
Burrito Chicken	1 (5 oz)	260	3	15
Burrito Red Chili	1 (5 oz)	270	6	10
Burritos Beef & Bean	1 (5 oz)	280	7	15
Burritos Beef & Bean Green Chili	1 (5 oz)	260	7	10
Burritos Beef & Bean Red Chili	1 (5 oz)	260	7	10
Enchilada Beef Dinner	1 meal (12 oz)	320	9	15
Enchilada Cheese Dinner	1 meal (12 oz)	330	10	15
Enchilada Chicken	1 pkg (12 oz)	380	9	25
Family Entree Beef Enchilada	2 (5.7 oz)	170	5	10
Family Entree Enchilada Beef	2 (5.3 oz)	250	8	15
Family Entree Enchilada Beef & Cheese	2 (5.3 oz)	250	9	20
Family Entree Enchilada Cheese	2 (5.7 oz)	170	4	10
Fiesta Dinner	1 meal (12 oz)	340	11	15
Mexican Dinner	1 meal (13.25 oz)	440	13	20
Salis Con Queso	1 pkg (11 oz)	390	10	40
Patio Britos				
Beef & Bean	10 (6 oz)	420	7	20
Nacho Beef	10 (6 oz)	410	5	20
Nacho Cheese	10 (6 oz)	360	3	15
Spicy Chicken	10 (6 oz)	400	3	25
Rudy's Farm				
Burrito Beef/Bean	1 (5 oz)	326	5	15
Burrito Hot Beef/Bean	1 (5 oz)	305	5	11

FOOD	PORTION	CALS.	FIB.	CHOL.
Senor Felix's				
Burrito Black Bean	1 (10 oz)	540	7	40
Burrito Black Bean Soy	1 (5 oz)	240	3	0
Burrito Chicken	1 (10 oz)	520	3	65
Burrito Hot Potato	1 (10 oz)	560	5	40
Burrito Soy Hot	1 (10 oz)	520	5	0
Burritos Charbroiled Chicken	1 + 4 tsp sauce (6.7 oz)	320	7	20
Burritos Sonora Style	1 + 4 tsp sauce (6.7 oz)	280	3	10
Burritos Yucatan Style	1 + 4 tsp sauce (6.7 oz)	310	5	10
Empanadas Chicken	1 (4.7 oz)	340	13	30
Empanadas Corn & Rice	1 (4.7 oz)	280	6	25
Empanadas Pumpkin & Mushroom	1 (4.7 oz)	260	6	25
Empanadas Spinach & Ricotta	1 (4.7 oz)	260	6	30
Enchilada Red Pepper	1 (10 oz)	420	8	25
Enchilada Soy Verde	1 (10 oz)	430	6	0
Enchilada Supreme Soy Cheese	1 (10 oz)	460	6	0
Enchilada Verde	1 (5 oz)	423	6	25
Tamales Blue Corn & Soy Cheese	2 + 4 tsp sauce (5.7 oz)	240	3	15
Tamales Chicken	2 + 4 tsp sauce (5.7 oz)	240	8	20
Tamales Gourmet Vegetarian	2 + 4 tsp sauce	240	8	20
Taquitos Blue Corn Soy	3 + 4 tsp sauce (5.2 oz)	230	3	0
Taquitos Chicken	2 + 4 tsp sauce (5.7 oz)	240	3	15
Stouffer's				
Cheese Enchilada	1 pkg (9.75 oz)	370	5	25
Chicken Enchilada	1 pkg (10 oz)	370	3	30
Today's Tamales				
Cheese & Chili	1 pkg (7 oz)	390	6	30
Del Sol	1 pkg (6.5 oz)	310	15	0
Original Bean	1 pkg (7 oz)	330	10	0
Spicy Taco	1 pkg (7 oz)	310	10	0
Weight Watchers				
Chicken Enchilada Suiza	1 pkg (9 oz)	250	4	25
Nacho Grande Chicken Enchiladas	1 pkg (9 oz)	290	4	20
MIX				
Gebhardt				
Menudo Mix	1 tsp	5	tr	0

FOOD	PORTION	CALS.	FIB.	CHOL.
Hain				
Taco Seasoning Mix	1/10 pkg	10	—	0
Old El Paso				
Burrito Seasoning Mix	2 tsp (6 g)	20	1	0
Dinner Kit Burrito as prep	1	280	3	66
Dinner Kit Soft Taco as prep	2	380	3	63
Dinner Kit Taco as prep	2	270	4	60
Enchilada Sauce Mix	2 tsp (4 g)	10	tr	0
Taco Mix 40% Less Sodium	2 tsp (6 g)	20	0	0
Taco Seasoning Mix	2 tsp (6 g)	20	0	0
Ortega				
Taco Meat Seasoning Mix Mild	1 filled taco	90	—	0
Quaker				
Masa Trigo	2 tortillas	149	1	0
READY-TO-EAT				
taco shell baked	1 med (1/2 oz)	61	tr	0
taco shell baked w/o salt	1 med (1/2 oz)	61	tr	0
Chi-Chi's				
Taco Shells White Corn	2 (1 oz)	130	2	0
Gebhardt				
Taco Shells	1	50	tr	0
Old El Paso				
Taco Shells Mini	7 (1.1 oz)	160	2	0
Taco Shells Regular	3 (1.1 oz)	170	2	0
Taco Shells Super	2 (1.3 oz)	190	2	0
Taco Shells White Corn	3 (1.1 oz)	170	2	0
Tostaco Shells	1 (0.8 oz)	130	1	0
Tostada Shells	3 (1.1 oz)	160	2	0
Rosarita				
Taco Shells	1 shell (11 g)	50	tr	0
Tostada Shells	1 shell (14 g)	60	tr	0
TAKE-OUT				
burrito w/ apple	1 lg (5.4 oz)	484	—	7
burrito w/ apple	1 sm (2.6 oz)	231	—	3
burrito w/ beans	2 (7.6 oz)	448	—	5
burrito w/ beans & cheese	2 (6.5 oz)	377	—	27
burrito w/ beans & chili peppers	2 (7.2 oz)	413	—	33
burrito w/ beans & meat	2 (8.1 oz)	508	—	48
burrito w/ beans cheese & beef	2 (7.1 oz)	331	—	125
burrito w/ beans cheese & chili peppers	2 (11.8 oz)	663	—	158
burrito w/ beef	2 (7.7 oz)	523	—	65
burrito w/ beef & chili peppers	2 (7.1 oz)	426	—	54
burrito w/ beef cheese & chili peppers	2 (10.7 oz)	634	—	170

FOOD	PORTION	CALS.	FIB.	CHOL.
burrito w/ cherry	1 sm (2.6 oz)	231	—	3
burrito w/ cherry	1 lg (5.4 oz)	484	—	7
chimichanga w/ beef	1 (6.1 oz)	425	—	9
chimichanga w/ beef & cheese	1 (6.4 oz)	443	—	51
chimichanga w/ beef & red chili peppers	1 (6.7 oz)	424	—	9
chimichanga w/ beef cheese & red chili peppers	1 (6.3 oz)	364	—	50
enchilada eggplant	1	142	—	7
enchilada w/ cheese	1 (5.7 oz)	320	—	44
enchilada w/ cheese & beef	1 (6.7 oz)	324	—	40
enchirito w/ cheese beef & beans	1 (6.8 oz)	344	—	49
frijoles w/ cheese	1 cup (5.9 oz)	226	—	36
nachos w/ cheese	6 to 8 (4 oz)	345	—	18
nachos w/ cheese & jalapeno peppers	6 to 8 (7.2 oz)	607	—	83
nachos w/ cheese beans ground beef & peppers	6 to 8 (8.9 oz)	568	—	21
nachos w/ cinnamon & sugar	6 to 8 (3.8 oz)	592	—	39
taco	1 sm (6 oz)	370	—	57
taco salad	1½ cups	279	—	44
taco salad w/ chili con carne	1½ cups	288	—	4
tostada w/ beans & cheese	1 (5.1 oz)	223	—	30
tostada w/ beans beef & cheese	1 (7.9 oz)	334	—	75
tostada w/ beef & cheese	1 (5.7 oz)	315	—	41
tostada w/ guacamole	2 (9.2 oz)	360	—	39

SPARE RIBS
(*see* PORK)

SPICES
(*see individual names*, HERBS/SPICES)

SPINACH
CANNED

FOOD	PORTION	CALS.	FIB.	CHOL.
spinach	½ cup	25	—	0
Del Monte				
50% Less Salt	½ cup (4 oz)	30	2	0
Chopped	½ cup (4 oz)	30	2	0
No Salt Added	½ cup (4 oz)	30	2	0
Whole Leaf	½ cup (4 oz)	30	2	0
Popeye				
Chopped	½ cup (4.1 oz)	40	4	0
Leaf	½ cup (4.2 oz)	45	4	0
Low Sodium	½ cup (4.2 oz)	35	3	0

FOOD	PORTION	CALS.	FIB.	CHOL.
S&W				
Northwest Premium	½ cup	25	—	0
Sunshine				
Chopped	½ cup (4.1 oz)	40	4	0
FRESH				
cooked	½ cup	21	2	0
mustard chopped cooked	½ cup	14	—	0
mustard raw chopped	½ cup	17	—	0
new zealand chopped cooked	½ cup	11	—	0
new zealand raw	½ cup	4	—	0
raw chopped	½ cup	6	1	0
raw chopped	1 pkg (10 oz)	46	—	0
Dole				
Spinach	3 oz	9	8	0
Fresh Express				
Spinach	1½ cups (3 oz)	40	5	0
FROZEN				
cooked	½ cup	27	—	0
Birds Eye				
Chopped	½ cup	20	3	0
Creamed	½ cup	90	1	15
Leaf	½ cup	20	3	0
Budget Gourmet				
Au Gratin	1 pkg (5.5 oz)	160	—	25
Green Giant				
Creamed	½ cup	70	—	2
Cut Leaf In Butter Sauce	½ cup	40	4	5
Harvest Fresh	½ cup	25	3	0
Spinach	½ cup	25	5	0
Stouffer's				
Creamed	½ cup (2.25 oz)	150	2	15
Souffle	½ cup (4 oz)	150	—	120
Tabatchnick				
Creamed	7.5 oz	60	2	5
TAKE-OUT				
indian saag	1 serv	28	1	0
spanakopita spinach pie	1 cup (6 oz)	196	4	30

SPINACH JUICE

juice	3½ oz	7	—	0

SPORTS DRINKS

(*see also* NUTRITIONAL SUPPLEMENTS)

Gatorade				
Citrus Cooler	1 cup (8 oz)	50	—	0

FOOD	PORTION	CALS.	FIB.	CHOL.
Gatorade (CONT.)				
Fruit Punch	1 cup (8 oz)	50	—	0
Grape	1 cup (8 oz)	50	—	0
Iced Tea Cooler	1 cup (8 oz)	50	—	0
Lemon-Lime	1 cup (8 oz)	50	—	0
Lemonade	1 cup (8 oz)	50	—	0
Orange	1 cup (8 fl oz)	50	—	0
Tropical Fruit	1 cup (8 oz)	50	—	0
PowerAde				
Fruit Punch	8 fl oz	72	—	0
Grape	8 fl oz	73	—	0
Lemon-Lime	8 fl oz	72	—	0
Orange	8 fl oz	72	—	0
Slice				
All Sport Diet Lemon Lime	8 fl oz	1	—	0
All Sport Lemon Lime	8 fl oz	72	—	0
All Sport Orange	8 fl oz	74	—	0
All Sport Punch	8 fl oz	81	—	0
Snapple				
Sport Fruit	1 bottle	80	—	0
Sport Lemon	1 bottle	80	—	0
Sport Lemon Lime	1 bottle	80	—	0
Sport Orange	1 bottle	80	—	0
Ultra Fuel				
Lemon Lime	16 fl oz	400	—	0
SQUAB				
breast w/o skin raw	1 (3.5 oz)	135	—	91
SQUASH				
(*see also* ZUCCHINI)				
CANNED				
crookneck sliced	½ cup	14	—	0
Allen				
Yellow	½ cup (4.2 oz)	25	2	0
Sunshine				
Yellow	½ cup (4.2 oz)	25	2	0
FRESH				
acorn cooked mashed	½ cup	41	3	0
acorn cubed baked	½ cup	57	2	0
butternut baked	½ cup	41	2	0
crookneck raw sliced	½ cup	12	1	0
crookneck sliced cooked	½ cup	18	1	0
hubbard baked	½ cup	51	3	0
hubbard cooked mashed	½ cup	35	3	0

FOOD	PORTION	CALS.	FIB.	CHOL.
scallop raw sliced	½ cup	12	1	0
scallop sliced cooked	½ cup	14	1	0
spaghetti cooked	½ cup	23	2	0
Nature's Pasta				
Spaghetti Squash	1 cup (5.5 oz)	20	2	0
FROZEN				
butternut cooked mashed	½ cup	47	3	0
crookneck sliced cooked	½ cup	24	—	0
Birds Eye				
Winter Cooked	½ cup	45	2	0
Southland				
Butternut	4 oz	45	—	0
SEEDS				
dried	1 oz	154	—	0
dried	1 cup	747	—	0
roasted	1 oz	148	—	0
roasted	1 cup	1184	—	0
salted & roasted	1 cup	1184	—	0
salted & roasted	1 oz	148	—	0
whole roasted	1 oz	127	—	0
whole roasted	1 cup	285	—	0
whole salted roasted	1 oz	127	—	0
whole salted roasted	1 cup	285	—	0

SQUID

FOOD	PORTION	CALS.	FIB.	CHOL.
fried	3 oz	149	—	221
raw	3 oz	78	—	198

SQUIRREL

FOOD	PORTION	CALS.	FIB.	CHOL.
roasted	3 oz	147	—	103

STAR FRUIT

FOOD	PORTION	CALS.	FIB.	CHOL.
fresh	1	42	—	0
Sonoma				
Dried	7-9 pieces (1.4 oz)	140	0	0

STRAWBERRIES
CANNED

FOOD	PORTION	CALS.	FIB.	CHOL.
in heavy syrup	½ cup	117	—	0
FRESH				
strawberries	1 cup	45	4	0
strawberries	1 pint	97	—	0
Dole				
Strawberries	8	50	3	0
FROZEN				
sweetened sliced	1 cup	245	—	0

FOOD	PORTION	CALS.	FIB.	CHOL.
sweetened sliced	1 pkg (10 oz)	273	—	0
unsweetened	1 cup	52	—	0
whole sweetened	1 cup	200	—	0
whole sweetened	1 pkg (10 oz)	223	—	0
Big Valley				
Strawberries	⅔ cup (4.9 oz)	50	2	0
Birds Eye				
Halved In Delicious Syrup	½ cup	120	2	0
Halved In Lite Syrup	½ cup	90	2	0
Whole In Lite Syrup	½ cup	80	2	0

STRAWBERRY JUICE
Juice Works
Drink	6 oz	100	—	0
Kern's				
Nectar	6 fl oz	110	—	0
Kool-Aid				
Strawberry	8 oz	98	—	0
Libby				
Nectar	1 can (11.5 fl oz)	210	—	0
Smucker's				
Juice	8 oz	130	—	0
Tang				
Strawberry	8.45 fl oz	121	—	0

STUFFING/DRESSING
HOME RECIPE
bread as prep w/ water & fat	½ cup	251	—	tr
bread as prep w/ water egg & fat	½ cup	107	—	75
MIX				
cornbread as prep	½ cup	179	—	0
Arnold				
All Purpose Seasoned	½ oz	50	1	0
Corn	½ oz	50	1	0
Herb Seasoned	½ oz	50	1	0
Sage & Onion	½ oz	50	1	0
Brownberry				
Corn	1 oz	103	2	0
Herb	1 oz	100	2	0
Sage & Onion	1 oz	97	2	0
Kellogg's				
Croutettes	1 cup (1.2 oz)	120	0	0
Stove Top				
Beef as prep	½ cup	178	—	tr
Chicken as prep	½ cup	176	—	1

FOOD	PORTION	CALS.	FIB.	CHOL.
Stove Top (CONT.)				
Chicken With Rice as prep	½ cup	182	—	1
Cornbread as prep	½ cup	175	—	tr
Flex Serve Chicken as prep	½ cup	173	—	1
Flex Serve Cornbread as prep	½ cup	181	—	tr
Flex Serve Homestyle Herb as prep	½ cup	173	—	1
Long Grain & Wild Rice as prep	½ cup	182	—	1
Select Wild Rice & Mushroom	½ cup	172	—	21
Wonder				
Seasoned Stuffing	1 cup (0.9 oz)	60	tr	0
TAKE-OUT				
bread	½ cup (3½ oz)	195	3	0
sausage	½ cup	292	1	12

SUCKER

white baked	3 oz	101	—	45

SUGAR

(*see also* FRUCTOSE, SUGAR SUBSTITUTES, SYRUP)

brown packed	1 cup (7.7 oz)	828	—	0
brown unpacked	1 cup (5.1 oz)	546	—	0
maple	1 piece (1 oz)	100	—	0
powdered	1 tbsp (0.3 oz)	31	—	0
powdered unsifted	1 cup (4.2 oz)	467	—	0
white	1 cup (7 oz)	773	—	0
white	1 packet (6 g)	25	—	0
white	1 tbsp	45	—	0
white	1 tsp (4 g)	15	—	0
C&H				
White	1 tsp	16	—	0
Domino				
White	1 tsp	16	—	0
Hain				
Turbinado	1 tbsp	50	—	0
Hollywood				
Turbinado	1 tbsp	50	—	0

SUGAR SUBSTITUTES

(*see also* FRUCTOSE)

Equal				
Packet	1 pkg	4	—	0
Mrs. Bateman's				
Sugarlike	1 tsp (4 g)	4	0	0
NatraTaste				
Packet	1 pkg (1 g)	0	—	0

FOOD	PORTION	CALS.	FIB.	CHOL.
S&W				
Liquid Table Sweetener	⅛ tsp	0	—	0
Sprinkle Sweet				
Sugar Substitute	1 tsp	2	—	0
Sweet One				
Packet	1 pkg (1 g)	4	—	0
Sweet'N Low				
Granulated	1 pkg (1g)	4	—	0
Sweet*10				
Granular	⅛ tsp	0	—	0
Weight Watchers				
Sweetener	1 measure (1 g)	5	0	0
SUGAR-APPLE				
fresh	1	146	—	0
fresh cut up	1 cup	236	—	0
SUNCHOKE				
fresh raw sliced	½ cup	57	—	0
SUNDAE TOPPINGS				
(*see* ICE CREAM TOPPINGS)				
SUNFISH				
pumpkinseed baked	3 oz	97	—	73
SUNFLOWER				
dried	1 oz	162	—	0
dried	1 cup	821	—	0
dry roasted	1 oz	165	—	0
dry roasted	1 cup	745	—	0
dry roasted salted	1 oz	165	—	0
dry roasted salted	1 cup	745	—	0
oil roasted	1 cup	830	—	0
oil roasted salted	1 cup	830	—	0
oil roasted salted	1 oz	175	—	0
sunflower butter	1 tbsp	93	—	0
sunflower butter w/o salt	1 tbsp	93	—	0
toasted	1 oz	176	—	0
toasted	1 cup	826	—	0
toasted salted	1 oz	176	—	0
toasted salted	1 cup	826	—	0
Fisher				
Seeds Oil Roasted	1 oz	170	—	0
Seeds Salted In Shell shelled	1 oz	160	—	0
Seeds Salted In Shell unshelled	1 oz	170	—	0

FOOD	PORTION	CALS.	FIB.	CHOL.
Frito Lay				
Seeds	1 oz	160	—	0
Planters				
Kernels	1 pkg (2 oz)	340	8	0
Kernels	1 pkg (1.7 oz)	290	7	0
Kernels Barbecue	1 pkg (1.7 oz)	290	6	0
Kernels Honey Roasted	1 pkg (1.7 oz)	280	6	0
Kernels Salted	1 oz	170	4	0
Munch'N Go Singles Dry Roasted	1 pkg	120	1	0
Nuts Dry Roasted	¼ cup (1.1 oz)	190	4	0
Original With Shell Dry Roasted	¾ cup	160	2	0
Stone-Buhr				
Seeds Raw	4 tsp (1 oz)	170	6	0

SUSHI
TAKE-OUT

california roll	1 piece (0.8 oz)	28	—	1
kim chi	⅓ cup (5.8 oz)	18	—	0
sashimi	1 serv (6 oz)	198	—	63
tuna roll	1 piece (0.7 oz)	23	—	3
vegetable roll	1 piece (1.2 oz)	27	—	0
vinegared ginger	⅓ cup (1.6 oz)	48	—	0
wasabi	2 tsp (0.3 oz)	5	—	0
yellowtail roll	1 piece (0.6 oz)	25	—	0

SWAMP CABBAGE

chopped cooked	½ cup	10	—	0
raw chopped	1 cup	11	—	0

SWEET POTATO
(*see also* YAM)
CANNED

in syrup	½ cup	106	—	0
pieces	1 cup	183	—	0
Princella				
Mashed	⅔ cup (5.1 oz)	120	3	0
Royal Prince				
Candied	½ cup (4.9 oz)	210	2	0
Halves	3 pieces (5.7 oz)	190	4	0
Orange Pineapple	½ cup (4.8 oz)	210	3	0
Sugary Sam				
Mashed	⅔ cup (5.1 oz)	120	3	0
FRESH				
baked w/ skin	1 (3½ oz)	118	3	0

FOOD	PORTION	CALS.	FIB.	CHOL.
leaves cooked	½ cup	11	—	0
mashed	½ cup	172	3	0
FROZEN				
cooked	½ cup	88	—	0
TAKE-OUT				
candied	3½ oz	144	—	0

SWEETBREADS
lamb braised	3 oz	199	—	340

SWISS CHARD
cooked	½ cup	18	—	0
raw chopped	½ cup	3	—	0

SWORDFISH
cooked	3 oz	132	—	43
raw	3 oz	103	—	33

SYRUP
(*see also* ICE CREAM TOPPINGS, PANCAKE/WAFFLE SYRUP)

corn	2 tbsp	122	—	0
corn dark	1 cup (11.5 oz)	925	—	0
corn dark	1 tbsp (0.7 oz)	56	—	0
corn light	1 tbsp (0.7 oz)	56	—	0
corn light	1 cup (11.5 oz)	925	—	0
malt	1 tbsp (0.8 oz)	76	—	0
malt	1 cup (13 oz)	1222	—	0
maple	1 tbsp (0.8 oz)	52	—	0
maple	1 cup (11.1 oz)	824	—	0
raspberry	3.5 oz	267	—	0
sorghum	1 tbsp (0.7 oz)	61	—	0
sorghum	1 cup (11.6 oz)	957	—	0
Eden				
Barley Malt Organic Syrup	1 tbsp (0.7 fl oz)	60	0	0
Estee				
Blueberry Lite	¼ cup (2.4 oz)	80	—	0
Home Brands				
Maple Rich	1 oz	110	—	0
Karo				
Corn Syrup Dark	1 tbsp (21 g)	60	—	0
Corn Syrup Dark	1 cup (331 g)	975	—	0
Corn Syrup Light	1 tbsp (21 g)	60	—	0
Corn Syrup Light	1 cup (331 g)	960	—	0
McIlhenny				
Cane	2 tbsp (1.4 oz)	130	tr	0

FOOD	PORTION	CALS.	FIB.	CHOL.
Red Wing				
Strawberry	2 tbsp (1.4 oz)	110	0	0
S&W				
Blueberry Diet	1 tbsp	4	—	0
Maple Flavored Diet	1 tbsp	4	—	0
Strawberry Diet	1 tbsp	4	—	0
Smucker's				
All Flavors Fruit Syrup	2 tbsp	100	—	0
Tree Of Life				
Maple	¼ cup (2.1 oz)	200	—	0

TACO
(*see* SPANISH FOOD)

TAHINI
(*see* SESAME)

TAMARIND

fresh	1	5	—	0
fresh cut up	1 cup	287	—	0

TANGERINE
CANNED

in light syrup	½ cup	76	—	0
juice pack	½ cup	46	—	0
FRESH				
sections	1 cup	86	—	0
tangerine	1	37	—	0
Dole				
Tangerine	2	70	2	0

TANGERINE JUICE

canned sweetened	1 cup	125	—	0
fresh	1 cup	106	—	0
frzn sweetened as prep	1 cup	110	—	0
frzn sweetened not prep	6 oz	344	—	0
After The Fall				
Juice	1 can (12 oz)	170	0	0
Dole				
Mandarin frzn as prep	8 fl oz	140	0	0
Fresh Samantha				
Fresh Juice	1 cup (8 oz)	106	1	0
Minute Maid				
Frozen	8 fl oz	120	—	0

TAPIOCA

pearl dry	⅓ cup	174	1	0

FOOD	PORTION	CALS.	FIB.	CHOL.
General Foods				
Minute Tapioca	1 tbsp	32	—	0
TARO				
chips	1 oz	141	—	0
chips	10 (0.8 oz)	115	—	0
leaves cooked	½ cup	18	—	0
raw sliced	½ cup	56	—	0
shoots sliced cooked	½ cup	10	—	0
sliced cooked	½ cup (2.3 oz)	94	—	0
tahitian sliced cooked	½ cup	30	—	0
TARRAGON				
ground	1 tsp	5	—	0
TEA/HERBAL TEA				
(*see also* ICED TEA)				
HERBAL				
Bigelow				
Almond Orange	5 fl oz	tr	—	0
Apple Orchard	5 fl oz	5	—	0
Apple Spice	5 fl oz	tr	—	0
Chamomile	5 fl oz	tr	—	0
Chamomile Mint	5 fl oz	tr	—	0
Cinnamon Orange	5 fl oz	tr	—	0
Early Riser	5 fl oz	3	—	0
Feeling Free	5 fl oz	1	—	0
Fruit & Almond	5 fl oz	1	—	0
Hibiscus & Rose Hips	5 fl oz	1	—	0
I Love Lemon	5 fl oz	1	—	0
Lemon & C	5 fl oz	tr	—	0
Looking Good	5 fl oz	1	—	0
Mint Blend	5 fl oz	tr	—	0
Mint Medley	5 fl oz	1	—	0
Orange & C	5 fl oz	tr	—	0
Orange & Spice	5 fl oz	1	—	0
Peppermint	5 fl oz	tr	—	0
Roasted Grains & Carob	5 fl oz	3	—	0
Spearmint	5 fl oz	tr	—	0
Sweet Dreams	5 fl oz	1	—	0
Take-A-Break	5 fl oz	3	—	0
Celestial Seasonings				
Almond Sunset	8 fl oz	3	—	0
Bengal Spice	8 fl oz	5	—	0
Caffeine Free	8 fl oz	2	—	0

FOOD	PORTION	CALS.	FIB.	CHOL.
Celestial Seasonings (CONT.)				
Chamomile	8 fl oz	2	—	0
Cinnamon Apple Spice	8 fl oz	<3	—	0
Cinnamon Rose	8 fl oz	<4	—	0
Country Peach Spice	8 fl oz	3	—	0
Cranberry Cove	8 fl oz	2	—	0
Emperor's Choice	8 fl oz	4	—	0
Ginseng Plus	8 fl oz	3	—	0
Grandma's Tummy Mint	8 fl oz	2	—	0
Lemon Mist	8 fl oz	3	—	0
Lemon Zinger	8 fl oz	4	—	0
Mama Bear's Cold Care	8 fl oz	6	—	0
Mandarin Orange Spice	8 fl oz	5	—	0
Mellow Mint	8 fl oz	2	—	0
Mint Magic	8 fl oz	1	—	0
Orange Zinger	8 fl oz	6	—	0
Peppermint	8 fl oz	2	—	0
Raspberry Patch	8 fl oz	4	—	0
Red Zinger	8 fl oz	4	—	0
Roastaroma	8 fl oz	10	—	0
Sleepytime	8 fl oz	4	—	0
Spearmint	8 fl oz	5	—	0
Strawberry Fields	8 fl oz	4	—	0
Sunburst C	8 fl oz	3	—	0
Tropical Escape	8 fl oz	1	—	0
Wild Forest Blackberry	8 fl oz	2	—	0
Lipton				
Tea Bag Almond Pleasure as prep	1 cup	0	0	0
Tea Bag Cinnamon Apple as prep	1 cup	0	0	0
Tea Bag Cinnamon Spice as prep	1 cup	0	0	0
Tea Bag Country Cranberry as prep	1 cup	0	0	0
Tea Bag Gentle Orange as prep	1 cup	0	0	0
Tea Bag Ginger Twist as prep	1 cup	0	0	0
Tea Bag Golden Honey & Lemon as prep	1 cup	0	0	0
Tea Bag Lemon Mint Refresher as prep	1 cup	0	0	0
Tea Bag Lemon Smoother as prep	1 cup	0	0	0
Tea Bag Moonlight Mint as prep	1 cup	0	0	0

FOOD	PORTION	CALS.	FIB.	CHOL.
Lipton (CONT.)				
Tea Bag Mountain Berry as prep	1 cup	0	0	0
Tea Bag Orange Refresher as prep	1 cup	0	0	0
Tea Bag Peppermint as prep	1 cup	0	0	0
Tea Bag Quietly Chamomile as prep	1 cup	0	0	0
Tea Bag Wildflower & Honey as prep	1 cup	0	—	0
REGULAR				
brewed tea	6 oz	2	—	0
instant unsweetened as prep w/ water	8 oz	2	—	0
Bigelow				
Chinese Fortune	5 fl oz	1	—	0
Cinnamon Stick	5 fl oz	1	—	0
Constant Comment	5 fl oz	1	—	0
Darjeeling Blend	5 fl oz	1	—	0
Earl Gray	5 fl oz	1	—	0
English Teatime	5 fl oz	1	—	0
Lemon Lift	5 fl oz	1	—	0
Orange Pekoe	5 fl oz	1	—	0
Peppermint Stick	5 fl oz	1	—	0
Plantation Mint	5 fl oz	1	—	0
Raspberry Royale	5 fl oz	1	—	0
Celestial Seasonings				
Cinnamon Vienna	8 fl oz	2	—	0
Earl Grey Extraordinary	8 fl oz	3	—	0
English Breakfast Classic	8 fl oz	3	—	0
Lemon	8 fl oz	7	—	0
Mint	8 fl oz	4	—	0
Morning Thunder	8 fl oz	3	—	0
Naturally Decaffeinated	8 fl oz	10	—	0
Orange Spice	8 fl oz	7	—	0
Orange Spice Decaff	8 fl oz	7	—	0
Organically Grown	8 fl oz	12	—	0
Raspberry	8 fl oz	7	—	0
Lipton				
English Blend as prep	1 cup	0	0	0
Family Size Bags Decaf as prep	1 qt	0	0	0
Family Size Bags as prep	1 qt	0	0	0
Instant as prep	1 serv	0	0	0
Instant Decaf as prep	1 serv	0	0	0
Instant Lemon as prep	1 serv	0	0	0

FOOD	PORTION	CALS.	FIB.	CHOL.
Lipton (cont.)				
Special Blends Amaretto as prep	1 cup	0	0	0
Special Blends Blackberry as prep	1 cup	0	0	0
Special Blends Cinnamon as prep	1 cup	0	0	0
Special Blends Earl Grey as prep	1 cup	0	0	0
Special Blends English Breakfast as prep	1 cup	0	0	0
Special Blends Honey & Cinnamon as prep	1 cup	0	0	0
Special Blends Honey & Lemon as prep	1 cup	0	0	0
Special Blends Honey & Orange as prep	1 cup	0	0	0
Special Blends Mint as prep	1 cup	0	0	0
Special Blends Orange & Spice as prep	1 cup	0	0	0
Special Blends Peach as prep	1 cup	0	0	0
Special Blends Raspberry as prep	1 cup	0	0	0
Tea Bag Decaf as prep	1	0	0	0
Tea Bag Green Tea as prep	1	0	0	0
Tea Bag as prep	1	0	0	0
Natural Touch				
Kaffree	8 fl oz	0	—	0
Nestea				
Tea Bag as prep	6 oz	0	—	0
TEFF				
Arrowhead				
Whole Grain	¼ cup (1.6 oz)	160	6	0
TEMPEH				
tempeh	½ cup	165	—	0
Lightlife				
Garden Vege	4 oz	142	2	0
Tempeh	4 oz	182	—	0
White Wave				
Burger	1 patty (3 oz)	110	6	0
Lemon Broil	1 patty (2 oz)	130	4	0
Organic Wild Rice	⅓ block (2.7 oz)	140	6	0
Teriyaki Burger	1 patty (3 oz)	110	6	0

FOOD	PORTION	CALS.	FIB.	CHOL.
THYME				
ground	1 tsp	4	—	0
Watkins				
Thyme	¼ tsp (0.5 oz)	0	0	0
TOFU				
firm	¼ block (3 oz)	118	1	0
firm	½ cup	183	2	0
fresh fried	1 piece (½ oz)	35	tr	0
fuyu salted & fermented	1 block (⅓ oz)	13	tr	0
koyadofu dried frozen	1 piece (½ oz)	82	tr	0
okara	½ cup	47	1	0
regular	¼ block (4 oz)	88	1	0
regular	½ cup	94	1	0
Casbah				
Gyro as prep w/ tofu	1 patty (2 oz)	105	tr	0
Jaclyn's				
Grilled In Black Bean Sauce	10.75 oz	270	—	0
Grilled In Peanut Sauce	10.75 oz	260	—	0
Mori-Nu				
Extra Firm	1 in slice (3 oz)	55	—	0
Firm	1 in slice (3 oz)	50	—	0
Lite Extra Firm	1 in slice (3 oz)	35	—	0
Lite Firm	1 in slice (3 oz)	35	—	0
Soft	1 in slice (3 oz)	45	—	0
Nasoya				
Chinese 5 Spice	¼ block (3 oz)	68	1	0
Extra Firm	⅕ block (3.2 oz)	92	tr	0
Firm	⅕ block (3.2 oz)	76	tr	0
French Country	⅕ block (3 oz)	68	1	tr
Silken	⅕ block (3.2 oz)	48	tr	0
Soft	⅕ block (3.2 oz)	63	tr	0
Spring Creek				
Baked Barbeque	2 oz	88	—	0
Baked Cajun	2 oz	87	—	0
Baked Teriyaki	2 oz	84	—	0
Great Balls Of Tofu!	2 (3 oz)	107	—	0
Nigari Firm	4 oz	140	3	0
Tofu Salads !Onion Dip	2 oz	46	—	0
Tofu Salads !Taco Dip	2 oz	46	—	0
Tofu Salads Missing Egg	2 oz	49	—	0
Tree Of Life				
Baked	⅕ block (3.2 oz)	150	0	0
Firm	⅕ block (3.2 oz)	100	0	0

FOOD	PORTION	CALS.	FIB.	CHOL.
Tree Of Life (CONT.)				
Raw Firm	⅕ block (3.2 oz)	100	0	0
Ready Ground Hot & Spicy	⅓ pkg (3 oz)	60	0	0
Ready Ground Original	⅓ pkg (3 oz)	60	0	0
Ready Ground Savory Garlic	⅓ pkg (3 oz)	60	0	0
Reduced Fat	⅕ block (3.2 oz)	90	2	0
Savory Baked	⅕ block (3.2 oz)	140	0	0
Smoked Hot'N Spicy	½ block (3 oz)	120	0	0
Smoked Original	½ block (3 oz)	120	0	0
White Wave				
Baked Tofus Teriyaki Oriental Style	¼ block (2 oz)	120	1	0
Hard	4 oz	120	—	0
International Baked Italian Garlic Herb	¼ pkg (2 oz)	120	1	0
International Baked Mexican Jalapeno	¼ pkg (2 oz)	120	1	0
International Baked Oriental Teriyaki	¼ pkg (2 oz)	120	1	0
International Baked Thai Sesame Peanut	¼ pkg (2 oz)	120	1	0
Soft	4 oz	120	—	0

TOMATILLO

fresh	1 (1.2 oz)	11	—	0
fresh chopped	½ cup	21	—	0

TOMATO

(*see also* PIZZA, SPAGHETTI SAUCE)

CANNED

paste	½ cup	110	6	0
puree	1 cup	102	6	0
puree w/o salt	1 cup	102	6	0
red whole	½ cup	24	—	0
sauce	½ cup	37	2	0
sauce spanish style	½ cup	40	2	0
sauce w/ mushrooms	½ cup	42	—	0
sauce w/ onion	½ cup	52	—	0
stewed	½ cup	34	—	0
w/ green chiles	½ cup	18	—	0
wedges in tomato juice	½ cup	34	—	0
Claussen				
Kosher	1	9	—	0
Contadina				
California Sliced	½ cup	40	—	0

FOOD	PORTION	CALS.	FIB.	CHOL.
Contadina (CONT.)				
Crushed	¼ cup	20	1	0
Italian Style Pear	½ cup	25	1	0
Italian Style Stewed	½ cup	40	1	0
Mexican Style Stewed	½ cup	40	1	0
Pasta Ready With Three Cheeses	½ cup	70	tr	<5
Paste	2 tbsp	30	1	0
Peeled Whole	½ cup	25	1	0
Puree	¼ cup	20	tr	0
Recipe Ready	½ cup	25	3	0
Stewed	½ cup	40	1	0
Del Monte				
Paste	2 tbsp (1.2 oz)	30	2	0
Peeled Diced	½ cup (4.4 oz)	25	2	0
Puree	¼ cup (2.2 oz)	30	1	0
Sauce	¼ cup (2.1 oz)	20	tr	0
Sauce No Salt Added	¼ cup (2.1 oz)	20	tr	0
Stewed Cajun Style	½ cup (4.4 oz)	35	2	0
Stewed Chunky Chili	½ cup (4.5 oz)	30	2	0
Stewed Chunky Pasta	½ cup (4.5 oz)	45	2	0
Stewed Chunky Pizza	½ cup (4.5 oz)	35	2	0
Stewed Chunky Salsa	½ cup (4.5 oz)	35	2	0
Stewed Italian Style	½ cup (4.4 oz)	30	2	0
Stewed Mexican Style	½ cup (4.4 oz)	35	2	0
Stewed Original	½ cup (4.4 oz)	35	2	0
Stewed Original No Salt Added	½ cup (4.4 oz)	35	2	0
Wedges	½ cup (4.4 oz)	35	2	0
Whole Peeled	½ cup (4.4 oz)	25	2	0
Eden				
Crushed Organic	¼ cup (2.1 oz)	20	1	0
Sauce Lightly Seasoned	¼ cup (2.1 oz)	25	1	0
Health Valley				
Sauce	1 cup	70	tr	0
Sauce Low Sodium	1 cup	70	1	0
Hebrew National				
Pickled	⅓ tomato (1 oz)	4	—	0
Hunt's				
Choice Cut	½ cup (4.2 oz)	22	1	0
Choice Cut Diced Tomatoes & Green Chiles	2 tbsp (0.4 oz)	1	tr	0
Choice Cut Diced Tomatoes & Roasted Garlic	½ cup (4.2 oz)	24	1	0
Crushed	½ cup (4.2 oz)	29	2	0

FOOD	PORTION	CALS.	FIB.	CHOL.
Hunt's (CONT.)				
Crushed Angela Mia	½ cup (4.2 oz)	27	2	0
Paste	2 tbsp (1.2 oz)	30	2	0
Paste Italian	2 tbsp (1.2 oz)	27	2	0
Paste No Salt Added	2 tbsp (1.2 oz)	30	2	0
Paste With Garlic	2 tbsp (1.2 oz)	28	2	0
Pear Shaped	½ cup (4.6 oz)	20	1	0
Puree	¼ cup (2.2 oz)	24	2	0
Ready Sauce Chunky Chili	¼ cup (2.2 oz)	22	1	0
Ready Sauce Chunky Italian	¼ cup (2.2 oz)	26	1	0
Ready Sauce Chunky Mexican	¼ cup (2.2 oz)	21	1	0
Ready Sauce Chunky Special	¼ cup (2.2 oz)	21	1	0
Ready Sauce Chunky Tomato	¼ cup (2.2 oz)	15	1	0
Ready Sauce Country Herb	¼ cup (2.2 oz)	33	1	0
Ready Sauce Garlic	¼ cup (2.2 oz)	29	2	0
Ready Sauce Garlic & Herb	¼ cup (2.2 oz)	26	1	0
Ready Sauce Meatloaf Fixins	¼ cup (2.2 oz)	23	1	0
Ready Sauce Original	¼ cup (2.2 oz)	30	1	0
Ready Sauce Salsa	¼ cup (2.2 oz)	18	1	0
Sauce	¼ cup (2.2 oz)	16	1	0
Sauce Italian	¼ cup (2.2 oz)	32	1	0
Sauce No Salt Added	¼ cup (2.2 oz)	16	1	0
Sauce With Herb	¼ cup (2.2 oz)	32	1	0
Stewed	½ cup (4.2 oz)	33	2	0
Stewed Italian	4 oz	40	tr	0
Tomatoes	½ cup (4.2 oz)	33	2	0
Whole	2 (5.2 oz)	22	1	0
Muir Glen				
Organic Chunky Sauce	¼ cup (2.3 oz)	20	1	0
Organic Crushed With Basil	¼ cup (2.3 oz)	25	1	0
Organic Diced	½ cup (4.5 oz)	25	1	0
Organic Diced No Salt Added	½ cup (4.5 oz)	25	1	0
Organic Ground Peeled	¼ cup (2.3 oz)	10	1	0
Organic Italian Style Diced	½ cup (4.4 oz)	25	1	0
Organic Paste	2 tbsp (1.2 oz)	30	1	0
Organic Puree	¼ cup (2.2 oz)	20	1	0
Organic Sauce	¼ cup (2.2 oz)	20	1	0
Organic Sauce No Salt Added	¼ cup (2.2 oz)	20	1	0
Organic Stewed	½ cup (4.5 oz)	30	tr	0
Organic Stewed Italian Style	½ cup (4.4 oz)	30	tr	0
Organic Stewed Mexican Style	½ cup (4.4 oz)	30	tr	0
Organic Whole Peeled	½ cup (4.6 oz)	30	1	0
Old El Paso				
Tomatoes & Jalapenos	¼ cup (2 oz)	15	1	0

FOOD	PORTION	CALS.	FIB.	CHOL.
Old El Paso (CONT.)				
Tomatoes & Green Chilies	¼ cup (2 oz)	10	0	0
Progresso				
Crushed	¼ cup (2.1 oz)	20	1	0
Paste	2 tbsp (1.2 oz)	30	1	0
Peeled Whole	½ cup (4.2 oz)	25	1	0
Peeled w/ Basil	½ cup (4.2 oz)	25	1	0
Puree	¼ cup (2.2 oz)	25	1	0
Puree Thick Style	¼ cup (2.2 oz)	30	1	0
Sauce	¼ cup (2.1 oz)	20	1	0
Ro-Tel				
Diced Tomatoes & Green Chilies	½ cup (4.4 oz)	20	1	0
Rosoff's				
Pickled	⅓ tomato (1 oz)	5	—	0
S&W				
Aspic Supreme	½ cup	60	—	0
Diced In Rich Puree	½ cup	35	—	0
Italian Stewed Sliced	½ cup	35	—	0
Italian Style w/ Basil	½ cup	25	—	0
Paste	6 oz	150	—	0
Peeled Ready Cut	½ cup	25	—	0
Puree	½ cup	60	—	0
Sauce	½ cup	40	—	0
Sauce Chunky	½ cup	45	—	0
Stewed 50% Salt Reduced	½ cup	35	—	0
Stewed Mexican Style	½ cup	40	—	0
Stewed Sliced	½ cup	35	—	0
Whole Diet	½ cup	25	—	0
Whole Peeled	½ cup	25	—	0
Schorr's				
Pickled	⅓ tomato (1 oz)	4	—	0
Sonoma				
Dried Spice Medley oil drained	1 tbsp (0.5 oz)	50	1	0
Pesto	¼ cup (2 oz)	110	1	2
Tapenade	1 tbsp (0.7 oz)	70	1	0
Tree Of Life				
Sauce	¼ cup (2 oz)	20	—	0
DRIED				
sun dried	1 piece	5	—	0
sun dried	1 cup	140	—	0
sun dried in oil	1 piece (3 g)	6	—	0
sun dried in oil	1 cup (4 oz)	235	—	0

FOOD	PORTION	CALS.	FIB.	CHOL.
Sonoma				
Bits	2-3 tsp (5 g)	15	1	0
Dried	2-3 halves (5 g)	15	1	0
Halves	2-3 halves (5 g)	15	1	0
Julienne	7-9 pieces (5 g)	15	1	0
Pasta Toss	½ cup (0.7 oz)	70	3	0
Season It	2-3 tsp (5 g)	20	1	0
FRESH				
cooked	½ cup	32	—	0
green	1	30	—	0
red	1 (4½ oz)	26	2	0
red chopped	1 cup	35	2	0
TAKE-OUT				
stewed	1 cup	80	—	0
TOMATO JUICE				
tomato juice	6 oz	32	—	0
tomato juice	½ cup	21	—	0
Campbell				
Juice	6 oz	40	—	0
Del Monte				
Snap-E-Tom	6 fl oz	40	1	0
Snap-E-Tom	10 fl oz	60	2	0
Snap-E-Tom	8 fl oz	50	2	0
Hunt's				
Juice	8 fl oz	22	1	0
No Salt Added	8 fl oz	34	2	0
Libby				
Juice	6 oz	35	—	0
Mott's				
Beefamato	8 fl oz	80	1	0
Clamato	8 fl oz	100	2	0
Clamato Caesar	8 fl oz	100	0	0
Muir Glen				
Organic	8 oz	40	tr	0
S&W				
California	6 oz	35	—	0
Diet	½ cup	35	—	0
TONGUE				
beef simmered	3 oz	241	—	91
lamb braised	3 oz	234	—	161
pork braised	3 oz	230	—	124

FOOD	PORTION	CALS.	FIB.	CHOL.

TOPPINGS
(see ICE CREAM TOPPINGS)

TORTILLA
(see also CHIPS TORTILLA, SPANISH FOOD)

FOOD	PORTION	CALS.	FIB.	CHOL.
corn	1 (6 in diam)	56	1	0
corn w/o salt	1 (0.9 oz) 6 in diam	56	1	0
flour w/o salt	1 (1.2 oz) 8 in diam	114	1	0
Alvarado St. Bakery				
Burrito Size	1 (2.2 oz)	170	1	0
Fajita Size	1 (1.6 oz)	130	1	0
El Charrito				
Corn	2	95	—	0
Flour	2	170	—	0
Old El Paso				
Flour	1 (1.4 oz)	150	0	0
Soft Taco Tortilla	2 (1.8 oz)	180	0	0
Tyson				
Burrito Style Flour	1	170	—	0
Burrito Style Hand Stretched Small Flour	1	106	—	0
Burrito Style Heat Pressed Large Flour	1	182	—	0
Enchilada Style Corn	1	54	—	0
Fajita Style Flour	1	89	—	0
Soft Taco Flour	1	121	—	0
Whole Wheat	1	120	—	0
Wonder				
Low Fat Wheat	1 (1.4 oz)	120	1	0
Low Fat White	1 (1.4 oz)	110	1	0
Zapata				
Tortilla	1 (1.2 oz)	100	tr	0

TORTILLA CHIPS
(see CHIPS)

TREE FERN
FOOD	PORTION	CALS.	FIB.	CHOL.
chopped cooked	½ cup	28	—	0

TRITICALE
FOOD	PORTION	CALS.	FIB.	CHOL.
dry	½ cup	323	17	0

TROUT
FOOD	PORTION	CALS.	FIB.	CHOL.
baked	3 oz	162	—	63
rainbow cooked	3 oz	129	—	62
sea trout baked	3 oz	113	—	90

FOOD	PORTION	CALS.	FIB.	CHOL.
Clear Springs				
Rainbow	3.5 oz	140	—	75
TRUFFLES				
fresh	3½ oz	25	—	0
TUNA				
(*see also* TUNA DISHES)				
CANNED				
light in oil	3 oz	169	—	15
light in oil	1 can (6 oz)	399	—	30
light in water	3 oz	99	—	25
light in water	1 can (5.8 oz)	192	—	49
white in oil	3 oz	158	—	26
white in oil	1 can (6.2 oz)	331	—	55
white in water	1 can (6 oz)	234	—	72
white in water	3 oz	116	—	35
Bumble Bee				
Chunk Light In Oil	2 oz	160	—	30
Chunk Light In Water	2 oz	60	—	30
Chunk White In Oil	2 oz	160	—	30
Chunk White In Water	2 oz	70	—	30
Solid White In Oil	2 oz	130	—	30
Solid White In Water	2 oz	70	—	30
Progresso				
In Olive Oil	¼ cup (2 oz)	160	0	30
Tree Of Life				
Tongol In Spring Water	2 oz	60	0	30
Tongol In Spring Water No Salt	2 oz	70	0	0
FRESH				
bluefin cooked	3 oz	157	—	42
bluefin raw	3 oz	122	—	32
skipjack baked	3 oz	112	—	51
yellowfin baked	3 oz	118	—	49
TUNA DISHES				
FROZEN				
Chefwich				
Tuna Melt	5 oz	360	—	23
MIX				
Bumble Bee				
Tuna Mix-ins Classic Italian	⅓ pkg (0.17 oz)	25	—	0
Tuna Mix-ins Garden & Herb	⅓ pkg (0.17 oz)	25	—	0
Tuna Mix-ins Lemon Herb	⅓ pkg (0.17 oz)	25	—	0

FOOD	PORTION	CALS.	FIB.	CHOL.
Bumble Bee (CONT.)				
Tuna Mix-ins Zesty Tomato	⅓ pkg (0.17 oz)	25	—	0
READY-TO-EAT				
The Spreadables				
Tuna Salad	¼ can	90	—	13
Wampler Longacre				
Salad	1 oz	60	—	5
TAKE-OUT				
tuna salad	1 cup	383	—	27
tuna salad	3 oz	159	—	11
tuna salad submarine sandwich w/ lettuce & oil	1	584	—	47

TURKEY

(*see also* DINNER, HOT DOG, TURKEY DISHES, TURKEY SUBSTITUTES)

CANNED

FOOD	PORTION	CALS.	FIB.	CHOL.
Armour				
Turkey Loaf	2 oz	110	—	40
Hormel				
Chunk	2 oz	70	0	35
Chunk Turkey Ham	2 oz	70	0	40
Chunk White	2 oz	60	0	25
Underwood				
Chunky Light	2.08 oz	75	—	25
FRESH				
back w/ skin roasted	½ back (9 oz)	637	—	238
breast w/ skin roasted	4 oz	212	—	83
dark meat w/ skin roasted	3.6 oz	230	—	93
dark meat w/o skin roasted	1 cup (5 oz)	262	—	119
dark meat w/o skin roasted	3 oz	170	—	78
ground cooked	3 oz	188	—	57
leg w/ skin roasted	2.5 oz	147	—	61
leg w/ skin roasted	1 (1.2 lbs)	1133	—	466
light meat w/ skin roasted	from ½ turkey (2.3 lbs)	2069	—	794
light meat w/ skin roasted	4.7 oz	268	—	103
light meat w/o skin roasted	4 oz	183	—	81
neck simmered	1 (5.3 oz)	274	—	186
skin roasted	1 oz	141	—	36
skin roasted	from ½ turkey (9 oz)	1096	—	281
w/ skin roasted	8.4 oz	498	—	196
w/ skin roasted	½ turkey (4 lbs)	3857	—	1514
w/ skin neck & giblets roasted	½ turkey (8.8 lbs)	4123	—	1920

FOOD	PORTION	CALS.	FIB.	CHOL.
w/o skin roasted	1 cup (5 oz)	238	—	107
w/o skin roasted	7.3 oz	354	—	159
wing w/ skin roasted	1 (6.5 oz)	426	—	150
Butterball				
Ground All White Meat	3 oz	100	—	45
Louis Rich				
Ground	3 oz	140	0	70
Mr. Turkey				
Ground 85% Fat Free	3.5 oz	210	—	110
Ground 91% Fat Free	3.5 oz	170	—	95
Perdue				
Breast Tenderloins Cooked	3 oz	110	—	55
Breast Boneless Cooked	3 oz	110	—	55
Breast Cutlets Thin Sliced Cooked	1 (2.5 oz)	90	—	50
Breast Fillets Cooked	3 oz	110	—	55
Burger Cooked	1 (3 oz)	170	—	110
Cubed Steak Cooked	3 oz	120	—	85
Dark Cooked	3 oz	200	—	95
Drumsticks Roasted	3 oz	150	—	100
Drumsticks Cooked	3 oz	150	—	100
Ground Cooked	3 oz	170	—	110
Ground Breast Cooked	3 oz	110	—	55
Half Breast Cooked	3 oz	170	—	65
Thighs Cooked	3 oz	180	—	100
Tom Wings Cooked	3 oz	160	—	90
White Cooked	3 oz	170	—	70
Whole Breast Cooked	3 oz	170	—	65
Wings Roasted	1 (3 oz)	180	—	95
Wings Drummettes Roasted	1 (3.5 oz)	180	—	100
Swift-Eckrich				
Ground All White	3 oz	100	—	45
The Turkey Store				
Seasoned Cuts Turkey Breast Roast	4 oz	110	—	45
Wampler Longacre				
Ground raw	1 oz	60	—	30
FROZEN				
roast boneless seasoned light & dark meat roasted	1 pkg (1.7 lbs)	1213	—	413
Empire				
Patties	1 (3.1 oz)	200	1	5
READY-TO-EAT				
bologna	1 oz	57	—	28

FOOD	PORTION	CALS.	FIB.	CHOL.
breast	1 slice (¾ oz)	23	—	9
poultry salad sandwich spread	1 oz	238	—	9
poultry salad sandwich spread	1 tbsp	109	—	4
prebasted breast w/ skin roasted	1 breast (3.8 lbs)	2175	—	718
prebasted breast w/ skin roasted	½ breast (1.9 lbs)	1087	—	359
prebasted thigh w/ skin roasted	1 thigh (11 oz)	494	—	194
roll light & dark meat	1 oz	42	—	16
roll light meat	1 oz	42	—	12
salami cooked	1 pkg (8 oz)	446	—	186
salami cooked	2 oz	111	—	46
turkey loaf breast meat	2 slices (1.5 oz)	47	—	17
turkey loaf breast meat	1 pkg (6 oz)	187	—	69
Alpine Lace				
Breast Fat Free	2 oz	50	—	0
Carl Buddig				
Honey Turkey	1 oz	40	—	15
Turkey	1 oz	50	0	15
Turkey Ham	1 oz	40	0	15
Empire				
Barbecue Whole	5 oz	250	0	100
Bologna	3 slices (1.8 oz)	90	0	30
Oven Prepared Breast Slices	3 slices (1.8 oz)	50	0	15
Pastrami	3 slices (1.8 oz)	60	1	30
Salami	3 slices (1.8 oz)	70	0	35
Smoked Breast Slices	3 slices (1.8 oz)	40	0	15
Falls				
BBQ	3 oz	140	—	55
Gourmet Breast	3 oz	80	—	35
Premium Cooked Breast	3 oz	100	—	40
Hansel n'Gretel				
Breast Gourmet	1 oz	28	—	9
Breast Gourmet Smoked	1 oz	31	—	11
Breast Honey	1 oz	28	—	9
Breast Lessalt Cooked	1 oz	25	—	9
Breast Oven Cooked	1 oz	26	—	8
Doubledecker Turkey Corned Beef	1 oz	30	—	12
Doubledecker Turkey Ham	1 oz	30	—	11
Healthy Choice				
Deli-Thin Honey Roast & Smoked	6 slices (2 oz)	70	0	25
Deli-Thin Roasted Breast	6 slices (2 oz)	60	0	25
Deli-Thin Smoked Breast	6 slices (2 oz)	60	0	25
Deli-Thin Turkey Ham	6 slices (2 oz)	60	0	40

FOOD	PORTION	CALS.	FIB.	CHOL.
Healthy Choice (CONT.)				
Fresh-Trak Honey Roast & Smoked Breast	1 slice (1 oz)	35	0	10
Fresh-Trak Oven Roasted Breast	1 slice (1 oz)	35	0	15
Honey Roasted & Smoked	1 slice (1 oz)	35	0	15
Oven Roasted Breast	1 slice (1 oz)	35	0	15
Smoked Breast	1 slice (1 oz)	30	0	10
Variety Pack Regular	3 slices (2.2 oz)	70	0	30
Hebrew National				
Deli Thin Hickory Smoked	1.8 oz	55	—	25
Deli Thin Lemon Garlic	1.8 oz	50	—	20
Deli Thin Oven Roasted	1.8 oz	80	—	20
Hormel				
Light & Lean 97 Breast Sliced	1 slice (1 oz)	30	0	10
Light & Lean 97 Breast Smoked	3 oz	80	0	35
Light & Lean 97 Cuts	16 pieces (1 oz)	30	0	15
Light & Lean 97 Cuts Smoked	16 pieces (1 oz)	30	0	15
Jordan's				
Healthy Trim Fat Free Oven Roasted Breast	1 slice (1 oz)	20	0	15
Healthy Trim Fat Free Oven Roasted Smoked Breast	1 slice (1 oz)	20	0	15
Louis Rich				
Bologna	1 slice (28 g)	50	0	20
Breaded Nuggets	4 (3.2 oz)	260	0	35
Breaded Patties	1 (3 oz)	220	0	35
Breaded Sticks	3 (3 oz)	230	0	35
Carving Board Oven Roasted Breast	2 slices (1.6 oz)	40	0	20
Carving Board Oven Roasted Thin Carved Breast	6 slices (2.1 oz)	60	0	25
Carving Board Smoked Breast	2 slices (1.6 oz)	40	0	20
Chopped Ham	1 slice (1 oz)	46	0	20
Cotto Salami	1 slice (28 g)	40	0	25
Deli-Thin Smoked Breast	4 slices (1.8 oz)	50	0	20
Fat Free Hickory Smoked Breast	1 slice (1 oz)	25	0	10
Fat Free Oven Roasted Breast	1 slice (28 g)	25	0	10
Ham Round	1 slice (28 g)	34	0	20
Ham Square	3 slices (2.2 oz)	70	0	45
Hickory Smoked Dinner Slices Breast	1 slice (2.8 oz)	80	0	35
Honey Cured Turkey Ham	3 slices (2.2 oz)	70	0	45
Honey Roasted Breast	1 slice (1 oz)	30	0	10

FOOD	PORTION	CALS.	FIB.	CHOL.
Louis Rich (CONT.)				
Honey Roasted Dinner Slices Breast	1 slice (2.8 oz)	80	0	35
Oven Roasted Breast	2 oz	60	0	25
Oven Roasted Breast	1 slice (1 oz)	30	0	10
Oven Roasted Deli-Thin Breast	4 slices (1.8 oz)	50	0	20
Oven Roasted Dinner Slices Breast	1 slice (2.8 oz)	70	0	35
Pastrami	2 slices (1.6 oz)	45	0	30
Salami	1 slice (28 g)	45	0	20
Skinless Barbecued Breast	2 oz	60	0	25
Skinless Hickory Smoked Breast	2 oz	60	0	25
Skinless Honey Roasted Breast	2 oz	60	0	25
Skinless Oven Roasted Breast	2 oz	50	0	25
Smoked Breast	1 slice (1 oz)	25	0	10
Smoked White	1 slice (1 oz)	30	0	15
Turkey Ham	4 slices (1.8 oz)	60	0	35
Mr. Turkey				
Deli Cuts Hardwood Smoked Breast	3 slices	30	—	13
Deli Cuts Honey Roasted Breast	3 slices	30	—	15
Deli Cuts Oven Roasted Breast	3 slices	30	—	13
Deli Cuts Turkey Ham	3 slices	35	—	20
Deli Cuts Turkey Pastrami	3 slices	35	—	20
Hardwood Smoked Breast	1 slice	30	—	15
Hardwood Smoked Turkey Ham	1 slice	35	—	20
Honey Cured Turkey Ham	1 slice	30	—	20
Oven Roasted Breast	1 slice	30	—	15
Smoked Breakfast Turkey Ham	1 oz	30	—	18
Turkey Bologna	1 slice	70	—	25
Turkey Cotto Salami	1 slice	50	—	20
Turkey Ham	1 slice	35	—	20
Turkey Pastrami	1 slice	30	—	15
Oscar Mayer				
Deli-Thin Roast	4 slices (1.8 oz)	50	0	20
Deli-Thin Smoked Honey Roasted	4 slices (1.8 oz)	60	0	20
Free Oven Roasted Breast	4 slices (1.8 oz)	40	—	15
Free Smoked Breast	4 slices (1.8 oz)	40	—	15
Healthy Favorites Oven Roasted Breast	4 slices (1.8 oz)	40	0	15
Healthy Favorites Smoked Breast	4 slices (1.8 oz)	40	0	15

FOOD	PORTION	CALS.	FIB.	CHOL.
Oscar Mayer (CONT.)				
Lunchables Fun Pack Turkey/ Pacific Cooler	1 pkg (11.2 oz)	460	tr	50
Lunchables Fun Pack Turkey/ Surger Cooler	1 pkg (11.2 oz)	440	0	45
Lunchables Turkey Oven Roasted/Green Onion Cheese	1 pkg (4.5 oz)	380	1	40
Lunchables Turkey Smoked/ Ranch & Herb Cheese	1 pkg (4.5 oz)	380	1	45
Lunchables Turkey/Cheddar	1 pkg (4.5 oz)	360	1	70
Perdue				
Nuggets Dinosaur	3 (3 oz)	200	2	35
Sara Lee				
Hardwood Smoked Breast Of Turkey	2 oz	60	—	20
Hardwood Smoked Turkey Ham	2 oz	60	—	40
Honey Roasted Breast Of Turkey	2 oz	60	—	20
Honey Roasted Turkey Ham	2 oz	70	—	40
Mesquite Smoked Breast Of Turkey	2 oz	60	—	30
Oven Roasted Breast Of Turkey	2 oz	60	—	25
Peppered Breast Of Turkey	2 oz	50	—	20
Seasoned Breast Of Turkey Pastrami	2 oz	60	—	30
Wampler Longacre				
Bologna	1 oz	60	—	20
Breast Chops	1 serv (4 oz)	120	—	50
Breast Sliced	1 slice (1 oz)	35	—	30
Breast Sliced Smoked	1 slice (0.75 oz)	20	—	10
Burger	1 (4 oz)	230	—	120
Burger	1 (3 oz)	170	—	90
Burger Barbecue	1 (4 oz)	240	—	120
Chef Select Breast Skinless	1 oz	35	—	15
Chef Select Breast Smoked	1 oz	35	—	15
Chunk Dark Smoked Cured	1 oz	45	—	25
Chunk Ham 12% Water Smoked	1 oz	45	—	15
Chunk Ham 20% Water	1 oz	40	—	20
Chunk Pastrami	1 oz	35	—	20
Cook-In-The-Bag Breast	1 oz	30	—	15
Cook-In-The-Bag Breast Mini	1 oz	30	—	10
Cook-In-The-Bag Combo Roast	1 oz	35	—	15

FOOD	PORTION	CALS.	FIB.	CHOL.
Wampler Longacre (CONT.)				
Cook-In-The-Bag Thigh Roast	1 oz	40	—	15
Dark Smoked Cured	1 oz	45	—	25
Deli Chef Breast And White Meat No Skin	1 oz	40	—	15
Gourmet Breast	1 oz	35	—	15
Gourmet Breast Mini	1 oz	35	—	15
Gourmet Breast Mini Smoked	1 oz	35	—	15
Gourmet Breast Smoked	1 oz	30	—	15
Gourmet Brown & Glazed Breast	1 oz	35	—	15
Gourmet Brown & Roasted Breast	1 oz	35	—	15
Gourmet Honey Cured Breast	1 oz	30	—	15
Lean-Lite Breast Skinless	1 oz	35	—	15
Lean-Lite Deli Breast	1 oz	35	—	15
Lean-Lite Deli Breast Smoked	1 oz	35	—	15
Old Fashioned Brown & Roasted Breast	1 oz	35	—	15
Pastrami	1 oz	35	—	20
Premium Breast Skinless	1 oz	30	—	15
Premium Brown & Roasted Breast Skinless	1 oz	16	—	15
Roll Combo	1 oz	44	—	17
Roll Sliced Breast	1 slice (0.75 oz)	30	—	30
Roll White	1 oz	45	—	15
Salami	1 oz	50	—	20
Salt Watchers Breast Skinless	1 oz	35	—	15
Seasoned Roast	1 oz	40	—	15
Sliced Salami	1 slice (0.8 oz)	45	—	20
Tenderlings BBQ	1 serv (4 oz)	110	—	40
Tenderlings Cajun	1 serv (4 oz)	110	—	40
Tenderlings Garlic & Pepper	1 serv (4 oz)	110	—	40
Tenderlings Original	1 serv (4 oz)	110	—	40
Turkey Ham 12% Water Baked	1 oz	45	—	15
Turkey Ham 20% Water Baked	1 oz	40	—	20
Unseasoned Roast	1 oz	40	—	15
Whole Browned & Roasted	1 oz	60	—	20
Weight Watchers				
Deli Thin Smoked Breast	5 slices (⅓ oz)	10	—	5
Oven Roasted Breast	2 slices (¾ oz)	25	—	10
Oven Roasted Turkey Ham	2 slices (¾ oz)	25	—	10

FOOD	PORTION	CALS.	FIB.	CHOL.
Weight Watchers (CONT.)				
Roasted & Smoked Breast	2 slices (¾ oz)	25	—	10

TURKEY DISHES

(*see also* DINNER, TURKEY SUBSTITUTES)

CANNED

Dinty Moore

| Stew | 1 cup (8.5 oz) | 140 | 2 | 15 |

FROZEN

Hot Pocket

| Stuffed Sandwich Turkey & Ham With Cheese | 1 (4.5 oz) | 320 | 1 | 35 |

Lean Pockets

| Stuffed Sandwich Turkey & Ham With Cheddar | 1 (4.5 oz) | 260 | 4 | 35 |
| Stuffed Sandwich Turkey Broccoli & Cheese | 1 (4.5 oz) | 260 | 4 | 35 |

Luigino's

| Gravy Dressing & Turkey | 1 pkg (8 oz) | 340 | 2 | 40 |

Weight Watchers

| Honey Dijon Turkey Pretzel Sandwich | 1 (4 oz) | 230 | 3 | 25 |

READY-TO-EAT

Spreadables

| Turkey Salad | ¼ can | 100 | — | 20 |

Wampler Longacre

Meatloaf Italian	1 serv (4 oz)	114	—	56
Meatloaf Mexican	1 serv (4 oz)	114	—	56
Meatloaf Original	1 serv (4 oz)	126	—	80
Salad	1 oz	60	—	10
Salad Turkey Ham	1 oz	50	—	10
Teriyaki	1 serv (4 oz)	112	—	25

SHELF-STABLE

Dinty Moore

| Microwave Cup Stew | 1 cup (7.5 oz) | 130 | 2 | 10 |

TURKEY SUBSTITUTES

Harvest Direct

| TVP Poultry Chunks | 3.5 oz | 280 | 18 | 0 |
| TVP Poultry Ground | 3.5 oz | 280 | 18 | 0 |

Soy Is Us

| Turkey Not! | ½ cup (1.75 oz) | 140 | 9 | 0 |

White Wave

| Meatless Sandwich Slices | 2 slices (1.6 oz) | 80 | 1 | 0 |

FOOD	PORTION	CALS.	FIB.	CHOL.

TURMERIC
ground	1 tsp	8	—	0

TURNIPS
CANNED
greens	½ cup	17	—	0

Allen
Chopped Greens And Diced Turnip	½ cup (4.2 oz)	30	tr	0
Greens	½ cup (4.2 oz)	25	2	0

Sunshine
Chopped Greens And Diced Turnip	½ cup (4.2 oz)	30	tr	0
Greens	½ cup (4.2 oz)	25	2	0

FRESH
cooked mashed	½ cup (4.2 oz)	47	—	0
cubed cooked	½ cup (3 oz)	33	—	0
greens chopped cooked	½ cup	15	2	0
greens raw chopped	½ cup	7	1	0
raw cubed	½ cup (2.4 oz)	25	—	0

FROZEN
greens cooked	½ cup	24	2	0

Southland
Rutabaga Yellow Turnips	4 oz	50	—	0

VANILLA
Virginia Dare
Vanilla Extract	1 tsp	10	—	0

VEAL
(see also DINNER, VEAL DISHES)
FRESH
cutlet lean only braised	3 oz	172	—	115
cutlet lean only fried	3 oz	156	—	91
ground broiled	3 oz	146	—	87
loin chop w/ bone lean & fat braised	1 chop (2.8 oz)	227	—	94
loin chop w/ bone lean only braised	1 chop (2.4 oz)	155	—	86
shoulder w/ bone lean only braised	3 oz	169	—	110
sirloin w/ bone lean & fat roasted	3 oz	171	—	87
sirloin w/ bone lean only roasted	3 oz	143	—	89

VEAL DISHES
TAKE-OUT
parmigiana	4.2 oz	279	2	136

FOOD	PORTION	CALS.	FIB.	CHOL.
VEGETABLE JUICE				
vegetable juice cocktail	6 fl oz	34	—	0
vegetable juice cocktail	½ cup	22	—	0
Mott's				
Vegetable Juice as prep	8 fl oz	60	2	0
Muir Glen				
Organic	8 oz	70	3	0
Organic Reduced Sodium	8 oz	70	3	0
Odwalla				
Vegetable Cocktail	8 fl oz	70	2	0
V8				
No Salt Added	6 fl oz	35	—	0
Original	6 fl oz	35	—	0
Spicy Hot	6 fl oz	35	—	0
VEGETABLES MIXED				
(see also individual vegetables, VEGETABLE JUICE)				
CANNED				
mixed vegetables	½ cup	39	—	0
peas & carrots	½ cup	48	—	0
peas & carrots low sodium	½ cup	48	—	0
peas & onions	½ cup	30	—	0
succotash	½ cup	102	—	0
Allen				
Green Beans And Potatoes	½ cup (4.2 oz)	35	2	0
Okra & Tomatoes	½ cup (4 oz)	25	3	0
Okra Tomatoes & Corn	½ cup (4.1 oz)	30	4	0
Chi-Chi's				
Diced Tomatoes & Green Chilies	¼ cup (2.5 oz)	20	0	0
Del Monte				
Mixed	½ cup (4.4 oz)	40	2	0
Peas And Carrots	½ cup (4.5 oz)	60	2	0
Green Giant				
Garden Medley	½ cup	40	1	0
Hanover				
Mixed	½ cup	110	—	0
Vegetable Salad	½ cup	90	—	0
House Of Tsang				
Vegetables & Sauce Cantonese Classic	½ cup (4.2 oz)	70	1	0
Vegetables & Sauce Hong Kong Sweet & Sour	½ cup (4.5 oz)	160	0	0
Vegetables & Sauce Szechuan Hot & Spicy	½ cup (4.2 oz)	70	1	0

FOOD	PORTION	CALS.	FIB.	CHOL.
House Of Tsang (CONT.)				
Vegetables & Sauce Tokyo Teriyaki	½ cup (4.4 oz)	100	0	0
Ka-Me				
Stir Fry	½ cup (4.5 oz)	20	2	0
La Choy				
Chop Suey Vegetables	½ cup	10	tr	0
S&W				
Garden Salad Marinated	½ cup	60	—	0
Mixed Vegetables Old Fashion Harvest Time	½ cup	35	—	0
Peas & Carrots Water Pack	½ cup	35	—	0
Succotash Country Style	½ cup	80	—	0
Sweet Peas & Diced Carrots	½ cup	50	—	0
Sweet Peas w/ Tiny Pearl Onions	½ cup	60	—	0
Seneca				
Peas & Carrots	½ cup	60	4	0
Succotash	½ cup	90	2	0
Sunshine				
Green Beans And Potatoes	½ cup (4.2 oz)	35	2	0
Trappey				
Okra & Tomatoes	½ cup (4 oz)	25	3	0
Okra Tomatoes & Corn	½ cup (4.1 oz)	30	4	0
FROZEN				
mixed vegetables cooked	½ cup	54	2	0
peas & carrots cooked	½ cup	38	—	0
peas & onions cooked	½ cup	40	—	0
succotash cooked	½ cup	79	—	0
Big Valley				
California Blend	¾ cup (3 oz)	25	3	0
Italian Blend	¾ cup (3 oz)	30	2	0
Oriental Blend	¾ cup (3 oz)	25	3	0
Stew Vegetables	⅔ cup (3 oz)	40	2	0
Winter Blend	¾ cup (3 oz)	25	2	0
Birds Eye				
Broccoli Cauliflower And Carrots With Cheese Sauce	½ pkg	80	4	10
Farm Fresh Broccoli And Cauliflower	¾ cup	30	3	0
Farm Fresh Broccoli Carrots And Water Chestnuts	¾ cup	40	3	0
Farm Fresh Broccoli Cauliflower And Carrots	¾ cup	35	3	0

FOOD	PORTION	CALS.	FIB.	CHOL.
Birds Eye (CONT.)				
Farm Fresh Broccoli Cauliflower And Red Peppers	¾ cup	30	3	0
Farm Fresh Broccoli Corn And Red Peppers	⅔ cup	60	3	0
Farm Fresh Broccoli Green Beans Pearl Onions and Red Peppers	¾ cup	35	3	0
Farm Fresh Broccoli Red Peppers Onions And Mushrooms	¾ cup	30	3	0
Farm Fresh Brussels Sprouts Cauliflower And Carrots	¾ cup	40	4	0
Farm Fresh Cauliflower Carrots And Snow Peas	⅔ cup	35	4	0
In Butter Sauce Broccoli Cauliflower And Carrots	½ cup	40	2	5
In Sauce Peas And Pearl Onions With Seasonings	½ cup	70	3	0
Internationals Austrian	3.3 oz	70	1	10
Internationals Bavarian	3.3 oz	90	2	25
Internationals California	3.3 oz	90	3	10
Internationals French Country	3.3 oz	70	2	10
Internationals Italian	3.3 oz	80	2	20
Internationals Japanese	3.3 oz	60	2	10
Internationals New England	3.3 oz	100	2	10
Mixed	½ cup	60	2	0
Peas And Potatoes With Cream Sauce	½ cup	100	1	10
Polybag	½ cup	60	2	0
Budget Gourmet				
Mandarin Vegetables	1 pkg (5.25 oz)	160	—	10
New England Recipe Vegetables	1 pkg (5.5 oz)	230	—	25
Spring Vegetables In Cheese Sauce	1 pkg (5 oz)	130	—	20
Green Giant				
American Mixtures California	½ cup	25	2	0
American Mixtures Heartland	½ cup	25	2	0
American Mixtures New England	½ cup	70	4	0
American Mixtures San Francisco	½ cup	25	2	0
American Mixtures Santa Fe	½ cup	70	2	0
American Mixtures Seattle	½ cup	25	2	0

FOOD	PORTION	CALS.	FIB.	CHOL.
Green Giant (CONT.)				
Broccoli Cauliflower And Carrots In Butter Sauce	½ cup	30	—	5
Broccoli Cauliflower And Carrots In Cheese Sauce	½ cup	60	2	2
Harvest Fresh Mixed Vegetables	½ cup	40	2	0
Mixed	½ cup	40	2	0
Mixed In Butter Sauce	½ cup	60	2	5
One Serve Broccoli Carrots & Rotini In Cheese Sauce	1 pkg	120	—	5
One Serve Broccoli Cauliflower And Carrots	1 pkg	25	3	0
Valley Combinations Broccoli & Cauliflower	½ cup	60	—	0
Hanover				
Broccoli Cut & Cauliflower Cut	½ cup	20	—	0
Caribbean Blend	½ cup	20	—	0
Garden Medley	½ cup	20	—	0
Mixed	½ cup	50	—	0
Oriental Blend	½ cup	25	—	0
Succotash	½ cup	80	—	0
Summer Vegetables	½ cup	35	—	0
Vegetables For Soup	½ cup	60	—	0
La Choy				
Mixed Fancy	½ cup	12	1	0
Ore Ida				
Stew Vegetables	⅔ cup (3 oz)	50	tr	0
Soglowek				
Golden Vegetarian Nuggets	4 pieces (2.5 oz)	190	1	0
Southland				
Peppers & Onions	2 oz	15	—	0
Soup Mix Vegetables	3.2 oz	50	—	0
Stew Vegetables	4 oz	60	—	0
Tree Of Life				
Mixed	½ cup (3 oz)	65	3	0
SHELF-STABLE				
Pantry Express				
Corn Green Beans Carrots Pasta In Tomato Sauce	½ cup	80	3	0
Green Beans Potatoes And Mushrooms In A Seasoned Sauce	½ cup	50	2	0
Mixed Vegetables	½ cup	35	1	0

FOOD	PORTION	CALS.	FIB.	CHOL.
TAKE-OUT				
caponata	¼ cup	28	—	0
gyoza potstickers vegetable	8 (4.9 oz)	210	5	0
succotash	½ cup	111	—	0
VENISON				
roasted	3 oz	134	—	95
Broken Arrow Ranch				
Antelope Chili Meat	3.5 oz	115	—	70
Antelope Ground Venison	3.5 oz	110	—	73
Antelope Stew Meat	3.5 oz	110	—	72
Nilgai Chili Meat	3.5 oz	115	—	70
Nilgai Leg	3.5 oz	100	—	65
Nilgai Stew Meat	3.5 oz	110	—	72
VINEGAR				
cider	1 tbsp	tr	—	0
Hain				
Cider	1 tbsp	2	—	0
Ka-Me				
Chinese Seasoned	1 tbsp (0.5 fl oz)	5	0	0
Rice Wine Chinese	1 tbsp (0.5 fl oz)	5	0	0
Rice Wine Japanese	1 tbsp (0.5 oz)	0	0	0
Seasoned Rice Japanese	1 tbsp (0.5 fl oz)	10	0	0
Nakano				
Rice	1 tbsp	0	—	0
Regina				
Red Wine	1 oz	4	—	0
Tree Of Life				
Apple Cider Organic	1 tbsp (0.5 oz)	0	—	0
Brown Rice	1 tbsp (0.5 oz)	2	—	0
White House				
Apple Cider	2 tbsp	2	0	0
Red Wine	2 tbsp	4	—	0
WAFFLES				
FROZEN				
Aunt Jemima				
Blueberry	2 (2.5 oz)	190	1	10
Buttermilk	2 (2.5 oz)	170	1	10
Cinnamon	2 (2.5 oz)	180	1	10
Oatmeal	2 (2.5 oz)	170	3	0
Whole Grain	2 (2.5 oz)	170	2	0
Belgian Chef				
Belgian	2 (2.5 oz)	140	1	0

FOOD	PORTION	CALS.	FIB.	CHOL.
Downyflake				
Blueberry	2	180	—	0
Buttermilk	2	190	—	0
Multi-Grain	2	250	4	0
Oat Bran	2	260	3	0
Regular	2	120	—	0
Regular Jumbo	2	170	—	0
Rice Bran	2	210	4	0
Roman Meal	2	280	3	4
Eggo				
Apple Cinnamon	2 (2.7 oz)	220	0	20
Blueberry	2 (2.7 oz)	220	0	20
Buttermilk	2 (2.7 oz)	220	0	25
Common Sense Oat Bran	2 (2.7 oz)	200	3	0
Common Sense Oat Bran With Fruit & Nut	2 (2.9 oz)	220	4	0
Homestyle	2 (2.7 oz)	220	0	25
Minis Blueberry	12 (3 oz)	240	0	25
Minis Cinnamon Toast	12 (3.2 oz)	280	0	25
Minis Homestyle	12 (1.8 oz)	240	0	25
Nut & Honey	2 (2.7 oz)	240	0	25
Nutri-Grain	2 (2.7 oz)	190	4	0
Nutri-Grain Multi-Bran	2 (2.7 oz)	180	6	0
Nutri-Grain Raisin & Bran	2 (3 oz)	210	5	0
Special K	2 (2 oz)	140	0	0
Strawberry	2 (2.7 oz)	220	0	20
Van's				
7 Grain Belgian	2	152	8	0
Belgian Original	2	145	2	0
Belgian Original Toaster	2	145	2	0
Blueberry Toaster	2	157	2	0
Blueberry Wheat Free Toaster	2	225	5	0
Fat Free	2	155	7	0
Mini	4	107	6	0
Multigrain Toaster	2	160	6	0
Organic Whole Wheat	2	190	6	0
Organic Whole Wheat Blueberry	2	190	6	0
Wheat Free Cinnamon Apple Toaster	2	220	5	0
Wheat Free Toaster	2	220	5	0
Weight Watchers				
Belgian	1 (1.5 oz)	120	—	5

FOOD	PORTION	CALS.	FIB.	CHOL.
HOME RECIPE				
plain	1 (7 in diam)	218	—	52
MIX				
plain as prep	1 (2.6 oz) 7 in diam	218	1	39
WALNUTS				
black dried	1 oz	172	1	0
black dried chopped	1 cup	759	—	0
english dried	1 oz	182	1	0
english dried chopped	1 cup	770	6	0
Planters				
Black	1 pkg (2 oz)	340	3	0
Gold Measure Halves	1 pkg (2 oz)	380	2	0
Halves	⅓ cup (1.2 oz)	220	1	0
Pieces	¼ cup (1 oz)	190	1	0
WATER				
(*see* MINERAL/BOTTLED WATER)				
WATER CHESTNUTS				
CANNED				
chinese sliced	½ cup	35	—	0
Empress				
Sliced	2 oz	14	—	0
Whole	2 oz	14	—	0
Ka-Me				
Whole In Water	½ cup (4.5 oz)	45	4	0
La Choy				
Sliced	¼ cup	18	tr	0
Whole	4	14	tr	0
FRESH				
sliced	½ cup	66	—	0
WATERCRESS				
(*see also* CRESS)				
raw chopped	½ cup	2	tr	0
WATERMELON				
FRESH				
cut up	1 cup	50	1	0
wedge	¹⁄₁₆	152	2	0
SEEDS				
dried	1 oz	158	—	0
dried	1 cup	602	—	0
WAX BEANS				
CANNED				
Del Monte				
Cut Golden	½ cup (4.3 oz)	20	2	0

FOOD	PORTION	CALS.	FIB.	CHOL.
Owatonna				
Cut	½ cup	20	—	0
S&W				
Golden Cut Premium	½ cup	20	—	0
Seneca				
Cuts Natural Pack	½ cup	25	2	0
Wax Beans	½ cup	25	2	0

WHEAT
(*see also* BRAN, BULGUR, CEREAL, COUSCOUS, FLOUR, WHEAT GERM)

FOOD	PORTION	CALS.	FIB.	CHOL.
sprouted	⅓ cup	71	—	0
Arrowhead				
Kamut Grain	¼ cup (1.7 oz)	140	5	0
Seitan Quick Mix	⅓ cup (1.4 oz)	150	2	0
Hodgson Mill				
Vital Wheat Gluten Plus Ascorbic Acid	1 tbsp (0.3 oz)	30	1	0
Near East				
Taboule Salad Mix as prep	⅔ cup	120	3	0
Wheat Pilaf as prep	1 cup	220	5	0
Sonoma				
Wheat Nuts Salted	2 tbsp (0.5 oz)	60	1	0
White Wave				
Seitan	½ pkg (4 oz)	140	1	0
Seitan Fajita Strips	⅓ cup (1.8 oz)	60	1	0
Seitan Marinated Slices	3 slices (1.8 oz)	60	1	0

WHEAT GERM

FOOD	PORTION	CALS.	FIB.	CHOL.
plain toasted	¼ cup	108	4	0
plain toasted	1 cup	431	—	0
plain untoasted	¼ cup	104	4	0
Arrowhead				
Wheat Germ	3 tbsp (0.5 oz)	50	2	0
Hodgson Mill				
Wheat Germ	2 tbsp (0.5 oz)	55	4	0
Kretschmer				
Honey Crunch	¼ cup	105	3	0
Original	¼ cup	103	3	0
Stone-Buhr				
Untoasted	2 tbsp (0.5 oz)	58	2	0

WHIPPED TOPPINGS
(*see also* CREAM)

FOOD	PORTION	CALS.	FIB.	CHOL.
cream pressurized	1 cup (2.1 oz)	154	—	46
cream pressurized	1 tbsp (3 g)	8	—	2

FOOD	PORTION	CALS.	FIB.	CHOL.
nondairy frzn	1 tbsp	13	—	0
nondairy powdered as prep w/ whole milk	1 cup	151	—	8
nondairy powdered as prep w/ whole milk	1 tbsp (4 g)	8	—	tr
nondairy pressurized	1 tbsp (4 g)	11	—	0
nondairy pressurized	1 cup	184	—	0
Cool Whip				
Extra Creamy	1 tbsp	13	—	tr
Lite	1 tbsp	9	—	tr
Non Dairy	1 tbsp	11	—	tr
D-Zerta				
As prep	1 tbsp	7	—	tr
Dream Whip				
As prep	1 tbsp	9	—	1
Hood				
Instant	2 tbsp	20	0	<5
Light Instant	2 tbsp	15	0	<5
Kraft				
Real Cream	2 tbsp (0.4 oz)	20	0	5
Whipped Topping	2 tbsp (0.4 oz)	20	0	0
La Creme				
Topping	1 tbsp	16	—	tr
Pet				
Whip	1 tbsp	14	—	0
Reddiwip				
Lite	2 tbsp (8 g)	15	—	0
Non-Dairy	2 tbsp (8 g)	20	—	0
Real Whipped Heavy Cream	2 tbsp (8 g)	30	—	10
Real Whipped Light Cream	2 tbsp (8 g)	20	—	<5

WHITE BEANS
CANNED
white beans	1 cup	306	—	0
Goya				
Spanish Style	7.5 oz	130	12	0
Progresso				
Cannellini	½ cup (4.6 oz)	100	5	0

DRIED
regular cooked	1 cup	249	—	0
small cooked	1 cup	253	—	0

WHITEFISH
baked	3 oz	146	—	65
smoked	3 oz	92	—	28
smoked	1 oz	39	—	9

FOOD	PORTION	CALS.	FIB.	CHOL.
WHITING				
cooked	3 oz	98	—	71
raw	3 oz	77	—	57
WILD RICE				
cooked	½ cup	83	—	0
Haddon House				
Extra Fancy	¼ cup (1.6 oz)	170	2	0
WINE				
(*see also* CHAMPAGNE, WINE COOLERS)				
red	3½ oz	74	—	0
rose	3½ oz	73	—	0
sherry	2 oz	84	—	0
sweet dessert	2 oz	90	—	0
vermouth dry	3½ oz	105	—	0
vermouth sweet	3½ oz	167	—	0
white	3½ oz	70	—	0
Boone's				
Country Kwencher	1 fl oz	24	—	0
Delicious Apple	1 fl oz	21	—	0
Sangria	1 fl oz	22	—	0
Snow Creek Berry	1 fl oz	18	—	0
Strawberry Hill	1 fl oz	22	—	0
Sun Peak Peach	1 fl oz	18	—	0
Wild Island	1 fl oz	18	—	0
Carlo Rossi				
Blush	1 fl oz	21	—	0
Burgundy	1 fl oz	22	—	0
Chablis	1 fl oz	21	—	0
Paisano	1 fl oz	23	—	0
Red Sangria	1 fl oz	24	—	0
Rhine	1 fl oz	21	—	0
Vin Rose	1 fl oz	21	—	0
White Grenache	1 fl oz	20	—	0
Fairbanks				
Cream Sherry	1 fl oz	42	—	0
Port	1 fl oz	44	—	0
Sherry	1 fl oz	34	—	0
White Port	1 fl oz	44	—	0
Gallo				
Blush Chablis	1 fl oz	22	—	0
Burgundy	1 fl oz	22	—	0
Cabernet Sauvignon	1 fl oz	22	—	0
Chablis Blanc	1 fl oz	20	—	0

FOOD	PORTION	CALS.	FIB.	CHOL.
Gallo (CONT.)				
Chardonnay	1 fl oz	23	—	0
Classic Burgundy	1 fl oz	21	—	0
French Colombard	1 fl oz	21	—	0
Hearty Burgundy	1 fl oz	22	—	0
Johannisbery Riesling '88	1 fl oz	20	—	0
Pink Chablis	1 fl oz	20	—	0
Red Rose	1 fl oz	23	—	0
Rhine	1 fl oz	22	—	0
Sauvignon Blanc '90	1 fl oz	20	—	0
White Grenache '92	1 fl oz	20	—	0
White Grenache New Vintage	1 fl oz	20	—	0
White Zinfandel '91	1 fl oz	18	—	0
White Zinfandel New Vintage	1 fl oz	18	—	0
Zinfandel '87	1 fl oz	23	—	0
Ka-Me				
Chinese Cooking	2 tbsp (1 fl oz)	20	0	0
Sheffield Cellars				
Sherry	1 fl oz	44	—	0
Tawny Port	1 fl oz	45	—	0
Vermouth Extra Dry	1 fl oz	28	—	0
Vermouth Sweet	1 fl oz	43	—	0
Very Dry Sherry	1 fl oz	32	—	0

WINE COOLERS

Bartles & Jaymes

Berry	12 fl oz	210	—	0
Margarita	12 fl oz	260	—	0
Original	12 fl oz	190	—	0
Peach	12 fl oz	210	—	0
Pina Colada	12 fl oz	280	—	0
Planter's Punch	12 fl oz	230	—	0
Strawberry	12 fl oz	210	—	0
Strawberry Daiquiri	12 fl oz	230	—	0
Tropical	12 fl oz	230	—	0

WINGED BEANS

dried cooked	1 cup	252	—	0

WOLFFISH

atlantic baked	3 oz	105	—	50

YAM

(*see also* SWEET POTATO)

CANNED

Allen

Cut	⅔ cup (5.8 oz)	160	3	0

FOOD	PORTION	CALS.	FIB.	CHOL.
Princella				
Cut	⅔ cup (5.8 oz)	160	3	0
Royal Prince				
Whole	4 pieces (5.9 oz)	200	4	0
S&W				
Candied	½ cup	180	—	0
Southern Whole In Extra Heavy Syrup	½ cup	139	—	0
Sugary Sam				
Cut	⅔ cup (5.8 oz)	160	3	0
Trappey				
Whole	4 pieces (5.9 oz)	200	4	0
FRESH				
mountain yam hawaii cooked	½ cup	59	—	0
yam cubed cooked	½ cup	79	—	0
YAMBEAN				
cooked	¾ cup	38	—	0
YARDLONG BEANS				
dried cooked	1 cup	202	—	0
YEAST				
baker's compressed	1 cake (0.6 oz)	18	2	0
baker's dry	1 pkg (¼ oz)	21	—	0
baker's dry	1 tbsp	35	3	0
brewer's dry	1 tbsp	25	—	0
Fleischmann's				
Active Dry	1 pkg (¼ oz)	20	—	0
Fresh Active	1 pkg (0.6 oz)	15	—	0
Household Yeast	½ oz	15	—	0
RapidRise	1 pkg (¼ oz)	20	—	0
Red Star				
Yeast	4 tbsp (0.5 oz)	47	4	0
Yeast Flakes	3 tbsp (0.5 oz)	47	4	0
YELLOW BEANS				
canned	½ cup	13	1	0
canned low sodium	½ cup	13	1	0
dried cooked	1 cup	254	—	0
fresh cooked	½ cup	22	—	0
fresh raw	½ cup	17	—	0
frozen cooked	½ cup	18	—	0
YELLOWEYE BEANS				
CANNED				
B&M				
Baked	½ cup (4.6 oz)	170	7	<5

FOOD	PORTION	CALS.	FIB.	CHOL.
DRIED				
Bean Cuisine				
Dried	½ cup	115	5	0
YOGURT				
(*see also* YOGURT FROZEN)				
coffee lowfat	8 oz	194	—	11
fruit lowfat	4 oz	113	—	5
fruit lowfat	8 oz	225	—	10
plain	8 oz	139	—	29
plain lowfat	8 oz	144	—	14
plain no fat	8 oz	127	—	4
vanilla lowfat	8 oz	194	—	11
Breyers				
1% Fat Black Cherry	8 oz	260	0	15
1% Fat Blueberry	8 oz	250	0	15
1% Fat Mixed Berry	8 oz	250	0	15
1% Fat Peach	8 oz	250	0	15
1% Fat Pineapple	8 oz	250	0	15
1% Fat Red Raspberry	8 oz	250	2	15
1% Fat Strawberry	8 oz	250	0	15
1% Fat Strawberry Banana	8 oz	250	tr	15
1.5% Fat Coffee	8 oz	220	0	20
1.5% Fat Plain	8 oz	130	0	20
1.5% Fat Vanilla	8 oz	220	0	20
Cabot				
All Flavors	8 oz	220	—	10
Plain	8 oz	140	—	14
Colombo				
Banana Strawberry	8 oz	210	0	15
Black Cherry	8 oz	200	0	15
Blueberry	8 oz	200	0	15
Fat Free Apples 'n Spice	8 oz	190	0	5
Fat Free Apricot	8 oz	190	0	5
Fat Free Banana Strawberry	8 oz	200	0	5
Fat Free Blueberry	8 oz	190	0	5
Fat Free Cappuccino	8 oz	180	0	<5
Fat Free Cherry	8 oz	190	0	5
Fat Free Cranberry Strawberry	8 oz	200	0	5
Fat Free French Roast	8 oz	180	0	<5
Fat Free Fruit Cocktail	8 oz	190	0	5
Fat Free Lemon	8 oz	170	0	<5
Fat Free Peach	8 oz	190	0	5
Fat Free Plain	8 oz	110	0	5

FOOD	PORTION	CALS.	FIB.	CHOL.
Colombo (CONT.)				
Fat Free Raspberry	8 oz	190	0	5
Fat Free Strawberry	8 oz	190	0	5
Fat Free Strawberry Pineapple Orange	8 oz	190	0	5
Fat Free Vanilla	8 oz	170	0	5
French Vanilla	8 oz	180	0	20
Light 100 Blueberry	8 oz	100	0	<5
Light 100 Cherry Vanilla	8 oz	100	0	<5
Light 100 Coffee & Cream	8 oz	100	0	<5
Light 100 Creamy Vanilla	8 oz	100	0	<5
Light 100 Fruit Medley	8 oz	100	0	<5
Light 100 Juicy Peach	8 oz	100	0	<5
Light 100 Lemon Creme	8 oz	100	0	<5
Light 100 Mandarin Orange	8 oz	100	0	<5
Light 100 Mixed Berries	8 oz	100	0	<5
Light 100 Raspberry	8 oz	100	0	<5
Light 100 Strawberry	8 oz	100	0	<5
Peach Melba	8 oz	200	0	15
Plain	8 oz	120	0	20
Raspberry	8 oz	200	0	15
Strawberry	8 oz	200	0	15
Dannon				
Blended Nonfat Blueberry	6 oz	160	0	<5
Blended Nonfat French Vanilla	6 oz	160	0	<5
Blended Nonfat Lemon Chiffon	6 oz	150	0	<5
Blended Nonfat Peach	6 oz	150	0	<5
Blended Nonfat Raspberry	6 oz	160	0	<5
Blended Nonfat Strawberry	6 oz	150	0	<5
Blended Nonfat Strawberry Banana	6 oz	150	0	<5
Danimals Lowfat Tropical Punch	4.4 oz	140	0	10
Danimals Lowfat Blueberry	4.4 oz	140	0	10
Danimals Lowfat Grape Lemonade	4.4 oz	130	0	10
Danimals Lowfat Lemon Ice	4.4 oz	130	0	10
Danimals Lowfat Orange Banana	4.4 oz	140	0	10
Danimals Lowfat Strawberry	4.4 oz	140	0	10
Danimals Lowfat Vanilla	4.4 oz	140	0	10
Danimals Lowfat Wild Raspberry	4.4 oz	130	0	10
Fruit On The Bottom Lowfat Apple Cinnamon	8 oz	240	1	15

FOOD	PORTION	CALS.	FIB.	CHOL.
Dannon (CONT.)				
Fruit On The Bottom Lowfat Blueberry	8 oz	240	1	15
Fruit On The Bottom Lowfat Boysenberry	8 oz	240	1	15
Fruit On The Bottom Lowfat Cherry	8 oz	240	1	15
Fruit On The Bottom Lowfat Mixed Berries	8 oz	240	1	15
Fruit On The Bottom Lowfat Orange	8 oz	240	0	15
Fruit On The Bottom Lowfat Peach	8 oz	240	1	15
Fruit On The Bottom Lowfat Pear	8 oz	240	1	15
Fruit On The Bottom Lowfat Raspberry	8 oz	240	1	15
Fruit On The Bottom Lowfat Strawberry	8 oz	240	1	15
Fruit On The Bottom Lowfat Strawberry Banana	8 oz	240	1	15
Light Nonfat Banana Cream Pie	4.4 oz	60	0	0
Light Nonfat Cherry Vanilla	1 cup (3.5 oz)	110	0	<5
Light Nonfat Lemon Chiffon	4.4 oz	60	0	0
Light Nonfat Peach	4.4 oz	50	0	0
Light Nonfat Strawberry	4.4 oz	50	0	0
Light Nonfat Strawberry	1 cup (3.5 oz)	110	0	<5
Light Nonfat Vanilla	1 cup (3.5 oz)	110	0	<5
Light 'N Crunchy Nonfat Cappuccino w/ Chocolate	1 pkg	150	0	<5
Light 'N Crunchy Nonfat Caramel Apple Crunch	1 pkg	150	0	<5
Light 'N Crunchy Nonfat Lemon Chiffon w/ Blueberry	1 pkg	140	0	<5
Light 'N Crunchy Nonfat Raspberry w/ Granola	1 pkg	150	0	<5
Light 'N Crunchy Nonfat Vanilla w/ Chocolate	1 pkg	150	1	<5
Light Nonfat Banana Cream Pie	8 oz	100	0	<5
Light Nonfat Blueberry	8 oz	100	0	<5
Light Nonfat Creme Caramel	8 oz	100	0	<5
Light Nonfat Lemon	8 oz	100	0	<5
Light Nonfat Peach	8 oz	100	0	<5
Light Nonfat Raspberry	8 oz	100	0	<5

FOOD	PORTION	CALS.	FIB.	CHOL.
Dannon (CONT.)				
Light Nonfat Strawberry	8 oz	100	0	<5
Light Nonfat Strawberry Banana	8 oz	100	0	<5
Light Nonfat Tropical Fruit	8 oz	100	0	<5
Light Nonfat Vanilla	8 oz	100	0	<5
Lowfat Coffee	8 oz	210	0	15
Lowfat Coffee	1 cup (8.7 oz)	230	0	20
Lowfat Cranberry Raspberry	8 oz	210	0	15
Lowfat Lemon	8 oz	210	0	15
Lowfat Lemon	1 cup (8.7 oz)	230	0	20
Lowfat Plain	1 cup (8.7 oz)	150	0	20
Lowfat Plain	8 oz	140	0	20
Lowfat Vanilla	8 oz	210	0	15
Lowfat Vanilla	1 cup (8.7 oz)	230	0	20
Minipack Blended Nonfat Blueberry	4.4 oz	120	0	<5
Minipack Blended Nonfat Cherry	4.4 oz	110	0	<5
Minipack Blended Nonfat Peach	4.4 oz	110	0	<5
Minipack Blended Nonfat Raspberry	4.4 oz	120	0	<5
Minipack Blended Nonfat Strawberry	4.4 oz	110	0	<5
Minipack Blended Nonfat Strawberry Banana	4.4 oz	110	0	<5
Nonfat Light Cherry Vanilla	8 oz	100	0	<5
Nonfat Light Strawberry Fruit Cup	8 oz	100	0	<5
Nonfat Plain	1 cup (8.7 oz)	120	0	0
Nonfat Plain	8 oz	110	0	5
Sprinkl'ins Banana	4.1 oz	140	0	10
Sprinkl'ins Cherry Vanilla	4.1 oz	140	0	10
Sprinkl'ins Crazy Crunch Cherry w/ Honey Grahams	4.4 oz	170	0	10
Sprinkl'ins Crazy Crunch Grape w/ Chocolate Grahams	4.4 oz	160	0	10
Sprinkl'ins Crazy Crunch Vanilla w/ Chocolate Grahams	4.4 oz	160	0	10
Sprinkl'ins Crazy Crunch Vanilla w/ Honey Grahams	4.4 oz	170	0	10
Sprinkl'ins Strawberry	4.1 oz	140	0	10
Sprinkl'ins Strawberry Banana	4.1 oz	140	0	10
Tropifruta Nonfat Banana	6 oz	150	0	5

FOOD	PORTION	CALS.	FIB.	CHOL.
Dannon (CONT.)				
Tropifruta Nonfat Guava	6 oz	150	0	5
Tropifruta Nonfat Mango	6 oz	150	0	5
Tropifruta Nonfat Papaya Pineapple	6 oz	150	0	5
Tropifruta Nonfat Pina Colada	6 oz	150	0	5
Tropifruta Nonfat Strawberry	6 oz	150	0	5
Tropifruta Nonfat Strawberry Banana	6 oz	150	0	5
Tropifruta Nonfat Strawberry Kiwi	6 oz	150	0	5
With Fruit Toppings Banana Creme Strawberry	6 oz	170	1	10
With Fruit Toppings Bavarian Creme Raspberry	6 oz	170	0	10
With Fruit Toppings Cheesecake Cherry	6 oz	170	0	10
With Fruit Toppings Cheesecake Strawberry	6 oz	170	1	10
With Fruit Toppings Vanilla Peach & Apricot	6 oz	170	0	10
With Fruit Toppings Vanilla Strawberry	6 oz	170	1	10
Friendship				
Coffee	8 oz	210	0	20
Fruit Crunch Blueberry	6 oz	190	0	10
Fruit Crunch Peach	6 oz	190	0	10
Fruit Crunch Strawberry	6 oz	190	0	10
Fruit Crunch Strawberry Banana	6 oz	190	0	10
Plain	8 oz	150	0	20
Hood				
Fat Free Blueberry	1 (8 oz)	190	1	5
Fat Free Cherry	1 (8 oz)	190	1	5
Fat Free Peach	1 (8 oz)	190	1	5
Fat Free Plain	1 (8 oz)	130	0	5
Fat Free Raspberry	1 (8 oz)	190	1	5
Fat Free Strawberry	1 (8 oz)	190	1	5
Fat Free Strawberry Banana	1 (8 oz)	190	1	5
Fat Free Swiss Blueberry	1 (8 oz)	210	0	5
Fat Free Swiss Lemon	1 (8 oz)	210	0	5
Fat Free Swiss Raspberry	1 (8 oz)	210	0	5
Fat Free Swiss Strawberry	1 (8 oz)	210	0	5
Fat Free Swiss Strawberry Banana	1 (8 oz)	210	0	5

FOOD	PORTION	CALS.	FIB.	CHOL.
Hood (CONT.)				
Fat Free Swiss Vanilla	1 (8 oz)	210	0	5
Fat Free Vanilla	1 (8 oz)	190	1	5
Knudsen				
1.5% Fat Creamy Lemon	8 oz	220	0	20
70 Calories Black Cherry	6 oz	70	0	<5
70 Calories Blueberry	6 oz	70	0	5
70 Calories Lemon	6 oz	70	tr	5
70 Calories Peach	6 oz	70	tr	5
70 Calories Pineapple	6 oz	70	0	5
70 Calories Red Raspberry	6 oz	70	0	5
70 Calories Strawberry	6 oz	70	0	5
70 Calories Strawberry Banana	6 oz	70	0	5
70 Calories Strawberry Fruit Basket	6 oz	70	0	5
70 Calories Vanilla	6 oz	70	0	5
Free Lemon	6 oz	160	0	5
Free Mixed Berry	6 oz	170	0	5
Free Peach	6 oz	170	0	5
Free Red Raspberry	6 oz	170	0	5
Free Strawberry	6 oz	170	0	5
Free Vanilla	6 oz	170	0	5
La Yogurt				
French Style Banana	6 oz	180	0	10
French Style Blueberry	6 oz	180	1	10
French Style Cherry	6 oz	180	0	10
French Style Cherry Vanilla	6 oz	190	0	10
French Style Guava	6 oz	180	1	10
French Style Key Lime	6 oz	180	0	10
French Style Mango	6 oz	180	0	10
French Style Mixed Berry	6 oz	180	0	10
French Style Nonfat Blueberry	6 oz	70	0	5
French Style Nonfat Cherry	6 oz	75	0	5
French Style Nonfat Raspberry	6 oz	70	0	5
French Style Nonfat Strawberry	6 oz	70	0	5
French Style Nonfat Strawberry Banana	6 oz	70	0	5
French Style Peach	6 oz	180	0	10
French Style Pina Colada	6 oz	180	0	10
French Style Raspberry	6 oz	180	1	10
French Style Strawberry	6 oz	180	0	10
French Style Strawberry Banana	6 oz	180	0	10

FOOD	PORTION	CALS.	FIB.	CHOL.
La Yogurt (CONT.)				
French Style Strawberry Fruit Cup	6 oz	180	0	10
French Style Tropical Orange	6 oz	180	0	10
French Style Vanilla	6 oz	170	0	15
Latin Style Banana	6 oz	190	0	10
Latin Style Guava	6 oz	190	0	10
Latin Style Mango	6 oz	190	0	10
Latin Style Papaya	6 oz	190	0	10
Latin Style Passion Fruit	6 oz	190	0	10
Latin Style Strawberry Kiwi	6 oz	180	0	10
Light N'Lively				
Free Blueberry	6 oz	190	0	5
Free Lemon	6 oz	170	0	5
Free Mixed Berry	6 oz	170	0	5
Free Peach	6 oz	170	0	5
Free Red Raspberry	6 oz	180	0	5
Free Strawberry	6 oz	180	0	5
Free Strawberry Fruit Cup	6 oz	170	0	5
Free Vanilla	6 oz	160	0	5
Free 50 Calories Blueberry	4.4 oz	50	0	<5
Free 50 Calories Peach	4.4 oz	50	0	<5
Free 50 Calories Red Raspberry	4.4 oz	50	0	<5
Free 50 Calories Strawberry	4.4 oz	50	0	<5
Free 50 Calories Strawberry Banana	4.4 oz	50	0	<5
Free 50 Calories Strawberry Fruit Cup	4.4 oz	50	0	<5
Free 70 Calories Black Cherry	6 oz	70	0	<5
Free 70 Calories Blueberry	6 oz	70	0	<5
Free 70 Calories Lemon	6 oz	70	0	<5
Free 70 Calories Peach	6 oz	70	0	<5
Free 70 Calories Red Raspberry	6 oz	70	0	<5
Free 70 Calories Strawberry	6 oz	70	0	<5
Free 70 Calories Strawberry Banana	6 oz	70	0	<5
Free 70 Calories Strawberry Fruit Cup	6 oz	70	0	<5
Kidpack Banana Berry	4.4 oz	130	0	10
Kidpack Berry Blue	4.4 oz	150	0	10
Kidpack Cherry	4.4 oz	140	0	10
Kidpack Grape	4.4 oz	130	0	10
Kidpack Outrageous Orange	4.4 oz	150	0	10
Kidpack Tropical Punch	4.4 oz	140	0	10

FOOD	PORTION	CALS.	FIB.	CHOL.
Light N'Lively (CONT.)				
Kidpack Wild Berry	4.4 oz	140	0	10
Kidpack Wild Strawberry	4.4 oz	140	0	10
Multipack Blueberry	4.4 oz	140	0	10
Multipack Peach	4.4 oz	140	0	10
Multipack Pineapple	4.4 oz	140	0	5
Multipack Red Raspberry	4.4 oz	130	0	10
Multipack Strawberry	4.4 oz	140	0	10
Multipack Strawberry Banana	4.4 oz	140	0	10
Multipack Strawberry Fruit Cup	4.4 oz	140	0	10
Weight Watchers				
Ultimate 90 Blueberries 'n Creme	1 cup	90	3	5
Ultimate 90 Cappuccino	1 cup	90	0	5
Ultimate 90 Cherries Jubilee	1 cup	90	3	5
Ultimate 90 Cranberry Raspberry	1 cup	90	0	5
Ultimate 90 Lemon Chiffon	1 cup	90	1	5
Ultimate 90 Peach	1 cup	90	0	5
Ultimate 90 Plain	1 cup	90	0	5
Ultimate 90 Raspberries 'n Creme	1 cup	90	0	5
Ultimate 90 Strawberry	1 cup	90	2	5
Ultimate 90 Strawberry Banana	1 cup	90	2	5
Ultimate 90 Vanilla	1 cup	90	0	5
Yoplait				
Custard Style Banana	6 oz	190	—	20
Custard Style Blueberry	6 oz	190	—	20
Custard Style Cherry	6 oz	180	—	20
Custard Style Lemon	6 oz	190	—	20
Custard Style Mixed Berry	6 oz	180	—	20
Custard Style Raspberry	6 oz	190	—	20
Custard Style Strawberry	4 oz	130	—	15
Custard Style Strawberry	6 oz	190	—	20
Custard Style Strawberry Banana	6 oz	190	—	20
Custard Style Strawberry Banana	4 oz	130	—	15
Custard Style Vanilla	4 oz	130	—	15
Custard Style Vanilla	6 oz	180	—	20
Fat Free Blueberry	6 oz	150	—	5
Fat Free Cherry	6 oz	150	—	5
Fat Free Mixed Berry	6 oz	150	—	5
Fat Free Peach	6 oz	150	—	5

FOOD	PORTION	CALS.	FIB.	CHOL.
Yoplait (CONT.)				
Fat Free Raspberry	6 oz	150	—	5
Fat Free Strawberry	6 oz	150	—	5
Fat Free Strawberry Banana	6 oz	150	—	5
Light Blueberry	4 oz	60	—	<5
Light Blueberry	6 oz	80	—	<5
Light Cherry	6 oz	80	—	<5
Light Cherry	4 oz	60	—	<5
Light Peach	4 oz	60	—	<5
Light Peach	6 oz	80	—	<5
Light Raspberry	6 oz	80	—	<5
Light Raspberry	4 oz	60	—	<5
Light Strawberry	6 oz	80	—	<5
Light Strawberry	4 oz	60	—	<5
Light Strawberry Banana	6 oz	80	—	<5
Light Strawberry Banana	4 oz	60	—	<5
Nonfat Plain	8 oz	120	—	5
Nonfat Vanilla	8 oz	180	—	5
Original Apple	6 oz	190	—	10
Original Blueberry	6 oz	190	—	10
Original Blueberry	4 oz	120	—	5
Original Boysenberry	6 oz	190	—	10
Original Cherry	6 oz	190	—	10
Original Lemon	6 oz	190	—	10
Original Mixed Berry	6 oz	190	—	10
Original Orange	6 oz	190	—	10
Original Peach	6 oz	190	—	10
Original Peach	4 oz	120	—	5
Original Pina Colada	6 oz	190	—	10
Original Pineapple	6 oz	190	—	10
Original Plain	6 oz	130	—	15
Original Raspberry	6 oz	190	—	10
Original Raspberry	4 oz	120	—	5
Original Strawberry	6 oz	190	—	10
Original Strawberry	4 oz	120	—	5
Original Strawberry Banana	6 oz	190	—	10
Original Strawberry Rhubarb	6 oz	190	—	10
Original Vanilla	6 oz	180	—	10

YOGURT FROZEN
(see also TOFU, YOGURT*)*

FOOD	PORTION	CALS.	FIB.	CHOL.
chocolate soft serve	½ cup (4 fl oz)	115	—	3
vanilla soft serve	½ cup (4 fl oz)	114	—	2
Bee-Lite				
Chocolate	4 oz	100	—	0

FOOD	PORTION	CALS.	FIB.	CHOL.
Bee-Lite (CONT.)				
Vanilla	4 oz	110	—	0
Ben & Jerry's				
Cherry Garcia	½ cup (3.7 oz)	170	0	10
Chocolate Fudge Brownie	½ cup (3.7 oz)	190	2	10
Coffee Almond Fudge	½ cup (3.7 oz)	200	1	15
English Toffee Crunch	½ cup (3.7 oz)	190	0	10
No Fat Cappuccino	½ cup (3.3 oz)	140	0	0
Pop Cherry Garcia	1 (3.8 oz)	290	2	20
Bresler's				
All Flavors	5 oz	145	—	9
All Flavors Lite	5 oz	135	—	0
Breyers				
Chocolate	½ cup (2.7 oz)	150	1	15
Light Fat Free Apple Pie A La Mode	1 cup (8 oz)	130	tr	5
Light Fat Free Black Cherry Jubilee	1 cup (8 oz)	130	tr	5
Light Fat Free Blueberries n' Cream	1 cup (8 oz)	130	tr	5
Light Fat Free Cherry Chocolate	1 cup (8 oz)	130	tr	5
Light Fat Free Classic Strawberry	1 cup (8 oz)	130	tr	5
Light Fat Free Key Lime Pie	1 cup (8 oz)	130	tr	5
Light Fat Free Lemon Chiffon	1 cup (8 oz)	130	tr	5
Light Fat Free Peaches n'Cream	1 cup (8 oz)	130	tr	5
Light Fat Free Strawberry Cheesecake	1 cup (8 oz)	130	tr	5
Red Raspberry	½ cup (2.7 oz)	140	0	15
Strawberry Banana	½ cup (2.7 oz)	140	0	15
Vanilla	½ cup (2.7 oz)	140	0	15
Dannon				
Coco-Nut Fudge	½ cup (3 oz)	160	0	15
Light Cappuccino	½ cup (2.8 oz)	80	0	0
Light Cherry Vanilla Swirl	½ cup (2.8 oz)	90	0	0
Light Chocolate	½ cup (2.7 oz)	80	1	0
Light Lemon Chiffon	½ cup (2.8 oz)	90	0	0
Light Peach Raspberry Melba	½ cup (2.8 oz)	90	0	0
Light Strawberry Cheesecake	½ cup (2.8 oz)	90	0	0
Light Vanilla	½ cup (2.8 oz)	80	0	0
Light Nonfat Cappuccino	8 oz	100	0	<5
Light'N Crunchy Banana Cream Pie	½ cup (2.8 oz)	110	0	0
Light'N Crunchy Mocha Chocolate Chunk	½ cup (2.8 oz)	110	0	0

FOOD	PORTION	CALS.	FIB.	CHOL.
Dannon (CONT.)				
Light'N Crunchy Peanut Chocolate Crunch	½ cup (2.8 oz)	110	0	0
Light'N Crunchy Triple Chocolate	½ cup (2.8 oz)	110	0	0
Light'N Crunchy Vanilla Blueberry Swirl	½ cup (2.8 oz)	110	0	0
Pure Indulgence Cherry Chocolate Cherry	½ cup (3 oz)	150	0	15
Pure Indulgence Chunky Chocolate Nut	½ cup (3 oz)	150	0	0
Pure Indulgence Cookies'n Cream	½ cup (3 oz)	150	0	0
Pure Indulgence Crunchy Expresso	½ cup (3 oz)	150	0	15
Pure Indulgence Heath Toffee Crunch	½ cup (3 oz)	150	0	5
Pure Indulgence Vanilla Raspberry Truffle	½ cup (3 oz)	150	1	15
Desserve				
All Flavors	4 oz	70	—	0
Dutch Chocolate	4 oz	80	—	0
Edy's				
Banana Strawberry	3 oz	80	—	5
Blueberry	3 oz	80	—	5
Cherry	3 oz	80	—	5
Chocolate	3 oz	80	—	5
Chocolate Chip	3 oz	100	—	5
Citrus Heights	3 oz	80	—	5
Cookies'N'Cream	3 oz	100	—	5
Marble Fudge	3 oz	100	—	5
Perfectly Peach	3 oz	80	—	5
Raspberry	3 oz	80	—	5
Raspberry Vanilla Swirl	3 oz	80	—	5
Strawberry	3 oz	80	—	5
Vanilla	3 oz	80	—	5
Elan				
Blueberry	4 oz	130	—	11
Caramel Almond Praline	4 oz	150	—	10
Chocolate	4 oz	130	—	10
Chocolate Almond	4 oz	160	—	10
Coffee	4 oz	130	—	11
Coffee Decaffeinated	4 oz	130	—	11
Peach	4 oz	130	—	10

FOOD	PORTION	CALS.	FIB.	CHOL.
Elan (CONT.)				
Rum Raisin	4 oz	135	—	12
Strawberry	4 oz	125	—	10
Vanilla	4 oz	130	—	11
Fi-Bar				
Chocolate	1	190	4	0
Strawberry	1	190	4	0
Vanilla	1	190	4	0
Friendly's				
Apple Bettie	½ cup (2.6 oz)	140	0	10
Fabulous Fudge Swirl	½ cup (2.6 oz)	140	0	10
Fudge Berry Swirl	½ cup (2.6 oz)	150	0	10
Lowfat Perfectly Peach	½ cup (2.6 oz)	110	0	10
Lowfat Purely Chocolate	½ cup (2.6 oz)	120	0	10
Lowfat Raspberry Delight	½ cup (2.6 oz)	120	0	10
Lowfat Simply Vanilla	½ cup (2.6 oz)	120	0	10
Lowfat Strawberry Patch	½ cup (2.6 oz)	110	0	10
Mint Chocolate Chip	½ cup (2.6 oz)	130	0	10
Strawberry Cheesecake Blast	½ cup (2.6 oz)	140	0	15
Toffee Almond Crunch	½ cup (2.6 oz)	160	tr	15
Good Humor				
Creamsicle Raspberry	1 (2.8 oz)	100	0	<5
Frista Cup	1 (6.2 oz)	220	1	15
Haagen-Dazs				
Banana Nut Blast	½ cup (3.5 oz)	220	1	40
Bars Cherry Chocolate Fudge	1 (2.6 oz)	240	1	35
Bars Peach	1 (2.5 oz)	90	0	15
Bars Pina Colada	1 (2.5 oz)	100	0	15
Bars Raspberry & Vanilla	1 (2.5 oz)	90	0	15
Bars Strawberry Daiquiri	1 (2.5 oz)	90	0	15
Chocolate	½ cup (3.4 oz)	160	tr	30
Coffee	½ cup (3.4 oz)	160	0	45
Fat Free Bar Raspberry & Vanilla	1 (2.5 oz)	90	0	0
Fat Free Cherry Vanilla	½ cup (3.3 oz)	140	0	<5
Fat Free Chocolate	½ cup (3.3 oz)	140	tr	<5
Fat Free Coffee	½ cup (3.3 oz)	140	0	<5
Fat Free Vanilla	½ cup (3.3 oz)	140	0	<5
Fat Free Vanilla Fudge	½ cup (3.3 oz)	160	0	<5
Orange Tango	½ cup (3.5 oz)	130	0	20
Pina Colada	½ cup (3.4 oz)	130	0	25
Raspberry Randevous	½ cup (3.5 oz)	130	1	20
Strawberry Cheesecake Craze	½ cup (3.6 oz)	220	0	65
Strawberry Duet	½ cup (3.4 oz)	130	tr	25

FOOD	PORTION	CALS.	FIB.	CHOL.
Haagen-Dazs (CONT.)				
Vanilla	½ cup (3.4 oz)	160	0	45
Hood				
Bavarian Truffle & Twist	½ cup (2.6 oz)	150	0	10
Coffee Toffee Chunk Sundae	½ cup (2.6 oz)	150	0	10
Combo Bars	1 (2.2 oz)	90	0	5
Cookies & Cream	½ cup (2.6 oz)	140	0	10
Grandma's Raisin Oatmeal Cookie Dough	½ cup (2.6 oz)	140	0	10
Mixed Berry Swirl	½ cup (2.6 oz)	120	0	10
Natural Strawberry	½ cup (2.6 oz)	110	0	10
Natural Strawberry Banana	½ cup (2.6 oz)	110	0	10
Natural Vanilla	½ cup (2.6 oz)	120	0	10
Nonfat Caramel & Brownie Sundae	½ cup (2.6 oz)	120	0	0
Nonfat Chocolate Marshmallow	½ cup (2.6 oz)	110	0	0
Nonfat Double Raspberry	½ cup (2.6 oz)	120	0	0
Nonfat Mocha Fudge	½ cup (2.6 oz)	120	0	0
Nonfat Olde Fashioned Vanilla	½ cup (2.6 oz)	110	0	0
Nonfat Peach Cobbler A La Mode	½ cup (2.6 oz)	110	0	0
Nonfat Strawberry	½ cup (2.6 oz)	100	0	0
Nonfat Vanilla Fudge	½ cup (2.6 oz)	120	0	0
Raspberry Swirl	½ cup (2.6 oz)	130	0	10
Sundae Cups Chocolate & Strawberry	1 (2.2 oz)	110	1	5
Vanilla Chocolate Strawberry	½ cup (2.6 oz)	120	0	10
Vanilla Swiss Almond Sundae	½ cup (2.6 oz)	150	0	10
Just 10				
All Flavors	1 oz	10	—	0
Kissed With Honey				
Chocolate	3.5 oz	100	—	9
Nonfat Chocolate	3.5 oz	85	—	0
Nonfat Vanilla	3.5 oz	85	—	0
Vanilla	3.5 oz	100	—	9
Sealtest				
Chocolate	½ cup (2.7 oz)	120	tr	5
Mocha Fudge	½ cup (2.6 oz)	130	tr	10
Vanilla	½ cup (2.6 oz)	120	0	10
Tofutti				
Better Than Yogurt Chocolate Fudge	4 fl oz	120	0	0
Better Than Yogurt Coffee Marshmallow Swirl	4 fl oz	100	0	0

FOOD	PORTION	CALS.	FIB.	CHOL.
Tofutti (CONT.)				
Better Than Yogurt Passion Island Fruit	4 fl oz	100	0	0
Better Than Yogurt Peach Mango	4 fl oz	100	0	0
Better Than Yogurt Strawberry Banana	4 fl oz	100	0	0
Better Than Yogurt Vanilla Fudge	4 fl oz	120	0	0
Turkey Hill				
Chocolate Cherry Cordial	½ cup (2.6 oz)	130	0	10
Chocolate Chip Cookie Dough	½ cup (2.6 oz)	140	0	10
Death By Chocolate	½ cup (2.6 oz)	150	0	10
Nonfat Chocolate Cherry Cordial	½ cup (2.4 oz)	100	0	0
Nonfat Chocolate Marshmallow	½ cup (2.4 oz)	130	0	0
Nonfat Coffee Cappuccino	½ cup (2.4 oz)	110	0	0
Nonfat Mint Cookie 'N Cream	½ cup (2.4 oz)	110	0	0
Nonfat Neapolitan	½ cup (2.4 oz)	100	0	0
Nonfat Raspberry Chocolate Bliss	½ cup (2.4 oz)	110	0	0
Nonfat Southern Lemon Pie	½ cup (2.4 oz)	110	0	0
Nonfat Vanilla Fudge	½ cup (2.4 oz)	110	0	0
Peach Raspberry	½ cup (2.6 oz)	110	0	10
Strawberry	½ cup (2.6 oz)	110	0	10
Tin Roof Sundae	½ cup (2.6 oz)	140	0	10
Vanilla & Chocolate	½ cup (2.6 oz)	110	0	10
Vanilla Bean	½ cup (2.6 oz)	110	0	10

ZUCCHINI
CANNED

FOOD	PORTION	CALS.	FIB.	CHOL.
italian style	½ cup	33	—	0
Del Monte				
With Italian Tomato Sauce	½ cup (4.2 oz)	30	1	0
Progresso				
Italian Style	½ cup (4.2 oz)	40	2	0
S&W				
Italian Style	½ cup	45	—	0
FRESH				
baby raw	1 (½ oz)	3	tr	0
raw sliced	½ cup	9	1	0
sliced cooked	½ cup	14	1	0
FROZEN				
cooked	½ cup	19	—	0

FOOD	PORTION	CALS.	FIB.	CHOL.
Big Valley				
Zucchini	¾ cup (3 oz)	10	1	0
Empire				
Breaded	1 (2.9 oz)	100	1	0
Southland				
Zucchini Sliced	3.2 oz	15	—	0
TAKE-OUT				
indian paalkora	1 serv	46	2	1

PART • TWO

RESTAURANT CHAINS

FOOD	PORTION	CALS.	FIB.	CHOL.
ARBY'S				
BEVERAGES				
2% Milk	0.5 oz	5	0	0
Chocolate Shake	1 (12 oz)	451	0	36
Coca-Cola Classic	1 serv (12 oz)	140	0	0
Coffee	1 serv (8 oz)	3	0	0
Diet Coke	1 serv (12 oz)	0	0	0
Diet Pepsi	1 serv (12 oz)	0	0	0
Diet Seven Up	1 serv (12 oz)	0	0	0
Dr. Pepper	1 serv (12 oz)	160	0	0
Hot Chocolate	1 serv (8 oz)	110	0	0
Iced Tea	1 serv (16 oz)	6	0	0
Jamocha Shake	1 (12 oz)	384	0	36
Nehi Orange	1 serv (12 oz)	195	0	0
Orange Juice	1 serv (6 oz)	82	0	0
Pepsi Cola	1 serv (12 oz)	150	0	0
RC Cola	1 serv (12 oz)	165	0	0
RC Diet Rite	1 serv (12 oz)	1	0	0
Seven Up	1 serv (12 oz)	144	0	0
Upper Ten	1 serv (12 oz)	169	0	0
Vanilla Shake	1 (12 oz)	360	0	36
BREAKFAST SELECTIONS				
Bacon	2 strips (0.53 oz)	90	0	15
Biscuit Plain	1 (2.9 oz)	280	1	0
Blueberry Muffin	1 (2.3 oz)	230	0	25
Cinnamon Nut Danish	1 (3.5 oz)	360	1	0
Croissant Plain	1 (2 oz)	220	0	25
Egg Portion	1 serv (1.6 oz)	95	0	180
Ham	1 serv (1.5 oz)	45	0	20
Sausage	1 (1.3 oz)	163	0	25
Swiss	1 serv (0.5 oz)	45	0	12
Table Syrup	1 serv (1 oz)	100	0	0
Toastix	6 pieces (4.4 oz)	430	3	0
DESSERTS				
Apple Turnover	1 (3.2 oz)	330	0	0
Cheesecake Plain	1 serv (3 oz)	320	0	95
Cherry Turnover	1 (3.2 oz)	320	0	0
Chocolate Chip Cookie	1 (1 oz)	125	0	10
Polar Swirl Butterfinger	1 (11.6 oz)	457	0	28
Polar Swirl Heath	1 (11.6 oz)	543	0	39
Polar Swirl Oreo	1 (11.6 oz)	329	0	35
Polar Swirl Peanut Butter Cup	1 (11.6 oz)	517	1	34
Polar Swirl Snickers	1 (11.6 oz)	511	1	33

FOOD	PORTION	CALS.	FIB.	CHOL.
MAIN MENU SELECTIONS				
Arby's Sauce	1 serv (0.5 oz)	15	0	0
Baked Potato Broccoli'n Cheddar	1 (15.7 oz)	571	9	12
Baked Potato Deluxe	1 (15.3 oz)	736	7	59
Baked Potato Plain	1 (11.5 oz)	355	7	0
Baked Potato w/ Margarine & Sour Cream	1 (14 oz)	578	7	25
Barbeque Sauce	1 serv (0.5 oz)	30	0	0
Beef Stock Au Jus	1 serv (2 oz)	10	0	0
Breaded Chicken Fillet	1 (7.2 oz)	536	5	45
Cheddar Cheese Sauce	1 serv (0.75 oz)	35	0	4
Cheddar Curly Fries	1 serv (4.25 oz)	333	0	3
Chicken Cordon Bleu	1 (8.5 oz)	623	5	77
Chicken Finger	2 (3.6 oz)	290	1	32
Curly Fries	1 serv (3.5 oz)	300	0	0
Fish Fillet Sandwich	1 (7.7 oz)	529	2	43
French Fries	1 serv (2.5 oz)	246	0	0
Garden Salad	1 (11.9 oz)	61	5	0
Grilled Chicken BBQ	1 (7.1 oz)	388	2	43
Grilled Chicken Deluxe	1 (8.1 oz)	430	3	61
Ham 'n Cheese Sandwich	1 (5.9 oz)	359	2	53
Ham 'n Cheese Melt	1 (4.9 oz)	329	2	40
Honey Mayonnaise Reduced Calorie	1 serv (0.5 oz)	70	0	20
Horsey Sauce	1 serv (0.5 oz)	60	0	5
Italian Sub	1 (10.1 oz)	675	2	836
Italian Sub Sauce	1 serv (0.5 oz)	70	0	0
Ketchup	1 serv (0.5 oz)	16	0	0
Light Roast Beef Deluxe	1 (6.4 oz)	296	6	42
Light Roast Chicken Deluxe	1 (6.8 oz)	276	4	33
Light Roast Chicken Salad	1 serv (14.4 oz)	149	5	29
Light Roast Turkey Deluxe	1 (6.8 oz)	260	4	33
Mayonnaise	1 serv (0.5 oz)	110	0	5
Mayonnaise Light Cholesterol Free	1 serv (0.25 oz)	12	1	0
Mustard German Style	1 serv (0.16 oz)	5	0	0
Parmesan Cheese Sauce	1 serv (0.5 oz)	70	0	5
Potato Cakes	2 (3 oz)	204	0	0
Roast Beef Arby's Melt w/ Cheddar	1 (5.2 oz)	368	2	31
Roast Beef Arby-Q	1 (6.4 oz)	431	3	37
Roast Beef Bac'n Cheddar Deluxe	1 (8.1 oz)	539	3	44
Roast Beef Beef'n Cheddar	1 (6.7 oz)	487	2	50
Roast Beef Giant	1 (8.1 oz)	555	5	71

FOOD	PORTION	CALS.	FIB.	CHOL.
Roast Beef Junior	1 (4.4 oz)	324	2	30
Roast Beef Regular	1 (5.4 oz)	388	3	43
Roast Beef Sub	1 (10.8 oz)	700	4	846
Roast Beef Super	1 (8.7 oz)	523	5	43
Roast Chicken Club	1 (8.5 oz)	546	2	58
Roast Chicken Deluxe	1 (7.6 oz)	433	2	34
Roast Chicken Santa Fe	1 (6.4 oz)	436	1	54
Side Salad	1 (5 oz)	23	2	0
Sub Roll French Dip	1 (6.8 oz)	475	3	55
Sub Roll Hot Ham 'n Swiss	1 (9.3 oz)	500	2	68
Sub Roll Philly Beef'n Swiss	1 (10.4 oz)	755	3	91
Sub Roll Triple Cheese Melt	1 (8.4 oz)	720	2	91
Tartar Sauce	1 serv (1 oz)	140	0	30
Turkey Sub	1 (9.8 oz)	550	2	65
SALAD DRESSINGS				
Blue Cheese	1 serv (2 oz)	290	0	50
Buttermilk Ranch Reduced Calorie	1 serv (2 oz)	50	0	0
Honey French	1 serv (2 oz)	280	0	0
Italian Reduced Calorie	1 serv (2 oz)	20	0	0
Red Ranch	1 serv (0.5 oz)	75	0	0
Thousand Island	1 serv (2 oz)	260	0	30
SOUPS				
Boston Clam Chowder	1 serv (8 oz)	190	1	25
Cream of Broccoli	1 serv (8 oz)	160	2	25
Lumberjack Mixed Vegetable	1 serv (8 oz)	90	1	5
Old Fashioned Chicken Noodle	1 serv (8 oz)	80	1	20
Potato w/ Bacon	1 serv (8 oz)	170	—	20
Timberline Chili	1 serv (8 oz)	220	7	30
Wisconsin Cheese	1 serv (8 oz)	280	2	35

AU BON PAIN
BAKED GOODS

FOOD	PORTION	CALS.	FIB.	CHOL.
Bagel Cinnamon Raisin	1 (4.9 oz)	360	3	0
Bagel Onion	1 (5.1 oz)	370	3	0
Bagel Plain	1 (4.8 oz)	350	3	0
Bagel Poppy Seed	1 (5.1 oz)	380	3	0
Baguette Loaf	1 slice (1.8 oz)	140	1	0
Braided Roll	1 (1.8 oz)	170	1	0
Cheese Loaf	1 slice (1.8 oz)	40	1	5
Country Seed Roll	1 (2.6 oz)	220	3	0
Croissant Almond	1 (4.3 oz)	560	4	105
Croissant Apple	1 (3.4 oz)	260	1	25
Croissant Chocolate	1 (3.1 oz)	390	3	30
Croissant Cinnamon Raisin	1 (3.7 oz)	380	2	35

FOOD	PORTION	CALS.	FIB.	CHOL.
Croissant Plain	1 (2.1 oz)	270	1	40
Croissant Raspberry Cheese	1 (3.5 oz)	380	1	60
Croissant Strawberry Cheese	1 (3.5 oz)	370	1	60
Croissant Sweet Cheese	1 (3.6 oz)	390	1	75
Four Grain Loaf	1 slice (1.8 oz)	130	1	0
French Sandwich Roll	1 (1.8 oz)	120	1	0
Hearth Roll	1 (2.8 oz)	220	2	0
Hearth Sandwich Roll	1 (1.8 oz)	140	2	0
Low Fat Muffin Cinnamon Cranapple	1 (4.6 oz)	280	2	25
Low Fat Muffin Pineapple	1 (4.2 oz)	280	1	25
Low Fat Muffin Triple Berry	1 (4.2 oz)	270	2	25
Muffin Blueberry	1 (4.5 oz)	410	1	85
Muffin Carrot	1 (5 oz)	480	3	55
Muffin Chocolate Chip	1 (4.5 oz)	490	2	35
Muffin Corn	1 (4.6 oz)	470	2	65
Multigrain Loaf	1 slice (1.8 oz)	130	1	0
Parisienne Loaf	1 slice (1.8 oz)	120	1	0
Petit Pain Roll	1 (2.5 oz)	200	1	0
Rye Loaf	1 slice (1.8 oz)	110	2	0
Sandwich Croissant	1 (2.6 oz)	310	1	40
Scone Blueberry	1 (4 oz)	430	1	155
Scone Cinnamon	1 (4.1 oz)	520	1	145
Scone Orange	1 (4.1 oz)	440	2	155
Sesame Roll	1 (5.1 oz)	390	4	0
BEVERAGES				
Hot Apple Cider	1 lg (20 oz)	350	0	0
Hot Apple Cider	1 med (16 oz)	310	0	0
Hot Apple Cider	1 sm (10 oz)	190	0	0
Hot Raspberry Mocha Blast	1 serv (20 oz)	350	0	30
Hot Raspberry Mocha Blast	1 serv (10 oz)	180	0	15
Hot Raspberry Mocha Blast	1 serv (16 oz)	300	0	25
Iced Caffee Latte	1 sm (9 oz)	130	0	20
Iced Caffee Latte	1 med (12 oz)	150	0	25
Iced Caffee Latte	1 lg (20.5 oz)	270	0	40
Iced Cappuccino	1 sm (9 oz)	110	0	15
Iced Cappuccino	1 lg (20.5 oz)	270	0	40
Iced Cappuccino	1 med (12 oz)	150	0	25
Iced Cocoa	1 lg (20.5 oz)	440	0	40
Iced Cocoa	1 med (12 oz)	280	0	25
Iced Cocoa	1 sm (9 oz)	200	0	20
Iced Mocha Blast	1 sm (9 oz)	180	0	20
Iced Mocha Blast	1 med (12 oz)	260	0	25
Iced Mocha Blast	1 lg (20.5 oz)	360	0	40

FOOD	PORTION	CALS.	FIB.	CHOL.
Iced Raspberry Mocha Blast	1 serv (16 oz)	210	0	20
Iced Raspberry Mocha Blast	1 serv (12 oz)	160	0	15
Iced Raspberry Mocha Blast	1 serv (24 oz)	330	0	25
Whipped Cream	1 serv (1.2 oz)	160	0	55
DESSERTS				
Biscotti	1 (1.5 oz)	200	1	35
Biscotti Chocolate	1 (1.7 oz)	240	2	35
Cookie Chocolate Chip	1 (2.1 oz)	280	2	40
Cookie Oatmeal Raisin	1 (2.1 oz)	250	2	30
Cookie Peanut Butter	1 (2.1 oz)	280	1	30
Cookie Shortbread	1 (2.4 oz)	390	1	65
Danish Raspberry	1 (3.6 oz)	370	2	65
Danish Sweet Cheese	1 (3.6 oz)	420	1	90
Pecan Roll	1 (6.8 oz)	900	4	50
SALAD DRESSINGS				
Bleu Cheese	3 oz	410	0	40
Buttermilk Ranch	3 oz	310	0	35
Caesar	3 oz	380	0	25
Fat Free Tomato Basil	3 oz	70	1	0
Greek	3 oz	440	0	0
Honey Mustard	3 oz	380	1	40
Lemon Basil Vinaigrette	3 oz	330	0	0
Lite Italian	3 oz	230	0	0
Mandarin Orange	3 oz	380	0	0
Sesame French	3 oz	370	1	0
SALADS AND SALAD BARS				
Antipasto	1 serv (12.9 oz)	410	11	55
Caesar	1 serv (8.9 oz)	270	5	20
Chicken Caesar	1 serv (11.4 oz)	360	5	65
Chicken Tarragon	1 serv (16 oz)	470	6	80
Garden	1 lg (10.6 oz)	160	6	0
Garden	1 sm (7.5 oz)	100	4	0
Greek	1 serv (10.5 oz)	300	7	50
Oriental Chicken	1 serv (14.2 oz)	230	7	45
Tuna	1 serv (15 oz)	490	7	45
SANDWICHES AND FILLINGS				
Brie	½ serv (1.5 oz)	140	0	45
Cheddar Cheese	½ serv (1.5 oz)	170	0	45
Chicken Cracked Pepper	1 serv (3.9 oz)	140	0	72
Chicken Tarragon	1 serv (4 oz)	240	0	65
Country Ham	1 serv (3.7 oz)	150	0	55
Grilled Chicken	1 serv (3.9 oz)	140	0	72
Herb Cheese	½ serv (1.5 oz)	150	0	45
Hot Croissant Ham & Cheese	1 (4.2 oz)	380	1	70

FOOD	PORTION	CALS.	FIB.	CHOL.
Hot Croissant Spinach & Cheese	1 (3.6 oz)	270	2	40
Hot Croissant Turkey & Cheddar	1 (4.2 oz)	390	1	65
Lite Cream Cheese	1 serv (1.9 oz)	110	0	25
Provolone	½ serv (1.5 oz)	150	0	30
Roast Beef	1 serv (3.7 oz)	140	0	50
Swiss	½ serv (1.5 oz)	160	0	40
Tuna Salad	1 serv (4.5 oz)	360	1	50
Turkey Breast	1 serv (3.7 oz)	120	0	20
SOUPS				
Beef Barley	1 serv (12 oz)	112	3	18
Beef Barley	1 serv (8 oz)	75	2	15
Beef Barley	1 serv (16 oz)	150	5	25
Beef Stew	1 serv (16 oz)	280	3	45
Beef Stew	1 serv (8 oz)	140	2	25
Beef Stew	1 serv (12 oz)	210	3	35
Broccoli & Cheddar	1 serv (16 oz)	520	2	100
Broccoli & Cheddar	1 serv (12 oz)	390	2	75
Broccoli & Cheddar	1 serv (8 oz)	260	1	50
Chicken & Sausage Gumbo	1 serv (12 oz)	230	2	20
Chicken & Sausage Gumbo	1 serv (16 oz)	310	3	30
Chicken & Sausage Gumbo	1 serv (8 oz)	160	1	15
Chicken Noodle	1 serv (8 oz)	80	1	15
Chicken Noodle	1 serv (12 oz)	120	2	25
Chicken Noodle	1 serv (16 oz)	170	2	35
Chicken Wild Rice	1 serv (12 oz)	130	1	25
Chicken Wild Rice	1 serv (16 oz)	180	2	30
Chicken Wild Rice	1 serv (8 oz)	90	1	15
Chili	1 serv (16 oz)	460	9	70
Chili	1 serv (8 oz)	230	5	35
Chili	1 serv (12 oz)	340	7	50
Clam Chowder	1 serv (16 oz)	540	1	125
Clam Chowder	1 serv (8 oz)	270	0	65
Clam Chowder	1 serv (12 oz)	400	1	95
Corn Chowder	1 serv (8 oz)	260	1	50
Corn Chowder	1 serv (12 oz)	390	2	70
Corn Chowder	1 serv (16 oz)	530	3	95
Cream Of Broccoli	1 serv (12 oz)	330	2	60
Cream Of Broccoli	1 serv (8 oz)	220	1	40
Cream Of Broccoli	1 serv (16 oz)	440	3	80
Cream Of Chicken With Wild Rice	1 serv (16 oz)	330	1	90
Cream Of Chicken With Wild Rice	1 serv (12 oz)	250	2	65
Cream Of Chicken With Wild Rice	1 serv (8 oz)	160	1	45
Garden Vegetable	1 serv (1 cup)	29	2	0
Garden Vegetable	1 serv (16 oz)	58	4	0

FOOD	PORTION	CALS.	FIB.	CHOL.
Garden Vegetable	1 serv (12 oz)	45	3	0
Seafood Gumbo	1 serv (12 oz)	190	2	25
Seafood Gumbo	1 serv (8 oz)	130	1	20
Seafood Gumbo	1 serv (16 oz)	260	3	35
Split Pea	1 serv (16 oz)	352	28	0
Split Pea	1 serv (12 oz)	265	21	0
Split Pea	1 serv (8 oz)	176	14	tr
Tomato Florentine	1 serv (16 oz)	122	3	5
Tomato Florentine	1 serv (12 oz)	90	2	5
Tomato Florentine	1 serv (8 oz)	61	2	5
Tomato Tortellini	1 serv (8 oz)	60	2	5
Tomato Tortellini	1 serv (12 oz)	90	2	5
Tomato Tortellini	1 serv (16 oz)	110	3	10
Vegetable Stew	1 serv (8 oz)	60	2	5
Vegetable Stew	1 serv (12 oz)	100	4	5
Vegetable Stew	1 serv (16 oz)	130	5	5
Vegetarian Chili	1 serv (12 oz)	210	3	0
Vegetarian Chili	1 serv (8 oz)	139	2	0
Vegetarian Chili	1 serv (16 oz)	278	4	0
Vegetarian Lentil	1 serv (8 oz)	130	2	0
Vegetarian Lentil	1 serv (12 oz)	200	4	0
Vegetarian Lentil	1 serv (16 oz)	270	5	0

BASKIN-ROBBINS

FOOD	PORTION	CALS.	FIB.	CHOL.
Sugar Cone	1	60	—	0
Waffle Cone	1	140	—	0
FROZEN YOGURT				
Cafe Mocha	½ cup (4 fl oz)	70	—	0
Chocolate Nonfat	½ cup	110	—	0
Chocolate Vanilla	½ cup	110	—	0
Dutch Chocolate Chip Bar	1	260	—	7
Pralines Vanilla Bar	1	250	—	7
Strawberry Low-Fat	½ cup (4 fl oz)	120	—	5
Strawberry Nonfat	½ cup	110	—	0
Wild Cherry	½ cup (4 fl oz)	70	—	0
ICE CREAM				
Almond Butter Crunch Light	½ cup	130	—	12
Butter Pecan	½ cup	160	—	25
Butterfinger	½ cup	170	—	15
Caramel Banana Fat Free	½ cup	100	—	1
Cherry Cordial Sugar Free	½ cup	100	—	3
Chewy Babyruth	½ cup	190	—	25
Chilly Burgers Vanilla	1	240	—	29
Chocolate	½ cup	150	—	20

FOOD	PORTION	CALS.	FIB.	CHOL.
Chocolate Almond	½ cup	170	—	20
Chocolate Chip	½ cup	150	—	25
Chocolate Chip Sugar Free	½ cup	100	—	4
Chocolate Fudge	½ cup	170	—	25
Chocolate Mousse Royale	½ cup	180	—	20
Chocolate Raspberry Truffle	½ cup	180	—	25
Chocolate Vanilla Fat Free	½ cup	100	—	0
Chocolate Wonder Fat Free	½ cup	120	—	1
Chunky Banana Sugar Free	½ cup	80	—	3
Coconut Caramel Nut Light	½ cup	130	—	8
Cookies N Cream	½ cup	160	—	20
Double Raspberry Light	½ cup	120	—	9
Espresso N Cream Light	½ cup	120	—	12
French Vanilla	½ cup	170	—	55
Fudge Brownie	½ cup	180	—	20
Gold Medal Ribbon	½ cup	150	—	20
Jamoca Almond Fudge	½ cup	150	—	20
Jamoca Swirl Fat Free	½ cup	100	—	2
Jamoca Swiss Almond Sugar Free	½ cup	90	—	4
Just Peachy Fat Free	½ cup	100	—	2
Kahlua N Cream	½ cup	160	—	10
Mint Chocolate Chip	½ cup	150	—	25
Peanut Butter Chocolate	½ cup	190	—	20
Pineapple Cheesecake Fat Free	½ cup	110	—	0
Pineapple Coconut Sugar Free	½ cup	90	—	3
Pistachio Almond	½ cup	160	—	20
Praline Dream Light	½ cup	130	—	11
Pralines N Cream	½ cup	160	—	20
Reeses Peanut Butter Cup	½ cup	170	—	20
Rocky Road	½ cup	170	—	20
Strawberry Royal Light	½ cup	110	—	9
Strawberry Sugar Free	½ cup	80	—	3
Thin Mint Chip Sugar Free	½ cup	90	—	4
Tiny Toon Adventures Toonwiches Chocolate	1	330	—	33
Tiny Toon Adventures Toonwiches Vanilla	1	340	—	34
Tiny Toon Adventures Bar Mint Chocolate Chip	1	230	—	17
Tiny Toon Adventures Bar Vanilla	1	210	—	18
Vanilla	½ cup	140	—	30
Vanilla Fudge Light	½ cup	110	—	11
Very Berry Strawberry	½ cup	120	—	15
World Class Chocolate	½ cup	160	—	20

FOOD	PORTION	CALS.	FIB.	CHOL.
ICES AND ICE POPS				
Daiquiri Ice	1 scoop	140	—	0
Rainbow Sherbet	1 scoop	160	—	6
Sorbet Strawberry	½ cup (4 fl oz)	100	—	0
BEN & JERRY'S				
Sugar Cone	1	48	tr	0
FROZEN YOGURT				
Cherry Garcia	½ cup (2.7 oz)	140	0	5
Chocolate Chip Cookie Dough	½ cup (2.7 oz)	180	0	10
Chocolate Fudge Brownie	½ cup (2.7 oz)	160	2	10
Coffee Almond Fudge	½ cup (2.7 oz)	180	1	10
English Toffee Crunch	½ cup (2.7 oz)	180	0	10
No Fat Cappuccino	½ cup (2.7 oz)	120	0	0
No Fat Chocolate	½ cup (2.7 oz)	120	0	0
No Fat Peach Melba	½ cup (2.7 oz)	110	1	0
No Fat Raspberry	½ cup (2.7 oz)	120	1	0
No Fat Strawberry	½ cup (2.7 oz)	120	1	0
No Fat Vanilla	½ cup (2.7 oz)	120	0	0
Strawberry Cheesecake	½ cup (2.7 oz)	140	0	10
Vanilla Fudge	½ cup (2.7 oz)	140	1	0
ICE CREAM				
Apple Pie	½ cup (2.7 oz)	200	0	55
Aztec Harvests Coffee	½ cup (2.7 oz)	180	0	70
Banana Walnut	½ cup (2.7 oz)	240	1	55
Butter Pecan	½ cup (2.7 oz)	250	1	80
Cappuccino Chocolate Chunk	½ cup (2.7 oz)	220	1	65
Cherry Garcia	½ cup (2.7 oz)	200	0	65
Cherry Vanilla	½ cup (2.7 oz)	180	0	65
Chocolate Amaretto	½ cup (2.7 oz)	180	2	45
Chocolate Chip Cookie Dough	½ cup (2.7 oz)	230	0	65
Chocolate Fudge Brownie	½ cup (2.7 oz)	200	2	40
Chocolate Orange Fudge	½ cup (2.7 oz)	190	1	45
Chocolate Peanut Butter Cookie Dough	½ cup (2.7 oz)	240	1	50
Chocolate Raspberry Swirl	½ cup (2.7 oz)	190	1	35
Chubby Hubby	½ cup (2.7 oz)	260	2	50
Chunky Monkey	½ cup (2.7 oz)	240	1	55
Cinnamon	½ cup (2.7 oz)	180	0	75
Coconut Almond Fudge Chip	½ cup (2.7 oz)	260	2	60
Coffee Toffee Crunch	½ cup (2.7 oz)	240	0	60
Deep Dark Chocolate	½ cup (2.7 oz)	200	2	45
Double Chocolate Fudge Swirl	½ cup (2.7 oz)	210	2	45
Egg Nog	½ cup (2.7 oz)	190	0	65

FOOD	PORTION	CALS.	FIB.	CHOL.
English Toffee Crunch	½ cup (2.7 oz)	240	0	65
Maple Walnut	½ cup (2.7 oz)	240	1	60
Mint Chocolate Chunk	½ cup (2.7 oz)	220	1	65
Mint Chocolate Cookie	½ cup (2.7 oz)	220	1	65
Mint Fudge Swirl	½ cup (2.7 oz)	200	0	70
Mocha Fudge	½ cup (2.7 oz)	200	0	60
New York Super Fudge Chunk	½ cup (2.7 oz)	240	2	40
Peach	½ cup (2.7 oz)	170	0	65
Peanut Butter Cup	½ cup (2.7 oz)	260	1	60
Pistachio Pistachio	½ cup (2.7 oz)	220	1	70
Praline Pecan	½ cup (2.7 oz)	250	1	70
Rain Forest Crunch	½ cup (2.7 oz)	240	0	70
Reverse Chocolate Chunk	½ cup (2.7 oz)	230	1	40
Rum Raisin	½ cup (2.7 oz)	200	1	60
Strawberry	½ cup (2.7 oz)	170	1	55
Sweet Cream Cookie	½ cup (2.7 oz)	220	1	65
Vanilla	½ cup (2.7 oz)	190	0	75
Vanilla Bean	½ cup (2.7 oz)	190	0	75
Vanilla Caramel Fudge	½ cup (2.7 oz)	180	0	70
Vanilla Chocolate Chunk	½ cup (2.7 oz)	220	1	65
Vanilla Fudge Brownie	½ cup (2.7 oz)	200	0	60
Wavy Gravy	½ cup (2.7 oz)	260	2	55
White Russian	½ cup (2.7 oz)	190	0	70
ICES				
Lemon Daiquiri	½ cup (2.7 oz)	120	0	0
Mandarin	½ cup (2.7 oz)	130	0	0
Marguerita Lime	½ cup (2.7 oz)	120	0	0
Pina Colada Sorbet	½ cup (2.7 oz)	120	0	0
Raspberry	½ cup (2.7 oz)	120	0	0

BIG BOY
ICE CREAM

FOOD	PORTION	CALS.	FIB.	CHOL.
Frozen Yogurt	1 serv	72	—	0
Frozen Yogurt Shake	1 serv	184	—	2
No-No Frozen Dessert	1 serv	75	—	0
MAIN MENU SELECTIONS				
Baked Cod Dinner	1 serv	392	—	76
Baked Cod Dijon Dinner	1 serv	455	—	76
Baked Potato	1	163	—	0
Bran Muffin	1	367	—	0
Breast of Chicken Dinner	1 serv	358	—	68
Breast of Chicken w/ Mozzarella Dinner	1 serv	379	—	79
Breast of Chicken w/ Mozzarella Sandwich	1	390	—	71

FOOD	PORTION	CALS.	FIB.	CHOL.
Broiled Cod Dijon Dinner	1 serv	455	—	76
Broiled Cod Dinner	1 serv	392	—	76
Cajun Chicken Dinner	1 serv	358	—	68
Cajun Cod Dinner	1 serv	392	—	76
Carrots	1 serv	35	—	0
Chicken Breast Salad w/ Dijon And Pita Bread	1 serv	377	—	60
Corn	1 serv	90	—	0
Dijon Sauce	1 serv	63	—	0
Dinner Salad	1	19	—	0
Green Beans	1 serv	28	—	0
Mixed Vegetables	1 serv	27	—	0
Peas	1 serv	77	—	0
Promise Margarine	1 pat (5 g)	35	—	0
Rice	1 serv	114	—	0
Roll	1	139	—	2
Spaghetti Marinara Dinner	1 serv	450	—	8
Stir Fry Vegetable	1 serv	408	—	0
Stir Fry Dinner Chicken 'n Vegetable	1 serv	562	—	68
Turkey Pita	1	224	—	75
Vegetable Pita	1	144	—	10
SALAD DRESSINGS				
Buttermilk	1 serv	36	—	10
SOUPS				
Cabbage	1 cup	37	—	1
Cabbage	1 bowl	43	—	1

BOJANGLES
BAKED SELECTIONS

FOOD	PORTION	CALS.	FIB.	CHOL.
Biscuit	1 (2.4 oz)	239	—	1
Cinnamon Twist	1 (3.5 oz)	431	—	0
MAIN MENU SELECTIONS				
Biscuit Sandwich Bacon	1 (2.6 oz)	294	—	9
Biscuit Sandwich Bacon & Cheese	1 (3 oz)	422	—	20
Biscuit Sandwich Bacon & Egg	1 (4.2 oz)	386	—	220
Biscuit Sandwich Bacon, Egg & Cheese	1 (4.6 oz)	428	—	331
Biscuit Sandwich Chicken Filet	1 (3.6 oz)	399	—	69
Biscuit Sandwich Chicken Filet & Cheese	1 (6 oz)	441	—	80
Biscuit Sandwich Chicken Filet & Egg	1 (7.2 oz)	491	—	280
Biscuit Sandwich Chicken Filet, Egg & Cheese	1 (7.6 oz)	533	—	291

FOOD	PORTION	CALS.	FIB.	CHOL.
Biscuit Sandwich Country Ham	1 (3.6 oz)	314	—	34
Biscuit Sandwich Country Ham & Cheese	1 (4 oz)	356	—	45
Biscuit Sandwich Country Ham & Egg	1 (5.2 oz)	406	—	245
Biscuit Sandwich Country Ham, Egg & Cheese	1 (5.6 oz)	448	—	256
Biscuit Sandwich Egg	1 (3.9 oz)	331	—	212
Biscuit Sandwich Egg & Cheese	1 (4.3 oz)	373	—	223
Biscuit Sandwich Sausage	1 (4.3 oz)	448	—	49
Biscuit Sandwich Sausage & Cheese	1 (4.7 oz)	490	—	60
Biscuit Sandwich Sausage & Egg	1 (5.9 oz)	540	—	260
Biscuit Sandwich Sausage, Egg & Cheese	1 (6.3 oz)	582	—	271
Biscuit Sandwich Steak	1 (5.1 oz)	488	—	72
Biscuit Sandwich Steak & Cheese	1 (5.5 oz)	530	—	83
Biscuit Sandwich Steak & Egg	1 (6.7 oz)	580	—	283
Biscuit Sandwich Steak, Egg & Cheese	1 (7.1 oz)	622	—	294
Bo*Biscuit Canadian Bacon, Egg & Cheese	1 (5.2 oz)	417	—	236
Cajun Pintos	1 serv (2.5 oz)	124		0
Cole Slaw	1 serv (3.6 oz)	105	—	0
Dirty Rice	1 serv (2.9 oz)	167	—	12
Mashed Potatoes & Gravy	1 serv (3.6 oz)	165	—	9
Sandwich Cajun Filet	1 serv (6.7 oz)	550	—	108
Sandwich Grilled Filet	1 serv (5.8 oz)	429	—	67
Sandwich Grilled Filet Deluxe	1 serv (6.2 oz)	502	—	78
Sandwich Grilled Filet w/o Mayonnaise	1 serv (5.2 oz)	329	—	59
Seasoned Fries	1 serv (4 oz)	252	—	0
Skinfree Southern Breast	1 serv (4.2 oz)	271	—	104
Skinfree Southern Leg	1 serv (1.9 oz)	128	—	54
Skinfree Southern Thigh	1 serv (3.4 oz)	264	—	88
Spiced Cajun Breast	1 serv (4.8 oz)	385	—	126
Spiced Cajun Leg	1 serv (3.2 oz)	245	—	105
Spiced Cajun Thigh	1 serv (3.7 oz)	335	—	125

BOSTON MARKET
DESSERTS

Brownie	1 (3.3 oz)	450	3	80
Cookie Chocolate Chip	1 (2.8 oz)	340	1	25
Cookie Oatmeal Raisin	1 (2.8 oz)	320	1	25

FOOD	PORTION	CALS.	FIB.	CHOL.
MAIN MENU SELECTIONS				
½ Chicken w/ Skin	1 serv (10 oz)	630	0	370
¼ Dark Meat Chicken w/ Skin	1 serv (4.6 oz)	330	0	180
¼ Dark Meat Chicken w/o Skin	1 serv (3.6 oz)	210	0	150
¼ White Meat Chicken w/ Skin	1 serv (5.4 oz)	330	0	175
¼ White Meat Chicken w/o Skin Or Wing	1 serv (3.6 oz)	160	0	95
BBQ Baked Beans	¾ cup (7.1 oz)	330	9	10
Buttered Corn	¾ cup (5.1 oz)	190	4	0
Butternut Squash	¾ cup (6.8 oz)	160	3	15
Caesar Salad Entree	1 serv (10 oz)	520	3	40
Caesar Salad w/o Dressing	1 serv (8 oz)	225	3	25
Caesar Side Salad	1 (4 oz)	210	1	20
Chicken Caesar Salad	1 serv (13 oz)	670	3	120
Chicken Gravy	1 serv (1 oz)	15	0	0
Chicken Salad Sandwich	1 (10.7 oz)	680	5	145
Chicken Sandwich w/ Cheese & Sauce	1 serv (12.4 oz)	760	5	160
Chicken Sandwich w/o Cheese & Sauce	1 (10 oz)	430	5	95
Chunky Chicken Salad	3.4 cup (5.5 oz)	390	1	145
Cole Slaw	¾ cup (6.5 oz)	280	3	25
Corn Bread	1 (2.4 oz)	200	1	25
Cranberry Relish	¾ cup (7.9 oz)	370	5	0
Creamed Spinach	¾ cup (6.4 oz)	300	2	75
Fruit Salad	¾ cup (5.5 oz)	70	2	0
Ham & Turkey Club w/ Cheese & Sauce	1 (13.3 oz)	890	4	150
Ham & Turkey Club w/o Cheese & Sauce	1 (9.3 oz)	430	4	55
Ham Sandwich w/ Cheese & Sauce	1 (11.8 oz)	760	5	100
Ham Sandwich w/o Cheese & Sauce	1 (9.3 oz)	450	4	45
Ham w/ Cinnamon Apples	1 serv (8 oz)	350	2	75
Homestyle Mashed Potatoes & Gravy	¾ cup (6.6 oz)	200	2	25
Hot Cinnamon Apples	¾ cup (6.4 oz)	250	3	0
Macaroni & Cheese	¾ cup (6.7 oz)	280	1	20
Mashed Potatoes	⅔ cup (5.6 oz)	180	2	25
Meat Loaf & Brown Gravy	1 serv (7 oz)	390	1	120
Meat Loaf & Chunky Tomato Sauce	1 serv (8 oz)	370	2	120
Meat Loaf Sandwich w/ Cheese	1 (13.8 oz)	860	6	165

FOOD	PORTION	CALS.	FIB.	CHOL.
Meat Loaf Sandwich w/o Cheese	1 (12.3 oz)	690	6	120
Mediterranean Pasta Salad	¾ cup (4.5 oz)	170	2	10
New Potatoes	¾ cup (4.6 oz)	140	2	0
Original Chicken Pot Pie	1 serv (14.9 oz)	750	9	115
Rice Pilaf	⅔ cup (5.1 oz)	180	2	0
Rotisserie Turkey Breast Skinless	1 serv (5 oz)	170	0	100
Steamed Vegetables	⅔ cup (3.7 oz)	35	3	0
Stuffing	¾ cup (6.1 oz)	310	3	0
Tortellini Salad	¾ cup (5.6 oz)	380	2	90
Turkey Sandwich w/ Cheese & Sauce	1 (11.8 oz)	710	4	110
Turkey Sandwich w/o Cheese & Sauce	1 (9.3 oz)	400	4	60
Zucchini Marinara	¾ cup (6.6 oz)	80	2	0
SOUPS				
Chicken	¾ cup (6.8 oz)	80	1	25
Chicken Tortilla	1 cup (8.4 oz)	220	2	35

BROWN'S CHICKEN

FOOD	PORTION	CALS.	FIB.	CHOL.
Breadsticks w/ Garlic Butter	1 serv (12 oz)	1593	—	1
Breast	3 oz	284	—	67
Coleslaw	3 oz	131	—	6
Corn Fritters	3 oz	415	—	4
Corn On Cob	3 oz	126	—	1
Fettucini Alfredo	1 serv (12 oz)	1507	—	51
French Fries	3 oz	503	—	1
Gizzard	3 oz	387	—	88
Leg	3 oz	287	—	52
Liver	3 oz	341	—	147
Mostaccioli w/ Meat	1 serv (12 oz)	835	—	17
Mostaccioli w/o Meat	1 serv (12 oz)	792	—	0
Mushrooms	3 oz	289	—	1
Potato Salad	3 oz	94	—	11
Ravioli w/ Meat	1 serv (12 oz)	865	—	17
Ravioli w/o Meat	1 serv (12 oz)	822	—	0
Shrimp	3 oz	277	—	31
Thigh	3 oz	355	—	63
Wing	3 oz	385	—	81

BURGER KING
BEVERAGES

FOOD	PORTION	CALS.	FIB.	CHOL.
Coca-Cola Classic	1 med (22 fl oz)	260	0	0
Coffee	1 serv (12 oz)	5	0	0
Diet Coke	1 med (22 fl oz)	1	0	0
Milk 2%	1 (8.6 oz)	120	0	20

FOOD	PORTION	CALS.	FIB.	CHOL.
Shake Chocolate	1 med (10 oz)	310	3	20
Shake Chocolate Syrup Added	1 med (12 oz)	460	1	20
Shake Strawberry Syrup Added	1 med (12 oz)	430	1	20
Shake Vanilla	1 med (10 oz)	310	1	20
Sprite	1 med (22 fl oz)	260	0	0
Tropicana Orange Juice	1 serv (11 oz)	140	0	0
BREAKFAST SELECTIONS				
AM Express Grape Jelly	1 serv (0.4 oz)	30	0	0
AM Express Strawberry Jam	1 serv (0.4 oz)	30	0	0
AM Express Dip	1 serv (1 oz)	80	0	0
Croissan'wich Bacon, Egg & Cheese	1 (4.1 oz)	350	tr	225
Croissan'wich Ham, Egg & Cheese	1 (5.1 oz)	351	tr	230
Croissan'wich Sausage, Egg & Cheese	1 (5.6 oz)	530	tr	255
French Toast Sticks	1 serv (4.9 oz)	500	1	0
Hash Browns	1 serv (2.5 oz)	220	2	0
Land O'Lakes Whipped Classic Blend	1 serv (0.4 oz)	65	0	0
MAIN MENU SELECTIONS				
American Cheese	1 slice (0.9 oz)	90	0	25
BK Big Fish Sandwich	1 (8.9 oz)	720	2	60
BK Broiler Chicken Sandwich	1 (8.7 oz)	540	2	80
Bacon Bits	1 serv (3 g)	15	0	5
Broiled Chicken Salad w/o Dressing	1 serv (10.6 oz)	200	3	60
Bull's Eye Barbecue Sauce	1 serv (0.5 oz)	20	0	0
Cheeseburger	1 (5 oz)	380	1	65
Chicken Sandwich	1 (8 oz)	700	2	60
Chicken Tenders	6 pieces (3.1 oz)	250	2	35
Croutons	1 serv (0.2 oz)	30	0	0
Dipping Sauce Barbecue	1 serv (1 oz)	35	0	0
Dipping Sauce Honey	1 serv (1 oz)	90	0	0
Dipping Sauce Ranch	1 serv (1 oz)	170	0	0
Dipping Sauce Sweet & Sour	1 serv (1 oz)	45	0	0
Double Cheeseburger	1 (7.5 oz)	600	1	135
Double Cheeseburger w/ Bacon	1 (7.8 oz)	540	1	145
Double Whopper	1 (12.3 oz)	870	3	170
Dutch Apple Pie	1 serv (4 oz)	310	2	0
French Fries	1 med (4.1 oz)	400	3	0
Garden Salad w/o Dressing	1 (7.5 oz)	90	0	15
Hamburger	1 (4.5 oz)	330	1	55
Ketchup	1 serv (0.5 oz)	15	0	0

FOOD	PORTION	CALS.	FIB.	CHOL.
Lettuce	1 leaf (0.7 oz)	0	0	0
Mayonnaise	1 serv (1 oz)	210	0	20
Mustard	1 serv (3 g)	0	0	0
Onion	1 serv (0.5 oz)	5	0	0
Onion Rings	1 serv (4.4 oz)	310	5	0
Pickles	1 serv (0.5 oz)	0	0	0
Side Salad w/o Dressing	1 (4.7 oz)	50	2	6
Tartar Sauce	1 serv (1 oz)	180	0	15
Tomato	1 serv (1 oz)	6	0	0
Whopper	1 (9.5 oz)	640	3	90
Whopper Double w/ Cheese	1 (13.2 oz)	960	3	195
Whopper Jr.	1 (5.9 oz)	420	2	60
Whopper Jr. w/ Cheese	1 (6.3 oz)	460	2	75
Whopper w/ Cheese	1 (10.3 oz)	730	3	115
SALAD DRESSINGS				
Bleu Cheese	1 serv (1 oz)	160	tr	30
French	1 serv (1 oz)	140	0	0
Light Italian Reduced Calorie	1 serv (1 oz)	15	0	0
Ranch	1 serv (1 oz)	180	tr	10
Thousand Island	1 serv (1 oz)	140	tr	15

CAPTAIN D'S
DESSERTS

FOOD	PORTION	CALS.	FIB.	CHOL.
Carrot Cake	1 piece (4 oz)	434	0	32
Cheesecake	1 piece (4 oz)	420	0	141
Chocolate Cake	1 piece (4 oz)	303	0	20
Lemon Pie	1 piece (4 oz)	351	0	45
Pecan Pie	1 piece (4 oz)	458	4	4
MAIN MENU SELECTIONS				
Baked Potato	1	278	—	0
Breadstick	1	113	—	0
Broiled Chicken Lunch	1 serv	503	—	82
Broiled Chicken Platter	1 serv	802	—	82
Broiled Chicken Sandwich	1 (8.2 oz)	451	—	105
Broiled Fish & Chicken Platter	1 serv	777	—	66
Broiled Fish & Chicken Lunch	1 serv	478	—	66
Broiled Fish Lunch	1 serv	435	—	49
Broiled Fish Platter	1 serv	734	—	49
Broiled Shrimp Lunch	1 serv	421	—	155
Broiled Shrimp Platter	1 serv	720	—	155
Cheese	1 slice (1 oz)	54	0	14
Cob Corn	1 serv (9.5 oz)	251	—	0
Cocktail Sauce	1 lg serv (4 fl oz)	137	0	0
Cocktail Sauce	1 serv (1 fl oz)	34	0	0

FOOD	PORTION	CALS.	FIB.	CHOL.
Cole Slaw	1 pt (16 oz)	633	8	66
Cole Slaw	1 serv (4 oz)	158	2	16
Crackers	4 (0.5 oz)	50	tr	3
Cracklins	1 serv (1 oz)	218	0	0
Dinner Salad w/o Dressing	1 (2.5 oz)	27	1	1
French Fried Potatoes	1 serv (3.5 oz)	302	0	0
Fried Okra	1 serv (4 oz)	300	0	0
Green Beans Seasoned	1 serv (4 oz)	46	1	4
Hushpuppies	6 (6.7 oz)	756	1	0
Hushpuppy	1 (1.1 oz)	126	tr	0
Imitation Sour Cream	1 serv	29	—	0
Margarine	1 serv	102	—	0
Non-Dairy Creamer	1 serv	14	0	0
Rice	1 serv (4 oz)	124	1	0
Sugar	1 pkg	18	0	0
Sweet & Sour Sauce	1 serv (1.8 fl oz)	52	0	0
Sweet & Sour Sauce	1 lg serv (4 fl oz)	206	0	0
Tartar Sauce	1 serv (1 fl oz)	75	0	10
Tartar Sauce	1 lg serv (4 fl oz)	298	0	41
Vegetable Medley	1 serv	36	—	0
White Beans	1 serv (4 oz)	126	3	2
SALAD DRESSINGS				
Blue Cheese	1 pkg (1 fl oz)	105	0	14
French	1 pkg (1 fl oz)	111	0	7
Light Italian	1 serv	16	—	0
Ranch	1 pkg (1 fl oz)	92	0	15

CARL'S JR.
BAKED SELECTIONS

FOOD	PORTION	CALS.	FIB.	CHOL.
Cheese Danish	1 (4.1 oz)	400	1	15
Cheesecake Strawberry Swirl	1 serv (3.5 oz)	300	0	55
Chocolate Cake	1 serv (3 oz)	300	4	13
Chocolate Chip Cookie	1 (2.5 oz)	370	1	25
Cinnamon Roll	1 (4.2 oz)	420	4	15
Muffin Blueberry	1 (4.2 oz)	340	1	40
Muffin Bran	1 (4.7 oz)	370	6	45
BEVERAGES				
Coca-Cola Classic	1 reg (16 fl oz)	190	0	0
Coffee	1 reg (12 oz)	10	0	0
Diet 7UP	1 reg (16 oz)	0	0	0
Diet Coke	1 reg (16 oz)	0	0	0
Dr. Pepper	1 reg (16 oz)	200	0	0
Hot Chocolate	1 reg (12 oz)	110	tr	<5
Iced Tea	1 reg (14 fl oz)	5	—	0

FOOD	PORTION	CALS.	FIB.	CHOL.
Milk 1%	1 (10 fl oz)	150	0	15
Minute Maid Orange Soda	1 reg (16 oz)	230	0	0
Orange Juice	1 (6 fl oz)	90	0	0
Ramblin' Root Beer	1 reg (16 oz)	230	0	0
Shake Chocolate	1 sm (13.5 oz)	390	0	30
Shake Strawberry	1 sm (13.5 oz)	400	0	30
Shake Vanilla	1 sm (13.5 fl oz)	330	0	35
Sprite	1 reg (16 fl oz)	190	0	0
BREAKFAST SELECTIONS				
Bacon	2 strips (0.3 oz)	40	0	10
Breakfast Burrito	1 (5.3 oz)	430	tr	460
Breakfast Quesadilla Cheese	1 (5.2 oz)	300	1	225
English Muffin w/ Margarine	1 (2.6 oz)	230	2	0
French Toast Dips w/o Syrup	1 serv (3.7 oz)	410	3	0
Grape Jelly	1 serv (0.5 oz)	35	0	0
Hash Brown Nuggets	1 serv (3.3 oz)	270	2	0
Sausage	1 patty (1.8 oz)	200	0	35
Scrambled Eggs	1 serv (3.5 oz)	160	0	425
Strawberry Jam	1 serv (0.5 oz)	35	0	0
Sunrise Sandwich	1 (4.6 oz)	370	2	225
Table Syrup	1 serv (1 oz)	90	0	0
MAIN MENU SELECTIONS				
American Cheese	1 slice (0.5 oz)	60	0	15
BBQ Chicken Sandwich	1 (6.7 oz)	310	3	55
BBQ Sauce	1 serv (1.1 oz)	50	0	0
Big Burger	1 (6.8 oz)	470	2	55
Breadstick	1 (0.3 oz)	35	1	0
Carl's Catch Fish Sandwich	1 (7.5 oz)	560	5	60
Chicken Club Sandwich	1 (8.8 oz)	550	3	85
Chicken Stars	6 pieces (3 oz)	230	0	85
CrissCut Fries	1 lg (5.7 oz)	550	3	0
Croutons	1 serv (7 g)	35	0	0
Double Western Bacon Cheeseburger	1 (11.5 oz)	970	2	145
Famous Big Star Hamburger	1 (8.6 oz)	610	2	70
French Fries	1 reg (4.4 oz)	370	3	0
Great Stuff Potato Bacon & Cheese	1 (14.2 oz)	630	6	40
Great Stuff Potato Broccoli & Cheese	1 (14.2 oz)	530	8	15
Great Stuff Potato Plain	1 (9.4 oz)	290	6	0
Great Stuff Potato Sour Cream & Chive	1 (10.9 oz)	430	6	10
Hamburger	1 (3.1 oz)	200	1	25

FOOD	PORTION	CALS.	FIB.	CHOL.
Honey Sauce	1 serv (1 oz)	90	0	0
Hot & Crispy Sandwich	1 (5 oz)	400	2	45
Mustard Sauce	1 serv (1 oz)	45	0	0
Onion Rings	1 serv (5.3 oz)	520	3	0
Salsa	1 serv (0.9 oz)	10	0	0
Santa Fe Chicken Sandwich	1 (7.9 oz)	530	3	85
Super Star Hamburger	1 (11.2 oz)	820	2	120
Sweet N'Sour Sauce	1 serv (1 oz)	50	0	0
Swiss Cheese	1 slice (0.5 oz)	45	0	10
Western Bacon Cheeseburger	1 (8.1 oz)	870	2	90
Zucchini	1 serv (5.9 oz)	380	3	0
SALAD DRESSINGS				
1000 Island	2 fl oz	250	0	20
Blue Cheese	2 fl oz	310	0	25
French Fat Free	2 fl oz	70	1	0
House	2 fl oz	220	0	20
Italian Fat Free	2 fl oz	15	0	0
SALADS AND SALAD BARS				
Salad-To-Go Charbroiled Chicken	1 serv (12 oz)	260	4	70
Salad-To-Go Garden	1 (4.8 oz)	50	2	5
CARVEL				
FROZEN YOGURT				
Vanilla No Sugar Added	4 fl oz	100	—	10
ICE CREAM				
Brown Bonnet Cone	1	380	—	40
Cake Cookies & Cream	1/12 cake (3.3 oz)	220	1	25
Chipsters	1	380	—	30
Chocolate	4 fl oz	180	—	40
Chocolate No Fat	4 fl oz	90	1	0
Flying Saucer Chocolate	1 (4 oz)	230	2	30
Flying Saucer Chocolate w/ Sprinkles	1 (4 oz)	330	2	30
Flying Saucer Vanilla	1 (4 oz)	240	1	40
Flying Saucer Vanilla w/ Sprinkles	1 (4 oz)	340	1	40
Ice Cream Cake	1 piece (4 oz)	230	—	35
Ice Cream Cupcakes	1	210	—	30
Vanilla	4 fl oz	190	—	50
Vanilla No Fat	4 fl oz	120	—	5
SHERBET				
Assorted Flavors	4 oz	150	—	5
CHICK-FIL-A				
BEVERAGES				
Coca-Cola Classic	1 serv (9 oz)	110	0	0

FOOD	PORTION	CALS.	FIB.	CHOL.
Diet Coke	1 serv (9 oz)	0	0	0
Diet Lemonade	1 serv (9 oz)	5	0	0
Iced Tea Sweetened	1 serv (9 oz)	150	0	0
Iced Tea Unsweetened	1 serv (9 fl oz)	0	0	0
Lemonade	1 serv (9 oz)	90	0	0
DESSERTS				
Cheesecake	1 slice (3.1 oz)	270	0	10
Cheesecake w/ Blueberry Topping	1 slice (4.1 oz)	290	0	10
Cheesecake w/ Strawberry Topping	1 slice (4.1 oz)	290	0	10
Fudge Nut Brownie	1 (2.6 oz)	350	0	30
Icedream Cone	1 sm (4.5 oz)	140	0	40
Icedream Cup	1 sm (7.5 oz)	350	0	70
Lemon Pie	1 slice (3.5 oz)	280	0	5
MAIN MENU SELECTIONS				
Carrot & Raisin Salad	1 sm (2.7 oz)	150	2	6
Chargrilled Chicken Club Sandwich w/o Dressing	1 (8.2 oz)	390	2	70
Chargrilled Chicken Deluxe Sandwich	1 (7.4 oz)	290	2	40
Chargrilled Chicken Garden Salad	1 serv (14 oz)	170	5	25
Chargrilled Chicken Sandwich	1 (5.3 oz)	280	1	40
Chargrilled Chicken w/o Bun or Pickles	1 piece (2.8 oz)	130	0	30
Chick-n-Q Sandwich	1 (6.1 oz)	370	1	20
Chick-n-Strips	4 (4.2 oz)	230	0	20
Chick-n-Strips Salad	1 serv (15.9 oz)	290	5	20
Chicken Sandwich	1 (5.9 oz)	290	1	50
Chicken Deluxe Sandwich	1 (8 oz)	300	2	50
Chicken Salad Plate	1 serv (16.5 oz)	290	6	35
Chicken Salad Sandwich On Whole Wheat	1 (5.9 oz)	320	1	10
Chicken w/o Bun or Pickles	1 piece (3.7 oz)	160	0	45
Cole Slaw	1 sm (2.8 oz)	130	1	15
Grilled 'n Lites	2 skewers (2.7 oz)	100	0	0
Hearty Breast of Chicken Soup	1 cup (7.6 oz)	110	1	45
Nuggets	8 (3.9 oz)	290	0	60
Tossed Salad	1 serv (4.6 oz)	70	1	0
Waffle Potato Fries	1 sm (3 oz)	290	0	5
Waffle Potato Fries w/o Salt	1 sm (3 oz)	290	0	5

CHILI'S

DESSERTS

FOOD	PORTION	CALS.	FIB.	CHOL.
Diet By Chocolate Cake	1 serv	370	8	0

FOOD	PORTION	CALS.	FIB.	CHOL.
Diet By Chocolate Cake w/ Yogurt	1 serv	465	8	3
Diet By Chocolate Cake w/ Yogurt & Fudge Topping	1 serv	534	8	3

MAIN MENU SELECTIONS

FOOD	PORTION	CALS.	FIB.	CHOL.
Guiltless Grill Chicken Fajitas	1 serv	726	24	44
Guiltless Grill Chicken Platter	1 serv	563	12	58
Guiltless Grill Chicken Salad w/ Dressing	1 serv	254	6	47
Guiltless Grill Chicken Sandwich	1	527	18	43
Guiltless Grill Veggie Pasta	1 serv	590	16	55
Guiltless Grill Veggie Pasta w/ Chicken	1 serv	696	17	97

CHURCH'S CHICKEN

FOOD	PORTION	CALS.	FIB.	CHOL.
Apple Pie	1 serv (3.1 oz)	280	1	<5
Biscuit	1 (2.1 oz)	250	1	<5
Breast	1 serv (2.8 oz)	200	0	65
Cajun Rice	1 serv (3.1 oz)	130	tr	5
Cole Slaw	1 serv (3 oz)	92	2	0
Corn On The Cob	1 serv (5.7 oz)	139	9	0
French Fries	1 serv (2.7 oz)	210	2	0
Leg	1 serv (2 oz)	140	0	45
Okra	1 serv (2.8 oz)	210	4	0
Potatoes & Gravy	1 serv (3.7 oz)	90	1	0
Tender Strip	1 (1.1 oz)	80	1	15
Thigh	1 serv (2.8 oz)	230	0	80
Wing	1 serv (3.1 oz)	250	0	60

COLOMBO FROZEN YOGURT

FOOD	PORTION	CALS.	FIB.	CHOL.
Alpine Strawberry Nonfat	4 fl oz	100	0	0
Banana Strawberry Nonfat	4 fl oz	50	—	0
Brazilian Banana Nonfat	4 fl oz	100	0	0
Butter Pecan Nonfat	4 fl oz	100	0	0
Cappuccino Nonfat	4 fl oz	100	0	0
Cherry Amaretto Nonfat	4 fl oz	50	—	0
Cherry Vanilla Nonfat	4 fl oz	100	0	0
Chocolate Nonfat	4 fl oz	50	—	0
Coconut Cooler Nonfat	4 fl oz	100	0	0
Cool Berry Blue Nonfat	4 fl oz	100	0	0
Country Pumpkin Nonfat	4 fl oz	100	0	0
Double Dutch Chocolate Nonfat	4 fl oz	100	0	0
Egg Nog Nonfat	4 fl oz	100	0	0
French Vanilla Lowfat	4 fl oz	110	0	5
French Vanilla Nonfat	4 fl oz	100	0	0
Georgia Peach Nonfat	4 fl oz	100	0	0

FOOD	PORTION	CALS.	FIB.	CHOL.
German Fudge Chocolate Nonfat	4 fl oz	100	0	0
Hawaiian Pineapple Nonfat	4 fl oz	100	0	0
Hazelnut Amaretto Nonfat	4 fl oz	100	0	0
Honey Almond Nonfat	4 fl oz	100	0	0
Irish Cream Nonfat	4 fl oz	100	0	0
New York Cheesecake Nonfat	4 fl oz	100	0	0
Old World Chocolate Lowfat	4 fl oz	110	0	5
Orange Bavarian Creme Nonfat	4 fl oz	100	0	0
Peanut Butter Lowfat	4 fl oz	110	0	5
Pecan Praline Nonfat	4 fl oz	100	0	0
Pina Colada Nonfat	4 fl oz	100	0	0
Raspberry Nonfat	4 fl oz	50	—	0
Rockin' Raspberry Nonfat	4 fl oz	100	0	0
Simply Vanilla Lowfat	4 fl oz	110	0	5
Simply Vanilla Nonfat	4 fl oz	100	0	0
Strawberry Nonfat	4 fl oz	50	—	0
Tropical Tango Nonfat	4 fl oz	100	0	0
Vanilla Nonfat	4 fl oz	50	—	0
White Chocolate Almond Nonfat	4 fl oz	100	0	0
Wild Strawberry Lowfat	4 fl oz	110	0	5

DAIRY QUEEN
FOOD SELECTIONS

FOOD	PORTION	CALS.	FIB.	CHOL.
Cheese Dog	1 (4 oz)	290	1	40
Chicken Breast Fillet Sandwich	1 (6.7 oz)	430	2	55
Chicken Breast Fillet Sandwich w/ Cheese	1 (7.2 oz)	480	2	70
Chicken Strip Basket w/ BBQ Sauce	1 serv (10.2 oz)	810	5	55
Chicken Strip Basket w/ Gravy	1 serv (13.1 oz)	860	5	55
Chili 'n' Cheese Dog	1 (5 oz)	330	2	45
Chili Dog	1 (4.5 oz)	280	2	35
DQ Homestyle Bacon Double Cheeseburger	1 (8.9 oz)	610	2	130
DQ Homestyle Cheeseburger	1 (5.3 oz)	340	2	55
DQ Homestyle Deluxe Double Cheeseburger	1 (8.5 oz)	540	2	115
DQ Homestyle Deluxe Double Hamburger	1 (7.4 oz)	440	2	90
DQ Homestyle Double Cheeseburger	1 (7.7 oz)	540	2	115
DQ Homestyle Hamburger	1 (4.8 oz)	290	2	45
DQ Homestyle Ultimate Burger	1 (9.4 oz)	670	2	135
Fish Fillet Sandwich	1 (6 oz)	370	2	45

FOOD	PORTION	CALS.	FIB.	CHOL.
Fish Fillet Sandwich w/ Cheese	1 (6.5 oz)	420	2	60
French Fries	1 reg (3.5 oz)	300	4	0
French Fries	1 lg (4.5 oz)	390	0	0
French Fries	1 sm (2.5 oz)	210	3	0
Grilled Chicken Breast Fillet Sandwich	1 (6.5 oz)	310	3	50
Hot Dog	1 (3.5 oz)	240	1	25
Onion Rings	1 serv (3 oz)	240	2	0
ICE CREAM				
Banana Split	1 (12.9 oz)	510	3	30
Blizzard Butterfinger	1 reg (16 oz)	750	1	50
Blizzard Butterfinger	1 sm (12 oz)	520	1	35
Blizzard Chocolate Sandwich Cookie	1 sm (12 oz)	520	1	40
Blizzard Chocolate Sandwich Cookie	1 reg (16 oz)	640	1	45
Blizzard Chocolate Chip Cookie Dough	1 reg (16 oz)	950	2	75
Blizzard Chocolate Chip Cookie Dough	1 sm (12 oz)	660	1	55
Blizzard Heath	1 reg (16 oz)	820	1	60
Blizzard Heath	1 sm (12 oz)	560	1	45
Blizzard Reese's Peanut Butter Cup	1 sm (12 oz)	590	1	45
Blizzard Reese's Peanut Butter Cup	1 reg (16 oz)	790	2	55
Blizzard Strawberry	1 sm (12 oz)	400	1	35
Blizzard Strawberry	1 reg (16 oz)	570	1	50
Breeze Heath	1 reg (16 oz)	710	1	20
Breeze Heath	1 sm (12 oz)	470	1	10
Breeze Strawberry	1 reg (16 oz)	460	1	10
Breeze Strawberry	1 sm (12 oz)	320	1	5
Buster Bar	1 (5.2 oz)	450	2	15
Cone Chocolate	1 reg (7.5 oz)	360	0	30
Cone Chocolate	1 sm (5 oz)	240	0	20
Cone Vanilla	1 lg (8.9 oz)	410	0	40
Cone Vanilla	1 reg (7.5 oz)	350	0	30
Cone Vanilla	1 sm (5 oz)	230	0	20
Cone Yogurt	1 reg (7.5 oz)	280	0	5
Cone Dipped	1 reg (8.2 oz)	510	1	30
Cone Dipped	1 sm (5.5 oz)	340	1	20
Cup Of Yogurt	1 reg (6.9 oz)	230	0	5
DQ Bar Caramel Nut	1 (2.8 oz)	260	0	15
DQ Bar Fudge	1 (2.3 oz)	50	0	0

FOOD	PORTION	CALS.	FIB.	CHOL.
DQ Bar Vanilla Orange	1 (2.3 oz)	60	0	0
DQ Heart Cake	1/10 of cake (4.8 oz)	270	1	20
DQ Lemon Freez'r	½ cup (3.2 oz)	80	0	0
DQ Log Cake Undecorated	1/8 of cake (4.7 oz)	280	1	15
DQ Nonfat Frozen Yogurt	½ cup (3 oz)	100	0	<5
DQ Round Cake 10 in	1/12 of cake (6.6 oz)	360	1	25
DQ Round Cake 8 in	1/8 of cake (6.2 oz)	340	1	25
DQ Sandwich	1 (2.1 oz)	150	1	5
DQ Sheet Cake Undecorated	1/20 of cake (6 oz)	350	1	20
DQ Soft Serve Chocolate	½ cup (3.3 oz)	150	0	15
DQ Soft Serve Vanilla	½ cup (3.3 oz)	140	0	15
DQ Treatzza Pizza Heath	1/8 of pie (2.3 oz)	180	1	5
DQ Treatzza Pizza M&M	1/8 of pie (2.4 oz)	190	1	5
DQ Treatzza Pizza Peanut Butter Fudge	1/8 of pie (2.5 oz)	220	1	5
DQ Treatzza Pizza Strawberry Banana	1/8 of pie (2.7 oz)	180	1	5
Dilly Bar Chocolate	1 (3 oz)	210	0	10
Dilly Bar Chocolate Mint	1 (2.7 oz)	190	0	15
Dilly Bar Toffee w/ Heath Pieces	1 (2.8 oz)	210	0	15
Fudge Nut Bar	1 (5 oz)	410	2	15
Malt Chocolate	1 sm (14.7 oz)	650	0	55
Malt Chocolate	1 reg (19.9 oz)	880	0	70
Misty Cooler Strawberry	1 (11.9 oz)	190	1	0
Misty Slush	1 reg (20.9 oz)	290	0	0
Misty Slush	1 sm (15.9 oz)	220	0	0
Peanut Buster Parfait	1 (10.7 oz)	730	2	35
Queen's Choice Big Scoop Chocolate	1 (4 oz)	250	0	55
Queen's Choice Big Scoop Vanilla	1 (4 oz)	250	0	55
Shake Chocolate	1 reg (18.9 oz)	770	0	70
Shake Chocolate	1 sm (13.9 oz)	560	0	50
Starkiss	1 (3 oz)	80	0	0
Strawberry Shortcake	1 (8.5 oz)	430	1	60
Sundae Chocolate	1 sm (6 oz)	290	0	25
Sundae Chocolate	1 reg (7.5 oz)	410	0	30
Yogurt Sundae Strawberry	1 reg (7.9 oz)	300	1	5

D'ANGELO SANDWICH SHOPS
SALADS AND SALAD BARS

FOOD	PORTION	CALS.	FIB.	CHOL.
D'Lite Chicken	1 serv	345	—	59
D'Lite Roast Beef	1 serv	355	—	48
D'Lite Tuna	1 serv	295	—	17
D'Lite Turkey	1 serv	355	—	79

FOOD	PORTION	CALS.	FIB.	CHOL.
SANDWICHES				
D'Lite Pocket Classic Vegetable	1	340	—	23
D'Lite Pocket Crunchy Vegetable	1	350	—	23
D'Lite Pocket Ginger Stir Fry Chicken	1	400	—	72
D'Lite Pocket Roast Beef	1	330	—	48
D'Lite Pocket Spicy Steak	1	425	—	41
D'Lite Pocket Steak	1	390	—	41
D'Lite Pocket Stuffed Turkey	1	510	—	82
D'Lite Pocket Turkey	1	350	—	79
D'Lite Small Sub Crunchy Vegetable	1	385	—	23
D'Lite Small Sub Roast Beef	1	365	—	48
D'Lite Small Sub Stuffed Turkey	1	545	—	82
D'Lite Small Sub Turkey	1	365	—	79
DELTACO				
BEVERAGES				
Coffee	1 serv	6	—	0
Coke Classic	1 sm	144	—	0
Coke Classic	1 med	198	—	0
Coke Classic	1 lg	287	—	0
Coke Classic Best Value	1 serv	395	—	0
Diet Coke	1 sm	1	—	0
Diet Coke	1 lg	2	—	0
Diet Coke	1 med	1	—	0
Diet Coke Best Value	1 serv	2	—	0
Iced Tea	1 lg	6	—	0
Iced Tea	1 med	4	—	0
Iced Tea	1 sm	3	—	0
Iced Tea Best Value	1 serv	8	—	0
M&M's Toppers	1 serv	256	—	19
Milk	1 serv	126	—	12
Mr Pibb	1 med	195	—	0
Mr Pibb	1 sm	142	—	0
Mr Pibb	1 lg	283	—	0
Mr Pibb Best Value	1 serv	390	—	0
Orange Juice	1 serv	83	—	0
Oreos Toppers	1 serv	257	—	19
Shake Chocolate	1 sm	549	—	40
Shake Chocolate	1 med	755	—	55
Shake Orange	1 sm	609	—	40
Shake Orange	1 med	837	—	55
Shake Strawberry	1 sm	486	—	40

FOOD	PORTION	CALS.	FIB.	CHOL.
Shake Strawberry	1 med	668	—	55
Shake Vanilla	1 sm	514	—	46
Shake Vanilla	1 med	707	—	63
Snickers Toppers	1 serv	254	—	18
Sprite	1 med	198	—	0
Sprite	1 sm	144	—	0
Sprite	1 lg	287	—	0
Sprite Best Value	1 serv	395	—	0
BREAKFAST SELECTIONS				
Burrito Beef And Egg	1	529	—	328
Burrito Breakfast	1	256	—	90
Burrito Egg And Cheese	1	443	—	305
Burrito Egg and Bean	1	470	—	305
Burrito Steak And Egg	1	500	—	337
CHILDREN'S MENU SELECTIONS				
Kid's Meal Hamburger	1 meal	617	—	29
Kid's Meal Taco	1 meal	532	—	16
MAIN MENU SELECTIONS				
American Cheese	1 slice	53	—	14
Beans And Cheese	1	122	—	9
Burrito Chicken	1	264	—	36
Burrito Combination	1	413	—	49
Burrito Del Beef	1	440	—	63
Burrito Deluxe Chicken	1	549	—	83
Burrito Deluxe Combo	1	453	—	59
Burrito Deluxe Del Beef	1	479	—	73
Burrito Green	1	229	—	15
Burrito Green Regular	1	330	—	22
Burrito Macho Beef	1	893	—	139
Burrito Macho Combo	1	774	—	100
Burrito Red	1	235	—	17
Burrito Red Regular	1	342	—	26
Burrito Spicy Chicken	1	392	—	35
Burrito The Works	1	448	—	27
Cheeseburger	1	284	—	42
Chicken Salad	1	254	—	58
Chicken Salad Deluxe	1	716	—	98
Del Burger	1	385	—	42
Del Cheeseburger	1	439	—	55
Double Del Cheeseburger	1	618	—	108
French Fries	1 sm	242	—	0
French Fries	1 lg	566	—	0
French Fries	1 reg	404	—	0
Fries Chili Cheese	1 serv	562	—	38

FOOD	PORTION	CALS.	FIB.	CHOL.
Fries Deluxe Chili Cheese	1 serv	600	—	48
Fries Nacho	1 serv	669	—	2
Guacamole	1 oz	60	—	0
Hamburger	1	231	—	29
Hot Sauce	1 pkg	2	—	0
Nacho Cheese Sauce	1 side order	100	—	2
Nachos	1 serv	390	—	2
Nachos Macho	1	1089	—	46
Quesadilla	1	257	—	30
Quesadilla Chicken	1	544	—	113
Quesadilla Regular	1	483	—	75
Quesadilla Spicy Jack	1	254	—	30
Quesadilla Spicy Jack Chicken	1	537	—	114
Quesadilla Spicy Jack Regular	1	476	—	76
Salsa	2 oz	14	—	tr
Salsa Dressing	1 oz	33	—	10
Soft Taco	1	146	—	16
Soft Taco Chicken	1	197	—	35
Soft Taco Deluxe Double Beef	1	211	—	35
Soft Taco Double Beef	1	178	—	25
Sour Cream	1 oz	60	—	20
Taco	1	140	—	16
Taco Chicken	1	186	—	35
Taco Deluxe Double Beef	1	205	—	35
Taco Double Beef	1	172	—	25
Taco Salad	1	235	—	31
Taco Salad Deluxe	1	741	—	83
Tostada	1	140	—	15

DENNY'S
BEVERAGES
Orange Juice	1 serv (10 oz)	130	—	0

BREAKFAST SELECTIONS
Applesauce	1 serv (2 oz)	40	—	0
Bacon	4 strips	145	—	20
Bagel	1	230	—	0
Banana	1	105	—	0
Banana Strawberry Medley	1 serv	95	—	0
Belgian Waffle	1	320	—	85
Biscuit Plain	1	215	—	1
Biscuit w/ Sausage Gravy	1 serv	465	—	15
Blueberry Topping	1 serv (3 oz)	110	—	0
Cantaloupe	¼	100	—	0
Chicken Fried Steak & Eggs w/o Bread	1 serv	650	—	460

FOOD	PORTION	CALS.	FIB.	CHOL.
Cream Cheese	1 oz	100	—	30
Egg	1	120	—	225
English Muffin	1	150	—	0
French Toast	1 serv	325	—	85
Grand Slam	1 serv	860	—	150
Grapefruit	½	40	—	0
Grapes	1 serv	50	—	0
Grits	1 serv	160	—	0
Ham	1 serv	170	—	50
Hashed Browns	1 serv	210	—	0
Honeydew	¼	125	—	0
Moon Over My Hammy	1 serv	980	—	265
Muffin Blueberry	1	310	—	0
Omelette Chili Cheese	1 serv	445	—	215
Omelette Denver	1 serv	735	—	650
Omelette Ham'n Cheddar	1 serv	490	—	240
Omelette Mexican	1 serv	550	—	245
Omelette Senior	1 serv	650	—	470
Omelette Ultimate	1 serv	745	—	670
Omelette Vegetable	1 serv	585	—	630
Pancakes Buttermilk	3	410	—	5
Sausage	4 links	225	—	20
Senior Grand Slam	1 serv	535	—	230
Senior Omelette	1 serv	640	—	470
Senior Starter	1 serv	550	—	235
Slams All-American w/o Bread	1 serv	980	—	265
Slams French	1 serv	915	—	235
Slams Harvest	1 serv	1055	—	445
Slams International	1 serv	975	—	235
Slams Scram w/o Bread	1 serv	1080	—	260
Slams Southern	1 serv	895	—	165
Steak & Eggs w/o Bread	1 serv	800	—	525
Strawberry Topping	1 serv (3 oz)	80	—	0
Syrup	1 serv (2 oz)	160	—	0
Toast w/o Butter	2 pieces	140	—	0
Whipped Butter	1 tbsp	65	—	20
Whipped Topping	1 serv (2 oz)	23	—	5
DESSERTS				
Apple Pie	1 serv	520	—	0
Apple Pie w/ Equal	1 serv	460	—	0
Banana Split	1 serv	850	—	90
Blueberry Cream Cheese Pie	1 serv	700	—	130
Cherry Cream Cheese Pie	1 serv	685	—	130
Cherry Pie	1 serv	635	—	0

FOOD	PORTION	CALS.	FIB.	CHOL.
Cherry Pie w/ Equal	1 serv	510	—	0
Chocolate Cake	1 serv	370	—	30
Coconut Cream Pie	1 serv	480	—	15
Double Dip Sundae	1 serv	545	—	60
French Silk Pie Cheese	1 serv	510	—	20
Hot Fudge Sundae	1 serv	495	—	60
Hot Fudge Cake Sundae	1 serv	730	—	60
Ice Cream Scoop	1 serv	135	—	30
Ice Cream Shake	1 serv	525	—	100
Key Lime Pie	1 serv	590	—	25
MAIN MENU SELECTIONS				
Buffalo Wings w/o Dressing	1 serv	350	—	200
Burger Bacon Swiss	1	745	—	125
Burger Patty Melt	1	780	—	120
Chicken Fried Steak	1 serv	465	—	80
Chicken Strips	1 serv	580	—	95
Chicken Strips w/o Dressing	1 serv	580	—	95
Chili Fries	1 serv	585	—	25
Club Sandwich	1	485	—	90
Coleslaw	1 serv	105	—	tr
Denny Burger	1	485	—	70
French Fries	1 serv	285	—	0
Fried Chicken	1 serv	460	—	185
Grilled Breast Of Chicken	1 serv (4 oz)	125	—	70
Grilled Breast Of Chicken	1 serv (6 oz)	190	—	105
Grilled Catfish	1 serv	475	—	80
Grilled Rainbow Trout	1 serv	490	—	115
Liver w/ Bacon & Onions	1 serv	585	—	545
Mozzarella Sticks	4	350	—	10
Nachos Supreme	1 serv	770	—	65
Prime Rib	1 serv (8 oz)	570	—	140
Quesadila	1 serv	460	—	35
Quesadila Chicken	1 serv	580	—	110
Roast Beef w/ Bread, Gravy, Potatoes	1 serv	600	—	165
Roast Turkey w/ Stuffing & Gravy	1 serv	490	—	40
Sandwich Bacon, Lettuce & Tomato	1	490	—	35
Sandwich Chicken Melt	1 serv	700	—	165
Sandwich French Dip	1 serv	575	—	85
Sandwich Grilled Cheese	1	715	—	100
Sandwich Grilled Chicken	1	665	—	70
Sandwich Mega Melt	1 serv	945	—	195
Sandwich Prime Time	1 serv	930	—	140

FOOD	PORTION	CALS.	FIB.	CHOL.
Sandwich Roast Beef Deluxe	1 serv	850	—	145
Sandwich Super Bird	1	585	—	115
Sandwich Tuna Melt Supreme	1	805	—	95
Sandwich Veggie Cheese Melt	1	565	—	70
Senior Chicken Fried Steak	1 serv	425	—	35
Senior Fried Chicken	1 serv	480	—	155
Senior Grilled Catfish Dinner w/o Vegetable	1 serv	450	—	55
Senior Grilled Cheese Sandwich	1 serv	360	—	50
Senior Grilled Chicken Dinner w/o Vegetable	1 serv	245	—	60
Senior Liver w/ Bacon & Onions	1 serv	435	—	250
Senior Roast Beef Dinner w/o Vegetable	1 serv	280	—	80
Senior Roast Turkey & Stuffing w/o Vegetable	1 serv	440	—	60
Senior Sirloin Tips w/o Vegetable	1 serv	220	—	50
Senior Spaghetti w/ Meatballs	1 serv	580	—	75
Senior Tuna Salad Sandwich	1	260	—	20
Senior Turkey Sandwich	1	340	—	75
Spaghetti w/ Meatballs	1 serv	1000	—	355
Spaghetti w/ Sauce	1 serv	605	—	0
Stir Fry Chicken w/ Vegetables & Rice Pilaf	1 serv	435	—	70
Works Burger	1	950	—	130
SALAD DRESSINGS				
Bleu Cheese	1 oz	120	—	20
Creamy Italian	1 oz	100	—	0
French	1 oz	100	—	5
French Reduced Calorie	1 oz	70	—	0
Italian Reduced Calorie	1 oz	16	—	0
Ranch	1 oz	110	—	10
Thousand Island	1 oz	120	—	10
SALADS AND SALAD BARS				
Caesar	1 serv	325	—	20
California Grilled Chicken	1 serv	290	—	75
Chef's	1 serv	370	—	320
Crispy Chicken Salad	1 serv	905	—	80
Crispy Chicken Salad w/o Tortilla Shell	1 serv	465	—	80
Garden Salad	1 serv	115	—	75
Grilled Chicken Caesar	1 serv	655	—	125
Taco Salad	1 serv	905	—	50
Taco Salad w/o Tortilla Shell	1 serv	470	—	50

FOOD	PORTION	CALS.	FIB.	CHOL.
SOUPS				
Cheese	1 serv	315	—	19
Chicken Noodle	1 serv	60	—	10
Chili With Beans	1 serv	160	—	20
Clam Chowder	1 serv	220	—	5
Cream Of Broccoli	1 serv	200	—	5
Cream of Potato	1 serv	230	—	15
Vegetable Beef	1 serv	80	—	5
DOMINO'S PIZZA				
12 INCH				
Deep Dish Cheese	2 slices (7.2 oz)	560	3	32
Deep Dish Ham	2 slices (7.7 oz)	577	3	38
Deep Dish Italian Sausage & Mushroom	2 slices (8.3 oz)	618	4	43
Deep Dish Pepperoni	2 slices (7.6 oz)	622	3	45
Deep Dish Veggie	2 slices (8.3 oz)	576	4	32
Deep Dish X-Tra Cheese & Pepperoni	2 slices (8.2 oz)	671	3	54
Hand-Tossed Cheese	2 slices (5.2 oz)	344	2	19
Hand-Tossed Ham	2 slices (5.6 oz)	362	2	26
Hand-Tossed Italian Sausage & Mushroom	2 slices (6.2 oz)	402	3	31
Hand-Tossed Pepperoni	2 slices (5.6 oz)	406	3	32
Hand-Tossed Veggie	2 slices (6.2 oz)	360	3	19
Hand-Tossed X-Tra Cheese & Pepperoni	2 slices (6.2 oz)	455	3	42
Thin Crust Cheese	⅓ pie (4.9 oz)	364	2	26
Thin Crust Ham	⅓ pie (5.6 oz)	388	2	35
Thin Crust Italian Sausage & Mushroom	⅓ pie (6.3 oz)	442	3	41
Thin Crust Pepperoni	⅓ pie (5.5 oz)	447	2	43
Thin Crust Veggie	⅓ pie (6.3 oz)	386	2	26
Thin Crust X-Tra Cheese & Pepperoni	⅓ pie (6.2 oz)	512	2	56
DUNKIN' DONUTS				
BAKED GOODS				
Bagel Cinnamon Raisin	1 (3 oz)	220	0	0
Bagel Onion	1 (3 oz)	200	0	0
Bagel Plain	1 (3 oz)	200	0	0
Bismark	1 (2.8 oz)	310	1	0
Bow Tie	1 (2.5 oz)	250	1	0
Brownie Blondie w/ Chocolate Chips	1 (2.4 oz)	300	1	25

FOOD	PORTION	CALS.	FIB.	CHOL.
Brownie Fudge	1 (2.4 oz)	290	tr	35
Brownie Peanut Butter Blondie	1 (2.4 oz)	330	1	25
Cake Donut Blueberry	1 (2.4 oz)	230	1	0
Cake Donut Blueberry Crumb	1 (2.6 oz)	260	1	0
Cake Donut Butternut	1 (2.6 oz)	340	2	0
Cake Donut Chocolate	1 (2.1 oz)	210	1	0
Cake Donut Chocolate Coconut	1 (2.4 oz)	250	2	0
Cake Donut Chocolate Glazed	1 (2.5 oz)	250	1	0
Cake Donut Cinnamon	1 (2.3 oz)	300	1	0
Cake Donut Coconut	1 (2.5 oz)	320	1	0
Cake Donut Double Chocolate	1 (2.6 oz)	260	1	0
Cake Donut Old Fashioned	1 (2.1 oz)	280	1	0
Cake Donut Peanut	1 (2.6 oz)	340	2	0
Cake Donut Powdered	1 (2.4 oz)	310	1	0
Cake Donut Sugared	1 (2.4 oz)	310	1	0
Cake Donut Toasted Coconut	1 (2.5 oz)	320	1	0
Cake Donut Whole Wheat Glazed	1 (2.7 oz)	230	2	0
Coffee Roll	1 (2.6 oz)	280	2	0
Coffee Roll Chocolate Frosted	1 (2.7 oz)	290	2	0
Coffee Roll Cinnamon Raisin	1 (3.1 oz)	330	3	0
Coffee Roll Maple Frosted	1 (2.7 oz)	300	2	0
Coffee Roll Vanilla Frosted	1 (2.7 oz)	300	2	0
Cookie Chocolate Chocolate Chunk	1 (1.5 oz)	200	1	30
Cookie Chocolate Chunk	1 (1.5 oz)	200	1	30
Cookie Chocolate Chunk w/ Nut	1 (1.5 oz)	200	1	30
Cookie Chocolate White Chocolate Chunk	1 (1.5 oz)	200	1	30
Cookie Oatmeal Raisin Pecan	1 (1.5 oz)	190	0	25
Cookie Peanut Butter Chocolate Chunk w/ Nuts	1 (1.5 oz)	210	1	25
Cookie Peanut Butter Chocolate Chunk w/ Peanuts	1 (1.5 oz)	210	3	30
Cream Cheese Plain	1 serv (1 oz)	100	0	30
Croissant Almond	1 (2.7 oz)	360	2	10
Croissant Cheese	1 (2.5 oz)	240	0	5
Croissant Chocolate	1 (2.5 oz)	370	1	10
Croissant Plain	1 (2.1 oz)	270	0	5
Crullers/Sticks Dunkin' Donut	1 (2.1 oz)	240	2	0
Crullers/Sticks Glazed	1 (3 oz)	340	2	0
Crullers/Sticks Glazed Chocolate	1 (3.2 oz)	410	3	0
Crullers/Sticks Jelly	1 (3.2 oz)	330	3	0
Crullers/Sticks Plain	1 (2.1 oz)	260	2	0
Crullers/Sticks Powdered	1 (2.3 oz)	290	2	0

FOOD	PORTION	CALS.	FIB.	CHOL.
Crullers/Sticks Sugar	1 (2.2 oz)	270	2	0
Eclair	1 (3.2 oz)	290	1	0
English Muffin	1 (2 oz)	130	1	0
French Roll	1 (2.1 oz)	140	1	0
Fritter Apple	1 (3.3 oz)	300	2	0
Fritter Glazed	1 (2.7 oz)	290	2	0
Muffin Banana Nut	1 (3.3 oz)	340	2	35
Muffin Blueberry	1 (3.3 oz)	310	2	35
Muffin Cherry	1 (3.3 oz)	330	1	35
Muffin Chocolate Chip	1 (3.3 oz)	400	2	35
Muffin Corn	1 (3.3 oz)	350	2	50
Muffin Cranberry Orange Nut	1 (3.5 oz)	310	2	30
Muffin Honey Raisin Bran	1 (3.3 oz)	330	4	15
Muffin Lemon Poppy Seed	1 (3.3 oz)	360	1	40
Muffin Oat Bran	1 (3.2 oz)	290	1	0
Muffin Lowfat Apple n' Spice	1 (3.3 oz)	220	1	0
Muffin Lowfat Banana	1 (3.3 oz)	240	1	0
Muffin Lowfat Blueberry	1 (3.3 oz)	230	1	0
Muffin Lowfat Bran	1 (3.3 oz)	260	4	0
Muffin Lowfat Cherry	1 (3.3 oz)	230	0	0
Muffin Lowfat Corn	1 (3.3 oz)	250	1	0
Muffin Lowfat Cranberry Orange	1 (3.3 oz)	230	1	0
Munchkins Butternut	3 (2 oz)	230	2	0
Munchkins Chocolate Glazed	3 (2 oz)	180	1	0
Munchkins Cinnamon	4 (2 oz)	240	1	0
Munchkins Coconut	3 (1.7 oz)	200	1	0
Munchkins Glazed Cake	3 (2.1 oz)	220	1	0
Munchkins Glazed Raised	4 (2.1 oz)	210	1	0
Munchkins Jelly	3 (1.9 oz)	170	1	0
Munchkins Lemon	3 (2 oz)	160	1	0
Munchkins Plain	4 (1.8 oz)	200	1	0
Munchkins Powdered Sugar	4 (2 oz)	240	1	0
Munchkins Sugar Raised	6 (1.9 oz)	210	1	0
Munchkins Toasted Coconut	3 (1.8 oz)	210	1	0
Tart Apple	1 (3.4 oz)	310	1	0
Tart Blueberry	1 (3.4 oz)	300	2	0
Tart Lemon	1 (3.4 oz)	280	1	0
Tart Raspberry	1 (3.4 oz)	310	2	0
Tart Strawberry	1 (3.4 oz)	310	1	0
Turnover Apple	1 (3.8 oz)	350	2	0
Turnover Blueberry	1 (3.8 oz)	370	2	0
Turnover Lemon	1 (3.8 oz)	350	2	0
Turnover Raspberry	1 (3.8 oz)	380	2	0
Turnover Strawberry	1 (3.8 oz)	380	2	0

FOOD	PORTION	CALS.	FIB.	CHOL.
Yeast Donut Apple Crumb	1 (2.6 oz)	250	1	0
Yeast Donut Apple n' Spice	1 (2.5 oz)	230	1	0
Yeast Donut Bavarian Kreme	1 (2.5 oz)	250	1	0
Yeast Donut Black Raspberry	1 (2.4 oz)	240	1	0
Yeast Donut Boston Kreme	1 (2.8 oz)	270	1	0
Yeast Donut Chocolate Kreme Filled	1 (2.6 oz)	320	1	0
Yeast Donut Chocolate Frosted	1 (2.1 oz)	210	1	0
Yeast Donut Glazed	1 (1.6 oz)	160	1	0
Yeast Donut Jelly Filled	1 (2.4 oz)	240	1	0
Yeast Donut Lemon	1 (2.5 oz)	240	1	0
Yeast Donut Maple Frosted	1 (2.1 oz)	210	1	0
Yeast Donut Marble Frosted	1 (2.1 oz)	210	1	0
Yeast Donut Strawberry	1 (2.4 oz)	240	1	0
Yeast Donut Strawberry Frosted	1 (2.1 oz)	220	1	0
Yeast Donut Sugar Raised	1 (1.6 oz)	170	1	0
Yeast Donut Vanilla Frosted	1 (2.1 oz)	220	1	0
BREAKFAST SELECTIONS				
Croissant Sandwich Egg & Cheese	1 (5 oz)	430	0	280
Croissant Sandwich Egg, Bacon & Cheese	1 (5.4 oz)	500	0	290
Croissant Sandwich Egg, Ham & Cheese	1 (6 oz)	530	0	295
Croissant Sandwich Egg, Sausage & Cheese	1 (6.9 oz)	630	0	320
COFFEE				
Cream	1 serv (1 oz)	60	0	20
Dark Roast	1 serv (10 oz)	5	0	0
Decaf	1 serv (10 oz)	0	0	0
French Vanilla	1 serv (10 oz)	5	0	0
Hazelnut	1 serv (10 oz)	5	0	0
Regular	1 serv (10 oz)	5	0	0
LUNCH SELECTIONS				
Croissant Sandwich Broccoli & Cheese	1 (6.1 oz)	370	2	20
Croissant Sandwich Chicken Salad	1 (7.6 oz)	540	1	75
Croissant Sandwich Ham & Cheese	1 (6.7 oz)	710	0	85
Croissant Sandwich Roast Beef & Cheese	1 (6 oz)	490	0	30
Croissant Sandwich Seafood Salad	1 (7.6 oz)	480	1	50
Croissant Sandwich Tuna Salad	1 (7.5 oz)	540	1	50

FOOD	PORTION	CALS.	FIB.	CHOL.
SOUPS				
Beef Barley	1 serv (8 oz)	90	0	10
Beef Noodle	1 serv (8 oz)	90	0	20
Chicken Noodle	1 serv (8 oz)	80	0	15
Chili	1 serv (8 oz)	170	0	20
Chili Con Carne w/ Beans	1 serv (8 oz)	300	0	45
Cream Of Broccoli	1 serv (8 oz)	200	0	25
Cream Of Potato	1 serv (8 oz)	190	1	25
Harvest Vegetable	1 serv (8 oz)	80	0	0
Manhattan Clam Chowder	1 serv (8 oz)	70	1	5
Minestrone	1 serv (8 oz)	100	2	0
New England Clam Chowder	1 serv (8 oz)	200	0	30
Split Pea w/ Ham	1 serv (8 oz)	190	0	15
EL POLLO LOCO				
DESSERTS				
Cheesecake	1 serv (3.5 oz)	310	0	60
Churro	1 serv (1.25 oz)	130	tr	5
MAIN MENU SELECTIONS				
Beans	1 serv (4 oz)	100	8	0
Burrito Bean, Rice & Cheese	1 (9 oz)	530	8	15
Burrito Chicken	1 (7 oz)	310	4	65
Burrito Classic Chicken	1 (9.5 oz)	560	4	75
Burrito Grilled Steak	1 (11 oz)	740	9	75
Burrito Loco Grande Chicken	1 (13 oz)	680	5	90
Burrito Spicy Hot Chicken	1 (10 oz)	570	4	75
Burrito Steak	1 (6 oz)	450	4	70
Burrito Vegetarian	1 (6 oz)	340	7	20
Burrito Whole Wheat Chicken	1 (10.5 oz)	510	5	60
Cheddar Cheese	1 serv (1 oz)	90	0	30
Chicken Breast	1 piece (3 oz)	160	0	110
Chicken Leg	1 piece (1.75 oz)	90	0	75
Chicken Thigh	1 piece (2 oz)	180	0	130
Chicken Wing	1 (1.5 oz)	110	0	80
Coleslaw	1 serv (3 oz)	100	1	10
Corn	1 serv (3 oz)	110	1	0
Fajita Meal Chicken	1 (17.5 oz)	780	17	60
Fajita Meal Steak	1 (17.5 oz)	1040	17	100
Guacamole	1 serv (1 oz)	60	0	0
Potato Salad	1 serv (4 oz)	180	1	10
Rice	1 serv (2 oz)	110	0	0
Salsa	1 serv (2 oz)	10	1	0
Sour Cream	1 serv (1 oz)	50	0	15
Taco Chicken	1 (5 oz)	180	2	35

FOOD	PORTION	CALS.	FIB.	CHOL.
Taco Steak	1 (4.5 oz)	250	2	40
Tortilla Corn	1 (1 oz)	60	tr	0
Tortilla Flour	1 (1 oz)	90	tr	0
SALAD DRESSINGS				
Blue Cheese	1 serv (1 oz)	80	0	5
Deluxe French	1 serv (1 oz)	60	0	0
Honey Dijon Mustard	1 serv (1 oz)	50	0	0
Italian Reduced Calorie	1 serv (1 oz)	25	0	0
Ranch	1 serv (1 oz)	75	0	0
Thousand Island	1 serv (1 oz)	110	0	5
SALADS AND SALAD BARS				
Chicken Salad	1 (12 oz)	160	4	45
Side Salad	1 (9 oz)	50	4	0

FRIENDLY'S
FROZEN YOGURT

FOOD	PORTION	CALS.	FIB.	CHOL.
Apple Bettie	½ cup (2.6 oz)	140	0	10
Chocolate Fudge Brownie	½ cup (2.6 oz)	160	0	10
Fabulous Fudge Swirl	½ cup (2.6 oz)	140	0	10
Fudge Berry Swirl	½ cup (2.6 oz)	150	0	10
Lowfat Perfectly Peach	½ cup (2.6 oz)	110	0	10
Lowfat Purely Chocolate	½ cup (2.6 oz)	120	0	10
Lowfat Raspberry Delight	½ cup (2.6 oz)	120	0	10
Lowfat Simply Vanilla	½ cup (2.6 oz)	120	0	10
Lowfat Strawberry Patch	½ cup (2.6 oz)	110	0	10
Mint Chocolate Chip	½ cup (2.6 oz)	130	0	10
Strawberry Cheesecake Blast	½ cup (2.6 oz)	140	0	15
Toffee Almond Crunch	½ cup (2.6 oz)	160	tr	15
ICE CREAM				
Black Raspberry	½ cup	150	0	30
Chocolate Almond Chip	½ cup	170	0	35
Forbidden Chocolate	½ cup	150	0	30
Fudge Nut Brownie	½ cup	200	0	25
Heath English Toffee	½ cup (2.7 oz)	190	0	30
Purely Pistachio	½ cup	160	0	35
Vanilla	½ cup	150	0	35
Vienna Mocha Chunk	½ cup	180	0	30

FRULLATI CAFE
BAKED GOODS

FOOD	PORTION	CALS.	FIB.	CHOL.
Muffin Banana Nut	1 (4 oz)	394	1	31
Muffin Cranberry Orange	1 (4 oz)	357	1	31
Muffin Fat Free Apple Streusel	1 (4 oz)	260	2	0
Muffin Fat Free Chocolate	1 (4 oz)	260	2	0
Muffin Fat Free Very Berry	1 (4 oz)	260	2	0

FOOD	PORTION	CALS.	FIB.	CHOL.
Muffin Sugar Free Blueberry	1 (4 oz)	308	1	12
Muffin Wild Blueberry	1 (4 oz)	344	1	31
BEVERAGES				
Apple Juice	1 serv (12 oz)	131	0	0
Carrot Juice	1 serv (12 oz)	111	2	0
Celery Juice	1 serv (12 oz)	22	2	0
Lemonade	1 serv	209	2	0
Lemonade Apple	1 serv	245	3	0
Lemonade Cherry	1 serv	237	2	0
Lemonade Orange	1 serv	270	5	0
Lemonade Strawberry	1 serv	234	2	0
Orange Banana Juice	1 serv (12 oz)	150	2	0
Orange Juice	1 serv (12 oz)	126	1	0
Smoothie A La Frullati	1 lg	426	3	20
Smoothie A La Frullati	1 sm	275	3	10
Smoothie Affinity	1 sm	226	2	10
Smoothie Affinity	1 lg	378	2	20
Smoothie Fiesta	1 lg	257	6	0
Smoothie Fiesta	1 sm	234	6	0
Smoothie Peach Banana	1 lg	289	5	0
Smoothie Peach Banana	1 sm	266	5	0
Smoothie Pina Colada	1 sm	236	2	10
Smoothie Pina Colada	1 lg	387	2	82
Smoothie Strawberry Banana	1 sm	165	4	0
Smoothie Strawberry Banana	1 lg	188	4	0
Smoothie Strawberry Blueberry	1 sm	90	3	0
Smoothie Strawberry Blueberry	1 lg	113	3	0
Smoothie Strawberry Fruit	1 lg	101	3	0
Smoothie Strawberry Fruit	1 sm	79	3	0
Smoothie Strawberry Watermelon	1 lg	123	2	0
Smoothie Strawberry Watermelon	1 sm	100	2	0
DESSERTS				
Frozen Yogurt	1 lg	263	0	3
Frozen Yogurt	1 reg	205	0	3
Frozen Yogurt	1 sm	146	0	2
Yogurt Smoothie Cappuccino	1 serv	472	0	17
Yogurt Smoothie Chocolate Fudge	1 serv	555	1	17
Yogurt Smoothie Fiesta	1 serv	432	3	17
Yogurt Smoothie Oreo Cookie	1 serv	566	2	19
Yogurt Smoothie Peach	1 serv	486	1	17
Yogurt Smoothie Peach Banana	1 serv	519	2	17
Yogurt Smoothie Peanut Butter	1 serv	630	2	17
Yogurt Smoothie Pina Colada	1 serv	519	1	5
Yogurt Smoothie Strawberry Banana	1 serv	514	2	17

FOOD	PORTION	CALS.	FIB.	CHOL.
Yogurt Smoothie Strawberry Fruit	1 serv	487	2	17
Yogurt Smoothie Strawberry Vanilla	1 serv	462	0	17
Yogurt Smoothie Strawberry Watermelon	1 serv	503	2	17
SALADS AND SALAD BARS				
Fruit Salad	1 lg	148	3	0
Fruit Salad	1 sm	99	2	0
Garden Salad	1 sm	56	2	0
Garden Salad w/ Italian Fat Free Dressing	1 lg	72	3	8
Pasta Salad	1 sm	179	0	0
Pasta Salad	1 lg	256	0	0
SANDWICHES				
Chicken On Croissant	1	481	4	109
Chicken On Honey Wheat	1	297	6	34
Chicken On Jewish Rye	1	261	5	34
Chicken On Pita	1	281	4	34
Chicken On White	1	291	4	35
Ham & Cheese On Croissant	1	797	3	192
Ham & Cheese On Honey Wheat	1	613	5	117
Ham & Cheese On Jewish Rye	1	577	4	117
Ham & Cheese On Pita	1	597	3	117
Ham & Cheese On White	1	607	3	118
Roast Beef On Croissant	1	631	3	155
Roast Beef On Honey Wheat	1	348	5	72
Roast Beef On Jewish Rye	1	312	4	72
Roast Beef On Pita	1	332	3	72
Roast Beef On White	1	342	3	72
Tuna On Croissant	1	480	4	90
Tuna On Honey Wheat	1	295	7	16
Tuna On Jewish Rye	1	259	5	16
Tuna On Pita	1	280	4	16
Tuna On White	1	289	4	16
Turkey On Croissant	1	566	3	122
Turkey On Honey Wheat	1	342	5	56
Turkey On Jewish Rye	1	306	4	56
Turkey On Pita	1	326	3	56
Turkey On White	1	338	3	57
Veggie On Croissant	1	510	4	83
Veggie On Honey Wheat	1	227	6	0
Veggie On Jewish Rye	1	191	5	0
Veggie On Pita	1	211	4	0
Veggie On White	1	221	4	0

FOOD	PORTION	CALS.	FIB.	CHOL.
GODFATHER'S PIZZA				
Golden Crust Cheese	⅒ lg (3.5 oz)	261	—	23
Golden Crust Cheese	⅛ med (3.1 oz)	229	—	19
Golden Crust Cheese	⅙ sm (3 oz)	213	—	19
Golden Crust Combo	⅙ sm (4.5 oz)	273	—	31
Golden Crust Combo	⅛ med (4.5 oz)	283	—	29
Golden Crust Combo	⅒ lg (5.1 oz)	322	—	34
Original Crust Cheese	⅙ sm (3.5 oz)	239	—	25
Original Crust Cheese	⅒ lg (4 oz)	271	—	28
Original Crust Cheese	⅛ med (3.5 oz)	242	—	22
Original Crust Cheese	¼ mini (2 oz)	138	—	13
Original Crust Combo	⅒ lg (5.5 oz)	332	—	39
Original Crust Combo	⅙ sm (5 oz)	299	—	37
Original Crust Combo	¼ mini (2.8 oz)	164	—	17
Original Crust Combo	⅛ med (5.2 oz)	318	—	38
GODIVA				
Almond Butter Dome	3 pieces (1.5 oz)	240	0	5
Bouchee Au Chocolat	1 piece (1.5 oz)	210	0	5
Bouchee Ivory Raspberry	1 piece (1 oz)	160	0	5
Gold Ballotin	3 pieces (1.5 oz)	210	0	5
Truffle Amaretto Di Saronno	2 pieces (1.5 oz)	210	0	5
Truffle Deluxe Liqueur	2 pieces (1.5 oz)	210	0	5
HAAGEN-DAZS				
FROZEN YOGURT				
Brownie Nut Blast	½ cup (3.5 oz)	215	1	41
Chocolate	½ cup (3.4 oz)	160	1	33
Coffee	½ cup (3.4 oz)	161	tr	45
Orange Tango	½ cup (3.5 oz)	132	tr	20
Pina Colada	½ cup (3.4 oz)	139	tr	25
Raspberry Randezvous	½ cup (3.5 oz)	132	1	20
Soft Serve Coffee	½ cup (3.3 oz)	145	tr	38
Soft Serve Nonfat Chocolate	½ cup (3.3 oz)	116	1	2
Soft Serve Nonfat Chocolate Mousse	½ cup (3.3 oz)	86	1	2
Soft Serve Nonfat Vanilla	½ cup (3.3 oz)	114	tr	2
Soft Serve Nonfat Vanilla Mousse	½ cup (3.3 oz)	78	tr	2
Strawberry Cheesecake Craze	½ cup (3.6 oz)	213	tr	64
Strawberry Duet	½ cup (3.4 oz)	135	1	25
Vanilla	½ cup (3.4 oz)	162	0	44
Vanilla Almond Crunch	½ cup (3.4 oz)	198	1	41
ICE CREAM				
Bar Chocolate	1 (2.7 oz)	247	1	108
Bar Coffee	1 (2.7 oz)	249	tr	111

FOOD	PORTION	CALS.	FIB.	CHOL.
Bar Vanilla	1 (2.7 oz)	251	0	111
Belgian Chocolate Chocolate	½ cup (3.6 oz)	315	3	84
Brownies A La Mode	½ cup (3.5 oz)	284	1	103
Butter Pecan	½ cup (3.7 oz)	304	1	100
Cappuccino Commotion	½ cup (3.6 oz)	305	1	98
Caramel Cone Explosion	½ cup (3.6 oz)	298	1	93
Chocolate	½ cup (3.7 oz)	249	1	110
Chocolate Chocolate Chip	½ cup (3.7 oz)	282	2	97
Chocolate Chocolate Mint	½ cup (3.6 oz)	285	1	94
Coffee	½ cup (3.7 oz)	251	tr	113
Coffee Chip	½ cup (3.6 oz)	285	1	98
Cookie Dough Dynamo	½ cup (3.6 oz)	298	tr	92
Cookies & Cream	½ cup (3.6 oz)	264	tr	107
Deep Chocolate Peanut Butter	½ cup (3.7 oz)	339	4	81
Macadamia Brittle	½ cup (3.7 oz)	282	tr	103
Macadamia Nut	½ cup (3.6 oz)	309	tr	109
Midnight Cookies & Cream	½ cup (3.6 oz)	285	1	89
Peanut Butter Burst	½ cup (2.6 oz)	314	1	91
Pralines & Cream	½ cup (3.6 oz)	278	tr	94
Rum Raisin	½ cup (3.7 oz)	256	tr	102
Strawberry	½ cup (3.7 oz)	242	1	91
Strawberry Cheesecake Craze	½ cup (3.7 oz)	273	1	97
Swiss Chocolate Almond	½ cup (3.6 oz)	288	2	97
Triple Brownie Overload	½ cup (3.5 oz)	298	1	91
Vanilla	½ cup (3.7 oz)	252	0	113
Vanilla Chip	½ cup (3.6 oz)	286	1	99
Vanilla Fudge	½ cup (3.7 oz)	268	tr	98
Vanilla Swiss Almond	½ cup (3.7 oz)	288	1	101
SORBET				
Mango	½ cup (4 oz)	107	1	0
Raspberry	½ cup (4 oz)	110	2	0
Soft Serve Lemonade	½ cup (3.3 oz)	113	1	0
Soft Serve Mango	½ cup (3.3 oz)	107	1	0
Soft Serve Raspberry	½ cup (3.3 oz)	108	2	0
Strawberry	½ cup (4 oz)	118	1	0
Zesty Lemon	½ cup (4 oz)	111	1	0

HARDEE'S
BEVERAGES

FOOD	PORTION	CALS.	FIB.	CHOL.
Orange Juice	1 serv (11 oz)	140	—	0
Shake Chocolate	1 (12.2 oz)	370	—	30
Shake Peach	1 (12.1 oz)	390	—	25
Shake Strawberry	1 (12.7 oz)	420	—	20
Shake Vanilla	1 (12.2 oz)	349	—	2

FOOD	PORTION	CALS.	FIB.	CHOL.
BREAKFAST SELECTIONS				
Bacon & Egg Biscuit	1 (4.4 oz)	490	—	155
Bacon, Egg & Cheese Biscuit	1 (4.8 oz)	530	—	155
Big Country Breakfast Bacon	1 (7.6 oz)	740	—	305
Big Country Breakfast Sausage	1 (9.6 oz)	930	—	340
Biscuit 'N' Gravy	1 (7.8 oz)	510	—	15
Cinnamon 'N' Raisin Biscuit	1 (2.8 oz)	370	—	0
Country Ham Biscuit	1 (3.8 oz)	430	—	25
Frisco Breakfast Sandwich Ham	1 (6.5 oz)	460	—	175
Ham Biscuit	1 (4 oz)	400	—	15
Ham, Egg & Cheese Biscuit	1 (5.6 oz)	500	—	170
Hash Rounds	1 serv (2.8 oz)	230	—	0
Rise 'N' Shine Biscuit	1 (2.9 oz)	390	—	0
Sausage & Egg Biscuit	1 (5.2 oz)	560	—	170
Sausage Biscuit	1 (4.1 oz)	510	—	25
Three Pancakes	1 serv (4.8 oz)	280	—	15
Three Pancakes w/ 1 Sausage Pattie	1 serv (6.2 oz)	430	—	40
Three Pancakes w/ 2 Bacon Strips	1 serv (5.3 oz)	350	—	25
Ultimate Omelet Biscuit	1 (4.9 oz)	530	—	175
ICE CREAM				
Cool Twist Sundae Hot Fudge	1 (5.5 oz)	290	—	20
Cool Twist Sundae Strawberry	1 (5.8 oz)	210	—	10
Cool Twist Cone Chocolate	1 (4.1 oz)	180	—	15
Cool Twist Cone Vanilla	1 (4.1 oz)	170	—	10
Cool Twist Cone Vanilla/ Chocolate	1 (4.1 oz)	180	—	10
MAIN MENU SELECTIONS				
Bacon Cheeseburger	1 (7.9 oz)	600	—	50
Big Cookie	1 (2.0 oz)	280	—	15
Big Deluxe Burger	1 (8.5 oz)	530	—	40
Cheeseburger	1 (4.2 oz)	300	—	25
Chicken Breast	1 piece (5.2 oz)	370	—	75
Chicken Fillet	1 (7.5 oz)	470	—	50
Chicken Leg	1 piece (2.4 oz)	170	—	45
Chicken Thigh	1 piece (4.2 oz)	330	—	60
Chicken Wing	1 piece (2.3 oz)	200	—	30
Cole Slaw	1 serv (4 oz)	240	—	10
Fisherman's Fillet	1 (7.6 oz)	500	—	60
French Fries	1 med (5.0 oz)	350	—	0
French Fries	1 sm (3.4 oz)	240	—	0
French Fries	1 lg (6.1 oz)	430	—	0
Frisco Burger	1 (8.5 oz)	760	—	70
Gravy	1 serv (1.5 fl oz)	20	—	0

FOOD	PORTION	CALS.	FIB.	CHOL.
Hamburger	1 (3.6 oz)	260	—	20
Hot Ham 'N' Cheese	1 (5.7 oz)	350	—	50
Marinated Chicken Grill	1 (7.1 oz)	202	—	65
Mashed Potatoes	1 serv (4 oz)	70	—	0
Mushroom 'N' Swiss Burger	1 (7.1 oz)	520	—	45
Quarter-Pound Cheeseburger	1 (6.5 oz)	490	—	35
Regular Roast Beef	1 (4.4 oz)	270	—	25
SALAD DRESSINGS				
French Fat Free	1 serv (2 oz)	70	—	0
Ranch	1 serv (2 oz)	290	—	25
Thousand Island	1 serv (2 oz)	250	—	35
SALADS AND SALAD BARS				
Garden Salad	1 (10.2 oz)	210	—	40
Grilled Chicken Salad	1 (11.5 oz)	150	—	60
Side Salad	1 (4.6 oz)	25	—	0

H.SALT SEAFOOD

FOOD	PORTION	CALS.	FIB.	CHOL.
Chicken	3 oz	108	—	69
Cod	3 oz	62	—	18
Hamburger	3 oz	228	—	65
Pork Loin	3 oz	254	—	55
Sirloin Steak	3 oz	239	—	58

IHOP

FOOD	PORTION	CALS.	FIB.	CHOL.
Pancake Buckwheat	1 (2.5 oz)	134	1	61
Pancake Buttermilk	1 (2 oz)	108	tr	31
Pancake Country Griddle	1 (2.25 oz)	134	1	38
Pancake Egg	1 (2 oz)	102	tr	66
Pancake Harvest Grain 'N Nut	1 (2.25 oz)	160	1	38
Waffle	1 (4 oz)	305	1	70
Waffle Belgian	1 (6 oz)	408	1	146
Waffle Belgian Harvest Grain 'N Nut	1 (6 oz)	445	3	147

JACK IN THE BOX
BEVERAGES

FOOD	PORTION	CALS.	FIB.	CHOL.
2% Milk	1 serv (8 fl oz)	120	0	20
Coca-Cola Classic	1 sm (16 fl oz)	190	0	0
Coffee	1 cup (8 fl oz)	5	0	0
Diet Coke	1 sm (16 fl oz)	0	0	0
Dr Pepper	1 sm (16 fl oz)	190	0	0
Iced Tea	1 sm (16 fl oz)	0	0	0
Milk Shake Chocolate	1 reg (11 fl oz)	390	tr	25
Milk Shake Strawberry	1 reg (10 fl oz)	330	0	30

FOOD	PORTION	CALS.	FIB.	CHOL.
Milk Shake Vanilla	1 reg (10 fl oz)	350	0	30
Orange Juice	1 serv (6 fl oz)	80	tr	0
Ramblin' Root Beer	1 sm (16 fl oz)	240	0	0
Sprite	1 sm (16 fl oz)	190	0	0
BREAKFAST SELECTIONS				
Breakfast Jack	1 (4.2 oz)	300	0	185
Country Crock Spread	1 pat (5 g)	25	0	0
Grape Jelly	1 serv (0.5 oz)	40	0	0
Hash Browns	1 serv (2 oz)	100	1	0
Pancake Platter	1 serv (5.6 oz)	400	3	30
Pancake Syrup	1 serv (1.5 fl oz)	120	0	0
Sausage Croissant	1 (6.4 oz)	670	2	250
Scrambled Egg Pocket	1 (6.4 oz)	430	0	355
Sourdough Breakfast Sandwich	1 (5.2 oz)	380	0	235
Supreme Croissant	1 (6 oz)	570	2	245
Ultimate Breakfast Sandwich	1 (8.5 oz)	620	tr	455
DESSERTS				
Cheesecake	1 serv (3.5 oz)	310	2	65
Chocolate Chip Cookie Dough Cheesecake	1 serv (3.6 oz)	360	1	45
Hot Apple Turnover	1 (3.9 oz)	350	0	0
MAIN MENU SELECTIONS				
¼ lb. Burger	1 (6 oz)	510	0	65
American Cheese	1 slice (0.4 oz)	45	0	10
Bacon & Cheddar Potato Wedges	1 serv (9.3 oz)	800	4	55
Bacon Bacon Cheeseburger	1 (8.5 oz)	710	0	115
Barbeque Dipping Sauce	1 serv (1 fl oz)	45	0	0
Cheeseburger	1 (3.9 oz)	320	0	35
Chicken Caesar Sandwich	1 (8.3 oz)	520	4	55
Chicken Fajita Pita	1 (6.9 oz)	290	3	35
Chicken Sandwich	1 (5.6 oz)	400	0	45
Chicken Strips Breaded	4 pieces (3.9 oz)	290	0	50
Chicken Strips Breaded	6 pieces (6.2 oz)	450	0	80
Chicken Supreme	1 (8.6 oz)	620	0	75
Chinese Hot Sauce	1 pkg (5 g)	10	0	0
Double Cheeseburger	1 (5.3 oz)	450	0	75
Egg Rolls	5 pieces (10 oz)	750	7	50
Egg Rolls	3 pieces (5.8 oz)	440	4	30
Fish Supreme	1 (8.6 oz)	590	0	70
French Fries	1 reg (6.7 oz)	350	4	0
French Fries	1 sm (2.4 oz)	220	3	0
Grilled Chicken Fillet	1 (7.4 oz)	430	0	65
Grilled Sourdough Burger	1 (7.8 oz)	670	0	110
Guacamole	1 serv (0.9 oz)	50	0	0

FOOD	PORTION	CALS.	FIB.	CHOL.
Hamburger	1 (3.4 oz)	280	0	25
Hot Sauce	1 pkg (0.5 fl oz)	5	tr	0
Jumbo Fries	1 serv (4.3 oz)	400	4	0
Jumbo Jack	1 (8 oz)	560	0	65
Jumbo Jack With Cheese	1 (8.5 oz)	650	0	90
Ketchup	1 pkg (0.3 oz)	10	0	0
Mayonnaise	1 pkg (0.7 oz)	150	0	15
Monterey Roast Beef Sandwich	1 (8.4 oz)	540	3	75
Mustard	1 pkg (6 g)	5	0	0
Onion Rings	1 serv (3.6 oz)	380	0	0
Salsa	1 serv (1 fl oz)	10	0	0
Seasoned Curly Fries	1 serv (3.8 oz)	360	4	0
Sour Cream	1 serv (1 oz)	60	0	20
Soy Sauce	1 serv (0.3 oz)	5	0	0
Spicy Crispy Chicken Sandwich	1 (7.9 oz)	560	0	50
Stuffed Jalapenos	7 pieces (4.8 oz)	420	3	55
Stuffed Jalapenos	10 pieces (6.8 oz)	600	4	75
Super Scoop French Fries	1 serv (6.5 oz)	590	6	0
Super Taco	1 (4.4 oz)	280	3	30
Sweet & Sour Dipping Sauce	1 serv (1 fl oz)	40	0	0
Swiss-Style Cheese	1 slice (0.4 oz)	40	0	10
Taco	1 (2.7 oz)	190	2	20
Tartar Dipping Sauce	1 pkg (1 oz)	150	0	10
Teriyaki Bowl Chicken	1 serv (15.4 oz)	580	6	30
The Colossus Burger	1 (10.1 oz)	1100	0	220
The Outlaw Burger	1 (8.2 oz)	720	0	95
The Really Big Chicken Sandwich	1 (12.5 oz)	900	1	120
Ultimate Cheeseburger	1 (9.8 oz)	1030	0	205
SALAD DRESSINGS				
Blue Cheese	1 serv (2 fl oz)	210	0	15
Buttermilk House	1 serv (2 fl oz)	290	0	20
Buttermilk House Dipping Sauce	1 serv (0.9 fl oz)	130	tr	10
Italian Low Calorie	1 serv (2 fl oz)	25	0	0
Thousand Island	1 serv (2 fl oz)	250	0	20
SALADS AND SALAD BARS				
Croutons	1 serv (0.4 oz)	50	0	0
Garden Chicken Salad	1 serv (8.9 oz)	200	3	65
Side Salad	1 (3.4 oz)	70	2	10

KENNY ROGERS ROASTERS
MAIN MENU SELECTIONS

½ Chicken w/ Skin	1 serv (9.06 oz)	515	—	301
½ Chicken w/o Skin & Wing	1 serv (7.03 oz)	313	—	221
¼ Chicken Dark Meat w/ Skin	1 serv (4.35 oz)	271	—	165

FOOD	PORTION	CALS.	FIB.	CHOL.
¼ Chicken Dark Meat w/o Skin & Wing	1 serv (3.29 oz)	169	—	130
¼ Chicken White Meat w/ Skin	1 serv (4.71 oz)	244	—	136
¼ Chicken White Meat w/o Skin & Wing	1 serv (3.74 oz)	144	—	92
Baked Sweet Potato	1 (9 oz)	263	1	0
Chicken Caesar Salad	1 serv (9.4 oz)	285	1	122
Cinnamon Apples	1 serv (5.27 oz)	199	3	13
Cole Slaw	1 serv (5.05 oz)	225	2	13
Corn Muffin	1 (2 oz)	175	1	0
Corn On The Cob	1 (2.25 oz)	68	2	0
Corn Stuffing	1 serv (7.1 oz)	326	tr	5
Creamy Parmesan Spinach	1 serv (5.3 oz)	119	tr	12
Garlic Parsley Potatoes	1 serv (6.5 oz)	259	3	16
Honey Baked Beans	1 serv (5 oz)	148	tr	0
Italian Green Beans	1 serv (6.1 oz)	116	tr	0
Macaroni & Cheese	1 serv (5.51 oz)	197	1	26
Pasta Salad	1 serv (5 oz)	236	1	40
Pita BBQ Chicken	1 (7.33 oz)	401	—	112
Pita Chicken Caesar	1 (9.2 oz)	606	1	122
Pita Roasted Chicken	1 (10.8 oz)	685	tr	159
Pot Pie Chicken	1 (12 oz)	708	tr	69
Potato Salad	1 serv (7.01 oz)	390	2	0
Real Mashed Potatoes	1 serv (8 oz)	295	1	2
Rice Pilaf	1 serv (5 oz)	173	0	0
Roasted Chicken Salad	1 serv (16.9 oz)	292	6	218
Sandwich Turkey	1 (9.2 oz)	385	1	88
Side Salad	1 serv (4.73 oz)	23	2	0
Sour Cream & Dill Pasta Salad	1 serv (5 oz)	233	1	16
Steamed Vegetables	1 serv (4.25 oz)	48	4	0
Sweet Corn Niblets	1 serv (5 oz)	112	1	0
Tomato Cucumber Salad	1 serv (6 oz)	123	1	0
Turkey Sliced Breast	1 serv (4.5 oz)	158	—	78
Zucchini & Squash Santa Fe	1 serv (5 oz)	70	1	0
SALAD DRESSINGS				
Blue Cheese	1 serv (2.47 oz)	370	0	65
Buttermilk Ranch	1 serv (2.47 oz)	430	0	10
Caesar	1 serv (2.47 oz)	340	0	15
Honey French	1 serv (2.47 oz)	350	0	0
Honey Mustard	1 serv (2.47 oz)	320	1	40
Italian Fat Free	1 serv (2.47 oz)	35	0	0
Thousand Island	1 serv (2.47 oz)	330	0	40
SOUPS				
Chicken Noodle	1 bowl (10 oz)	91	tr	22
Chicken Noodle	1 cup (6 oz)	55	1	13

FOOD	PORTION	CALS.	FIB.	CHOL.
KFC				
BAKED SELECTIONS				
Biscuit	1 (2.0 oz)	200	1	2
Cornbread	1 (2 oz)	228	1	42
MAIN MENU SELECTIONS				
BBQ Baked Beans	1 serv (3.9 oz)	132	4	3
Chicken Pot Pie	1 (13.4 oz)	700	5	85
Cole Slaw	1 serv (3.2 oz)	114	—	<5
Colonel's Chicken Sandwich	1 (5.9 oz)	482	—	47
Corn On The Cob	1 ear (5.3 oz)	222	8	0
Crispy Strips	4 (4 oz)	323	—	50
Extra Tasty Crispy Breast	1 (5.9 oz)	470	1	80
Extra Tasty Crispy Drumstick	1 (2.4 oz)	190	tr	60
Extra Tasty Crispy Thigh	1 (4.2 oz)	370	2	70
Extra Tasty Crispy Whole Wing	1 (1.9 oz)	200	tr	45
Garden Rice	1 serv (3.8 oz)	75	1	0
Green Beans	1 serv (3.6 oz)	36	2	3
Hot & Spicy Breast	1 (6.5 oz)	530	2	110
Hot & Spicy Drumstick	1 (2.3 oz)	190	tr	50
Hot & Spicy Thigh	1 (3.8 oz)	370	1	90
Hot & Spicy Whole Wing	1 (1.9 oz)	210	tr	50
Hot Wings	6 (4.8 oz)	471	—	150
Kentucky Nuggets	6 (3.4 oz)	284	—	66
Macaroni & Cheese	1 serv (4 oz)	162	0	16
Mashed Potatoes With Gravy	1 serv (4.2 oz)	109	2	tr
Mean Greens	1 serv (3.9 oz)	52	3	6
Original Chicken Sandwich	1 (7.2 oz)	497	—	52
Original Recipe Breast	1 (4.8 oz)	360	1	115
Original Recipe Drumstick	1 (1.8 oz)	130	0	70
Original Recipe Thigh	1 (3.3 oz)	260	1	110
Original Recipe Whole Wing	1 (1.7 oz)	150	0	40
Potato Salad	1 serv (4.4 oz)	180	2	11
Potato Wedges	1 serv (3.3 oz)	192	3	3
Red Beans & Rice	1 serv (3.9 oz)	114	3	4
Value BBQ Chicken Sandwich	1 (5.3 oz)	296	2	57
KRYSTAL				
BEVERAGES				
Chocolate Shake	1 (16 fl oz)	275	—	32
BREAKFAST SELECTIONS				
Biscuit	1 (2.5 oz)	244	—	2
Biscuit Bacon	1 (2.9 oz)	306	—	14
Biscuit Bacon, Egg & Cheese	1 (4.7 oz)	421	—	153
Biscuit Country Ham	1 (3.7 oz)	334	—	23

FOOD	PORTION	CALS.	FIB.	CHOL.
Biscuit Egg	1 (4 oz)	327	—	134
Biscuit Gravy	1 (7.5 oz)	419	—	23
Biscuit Sausage	1 (4.1 oz)	437	—	49
Sunriser	1 (3.8 oz)	259	—	162
DESSERTS				
Apple Pie	1 serv (4.5 oz)	300	—	0
Donut Plain	1 (1.3 oz)	150	—	5
Donut w/ Chocolate Icing	1 (1.8 oz)	212	—	5
Donut w/ Vanilla Icing	1 (1.8 oz)	198	—	5
Lemon Meringue Pie	1 serv (4 oz)	340	—	50
Pecan Pie	1 serv (4 oz)	450	—	55
MAIN MENU SELECTIONS				
Bacon Cheeseburger	1 (7.4 oz)	521	—	89
Big K	1 (8 oz)	540	—	93
Burger Plus	1 (6.5 oz)	415	—	63
Burger Plus w/ Cheese	1 (7.1 oz)	473	—	77
Cheese Krystal	1 (2.5 oz)	187	—	29
Chili	1 lg (12 oz)	327	—	28
Chili	1 reg (8 oz)	218	—	19
Chili Cheese Pup	1 (2.7 oz)	211	—	31
Chili Pup	1 (2.5 oz)	182	—	24
Corn Pup	1 (2.3 oz)	214	—	24
Crispy Crunchy Chicken Sandwich	1 (5.75 oz)	467	—	56
Double Cheese Krystal	1 (4.5 oz)	337	—	57
Double Krystal	1 (4 oz)	277	—	43
Fries	1 lg (5.3 oz)	463	—	16
Fries	1 reg (4.1 oz)	358	—	12
Fries	1 sm (3 oz)	262	—	9
Krys Kross Fries	1 serv (4.3 oz)	486	—	31
Krys Kross Fries Chili Cheese	1 serv (6.8 oz)	625	—	61
Krys Kross Fries w/ Cheese	1 serv (5.3 oz)	515	—	31
Krystal	1 (2.2 oz)	158	—	22
Plain Pup	1 (1.9 oz)	160	—	20

LITTLE CAESARS
MAIN MENU SELECTIONS

FOOD	PORTION	CALS.	FIB.	CHOL.
Crazy Bread	1 piece (1.4 oz)	106	1	0
Crazy Sauce	1 serv (6 oz)	170	5	0
Deli-Style Sandwich Ham & Cheese	1 (11.6 oz)	728	3	54
Deli-Style Sandwich Italian	1 (11.9 oz)	740	3	62
Deli-Style Sandwich Veggie	1 (11.9 oz)	647	4	29
Hot Oven-Baked Sandwich Cheeser	1 (12.1 oz)	822	5	580

FOOD	PORTION	CALS.	FIB.	CHOL.
Hot Oven-Baked Sandwich Meatsa	1 (15 oz)	1036	5	130
Hot Oven-Baked Sandwich Pepperoni	1 (11.2 oz)	899	4	58
Hot Oven-Baked Sandwich Supreme	1 (13.1 oz)	894	5	700
Hot Oven-Baked Sandwich Veggie	1 (13.7 oz)	669	6	58
PIZZA				
Baby Pan!Pan!	1 serv (8.4 oz)	616	4	47
Pan!Pan! Cheese	1 med slice (2.9 oz)	181	1	15
Pan!Pan! Pepperoni	1 med slice (3 oz)	199	1	15
Pizza!Pizza! Cheese	1 med slice (3.2 oz)	201	1	17
Pizza!Pizza! Pepperoni	1 med slice (3.3 oz)	220	1	17
SALAD DRESSINGS				
1000 Island	1 serv (1.5 oz)	183	—	30
Blue Cheese	1 serv (1.5 oz)	160	—	17
Caesar	1 serv (1.5 oz)	255	—	13
French	1 serv (1.5 oz)	166	—	0
Greek	1 serv (1.5 oz)	268	—	9
Italian	1 serv (1.5 oz)	200	—	12
Italian Fat Free	1 serv (1.5 oz)	15	—	0
Ranch	1 serv (1.5 oz)	221	—	18
SALADS AND SALAD BARS				
Antipasto Salad	1 serv (8.4 oz)	176	2	19
Caesar Salad	1 serv (5 oz)	140	2	11
Greek Salad	1 serv (10.3 oz)	168	3	37
Tossed Salad	1 serv (8.5 oz)	116	3	0

LONG JOHN SILVER'S
BEVERAGES
Diet Coke	1 serv (8 oz)	1	—	0
DESSERTS				
Apple Crumb Cheesecake	1 serv (3.5 oz)	300	0	25
Chocolate Cream Pie	1 serv (2.6 oz)	280	0	15
Double Lemon Pie	1 serv (3.4 oz)	350	0	40
Key Lime Cream Cheese Pie	1 serv (3 oz)	310	0	20
Pineapple Cream Cheesecake	1 serv (3.2 oz)	310	0	5
MAIN MENU SELECTIONS				
Baked Potato	1 (8 oz)	210	3	0
Battered Chicken	1 piece (2 oz)	120	3	15
Battered Clams	1 serv (3 oz)	300	5	40
Battered Fish	1 piece (2.9 oz)	170	5	30
Battered Shrimp	1 piece (0.4 oz)	35	0	10
Cheese Sticks	1 serv (1.6 oz)	160	tr	10
Coleslaw	1 serv (3.4 oz)	140	3	0

FOOD	PORTION	CALS.	FIB.	CHOL.
Corn Cobbette	1 piece (3.3 oz)	140	0	0
Corn Cobbette w/o Butter	1 (3.1 oz)	80	0	0
Flavorbaked Chicken	1 piece (3.5 oz)	150	tr	75
Flavorbaked Fish	1 piece (3.1 oz)	120	tr	45
Fries	1 serv (3 oz)	250	3	0
Green Beans	1 serv (3.5 oz)	30	2	<5
Honey Mustard Sauce	1 serv (0.4 fl oz)	20	0	0
Hushpuppy	1 (0.8 oz)	60	0	0
Ketchup	1 serv (0.32 oz)	10	0	0
Lettuce	1 serv (0.5 oz)	8	—	0
Margarine	1 serv (0.2 oz)	35	—	0
Mayonnaise	1 serv (0.5 oz)	100	—	8
Monterey Jack Cheese	1 serv (0.5 oz)	50	—	15
Popcorn Chicken	1 serv (3.3 oz)	250	1	35
Popcorn Fish	1 serv (3.6 oz)	290	1	20
Popcorn Shrimp	1 serv (3.3 oz)	280	1	85
Rice Pilaf	1 serv (3 oz)	140	tr	0
Sandwich Batter Dipped Fish No Sauce	1 (5.4 oz)	320	6	30
Sandwich Flavorbaked Chicken	1 (5.8 oz)	290	2	60
Sandwich Flavorbaked Fish	1 (6 oz)	320	2	55
Sandwich Ultimate Fish	1 (6.4 oz)	430	3	35
Sandwich Bun	1 (1.7 oz)	130	—	tr
Shrimp Sauce	1 serv (0.4 oz)	15	0	0
Sour Cream	1 serv (1 oz)	60	0	15
Sweet'N'Sour Sauce	1 serv (0.4 fl oz)	20	0	0
Tartar Sauce	1 serv (0.4 fl oz)	35	0	0
Tomato	1 serv (0.7 oz)	6	—	0
SALAD DRESSINGS				
Fat-Free French	1 serv (1.5 oz)	50	—	0
Fat-Free Ranch	1 serv (1.5 fl oz)	50	—	0
Italian	1 serv (1 oz)	130	—	0
Malt Vinegar	1 serv (0.3 fl oz)	0	0	0
Ranch Dressing	1 serv (1 fl oz)	170	—	5
Thousand Island	1 serv (1 oz)	110	—	15
SALADS AND SALAD BARS				
Ocean Chef Salad	1 serv (8.1 oz)	100	1	40
Side Salad	1 (4.3 oz)	25	tr	0

LYONS RESTAURANTS
MAIN MENU SELECTIONS

FOOD	PORTION	CALS.	FIB.	CHOL.
Light & Healthy Halibut Brochette	1 serv	502	—	47
Light & Healthy Lime & Cilantro Chicken	1 serv	511	—	101

FOOD	PORTION	CALS.	FIB.	CHOL.

MACHEEZMO MOUSE
CHILDREN'S MENU SELECTIONS

FOOD	PORTION	CALS.	FIB.	CHOL.
El Bento Kid	1 serv (7 oz)	235	—	63
Quesadilla Kid Cheese	1 serv (5 oz)	360	—	40
Quesadilla Kid Chicken	1 serv (7 oz)	430	—	100
Taco Kid Cheese	1 serv (6 oz)	285	—	20
Taco Kid Chicken	1 (8 oz)	355	—	80

MAIN MENU SELECTIONS

FOOD	PORTION	CALS.	FIB.	CHOL.
Beans	1 oz	35	—	0
Bento Stick	1 oz	30	—	63
Boss Sauce	1 oz	30	—	0
Broccoli	1 oz	4	—	0
Burrito Chicken	1 (13 oz)	580	—	110
Burrito Combo	1 (14 oz)	630	—	124
Burrito Vegetarian	1 (14 oz)	655	—	20
Cheese	1 oz	81	—	20
Chicken	1 oz	35	—	30
Chili	1 oz	43	—	22
Chips	1 oz	140	—	0
Cilantro	1 oz	8	—	0
Dinner Rice, Beans, Broccoli	1 serv (10 oz)	328	—	0
Dinner Rice, Beans, Salad	1 serv (12 oz)	344	—	0
El Bento	1 serv (16 oz)	600	—	63
El Bento Deluxe	1 serv (20 oz)	740	—	65
Enchilada Chicken	1 (12 oz)	533	—	92
Enchilada Chili	1 (12 oz)	549	—	76
Enchilada Veggie	1 (14 oz)	623	—	32
Enchilada Sauce	1 oz	6	—	0
Fresh Greens	1 oz	2	—	0
Green Sauce	1 oz	5	—	0
Guacamole	1 oz	100	—	0
Marinated Veggies	1 oz	10	—	0
Mexican Cheese	1 oz	100	—	24
Mustard Dressing	1 oz	25	—	0
Power Salad Chicken	1 serv (16 oz)	275	—	63
Power Salad Veggie	1 serv (13 oz)	200	—	0
Rice	1 oz	45	—	0
Salad Chicken	1 serv (15 oz)	430	—	110
Salad Veggie Taco	1 serv (16 oz)	655	—	20
Salsa	1 oz	4	—	0
Snack Famouse #5	1 serv (14 oz)	585	—	20
Snack Nacho Grande	1 serv (9 oz)	841	—	62
Snack Quesadilla Cheese	1 serv (6 oz)	377	—	42

FOOD	PORTION	CALS.	FIB.	CHOL.
Snack Quesadilla Chicken	1 serv (10 oz)	450	—	102
Snack Tacos Chicken	1 serv (6 oz)	290	—	82
Snack Tacos Chili	1 serv (6 oz)	314	—	66
Snack Tacos Veggie	1 serv (6 oz)	290	—	22
Sour Cream	1 oz	23	—	0
Tortilla Corn	3 (1 oz)	60	—	0
Tortilla Flour	1 oz	80	—	0
Tortilla Wheat	1 oz	80	—	0
Veggie Deluxe	1 serv (18 oz)	665	—	2
Yogurt Nonfat	1 oz	20	—	0

MANHATTAN BAGEL

FOOD	PORTION	CALS.	FIB.	CHOL.
Blueberry	1 (4 oz)	260	2	0
Cheddar Cheese	1 (4 oz)	270	2	10
Chocolate Chip	1 (4 oz)	290	2	0
Cinnamon Raisin	1 (4 oz)	280	3	0
Egg	1 (4 oz)	270	2	0
Everything	1 (4 oz)	290	3	0
Garlic	1 (4 oz)	270	2	0
Marble	1 (4 oz)	260	3	0
Oat Bran Raisin Walnut	1 (4 oz)	270	3	0
Onion	1 (4 oz)	270	2	0
Plain	1 (4 oz)	260	2	0
Poppy	1 (4 oz)	300	5	0
Pumpernickel	1 (4 oz)	250	3	0
Rye	1 (4 oz)	260	3	0
Salt	1 (4 oz)	260	2	0
Sesame	1 (4 oz)	310	3	0
Spinach	1 (4 oz)	270	3	0
Whole Wheat	1 (4 oz)	260	3	0

MAX & IRMA'S
MAIN MENU SELECTIONS

FOOD	PORTION	CALS.	FIB.	CHOL.
Cocktail Sauce	1 oz	33	—	0
Fruit Smoothie	1 serv (10 oz)	114	—	0
Garden Burger	1 serv (14 oz)	467	—	12
Gourmet Garden Burger	1 serv (15 oz)	484	—	12
Grilled Zucchini & Mushroom Pasta	1 serv (15 oz)	448	—	13
Grilled Zucchini & Mushroom Pasta With Chicken	1 serv (18 oz)	621	—	78
Peel & Eat Shrimp	1 serv (6 oz)	166	—	191
Ranch Mayonnaise Low Fat	1 serv (1 oz)	22	—	0

MCDONALD'S
BAKED SELECTIONS

FOOD	PORTION	CALS.	FIB.	CHOL.
Apple Pie Baked	1 (2.7 oz)	260	tr	0

FOOD	PORTION	CALS.	FIB.	CHOL.
Chocolate Chip Cookie	1 (1.2 oz)	170	1	20
Cinnamon Roll	1 (3.3 oz)	400	2	75
Danish Apple	1 (3.7 oz)	360	1	40
Danish Cheese	1 (3.7 oz)	410	0	70
Lowfat Muffin Apple Bran	1 (4 oz)	300	3	0
BEVERAGES				
Coca-Cola Classic	1 sm (16 oz)	150	—	0
Coca-Cola Classic	1 child serv (12 oz)	110	—	0
Coca-Cola Classic	1 med (21 oz)	210	—	0
Coca-Cola Classic	1 lg (32 oz)	310	—	0
Diet Coke	1 sm (16 oz)	1	—	0
Diet Coke	1 lg (32 oz)	0	—	0
Diet Coke	1 child serv (12 oz)	0	—	0
Diet Coke	1 med (21 oz)	0	—	0
Hi-C Orange	1 sm (16 oz)	160	—	0
Hi-C Orange	1 child serv (12 oz)	120	—	0
Hi-C Orange	1 med (21 oz)	240	—	0
Hi-C Orange	1 lg (32 oz)	350	—	0
Milk 1%	1 serv (8 oz)	100	0	10
Orange Juice	1 serv (6 oz)	80	0	0
Shake Chocolate	1 sm (14.5 oz)	340	1	25
Shake Strawberry	1 sm (14.5 oz)	340	0	25
Shake Vanilla	1 sm (14.5 oz)	340	0	25
Sprite	1 sm (16 fl oz)	150	—	0
Sprite	1 med (21 oz)	210	—	0
Sprite	1 child serv (12 oz)	110	—	0
Sprite	1 lg (32 oz)	310	—	0
BREAKFAST SELECTIONS				
Bacon Egg & Cheese Biscuit	1 (5.3 oz)	440	1	235
Biscuit	1 (2.7 oz)	260	1	0
Breakfast Burrito	1 (4.1 oz)	320	1	195
Egg McMuffin	1 (4.8 oz)	290	1	235
English Muffin	1 (1.9 oz)	140	1	0
Hash Browns	1 serv (1.9 oz)	130	1	0
Hotcakes Margarine & Syrup	2 serv (7.8 oz)	580	2	15
Hotcakes Plain	1 serv (5.3 oz)	310	2	15
Sausage	1 (1.5 oz)	170	0	35
Sausage Biscuit	1 (4.2 oz)	430	1	35
Sausage Biscuit With Egg	1 (6 oz)	510	1	245
Sausage McMuffin	1 (3.9 oz)	360	1	45
Sausage McMuffin With Egg	1 (5.7 oz)	440	1	255
Scrambled Eggs	2 (3.6 oz)	160	0	425
DESSERTS				
Lowfat Ice Cream Cone Vanilla	1 (3.2 oz)	120	0	5

FOOD	PORTION	CALS.	FIB.	CHOL.
Lowfat Sundae Hot Caramel	1 (6.4 oz)	300	tr	5
Lowfat Sundae Strawberry	1 (6.2 oz)	240	tr	5
McDonaldland Cookies	1 pkg (1.5 oz)	180	1	0
Nuts For Sundaes	1 serv (7 g)	40	0	0
Sundae Hot Fudge	1 (6.3 oz)	290	2	5
MAIN MENU SELECTIONS				
Arch Deluxe	1 (8.7 oz)	570	4	90
Arch Deluxe With Bacon	1 (8.9 oz)	610	4	100
Barbeque Sauce	1 pkg (1 oz)	45	0	0
Big Mac	1 (7.5 oz)	530	3	80
Cheeseburger	1 (4.2 oz)	320	2	45
Chicken McNuggets	6 pieces (3.7 oz)	290	0	60
Chicken McNuggets	4 pieces (2.5 oz)	190	0	40
Chicken McNuggets	9 pieces (5.6 oz)	430	0	90
Crispy Chicken Deluxe	1 (8.1 oz)	530	4	60
Fish Filet Deluxe	1 (8.3 oz)	510	5	50
French Fries	1 lg (5.2 oz)	450	5	0
French Fries	1 sm (2.4 oz)	210	2	0
French Fries	1 super (6.2 oz)	540	6	0
Grilled Chicken Deluxe	1 (7.5 oz)	330	4	50
Grilled Chicken Salad Deluxe	1 serv (7.5 oz)	110	2	45
Hamburger	1 (3.7 oz)	270	2	30
Honey Mustard	1 pkg (0.5 oz)	40	0	10
Hot Mustard	1 pkg (1 oz)	60	tr	5
McNuggets Sauce Honey	1 pkg (0.5 oz)	45	0	0
Quarter Pounder	1 (6 oz)	430	2	70
Quarter Pounder With Cheese	1 (7 oz)	530	2	95
Sweet 'N Sour Sauce	1 pkg (1 oz)	50	0	0
SALAD DRESSINGS				
Caesar	1 pkg (2.1 oz)	160	0	20
Fat Free Herb Vinaigrette	1 pkg (2.1 oz)	50	0	0
Ranch	1 pkg (2.1 oz)	230	0	20
Reduced Calorie Red French	1 pkg (2.1 oz)	160	0	0
SALADS AND SALAD BARS				
Croutons	1 pkg (0.4 oz)	50	tr	0
Garden Salad	1 serv (6.2 oz)	35	2	0

MY FAVORITE MUFFIN

FOOD	PORTION	CALS.	FIB.	CHOL.
Basic Muffin	⅓ muffin	220	0	0
Double Chocolate	⅓ muffin	190	2	0
Fat Free Bavarian	⅓ muffin	100	1	0
Fat Free Bavarian Chocolate	⅓ muffin	130	3	0

NATHAN'S
BEVERAGES

FOOD	PORTION	CALS.	FIB.	CHOL.
Lemonade	32 fl oz	378	—	0

FOOD	PORTION	CALS.	FIB.	CHOL.
Lemonade	16 fl oz	189	—	0
Lemonade	22 fl oz	260	—	0
MAIN MENU SELECTIONS				
Breaded Chicken Sandwich	1 (7.2 oz)	510	—	56
Charbroiled Chicken Sandwich	1 (4.5 oz)	288	—	53
Cheese Steak Sandwich	1 (6.1 oz)	485	—	73
Chicken 2 Pieces	1 serv (7.1 oz)	693	—	211
Chicken 4 Pieces	1 serv (14.2 oz)	1382	—	422
Chicken Platter 2 Pieces	1 serv (14.8 oz)	1096	—	212
Chicken Platter 4 Pieces	1 serv (21.9 oz)	1788	—	425
Chicken Salad	1 serv (12.7 oz)	154	—	49
Double Burger	1 (7.3 oz)	671	—	154
Filet of Fish Platter	1 serv (22 oz)	1455	—	147
Filet of Fish Sandwich	1 (5.2 oz)	403	—	32
Frank Nuggets	15 pieces (6.9 oz)	764	—	99
Frank Nuggets	11 pieces (5.1 oz)	563	—	73
Frank Nuggets	7 pieces (3.2 oz)	357	—	46
Frankfurter	1 (3.2 oz)	310	—	45
French Fries	1 serv (8.6 oz)	514	—	0
Fried Clam Platter	1 serv (13.1 oz)	1024	—	49
Fried Clam Sandwich	1 (5.4 oz)	620	—	44
Fried Shrimp	1 serv (4.4 oz)	348	—	71
Fried Shrimp Platter	1 serv (12.6 oz)	796	—	83
Hamburger	1 (4.7 oz)	434	—	77
Knish	1 (5.9 oz)	318	—	2
Pastrami Sandwich	1 (4.1 oz)	325	—	48
Sauteed Onions	1 serv (3.5 oz)	39	—	0
Super Burger	1 (7.6 oz)	533	—	86
Turkey Sandwich	1 (4.9 oz)	270	—	27
SALADS AND SALAD BARS				
Garden Salad	1 serv (10.9 oz)	193	—	36

OLIVE GARDEN

Baked Lasagna	1 lunch serv	330	—	60
Breadstick	1	70	—	0
Breadstick w/o margarine	1	30	—	0
Breadstick w/o margarine & garlic salt	1	30	—	0
Eggplant Parmigiana	1 lunch serv	220	—	45
Fettuccine Alfredo	1 lunch serv	790	—	160
Garden Fare Dinner Capellini Pomodoro	1 serv (16.6 oz)	420	—	10
Garden Fare Dinner Capellini Primavera	1 serv (18.1 oz)	380	—	15

FOOD	PORTION	CALS.	FIB.	CHOL.
Garden Fare Dinner Chicken Giardino	1 serv (18.6 oz)	480	—	100
Garden Fare Dinner Grilled Herb Chicken w/ Peppers	1 serv (17.5 oz)	470	—	75
Garden Fare Dinner Shrimp Primavera	1 serv (17.5 oz)	420	—	110
Garden Fare Dinner Spaghetti w/ Marinara Sauce	1 serv (16.2 oz)	500	—	0
Garden Fare Dinner Spaghetti w/ Sicilian Sauce	1 serv (15.9 oz)	530	—	0
Garden Fare Dinner Venetian Grilled Chicken	1 serv (9.5 oz)	360	—	115
Garden Fare Lunch Capellini Pomodoro	1 serv (10.2 oz)	290	—	5
Garden Fare Lunch Capellini Primavera	1 serv (12.1 oz)	270	—	10
Garden Fare Lunch Shrimp Primavera	1 serv (11.6 oz)	320	—	60
Garden Fare Lunch Spaghetti w/ Marinara Sauce	1 serv (11.2 oz)	350	—	0
Garden Fare Lunch Spaghetti w/ Sicilian Sauce	1 serv (11.2 oz)	370	—	0
Garden Salad	1 serv	230	—	4
Minestrone Soup	1 serv (6 oz)	80	—	0
Pasta e Fagioli	6 fl oz	140	—	15
Raspberry Sorbetto	1 serv (6 oz)	170	—	0
Salad Dressing	1 tbsp	60	—	2
Veal Marsala	1 dinner serv	330	—	100
Veal Parmigiana	1 dinner serv	590	—	150
Veal Piccata	1 dinner serv	230	—	45

PICCADILLY CAFETERIA
BAKED SELECTIONS

FOOD	PORTION	CALS.	FIB.	CHOL.
Corn Sticks	1 (2 oz)	165	tr	26
French Bread	1 slice	132	4	6
Garlic Bread	1 serv (15.8 oz)	1154	34	48
Mexican Corn Bread	1 piece	220	1	31
Roll	1 (2 oz)	130	4	0
Roll Whole Wheat	1 (1.7 oz)	117	3	19
Texas Toast	1 serv (15.5 oz)	1088	34	48

BEVERAGES

FOOD	PORTION	CALS.	FIB.	CHOL.
Iced Tea	1 serv (6.5 oz)	2	0	0
Punch	1 serv (9 oz)	133	0	0

DESSERTS

FOOD	PORTION	CALS.	FIB.	CHOL.
Apple Pie	1 slice (7.2 oz)	439	3	0

FOOD	PORTION	CALS.	FIB.	CHOL.
Cantaloupe	1 serv (9 oz)	89	3	0
Cantaloupe	1 serv (5.5 oz)	55	2	0
Chocolate Cream Pie	1 slice (7.5 oz)	512	tr	66
Custard	1 cup (5.4 oz)	183	0	25
Custard Pie	1 slice (6.2 oz)	412	tr	18
Dole Whip Topping	1 serv (3 oz)	68	0	0
Fresh Fruit Plate	1 serv (21.1 oz)	389	9	11
Gelatin	1 serv (4.75 oz)	128	0	14
Honeydew Melon	1 serv (5.5 oz)	55	1	0
Honeydew Melon	1 serv (9 oz)	89	2	0
Lemon Chiffon Pie	1 slice (6.3 oz)	481	tr	32
Pound Cake	1 slice (3.8 oz)	371	0	76
Watermelon	1 serv (11 oz)	100	1	0
MAIN MENU SELECTIONS				
Au Jus	1 serv (3 oz)	5	0	0
Baby Lima Beans	1 serv (4.5 oz)	151	4	0
Baked Potato	1	218	4	0
Baked Potato w/ Topping	1	350	4	33
Beef Chopped Steak Fried	1 serv (4 oz)	311	0	59
Beef Leg Roast	1 serv (4 oz)	311	tr	92
Beef Liver Fried	1 serv (4.5 oz)	430	2	418
Beef Tips Braised	1 serv (10 oz)	470	3	56
Black-eyed Peas w/ Pork Jowls	1 serv (4 oz)	108	0	7
Broccoli Buttered	1 serv (4 oz)	77	3	0
Broccoli & Rice Au Gratin	½ cup	184	1	18
Carrots Young Buttered	½ cup	90	1	0
Cauliflower Buttered	1 serv	80	2	0
Chicken Baked w/o Skin	¼ chicken	352	0	168
Chicken Teriyaki	1 serv (4 oz)	445	tr	124
Chicken Teriyaki Polynesian	1 serv (4 oz)	537	1	104
Corn	1 serv (4.5 oz)	128	0	0
Cornbread Stuffing	1 serv (4.5 oz)	164	tr	26
Cranberry Sauce	1 serv (1.5 oz)	64	tr	0
Eggplant Escalloped	½ cup	180	1	15
Fish Baked	1 serv (7 oz)	195	tr	54
Green Beans	1 serv (4.5 oz)	77	1	7
Ham Baked	1 serv (4 oz)	224	0	67
Macaroni & Cheese	½ cup	317	2	22
Mashed Potatoes	1 serv (4.8 oz)	120	0	0
Meatballs Baked & Spaghetti	1 serv (11.5 oz)	108	tr	23
New Potatoes Boiled	½ cup	148	tr	0
Okra Smothered	1 serv (4 oz)	121	1	0
Onion Sauce	1 serv (4 oz)	152	1	0
Rice	½ cup	99	tr	0

FOOD	PORTION	CALS.	FIB.	CHOL.
Rice Polynesian	1 serv (4 oz)	140	tr	0
Spaghetti Baked	1 serv (9.5 oz)	256	2	13
Squash Baked Italian	1 serv (4.75 oz)	73	1	8
Squash Mixed Yellow & Zucchini	1 serv (4 oz)	72	1	0
Squash Yellow Baked French Style	⅓ cup	86	1	5
Vegetables Unseasoned	1 serv (5 oz)	29	2	0
SALADS AND SALAD BARS				
Broccoli Salad	1 serv (4 oz)	202	2	13
Cabbage Combination Salad	1 serv (4.5 oz)	50	1	0
Carrot & Raisin Salad	1 serv (4.5 oz)	321	2	10
Cole Slaw w/ Cream	1 serv (4 oz)	182	1	9
Cucumber & Celery Salad	1 serv (4 oz)	82	1	0
Fruit Salad	1 serv (6 oz)	59	2	0
Neptune Salad	1 serv	361	1	25
Spinach Tossed Salad	1 serv (4 oz)	88	2	44
Spring Salad Bowl	1 serv (4 oz)	22	1	0
SOUPS				
Gumbo Chicken	1 serv (8 oz)	92	1	22
Gumbo Seafood	1 serv (8 oz)	98	1	45
Vegetable	1 serv (8 oz)	49	tr	0
PIZZA HUT				
Bigfoot Cheese	1 slice (2.7 oz)	186	2	16
Bigfoot Pepperoni	1 slice (2.8 oz)	205	2	20
Bigfoot Pepperoni Mushroom Italian Sausage	1 slice (3.2 oz)	214	2	21
Hand Tossed Medium Beef	1 slice (4.2 oz)	260	2	26
Hand Tossed Medium Cheese	1 slice (3.8 oz)	235	2	25
Hand Tossed Medium Ham	1 slice (3.7 oz)	213	2	21
Hand Tossed Medium Italian Sausage	1 slice (4.1 oz)	267	2	31
Hand Tossed Medium Meat Lovers	1 slice (4.6 oz)	314	2	38
Hand Tossed Medium Pepperoni	1 slice (3.6 oz)	238	2	24
Hand Tossed Medium Pepperoni Lover's	1 slice (4.3 oz)	306	2	40
Hand Tossed Medium Pork Topping	1 slice (4.2 oz)	268	2	26
Hand Tossed Medium Super Supreme	1 slice (5 oz)	296	3	34
Hand Tossed Medium Supreme	1 slice (4.8 oz)	284	3	30
Hand Tossed Medium Veggie Lover's	1 slice (4.7 oz)	216	3	17
Pan Medium Beef	1 slice (4.2 oz)	286	2	26

FOOD	PORTION	CALS.	FIB.	CHOL.
Pan Medium Cheese	1 slice (3.8 oz)	261	2	25
Pan Medium Ham	1 slice (3.7 oz)	239	2	21
Pan Medium Italian Sausage	1 slice (4.1 oz)	293	2	31
Pan Medium Meat Lover's	1 slice (4.6 oz)	340	2	38
Pan Medium Pepperoni	1 slice (3.6 oz)	265	2	24
Pan Medium Pepperoni Lover's	1 slice (4.3 oz)	332	2	40
Pan Medium Pork Topping	1 slice (4.2 oz)	294	2	26
Pan Medium Super Supreme	1 slice (5 oz)	323	3	34
Pan Medium Supreme	1 slice (4.8 oz)	311	3	30
Pan Medium Veggie Lover's	1 slice (4.7 oz)	243	3	17
Personal Pan Pepperoni	1 pie (9 oz)	637	5	55
Personal Pan Supreme	1 pie (11.5 oz)	722	6	66
Thin 'N Crispy Medium Beef	1 slice (3.5 oz)	229	2	26
Thin 'N Crispy Medium Cheese	1 slice (3 oz)	205	2	25
Thin 'N Crispy Medium Ham	1 slice (3 oz)	184	1	22
Thin 'N Crispy Medium Italian Sausage	1 slice (3.3 oz)	236	2	31
Thin 'N Crispy Medium Meat Lover's	1 slice (3.9 oz)	288	2	39
Thin 'N Crispy Medium Pork Topping	1 slice (3.5 oz)	237	2	26
Thin 'N Crispy Medium Super Supreme	1 slice (4.3 oz)	270	2	35
Thin 'N Crispy Medium Supreme	1 slice (4.1 oz)	257	2	31
Thin 'N Crispy Medium Supreme	1 slice (2.9 oz)	215	1	25
Thin 'N Crispy Medium Veggie Lover's	1 slice	186	2	17
Thin N' Crispy Medium Pepperoni Lover's	1 slice (3.7 oz)	289	2	42

PONDEROSA
BEVERAGES

Cherry Coke	6 oz	77	—	0
Chocolate Milk	8 oz	208	—	33
Coca-Cola	6 oz	72	—	0
Coffee Black	6 oz	2	—	0
Diet Coke	6 oz	tr	—	0
Diet Coke Caffeine Free	6 oz	tr	—	0
Diet Sprite	6 oz	2	—	0
Dr Pepper	6 oz	72	—	0
Lemonade	6 oz	68	—	0
Milk	8 oz	159	—	34
Mr. Pibb	6 oz	71	—	0
Orange Soda	6 oz	82	—	0

FOOD	PORTION	CALS.	FIB.	CHOL.
Root Beer	6 oz	80	—	0
Sprite	6 oz	72	—	0
Tea	6 oz	2	—	0
ICE CREAM				
Ice Milk Chocolate	3.5 oz	152	—	22
Ice Milk Vanilla	3.5 oz	150	—	20
Topping Caramel	1 oz	100	—	2
Topping Chocolate	1 oz	89	—	0
Topping Strawberry	1 oz	71	—	0
Topping Whippped	1 oz	80	—	0
MAIN MENU SELECTIONS				
BBQ Sauce	1 tbsp	25	—	0
Bake 'R Broil Fish	1 serv (5.2 oz)	230	—	50
Baked Potato	1 (7.2 oz)	145	—	0
Beans Baked	1 serv (4 oz)	170	—	0
Beans Green	1 serv (3.5 oz)	20	—	0
Breaded Cauliflower	1 serv (4 oz)	115	—	1
Breaded Okra	1 serv (4 oz)	124	—	1
Breaded Onion Rings	1 serv (4 oz)	213	—	2
Breaded Zucchini	1 serv (4 oz)	102	—	1
Carrots	1 serv (3.5 oz)	31	—	0
Cheese Herb Garlic Spread	1 tbsp	100	—	0
Cheese Sauce	2 oz	52	—	4
Chicken Breast	1 serv (5.5 oz)	90	—	54
Chicken Wings	2	213	—	75
Chopped Steak	4 oz	225	—	80
Chopped Steak	5.3 oz	296	—	105
Corn	1 serv (3.5 oz)	90	—	0
Fish Fried	1 serv (3.2 oz)	190	—	15
Fish Nuggets	1	31	—	8
French Fries	1 serv (3 oz)	120	—	3
Gravy Brown	2 oz	25	—	0
Gravy Turkey	2 oz	25	—	0
Hot Dog	1	144	—	27
Italian Breadsticks	1	100	—	0
Kansas City Strip	5 oz	138	—	76
Macaroni And Cheese	4 oz	67	—	4
Margarine Liquid	1 tbsp	100	—	0
Mashed Potatoes	1 serv (4 oz)	62	—	20
Meatballs	1	58	—	11
Mini Shrimp	6	47	—	22
New York Strip Choice	10 oz	314	—	50
New York Strip Choice	8 oz	384	—	62
Pasta Shells Plain	2 oz	78	—	0

FOOD	PORTION	CALS.	FIB.	CHOL.
Peas	1 serv (3.5 oz)	67	—	0
Porterhouse	13 oz	441	—	67
Porterhouse Choice	16 oz	640	—	82
Ribeye	5 oz	219	—	75
Ribeye Choice	6 oz	281	—	60
Rice Pilaf	1 serv (4 oz)	160	—	22
Roll Dinner	1	184	—	0
Roll Sourdough	1	110	—	0
Roughy Broiled	1 serv (5 oz)	139	—	28
Salmon Broiled	1 serv (6 oz)	192	—	60
Sandwich Steak	4 oz	408	—	62
Scrod Baked	1 serv (7 oz)	120	—	65
Shrimp Fried	7 pieces	231	—	105
Sirloin Choice	7 oz	241	—	63
Sirloin Tips Choice	5 oz	473	—	72
Spaghetti Plain	2 oz	78	—	0
Spaghetti Sauce	4 oz	110	—	0
Steak Kabobs Meat Only	3 oz	153	—	67
Stuffing	4 oz	230	—	22
Sweet/Sour Sauce	1 oz	37	—	0
Swordfish Broiled	1 serv (6 oz)	271	—	85
T-Bone	8 oz	176	—	71
T-Bone Choice	10 oz	444	—	80
Teriyaki Steak	5 oz	174	—	64
Tortilla Chips	1 oz	150	—	0
Trout Broiled	1 serv (5 oz)	228	—	110
Winter Mix	1 serv (3.5 oz)	25	—	0
SALAD DRESSINGS				
Blue Cheese	1 oz	130	—	27
Cole Slaw	1 oz	150	—	31
Creamy Italian	1 oz	103	—	0
Cucumber Reduced Calorie	1 oz	69	—	tr
Italian Reduced Calorie	1 oz	31	—	0
Parmesan Pepper	1 oz	150	—	9
Ranch	1 oz	147	—	3
Salad Oil	1 tbsp	120	—	0
Sour Cream	1 tbsp	26	—	5
Sweet-N-Tangy	1 oz	122	—	1
Thousand Island	1 oz	113	—	1
SALADS AND SALAD BARS				
Alfalfa Sprouts	1 oz	10	—	0
Apple	1	80	—	0
Apples Canned	4 oz	90	—	0
Applesauce	4 oz	80	—	0

FOOD	PORTION	CALS.	FIB.	CHOL.
Banana	1	87	—	0
Banana Chips	0.2 oz	25	—	0
Banana Pudding	1 oz	52	—	0
Bean Sprouts	1 oz	10	—	0
Beets Diced	4 oz	55	—	0
Breadsticks Sesame	2	35	—	0
Broccoli	1 oz	9	—	0
Cabbage Green	1 oz	9	—	0
Cabbage Red	1 oz	1	—	0
Cantaloupe	1 wedge	13	—	0
Carrots	1 oz	12	—	0
Cauliflower	1 oz	8	—	0
Celery	1 oz	4	—	0
Cheese Imitation Shredded	1 oz	90	—	5
Cheese Spread	1 oz	98	—	26
Cherry Peppers	2 pieces	7	—	0
Chicken Salad	3.5 oz	212	—	42
Chow Mein Noodles	0.2 oz	25	—	0
Cocktail Sauce	1 oz	34	—	0
Coconut Shredded	0.2 oz	25	—	0
Cottage Cheese	4 oz	120	—	17
Croutons	1 oz	115	—	0
Cucumber	1 oz	4	—	0
Eggs Diced	2 oz	94	—	260
Fruit Cocktail	4 oz	97	—	0
Garbanzo Beans	1 oz	102	—	0
Gelatin Plain	4 oz	71	—	0
Granola	0.2 oz	24	—	0
Grapes	10	34	—	0
Green Onion	1	7	—	0
Green Pepper	1 oz	6	—	0
Ham Diced	2 oz	120	—	76
Honeydew	1 wedge	24	—	0
Lemon	1 wedge	3	—	0
Lettuce	1 oz	5	—	0
Macaroni Salad	3.5 oz	335	—	9
Margarine Whipped	1 tbsp	34	—	0
Meal Mates Sesame Crackers	2	45	—	0
Melba Snacks	2	18	—	0
Mousse Chocolate	1 oz	78	—	0
Mousse Strawberry	1 oz	74	—	0
Mushrooms	1 oz	8	—	0
Olives Black	1	4	—	0
Olives Green	1	3	—	0

FOOD	PORTION	CALS.	FIB.	CHOL.
Onions Red & Yellow	1 oz	11	—	3
Orange	1	45	—	0
Pasta Salad	3.5 oz	269	—	tr
Peaches Canned	4 oz	70	—	0
Peanuts Chopped	0.2 oz	30	—	0
Pears Canned	4 oz	98	—	0
Pickles Dill Spears	0.14 oz	tr	—	0
Pickles Sweet Chips	0.14 oz	4	—	0
Pineapple Tidbits	4 oz	95	—	0
Pineapple Fresh	1 wedge	11	—	0
Potato Salad	3.5 oz	126	—	7
Radishes	1 oz	4	—	0
Ritz	2	40	—	0
Saltine Crackers	2	25	—	0
Spiced Apple Rings	4 oz	100	—	0
Spinach	1 oz	7	—	0
Strawberries	2 oz	14	—	0
Sunflower Seeds	0.2 oz	31	—	0
Tartar Sauce	1 oz	85	—	9
Tomatoes	1 oz	6	—	0
Turkey Ham Salad	3.5 oz	186	—	12
Turkey Julienne	1 oz	29	—	15
Vanilla Wafer	2	35	—	5
Watermelon	1 wedge	111	—	0
Yogurt Fruit	4 oz	115	—	5
Yogurt Vanilla	4 oz	110	—	6
Zucchini	1 oz	5	—	0

POPEYES

FOOD	PORTION	CALS.	FIB.	CHOL.
Apple Pie	1 serv (3.1 oz)	290	2	10
Biscuit	1 serv (2.3 oz)	250	1	<5
Breast Mild	1 (3.7 oz)	270	2	60
Breast Spicy	1 (3.7 oz)	270	2	60
Cajun Rice	1 serv (3.9 oz)	150	3	25
Cole Slaw	1 serv (4 oz)	149	3	3
Corn On The Cob	1 serv (5.2 oz)	127	9	0
French Fries	1 serv (3 oz)	240	3	10
Leg Mild	1 (1.7 oz)	120	0	40
Leg Spicy	1 (1.7 oz)	120	0	40
Nuggets	1 serv (4.2 oz)	410	3	55
Nuggets Mild Tender	1 (1.2 oz)	110	1	15
Nuggets Spicy Tender	1 (1.2 oz)	110	1	15
Onion Rings	1 serv (3.1 oz)	310	2	25
Potatoes & Gravy	1 serv (3.8 oz)	100	3	<5

FOOD	PORTION	CALS.	FIB.	CHOL.
Red Beans & Rice	1 serv (5.9 oz)	270	7	10
Shrimp	1 serv (2.8 oz)	250	3	110
Thigh Mild	1 (3.1 oz)	300	tr	70
Thigh Spicy	1 (3.1 oz)	300	tr	70
Wing Mild	1 (1.6 oz)	160	0	40
Wing Spicy	1 (1.6 oz)	160	0	40

PUDGIE'S FAMOUS CHICKEN

Fried Chicken	3.5 oz	233	—	81

QUINCY'S
BAKED SELECTIONS

Banana Nut	1 serv (2 oz)	165	—	5
Cornbread	1 serv (2 oz)	140	—	10
Yeast Roll	1 (1.5 oz)	160	—	0

BREAKFAST SELECTIONS

Bacon	1 serv (0.25 oz)	35	—	5
Corned Beef Hash	1 serv (4.5 oz)	210	—	45
Country Ham	1 serv (1.5 oz)	90	—	35
Escalloped Apples	1 serv (3.5 oz)	120	—	0
Oatmeal	1 serv	175	—	0
Pancakes	1 (1.5 oz)	95	—	30
Sausage Gravy	1 serv (4 oz)	70	—	10
Sausage Links	1 (2 oz)	225	—	20
Sausage Patties	1 (2 oz)	230	—	45
Scrambled Eggs	1 serv (2 oz)	95	—	215
Steak Fingers	1 serv (3.5 oz)	360	—	50
Syrup	1 oz	75	—	0

DESSERTS

Banana Pudding	1 serv (5 oz)	240	—	10
Brownie Pudding Cake	1 serv (4 oz)	310	—	0
Chocolate Chip Cookies	1 (0.5 oz)	60	—	5
Cobbler Apple	1 serv (6 oz)	255	—	5
Cobbler Cherry	1 serv (6 oz)	410	—	5
Cobbler Peach	1 serv (6 oz)	305	—	5
Frozen Yogurt	1 serv (4 oz)	135	—	5
Hot Toppings Caramel	1 serv (1 oz)	105	—	0
Hot Toppings Fudge	1 serv (1 oz)	105	—	0
Hot Toppings Pineapple	1 serv (1 oz)	70	—	0
Sugar Cookie	1 (0.5 oz)	60	—	5

MAIN MENU SELECTIONS

Baked Potato	1 (12 oz)	370	—	0
Beef Chopped Steak	1 serv (5.75 oz)	470	—	175
Beef Filet	1 (5.5 oz)	330	—	130
Blackeyed Peas	1 serv (4 oz)	75	—	3

FOOD	PORTION	CALS.	FIB.	CHOL.
Broccoli & Rice Casserole	1 serv (4 oz)	100	—	5
Broccoli w/ Cheese Sauce	1 serv (12 oz)	250	—	25
Cabbage Steamed	1 serv (4 oz)	85	—	0
Candied Yams	1 serv (4 oz)	250	—	0
Carrots Steamed	1 serv (4 oz)	85	—	0
Corn On The Cob	1 serv (6 oz)	140	—	0
Corn Whole Kernel	1 serv (4 oz)	110	—	0
Country Style Steak	1 serv (5 oz)	380	—	60
Country Style Steak Sandwich	1 serv (9 oz)	520	—	80
Green Beans	1 serv (4 oz)	25	—	1
Green Peas	1 serv (4 oz)	60	—	0
Grilled Chicken Large	1 serv (9.5 oz)	250	—	155
Grilled Chicken Regular	4.75 oz	125	—	80
Grilled Chicken Sandwich	1 serv (8.5 oz)	305	—	80
Grilled Trout	6 oz	300	—	115
Hashrounds	1 serv (2.75 oz)	230	—	0
Homestyle Chicken Filet	1 serv (6 oz)	410	—	95
Macaroni & Cheese	1 serv (4 oz)	165	—	10
Mashed Potatoes	1 serv (4 oz)	70	—	0
Mushrooms	1 serv (3 oz)	115	—	0
New Potatoes	1 serv (4 oz)	190	—	0
Pinto Beans	1 serv (4 oz)	70	—	0
Prime Rib	1 serv (8 oz)	570	—	140
Prime Rib	1 serv (16 oz)	1145	—	275
Quarter Pound Hamburger	1 serv (7.5 oz)	410	—	55
Refried Beans	1 serv (4 oz)	140	—	0
Ribeye	9.5 oz	870	—	220
Ribeye	1 serv (7.25 oz)	670	—	165
Rice Pilaf	1 serv (3.5 oz)	105	1	0
Sirloin Large	7.75 oz	850	—	200
Sirloin Petite	4 oz	450	—	100
Sirloin Regular	5.75 oz	650	—	145
Sirloin Strip	1 serv (9.5 oz)	595	—	200
Sirloin Tips	1 serv (4 oz)	240	—	100
Squash	1 serv (4 oz)	110	—	0
Stir Fry Beef	1 serv (16 oz)	950	5	125
Stir Fry Chicken	1 serv (15.75 oz)	780	5	80
T-Bone	14 oz	1610	—	330
Turnip Greens	1 serv (4 oz)	75	—	0
Vegetable Medley	1 serv (4 oz)	35	—	0
SALAD DRESSINGS				
Blue Cheese	1 serv (1 oz)	155	—	10
French	1 serv (1 oz)	125	—	0
Honey Mustard	1 serv (1 oz)	100	—	0

FOOD	PORTION	CALS.	FIB.	CHOL.
Italian	1 serv (1 oz)	134	—	0
Light 1000 Island	1 serv (1 oz)	65	—	20
Light Creamy Italian	1 serv (1 oz)	65	—	0
Light French	1 serv (1 oz)	85	—	0
Light Italian	1 serv (1 oz)	20	—	0
Parmesan Peppercorn	1 serv (1 oz)	150	—	0
Ranch	1 serv (1 oz)	110	—	10
SOUPS				
Chili With Beans	1 serv (6 oz)	235	—	15
Clam Chowder	1 serv (6 oz)	180	—	0
Cream Of Broccoli	1 serv (6 oz)	170	—	0
Vegetable Beef	1 serv (6 oz)	90	—	0
RAX				
BEVERAGES				
Chocolate Shake	1 (11 fl oz)	445	—	35
Coke	16 fl oz	205	—	0
Diet Coke	16 fl oz	1	—	0
DESSERTS				
Chocolate Chip Cookie	1 (2 oz)	262	—	6
MAIN MENU SELECTIONS				
Bacon	1 slice (0.1 oz)	14	—	2
Baked Potato	1 (10 oz)	264	—	0
Baked Potato w/ 1 Tbsp Margarine	1 (10.5 oz)	364	—	0
Barbecue Sauce	1 pkg (0.4 oz)	11	—	0
Beef Bacon 'N Cheddar	1 (6.7 oz)	523	—	42
Cheddar Cheese Sauce	1 fl oz	29	—	0
Country Fried Chicken Breast Sandwich	1 (7.4 oz)	618	—	45
Deluxe Roast Beef	1 (7.9 oz)	498	—	36
French Fries	1 serv (3.25 oz)	282	—	3
Grilled Chicken Breast Sandwich	1 (6.9 oz)	402	—	69
Grilled Chicken Garden Salad w/ French Dressing	1 serv (12.7 oz)	477	—	32
Grilled Chicken Garden Salad w/ Lite Italian Dressing	1 serv (12.7 oz)	264	—	32
Mushroom Sauce	1 fl oz	16	—	0
Philly Melt	1 (8.2 oz)	396	—	27
Regular Rax	1 (4.7 oz)	262	—	15
Swiss Slice	1 slice (0.4 oz)	42	—	10
SALAD DRESSINGS				
French	2 fl oz	275	—	0
Lite Italian	2 fl oz	63	—	0
SALADS AND SALAD BARS				
Gourmet Garden Salad w/ French Dressing	1 serv (10.7 oz)	409	—	10

FOOD	PORTION	CALS.	FIB.	CHOL.
Gourmet Garden Salad w/ Lite Italian Dressing	1 serv (10.7 oz)	305	—	2
Gourmet Garden Salad w/o Dressing	1 serv (8.7 oz)	134	—	2
Grilled Chicken Garden Salad w/o Dressing	1 serv (10.7 oz)	202	—	32

RED LOBSTER
CHILDREN'S MENU SELECTIONS

FOOD	PORTION	CALS.	FIB.	CHOL.
Cheeseburger	1 serv	1040	—	130
Fried Chicken Fingers	1 serv	680	—	35
Fried Shrimp	1 serv	650	—	80
Grilled Chicken Tenders	1 serv	580	—	55
Hamburger	1 serv	920	—	100
Popcorn Shrimp	1 serv	650	—	120
Popcorn Shrimp & Cheesesticks	1 serv	750	—	125
Spaghetti & Cheesesticks	1 serv	830	—	5

DESSERTS

FOOD	PORTION	CALS.	FIB.	CHOL.
Fudge Overboard	1 serv	620	—	105
Ice Cream	1 serv (4.5 oz)	140	—	30
Sensational 7	1 serv	790	—	140

MAIN MENU SELECTIONS

FOOD	PORTION	CALS.	FIB.	CHOL.
Admiral's Feast	1 serv	1060	—	265
Appetizer Calamari	1 serv	350	—	190
Appetizer Chicken Fingers	1 serv	390	—	65
Appetizer Chilled Shrimp In The Shell	1 serv (6 oz)	110	—	235
Appetizer Crab & Shrimp Cakes	1 serv	480	—	80
Appetizer Crab Add-On	1 serv	60	—	55
Appetizer Fresh Fried Mushrooms	1 serv	790	—	<5
Appetizer Lobster Quesadilla	1 serv	760	—	160
Appetizer Lobster Stuffed Mushroom	1 serv	400	—	100
Appetizer Mozzarella Cheesesticks	1 serv	730	—	50
Appetizer Parmesan Zucchini	1 serv	620	—	10
Appetizer Shrimp Cocktail	1 serv	50	—	105
Appetizer Stuffed Mushrooms	1 serv	420	—	90
Applesauce	1 serv (4 oz)	90	—	0
Atlantic Cod	1 serv (8 oz)	200	—	105
Atlantic Cod	1 lunch serv (5 oz)	110	—	60
Atlantic Salmon	1 lunch serv (5 oz)	200	—	80
Atlantic Salmon	1 serv (8 oz)	340	—	135
Baked Atlantic Cod	1 serv	220	—	100
Baked Atlantic Haddock	1 serv	220	—	100

FOOD	PORTION	CALS.	FIB.	CHOL.
Baked Flounder	1 lunch serv	190	—	90
Baked Potato	1 (8 oz)	130	—	0
Broccoli	1 serv (3 oz)	25	—	0
Broiled Fisherman's Platter	1 serv	600	—	250
Broiled Rock Lobster Tail	1 tail	190	—	110
Broiled Seafarer's Platter	1 serv	450	—	190
Caesar Salad w/ Dressing	1 serv	240	—	15
Catfish	1 serv (8 Oz)	220	—	130
Catfish	1 lunch serv (5 oz)	130	—	75
Catfish Santa Fe	1 serv	340	—	165
Catfish Santa Fe	1 lunch serv	180	—	85
Chicken Fingers	1 lunch serv	390	—	64
Chicken Fresco	1 serv	1320	—	240
Chicken Fresco	1 lunch serv	660	—	120
Clam Strips	1 lunch serv	360	—	15
Clam Strips	1 serv	720	—	35
Cocktail Sauce	1 oz	30	—	0
Cole Slaw	1 serv (4 oz)	190	—	25
Crab Alfredo	1 serv	1170	—	270
Crab Alfredo	1 lunch serv	590	—	135
Fish & Shrimp Combo	1 serv	730	—	230
Fish Nuggets	1 lunch serv	320	—	95
Fish Seasoning Add On For Blackened Dinner	1 serv	70	—	0
Fish Seasoning Add On For Blackened Lunch	1 serv	50	—	0
Fish Seasoning Add On For Broiled Dinner	1 serv	45	—	0
Fish Seasoning Add On For Broiled Lunch	1 serv	35	—	0
Fish Seasoning Add On For Grilled Dinner	1 serv	35	—	0
Fish Seasoning Add On For Grilled Lunch	1 serv	25	—	0
Fish Seasoning Add On For Lemon Pepper Dinner	1 serv	35	—	0
Fish Seasoning Add On For Lemon Pepper Lunch	1 serv	30	—	0
Fish Seasoning Add On For Santa Fe Style Dinner	1 serv	60	—	0
Fish Seasoning Add On For Santa Fe Style Lunch	1 serv	40	—	0
Flounder	1 lunch serv (5 oz)	130	—	75
Flounder	1 serv (8 oz)	220	—	130

FOOD	PORTION	CALS.	FIB.	CHOL.
French Fries	1 serv (4 oz)	350	—	0
Fried Flounder	1 lunch serv	230	—	60
Fried Shrimp	12 lg	500	—	290
Fried Shrimp	1 lunch serv	270	—	115
Garden Salad w/o Dressing	1 serv	50	—	0
Garlic Cheese Biscuit	1	140	—	5
Grilled Cheeseburger	1	580	—	130
Grilled Chicken Breasts	1 serv	230	—	105
Grilled Chicken Salad w/o Dressing	1 serv	320	—	70
Grouper	1 serv (8 oz)	220	—	90
Grouper	1 lunch serv (5 oz)	130	—	50
Haddock	1 serv (8 oz)	210	—	140
Haddock	1 lunch serv (5 oz)	120	—	80
Halibut	1 lunch serv (5 oz)	150	—	45
Halibut	1 serv (8 oz)	260	—	75
King Salmon	1 lunch serv (5 oz)	250	—	95
King Salmon	1 serv (8 oz)	420	—	160
Lake Trout	1 serv (8 oz)	340	—	140
Lake Trout	1 lunch serv (5 oz)	200	—	80
Lemon Pepper Grilled Mahi Mahi	1 serv	240	—	130
Lobster Shrimp & Scallop Scampi	1 lunch serv	430	—	80
Lobster Shrimp & Scallop Scampi	1 serv	870	—	135
Mahi Mahi	1 lunch serv (5 oz)	130	—	75
Mahi Mahi	1 serv (8 oz)	220	—	130
Maine Lobster Steamed	1 serv (1.25 lb)	160	—	125
Maine Lobster Stuffed	1 serv (2 lb)	430	—	210
Marinara Sauce	1 serv	50	—	0
Melted Butter	1 oz	200	—	60
Neptune's Feast	1 serv	1210	—	290
New York Strip Steak	1 serv	560	—	180
Perch	1 serv (8 oz)	220	—	130
Perch	1 lunch serv (5 oz)	130	—	75
Pollack	1 lunch serv (5 oz)	120	—	100
Pollack	1 serv (8 oz)	120	—	100
Popcorn Shrimp	1 serv	580	—	360
Popcorn Shrimp	1 lunch serv	380	—	235
Red Rockfish	1 serv (8 oz)	230	—	85
Red Rockfish	1 lunch serv (5 oz)	130	—	50
Red Snapper	1 serv (8 oz)	240	—	90
Red Snapper	1 lunch serv (5 oz)	140	—	50
Rice Pilaf	1 serv (4 oz)	180	—	0
Roasted Vegetables	1 serv (6 oz)	120	—	0
Roasted Vegetables	1 lunch serv (4 oz)	80	—	0

FOOD	PORTION	CALS.	FIB.	CHOL.
Sailor's Platter	1 lunch serv	250	—	170
Sandwich Blackened Catfish	1	340	—	85
Sandwich Broiled Fish	1	300	—	80
Sandwich Cajun Grilled Chicken	1	370	—	55
Sandwich Classic Fish	1	520	—	90
Sandwich Grilled Chicken	1	290	—	50
Sassy Sauce	1 oz	80	—	5
Seafood Broil	1 lunch serv	310	—	110
Shrimp & Chicken	1 serv	340	—	225
Shrimp Caesar Salad w/o Dressing	1 serv	240	—	110
Shrimp Carbonara	1 lunch serv	650	—	155
Shrimp Carbonara	1 serv	1290	—	310
Shrimp Combo	1 serv	380	—	210
Shrimp Feast	1 serv	470	—	390
Shrimp Milano	1 serv	1190	—	340
Shrimp Milano	1 lunch serv	590	—	170
Shrimp Scampi	1 lunch serv	110	—	100
Smothered Chicken	1 serv	530	—	170
Snow Crab Legs	1 serv	110	—	115
Sockeye Salmon	1 lunch serv (5 oz)	240	—	95
Sockeye Salmon	1 serv (8 oz)	410	—	165
Sole	1 serv (8 oz)	220	—	130
Sole	1 lunch serv (5 oz)	130	—	75
Soup Bread Salad w/o Dressing	1 lunch serv	430	—	40
Steak & Fried Shrimp	1 serv	780	—	340
Steak & Rock Lobster Tail	1 serv	570	—	220
Swordfish	1 serv (8 oz)	290	—	115
Swordfish	1 lunch serv (5 oz)	170	—	70
Tartar Sauce	1 oz	160	—	15
Teriyaki Grilled Chicken Breast	1 serv	240	—	105
Twice Baked Potato	1	430	—	60
Walleye	1 serv (8 oz)	210	—	205
Walleye	1 lunch serv (5 oz)	120	—	120
Yellow Lake Perch	1 serv (8 oz)	220	—	130
Yellow Lake Perch	1 lunch serv (5 oz)	130	—	75
SALAD DRESSINGS				
Blue Cheese	1 serv	170	—	30
Buttermilk Ranch	1 serv	110	—	15
Caesar	1 serv	170	—	10
Dijon Honey Mustard	1 serv	140	—	20
Fat Free Ranch	1 serv	50	—	0
Lite Red Wine Vinaigrette	1 serv	50	—	0

FOOD	PORTION	CALS.	FIB.	CHOL.
SOUPS				
Bayou Style Gumbo	1 serv (6 oz)	120	—	65
Broccoli Cheese	1 serv	160	—	25
Clam Chowder	1 serv (6 oz)	130	—	20
ROY ROGERS				
BEVERAGES				
Orange Juice	11 fl oz	140	—	0
BREAKFAST SELECTIONS				
3 Pancakes	1 serv (4.8 oz)	280	—	15
3 Pancakes w/ 1 Sausage	1 serv (6.2 oz)	430	—	40
3 Pancakes w/ 2 Bacon	1 serv (5.3 oz)	350	—	25
Bagel Cinnamon Raisin	1 (4 oz)	300	—	0
Bagel Plain	1 (4 oz)	300	—	0
Big Country Platters w/ Bacon	1 serv (7.6 oz)	740	—	305
Big Country Platters w/ Ham	1 serv (9.4 oz)	710	—	330
Big Country Platters w/ Sausage	1 serv (9.6 oz)	920	—	340
Biscuit	1 (2.9 oz)	390	—	0
Biscuit Bacon	1 (3.1 oz)	420	—	5
Biscuit Bacon & Egg	1 (4.2 oz)	470	—	150
Biscuit Cinnamon 'N' Raisin	1 (2.8 oz)	370	—	0
Biscuit Ham & Cheese	1 (4.5 oz)	450	—	25
Biscuit Ham & Egg	1 (5.1 oz)	460	—	165
Biscuit Ham, Egg & Cheese	1 (5.6 oz)	500	—	170
Biscuit Sausage	1 (4.1 oz)	510	—	25
Biscuit Sausage & Egg	1 (5.2 oz)	560	—	170
Hashrounds	1 serv (2.8 oz)	230	—	0
Sourdough Ham, Egg & Cheese	1 (6.8 oz)	480	—	185
DESSERTS				
Strawberry Shortcake	1 serv (6.6 oz)	480	—	40
ICE CREAM				
Ice Cream Cone	1 (4.1 oz)	180	—	15
Sundae Hot Fudge	1 (6 oz)	320	—	25
Sundae Strawberry	1 (5.5 oz)	260	—	15
MAIN MENU SELECTIONS				
¼ Roaster Dark Meat	7.4 oz	490	—	225
¼ Roaster Dark Meat w/ Skin Off	4 oz	190	—	110
¼ Roaster White Meat	8.6 oz	500	—	240
¼ Roaster White Meat w/ Skin Off	4.7 oz	190	—	100
Baked Beans	1 serv (5 oz)	160	—	10
Baked Potato	1 (3.9 oz)	130	—	0
Baked Potato w/ Margarine	1 (4.4 oz)	240	—	0
Baked Potato w/ Margarine & Sour Cream	1 (5.4 oz)	300	—	15

FOOD	PORTION	CALS.	FIB.	CHOL.
Cheeseburger	1 (4.2 oz)	300	—	25
Chicken Fillet Sandwich	1 (8.3 oz)	500	—	20
Cole Slaw	1 serv (5 oz)	295	—	15
Cornbread	1 serv (2.7 oz)	310	—	30
Fisherman's Fillet	1 (6.5 oz)	490	—	15
Fried Chicken Breast	1 (5.2 oz)	370	—	75
Fried Chicken Leg	1 (2.4 oz)	170	—	45
Fried Chicken Thigh	1 (4.2 oz)	330	—	60
Fried Chicken Wing	1 (2.3 oz)	200	—	30
Fry	1 lg (6.1 oz)	430	—	0
Fry	1 reg (5 oz)	350	—	0
Gravy	1 serv (1.5 fl oz)	20	—	0
Grilled Chicken Sandwich	1 (8.3 oz)	340	—	30
Hamburger	1 (3.8 oz)	260	—	20
Mashed Potatoes	1 serv (5 oz)	92	—	0
Nuggets	6 (4 oz)	290	—	15
Nuggets	9 (6.2 oz)	460	—	25
Pizza	1 serv (4.75 oz)	282	1	14
Roast Beef Sandwich	1 (5.7 oz)	260	—	60
Sourdough Grilled Chicken	1 (10.1 oz)	500	—	45
SALADS AND SALAD BARS				
Garden Salad	1 (9.3 oz)	190	—	40
Grilled Chicken Salad	1 serv (9.8 oz)	120	—	60
Side Salad	1 (4.9 oz)	20	—	0

SHAKEY'S
PIZZA

FOOD	PORTION	CALS.	FIB.	CHOL.
Homestyle Crust Cheese	1 slice	303	—	21
Homestyle Crust Onion, Green Pepper, Black Olives, Mushrooms	1 slice	320	—	21
Homestyle Crust Pepperoni	1 slice	343	—	27
Homestyle Crust Sausage, Mushroom	1 slice	343	—	24
Homestyle Crust Sausage, Pepperoni	1 slice	374	—	24
Homestyle Crust Shakey's Special	1 slice	384	—	29
Thick Crust Cheese	1 slice	170	—	13
Thick Crust Green Pepper, Black Olives, Mushrooms	1 slice	162	—	13
Thick Crust Pepperoni	1 slice	185	—	17
Thick Crust Sausage, Mushrooms	1 slice	179	—	15
Thick Crust Sausage, Pepperoni	1 slice	177	—	19
Thick Crust Shakey's Special	1 slice	208	—	18

FOOD	PORTION	CALS.	FIB.	CHOL.
Thin Crust Cheese	1 slice	133	—	14
Thin Crust Onion, Green Pepper, Black Olives, Mushrooms	1 slice	125	—	11
Thin Crust Pepperoni	1 slice	148	—	14
Thin Crust Sausage, Mushroom	1 slice	141	—	13
Thin Crust Sausage, Pepperoni	1 slice	166	—	17
Thin Crust Shakey's Special	1 slice	171	—	16

SHONEY'S
BEVERAGES

Clear Soda	1 lg	105	0	0
Clear Soda	1 sm	52	0	0
Coffee Regular & Decaf	1 cup	8	0	0
Cola	1 sm	69	0	0
Cola	1 lg	139	0	0
Creamer	⅜ oz	14	0	0
Hot Chocolate	1 cup	110	0	154
Hot Tea	1 cup	0	0	0
Milk 2%	1 cup	121	0	18
Orange Juice	4 oz	54	0	0
Sugar	1 pkg	13	0	0

BREAKFAST SELECTIONS

100% Natural	½ cup	244	2	0
Ambrosia Salad	¼ cup	75	1	0
Apple	1	81	3	0
Apple Butter	1 tbsp	37	—	0
Apple Grape Surprise	¼ cup	19	tr	0
Apple Ring	1	15	—	0
Apple Sliced	1 slice	13	1	0
Bacon	1 strip	36	0	5
Biscuit	1	170	—	0
Blueberries	¼ cup	21	1	0
Blueberry Muffin	1	107	1	17
Bread Pudding	1 sq	305	0	80
Breakfast Ham	1 slice	26	0	14
Brunch Cake Apple	1 sq	160	0	0
Brunch Cake Banana	1 sq	152	0	0
Brunch Cake Carrot	1 sq	150	0	0
Brunch Cake Pineapple	1 sq	147	0	0
Brunch Cake Sour Cream	1 sq	160	0	0
Buttered Toast	2 slices	163	1	0
Cantaloupe Sliced	1 slice	8	tr	0
Cantaloupe Diced	½ cup	28	tr	0
Captain Crunch Berry	½ cup	73	tr	0

FOOD	PORTION	CALS.	FIB.	CHOL.
Cheese Sauce	1 ladle	26	0	0
Chocolate Pudding	¼ cup	81	0	7
Cinnamon Honey Bun	1	344	0	0
Cottage Cheese	1 tbsp	12	0	1
Cottage Fries	¼ cup	62	0	0
Country Gravy	¼ cup	82	0	1
Croissant	1	260	0	2
Donut Mini Cinnamon	1 (14 g)	56	0	0
DoughNugget	1	157	0	0
Egg Fried	1	159	0	274
Egg Scrambled	¼ cup	95	0	248
English Muffin w/ margarine	1	140	1	0
Fluff	¼ cup	16	0	0
French Toast	1 slice	69	0	0
Fruit Delight	¼ cup	54	1	0
Fruit Topping All Flavors	1 tbsp	24	tr	0
Glaced Fruit	¼ cup	51	1	0
Golden Pound Cake	1 slice	134	0	13
Grape Jelly	1 tbsp	60	0	0
Grapefruit Canned	¼ cup	24	tr	0
Grapes	25	57	1	0
Grits	¼ cup	57	1	0
Hashbrowns	¼ cup	43	0	0
Home Fries	¼ cup	53	0	0
Honey Bun	1	265	0	3
Honeydew Sliced	1 slice	13	tr	0
Jelly Packet	1	40	0	0
Jr. Bun Chocolate	1	141	0	0
Jr. Bun Honey	1	141	0	0
Jr. Bun Maple	1	141	0	0
Kiwi Sliced	1 slice	11	tr	0
Marble Cake w/ Icing	1 slice	136	0	0
Mixed Fruit	¼ cup	37	tr	0
Mushroom Topping	1 oz	25	tr	0
Oleo Whipped	1 tbsp	70	0	0
Omelette Topping	1 spoonful	23	tr	3
Orange	1 med	65	1	0
Orange Sections	1 section	7	tr	0
Oriental Salad	¼ cup	79	1	1
Pancake	1	41	0	0
Pear	1	98	4	0
Pineapple Bits	1 tbsp	9	0	0
Pineapple Fresh Sliced	1 slice	10	tr	0
Pistachio Pineapple Salad	¼ cup	98	0	3

FOOD	PORTION	CALS.	FIB.	CHOL.
Prunes	1 tbsp	19	1	0
Raisin Bran	½ cup	87	3	0
Raisin English Muffin w/ Margarine	1	158	0	0
Sausage Link	1	91	0	13
Sausage Patty	1	136	0	2
Sausage Rice	¼ cup	110	tr	8
Shortcake	1	60	0	0
Sirloin Steak Charbroiled	6 oz	357	0	99
Smoked Sausage	1	103	0	13
Snow Salad	¼ cup	72	tr	0
Strawberries	5	23	1	0
Syrup Light	1 ladle	60	0	0
Syrup Low-Cal	2.2 oz	98	0	0
Tangerine	1	37	tr	0
Trix	½ cup	54	tr	0
Waldorf Salad	¼ cup	81	1	2
Watermelon Diced	½ cup	50	tr	0
Watermelon Sliced	1 slice	9	tr	0
Whipped Topping	1 scoop	10	0	0
CHILDREN'S MENU SELECTIONS				
Jr. Burger All-American	1 serv	234	0	30
Kid's Chicken Dinner (fried)	1 serv	244	0	40
Kid's Fish N' Chips (includes fries)	1 serv	337	2	41
Kid's Fried Shrimp	1 serv	194	0	70
Kid's Spaghetti	1 serv	247	1	27
DESSERTS				
Apple Pie A·La Mode	1 slice	492	—	35
Carrot Cake	1 slice	500	0	37
Strawberry Pie	1 slice	332	2	0
Walnut Brownie A La Mode	1	576	0	35
ICE CREAM				
Hot Fudge Cake	1 slice	522	0	27
Hot Fudge Sundae	1	451	0	60
Strawberry Sundae	1	380	tr	69
MAIN MENU SELECTIONS				
All-American Burger	1	501	1	86
BBQ Sauce	1 souffle cup	41	0	0
Bacon Burger	1	591	1	86
Baked Fish	1 serv	170	0	83
Baked Fish Light	1 serv	170	0	83
Baked Ham Sandwich	1	290	2	42
Baked Potato	10 oz	264	7	0
Beef Patty Light	1 serv	289	0	82

FOOD	PORTION	CALS.	FIB.	CHOL.
Charbroiled Chicken	1 serv	239	0	85
Charbroiled Chicken Sandwich	1	451	1	90
Chicken Fillet Sandwich	1	464	1	51
Chicken Tenders	1 serv	388	0	64
Cocktail Sauce	1 souffle cup	36	0	0
Country Fried Sandwich	1	588	1	29
Country Fried Steak	1 serv	449	1	27
Fish N' Chips (includes fries)	1 serv	639	3	103
Fish N' Shrimp	1 serv	487	tr	127
Fish Sandwich	1	323	tr	21
French Fries	4 oz	252	4	0
French Fries	3 oz	189	3	0
Fried Fish Light	1 serv	297	tr	65
Grecian Bread	1 slice	80	0	0
Grilled Bacon & Cheese Sandwich	1	440	1	36
Grilled Cheese Sandwich	1	302	1	36
Half O'Pound	1 serv	435	0	123
Ham Club On Whole Wheat	1	642	10	78
Hawaiian Chicken	1 serv	262	tr	85
Italian Feast	1 serv	500	1	74
Lasagna	1 serv	297	3	26
Liver N' Onions	1 serv	411	1	529
Mushroom Swiss Burger	1	616	1	106
Old-Fashioned Burger	1	470	1	82
Onion Rings	1	52	tr	2
Patty Melt	1	640	7	171
Philly Steak Sandwich	1	673	tr	103
Reuben Sandwich	1	596	6	138
Ribeye	6 oz	605	0	141
Rice	3.5 oz	137	tr	1
Sauteed Mushrooms	3 oz	75	1	0
Sauteed Onions	2.5 oz	37	1	0
Seafood Platter	1 serv	566	tr	127
Shoney Burger	1	498	tr	79
Shrimp Bite-Size	1 serv	387	0	140
Shrimp Broiled	1 serv	93	0	182
Shrimp Charbroiled	1 serv	138	0	162
Shrimp Sampler	1 serv	412	tr	217
Shrimper's Feast	1 serv	383	tr	125
Shrimper's Feast Large	1 serv	575	tr	188
Sirloin	6 oz	357	0	99
Slim Jim Sandwich	1	484	1	57
Spaghetti	1 serv	496	2	55
Steak N' Shrimp (charbroiled shrimp)	1 serv	361	0	141

FOOD	PORTION	CALS.	FIB.	CHOL.
Steak N' Shrimp (fried shrimp)	1 serv	507	tr	150
Sweet N' Sour Sauce	1 souffle cup	58	0	0
Tartar Sauce	1 souffle cup	84	0	11
Turkey Club On Whole Wheat	1	635	10	100
SALAD DRESSINGS				
Biscayne Lo-Cal	2 tbsp	62	0	0
Blue Cheese	2 tbsp	113	0	15
Creamy Italian	2 tbsp	135	0	0
French	2 tbsp	124	0	12
Golden Italian	2 tbsp	141	0	0
Honey Mustard	2 tbsp	165	0	18
Ranch	2 tbsp	95	0	15
Rue French	2 tbsp	122	0	0
Thousand Island	2 tbsp	130	0	12
W.W. Italian	2 tbsp	10	0	0
SALADS AND SALAD BARS				
Ambrosia Salad	¼ cup	75	1	0
Apple Grape Surprise	¼ cup	19	tr	0
Apple Ring	1	15	—	0
Beet Onion Salad	¼ cup	25	1	0
Broccoli	¼ cup	4	tr	0
Broccoli Cauliflower Carrot Salad	¼ cup	53	1	1
Broccoli Cauliflower Ranch	¼ cup	65	1	9
Broccoli & Cauliflower	¼ cup	98	1	0
Carrot	¼ cup	10	1	0
Carrot Apple Salad	¼ cup	99	1	8
Cauliflower	¼ cup	8	1	0
Celery	1 tbsp	5	tr	0
Cheese Shredded	1 tbsp	21	0	2
Chocolate Pudding	¼ cup	81	0	7
Chow Mein Noodles	1 spoonful	13	tr	0
Cole Slaw	¼ cup	69	1	7
Cottage Cheese	1 tbsp	12	0	1
Croutons	1 spoonful	13	0	0
Cucumber	1 tbsp	1	tr	0
Cucumber Lite	¼ cup	12	tr	0
Don's Pasta	¼ cup	82	tr	0
Egg Diced	1 tbsp	15	0	54
Fruit Delight	¼ cup	54	1	0
Fruit Topping All Flavors	¼ cup	64	tr	0
Glaced Fruit	¼ cup	51	1	0
Granola	1 spoonful	25	—	0
Grapefruit	¼ cup	24	tr	0
Green Pepper	1 tbsp	1	tr	0

FOOD	PORTION	CALS.	FIB.	CHOL.
Italian Vegetable	¼ cup	11	1	0
Jell-O	¼ cup	40	0	0
Jell-O Fluff	¼ cup	16	0	0
Kidney Bean Salad	¼ cup	55	2	2
Lettuce	1.8 oz	7	tr	0
Macaroni Salad	¼ cup	207	tr	14
Margarine Whipped	1 tsp	23	0	0
Melba Toast	2	20	0	0
Mixed Fruit Salad	¼ cup	37	tr	0
Mixed Squash	¼ cup	49	tr	0
Mushrooms	1 tbsp	1	tr	0
Oil	1 tsp	45	0	0
Olives Black	2	10	0	0
Olives Green	2	8	0	0
Onion Sliced	1 tbsp	1	tr	0
Oriental Salad	¼ cup	79	1	1
Pea Salad	¼ cup	73	2	42
Pickle Chips	1 slice	5	0	0
Pickle Spear	1 spear	2	0	0
Pineapple Bits	1 tbsp	9	—	0
Pistachio Pineapple Salad	¼ cup	98	0	0
Prunes	1 tbsp	19	1	0
Radish	1 tbsp	1	tr	0
Raisins	1 spoonful	26	1	0
Rotelli Pasta	¼ cup	78	tr	0
Seign Salad	¼ cup	72	1	5
Snow Delight	¼ cup	72	tr	0
Spaghetti Salad	¼ cup	81	tr	0
Spinach	¼ cup	1	tr	0
Spring Pasta	¼ cup	38	1	0
Summer Salad	¼ cup	114	1	0
Sunflower Seeds	1 spoonful	40	0	0
Three Bean Salad	¼ cup	96	1	0
Trail Mix	1 spoonful	30	tr	0
Turkey Ham	1 tbsp	12	0	1
Waldorf	¼ cup	81	1	2
Wheat Bread	1 slice	71	1	0
SOUPS				
Bean	6 fl oz	63	1	4
Beef Cabbage	6 fl oz	86	2	13
Broccoli Cauliflower	6 fl oz	124	1	12
Cheese Florentine Ham	6 fl oz	110	1	11
Chicken Noodle	6 fl oz	62	—	14
Chicken Rice	6 fl oz	72	1	6

FOOD	PORTION	CALS.	FIB.	CHOL.
Clam Chowder	6 fl oz	94	0	0
Cream Of Broccoli	6 fl oz	75	tr	1
Cream Of Chicken	6 fl oz	136	tr	11
Onion	6 fl oz	29	tr	1
Potato	6 fl oz	102	2	0
Tomato Florentine	6 fl oz	63	0	0
Tomato Vegetable	6 fl oz	46	tr	0
Vegetable Beef	6 fl oz	82	tr	5

SIZZLER
DESSERTS

Chocolate & Vanilla Soft Serve	4 oz	136	0	0
Chocolate Syrup	1 oz	90	0	0
Strawberry Topping	1 oz	70	0	0
Whipped Topping	1 tbsp	12	0	0

HOT BUFFET

Broccoli Cheese Soup	1 serv (4 oz)	139	0	8
Chicken Noodle Soup	1 serv (4 oz)	31	0	7
Chicken Wings	1 oz	73	0	20
Clam Chowder	1 serv (4 oz)	118	0	6
Fettucine	2 oz	80	0	5
Focaccia Bread	2 pieces	108	0	1
Marinara Sauce	1 oz	13	0	0
Meatballs	4	157	1	30
Minestrone Soup	1 serv (4 oz)	36	2	1
Nacho Cheese Soup	1 serv (4 oz)	120	0	30
Potato Skins	2 oz	160	3	0
Refried Beans	¼ cup	62	3	5
Saltine Crackers	2	25	0	2
Spaghetti	2 oz	80	1	0
Taco Filling	2 oz	103	1	16
Taco Shells	1	50	1	0
Vegetable Sirloin Soup	1 serv (4 oz)	60	0	10

MAIN MENU SELECTIONS

Buttery Dipping Sauce	1 serv (1.5 oz)	330	0	0
Cheese Toast	1 piece	273	1	5
Cocktail Sauce	1 serv (1.5 oz)	40	0	0
Dakota Ranch Steak	1 (6 oz)	316	—	101
Dakota Ranch Steak	1 (8 oz)	421	—	135
Dakota Ranch Steak	1 (9.5 oz)	500	—	160
French Fries	1 serv (4 oz)	358	4	0
Hamburger	1	626	1	142
Hibachi Chicken Breast w/ Pineapple	5 oz	193	1	65

FOOD	PORTION	CALS.	FIB.	CHOL.
Hibachi Sauce	1 serv (1.5 oz)	57	0	0
Lemon Herb Chicken Breast	5 oz	140	0	65
Malibu Chicken Patty	1	310	0	75
Malibu Sauce	1 serv (1.5 oz)	283	0	28
Margarine Whipped	1½ tbsp	105	0	0
Potato Baked Plain	1 (4 oz)	105	2	0
Rice Pilaf	1 serv (6 oz)	256	1	0
Salmon	8 oz	110	0	41
Santa Fe Chicken Breast	5 oz	150	0	65
Shrimp Broiled	5 oz	150	0	218
Shrimp Fried	4 pieces	223	2	118
Shrimp Mini	4 oz	152	1	80
Shrimp Scampi	5 oz	143	0	150
Sour Dressing	2 tbsp	60	0	0
Swordfish	8 oz	315	0	89
Tartar Sauce	1 serv (1.5 oz)	170	0	14
SALAD DRESSINGS				
Blue Cheese	1 oz	111	0	8
Honey Mustard	1 oz	160	0	10
Italian Lite	1 oz	14	0	0
Japanese Rice Vinegar Fat Free	1 oz	10	0	0
Parmesan Italian	1 oz	100	0	0
Ranch	1 oz	120	0	10
Ranch Reduced Calorie	1 oz	90	0	10
Thousand Island	1 oz	143	0	11
SALADS AND SALAD BARS				
Alfalfa Sprouts	¼ cup	2	0	0
Avocado	½	153	3	0
Bean Sprouts	¼ cup	8	0	0
Beets	¼ cup	13	1	0
Bell Peppers	2 oz	8	1	0
Broccoli	½ cup	12	1	0
Cabbage Red	¼ cup	5	0	0
Cantaloupe	½ cup	28	1	0
Carrot & Raisin Salad	2 oz	130	1	10
Carrots	¼ cup	12	1	0
Chinese Chicken Salad	2 oz	54	1	10
Chives	1 oz	62	1	0
Cottage Cheese	2 oz	51	0	5
Cucumber	2 oz	7	1	0
Eggs	1 oz	44	0	122
Garbanzo Beans	¼ cup	63	3	0
Grapes	½ cup	29	1	0
Guacamole	1 oz	42	0	0

FOOD	PORTION	CALS.	FIB.	CHOL.
Honeydew Melon	½ cup	30	1	0
Iceberg Lettuce	1 cup	7	1	0
Jicama	2 oz	13	0	0
Kidney Beans	¼ cup	52	4	0
Kiwifruit	2 oz	35	2	0
Mediterranean Minted Fruit Salad	2 oz	29	0	0
Mexican Fiesta Salad	2 oz	54	1	0
Mushrooms	¼ cup	4	0	0
Old Fashioned Potato Salad	2 oz	84	1	6
Onions Red	2 tbsp	8	0	0
Peaches	¼ cup	34	1	0
Peas	¼ cup	31	2	0
Pineapple	½ cup	38	1	0
Real Bacon Bits	1 tbsp	27	1	0
Red Herb Potato Salad	2 oz	121	1	9
Romaine Lettuce	1 cup	9	1	0
Salsa	1 oz	7	0	0
Seafood Louis Pasta Salad	2 oz	64	1	17
Seafood Salad	2 oz	56	0	7
Spicy Jicama Salad	2 oz	16	0	0
Spinach	½ cup	6	1	0
Strawberries	½ cup	22	2	0
Teriyaki Beef Salad	2 oz	49	1	7
Tomatoes Cherry	¼ cup	12	1	0
Tuna Pasta Salad	2 oz	133	0	10
Turkey Ham	1 oz	62	0	19
Watermelon	½ cup	26	0	0
Zucchini	¼ cup	5	1	0

SKIPPER'S
BEVERAGES

Coke Classic	1 (12 fl oz)	144	—	0
Coke Diet	1 (12 fl oz)	2	—	0
Milk Lowfat	1 (12 fl oz)	181	—	0
Root Beer	1 (12 fl oz)	154	—	0
Root Beer Float	1 (12 oz)	302	—	10
Sprite	1 (12 fl oz)	142	—	0

DESSERTS

Jell-O	1 serv (2.75 oz)	55	—	0

MAIN MENU SELECTIONS

Baked Fish With Margarine & Seasoning	1 serv (4.4 oz)	147	—	85
Baked Potato	1 (6 oz)	145	—	0
Captain's Cut	1 piece (2.6 oz)	160	—	29

FOOD	PORTION	CALS.	FIB.	CHOL.
Cocktail Sauce	1 tbsp	20	—	0
Coleslaw	1 serv (5 oz)	289	—	50
Corn Muffin	1 (2 oz)	91	—	16
French Fries	1 serv (3.5 oz)	239	—	3
Green Salad (no dressing)	1 serv (4 oz)	24	—	0
Ketchup	1 tbsp	17	—	0
Margarine	1 serv (0.5 oz)	50	—	0
Shrimp Fried Cajun	1 serv (4 oz)	342	—	64
Shrimp Fried Jumbo	1 piece (0.65 oz)	51	—	9
Shrimp Fried Original	1 serv (4 oz)	266	—	54
Tartar Original	1 tbsp	65	—	4
SOUPS				
Clam Chowder	1 pint (12 fl oz)	200	—	24
Clam Chowder	1 cup (6 fl oz)	100	—	12

SONIC DRIVE-IN

FOOD	PORTION	CALS.	FIB.	CHOL.
#1 Hamburger	1 (6.6 oz)	409	—	58
#2 Hamburger	1 (6.6 oz)	323	—	50
B-L-T Sandwich	1 (6.1 oz)	327	—	9
Bacon Cheeseburger	1 (7.2 oz)	548	—	87
Chicken Sandwich Breaded	1 (7.4 oz)	455	—	42
Chili Pie	1 (3.7 oz)	327	—	28
Corn Dog	1 (3 oz)	280	—	35
Extra Long Cheese Coney	1 (8.9 oz)	635	—	65
Extra Long Cheese Coney w/ Onions	1 (9.4 oz)	640	—	65
Fish Sandwich	1 (6.1 oz)	277	—	6
French Fries	1 lg (6.7 oz)	315	—	11
French Fries	1 reg (5 oz)	233	—	8
French Fries w/ Cheese	1 lg (7.7 oz)	219	—	38
Grilled Cheese Sandwich	1 (2.8 oz)	288	—	36
Grilled Chicken Sandwich w/o Dressing	1 (6.4 oz)	215	—	4
Hickory Burger	1 (5.1 oz)	314	—	50
Jalapeno Burger Double Meat & Cheese	1 (9.1 oz)	638	—	136
Mini Burger	1 (3.5 oz)	246	—	36
Mini Cheeseburger	1 (3.9 oz)	281	—	45
Regular Cheese Coney	1 (5 oz)	358	—	40
Regular Cheese Coney w/ Onions	1 (5.3 oz)	361	—	40
Regular Hot Dog	1 (3.5 oz)	258	—	23
Steak Sandwich Breaded	1 (3.9 oz)	631	—	50
Super Sonic Burger w/ Mustard Double Meat & Cheese	1 (10.1 oz)	644	—	136

FOOD	PORTION	CALS.	FIB.	CHOL.
Super Sonic Burger w/ Mayo Double Meat & Cheese	1 (10.1 oz)	730	—	144
Tater Tots	1 serv (3 oz)	150	—	10
Tater Tots w/ Cheese	1 serv (3.6 oz)	220	—	28

STARBUCKS

FOOD	PORTION	CALS.	FIB.	CHOL.
Americano Grande	1 serv	10	—	0
Americano Short	1 serv	5	—	0
Americano Tall	1 serv	5	—	0
Cappuccino Grande Lowfat Milk	1 serv	110	—	15
Cappuccino Grande Nonfat Milk	1 serv	80	—	5
Cappuccino Grande Whole Milk	1 serv	140	—	30
Cappuccino Short Lowfat Milk	1 serv	60	—	10
Cappuccino Short Nonfat Milk	1 serv	40	—	0
Cappuccino Short Whole Milk	1 serv	70	—	15
Cappuccino Tall Lowfat Milk	1 serv	80	—	15
Cappuccino Tall Nonfat Milk	1 serv	60	—	5
Cappuccino Tall Whole Milk	1 serv	110	—	25
Cocoa w/ Whipping Cream Grande Lowfat Milk	1 serv	350	—	70
Cocoa w/ Whipping Cream Grande Nonfat Milk	1 serv	310	—	50
Cocoa w/ Whipping Cream Grande Whole Milk	1 serv	400	—	90
Cocoa w/ Whipping Cream Short Lowfat Milk	1 serv	180	—	40
Cocoa w/ Whipping Cream Short Nonfat Milk	1 serv	160	—	30
Cocoa w/ Whipping Cream Short Whole Milk	1 serv	210	—	45
Cocoa w/ Whipping Cream Tall Lowfat Milk	1 serv	270	—	55
Cocoa w/ Whipping Cream Tall Nonfat Milk	1 serv	230	—	35
Cocoa w/ Whipping Cream Tall Whole Milk	1 serv	300	—	70
Drip Coffee Grande	1 serv	10	—	0
Drip Coffee Short	1 serv	5	—	0
Drip Coffee Tall	1 serv	10	—	0
Espresso Doppio	1 serv	5	—	0
Espresso Macchiato Doppio Lowfat Milk	1 serv	15	—	0
Espresso Macchiato Doppio Nonfat Milk	1 serv	15	—	0

FOOD	PORTION	CALS.	FIB.	CHOL.
Espresso Macchiato Doppio Whole Milk	1 serv	15	—	0
Espresso Macchiato Solo Lowfat Milk	1 serv	10	—	0
Espresso Macchiato Solo Nonfat Milk	1 serv	10	—	0
Espresso Macchiato Solo Whole Milk	1 serv	15	—	0
Espresso Solo	1 serv	5	—	0
Espresso Con Panna Doppio	1 serv	45	—	15
Espresso Con Panna Solo	1 serv	40	—	15
Latte Grande Lowfat Milk	1 serv	170	—	25
Latte Grande Nonfat Milk	1 serv	130	—	5
Latte Grande Whole Milk	1 serv	220	—	45
Latte Short Lowfat Milk	1 serv	80	—	10
Latte Short Nonfat Milk	1 serv	60	—	5
Latte Short Whole Milk	1 serv	100	—	20
Latte Tall Lowfat Milk	1 serv	140	—	20
Latte Tall Nonfat Milk	1 serv	110	—	5
Latte Tall Whole Milk	1 serv	180	—	40
Latte Iced Grande Lowfat Milk	1 serv	170	—	25
Latte Iced Grande Nonfat Milk	1 serv	130	—	5
Latte Iced Grande Whole Milk	1 serv	210	—	45
Latte Iced Short Lowfat Milk	1 serv	90	—	15
Latte Iced Short Nonfat Milk	1 serv	70	—	5
Latte Iced Short Whole Milk	1 serv	120	—	25
Latte Iced Tall Lowfat Milk	1 serv	120	—	20
Latte Iced Tall Nonfat Milk	1 serv	90	—	5
Latte Iced Tall Whole Milk	1 serv	150	—	35
Mocha w/ Whipping Cream Grande Lowfat Milk	1 serv	350	—	70
Mocha w/ Whipping Cream Grande Nonfat Milk	1 serv	310	—	50
Mocha w/ Whipping Cream Grande Whole Milk	1 serv	390	—	85
Mocha w/ Whipping Cream Short Lowfat Milk	1 serv	170	—	35
Mocha w/ Whipping Cream Short Nonfat Milk	1 serv	150	—	30
Mocha w/ Whipping Cream Short Whole Milk	1 serv	180	—	45
Mocha w/ Whipping Cream Tall Lowfat Milk	1 serv	260	—	50
Mocha w/ Whipping Cream Tall Nonfat Milk	1 serv	230	—	35

FOOD	PORTION	CALS.	FIB.	CHOL.
Mocha w/ Whipping Cream Tall Whole Milk	1 serv	290	—	65
Mocha w/o Whipping Cream Grande Lowfat Milk	1 serv	230	—	20
Mocha w/o Whipping Cream Grande Nonfat Milk	1 serv	190	—	5
Mocha w/o Whipping Cream Grande Whole Milk	1 serv	260	—	40
Mocha w/o Whipping Cream Short Lowfat Milk	1 serv	120	—	15
Mocha w/o Whipping Cream Short Nonfat Milk	1 serv	100	—	5
Mocha w/o Whipping Cream Short Whole Milk	1 serv	150	—	25
Mocha w/o Whipping Cream Tall Lowfat Milk	1 serv	170	—	15
Mocha w/o Whipping Cream Tall Nonfat Milk	1 serv	140	—	5
Mocha w/o Whipping Cream Tall Whole Milk	1 serv	190	—	30
Mocha Syrup Grande	1 serv (2 oz)	80	—	0
Mocha Syrup Short	1 serv (1 oz)	40	—	0
Mocha Syrup Tall	1 serv (1.5 oz)	60	—	0
Steamed Lowfat Milk Grande	1 serv	180	—	30
Steamed Lowfat Milk Short	1 serv	90	—	15
Steamed Lowfat Milk Tall	1 serv	140	—	20
Steamed Nonfat Milk Grande	1 serv	130	—	5
Steamed Nonfat Milk Short	1 serv	60	—	5
Steamed Nonfat Milk Tall	1 serv	100	—	5
Steamed Whole Milk Grande	1 serv	230	—	50
Steamed Whole Milk Short	1 serv	110	—	25
Steamed Whole Milk Tall	1 serv	180	—	40
Whipping Cream Grande	1 serv (1.1 oz)	110	—	45
Whipping Cream Short	1 serv (0.7 oz)	70	—	25
Whipping Cream Tall	1 serv (0.8 oz)	80	—	35

STUFF'N TURKEY

FOOD	PORTION	CALS.	FIB.	CHOL.
Chef's Salad	1 serv	288	3	58
Grilled Turkey Breast	1 serv	244	5	23
Homemade Turkey Salad	1 serv	651	9	110
Real Fresh Roasted Turkey Breast	1 serv	384	8	29
Rotisserie Turkey Breast	1 serv	251	4	48
Thanksgiving Dinner On A Sandwich	1 serv	605	10	33

FOOD	PORTION	CALS.	FIB.	CHOL.
Turkey Barbecue	1 serv	478	8	48
Turkey Powerhouse	1 serv	482	10	50

SUBWAY
COOKIES

FOOD	PORTION	CALS.	FIB.	CHOL.
Chocolate Chip	1 (1.3 oz)	161	—	12
Chocolate Chip M&M	1 (1.3 oz)	162	—	12
Chocolate Chip Walnut	1 (1.3 oz)	165	—	9
Chocolate Chunk	1 (1.3 oz)	160	—	10
Double Chocolate Brazil Nut	1 (1.3 oz)	200	—	10
Oatmeal Raisin	1 (1.3 oz)	147	—	10
Peanut Butter	1 (1.3 oz)	169	—	0
Sugar	1 (1.3 oz)	178	—	27
Toffee Crunch	1 (1.3 oz)	153	—	9
White Chocolate Chip	1 (1.3 oz)	166	—	10
White Chocolate Macadamia Nut	1 (1.3 oz)	174	—	17

SALAD DRESSINGS

FOOD	PORTION	CALS.	FIB.	CHOL.
Creamy Italian	1 tbsp	65	—	4
Fat Free French	1 tbsp	15	—	0
Fat Free Italian	1 tbsp	5	—	0
Fat Free Ranch	1 tbsp	12	—	0
French	1 tbsp	65	—	0
Ranch	1 tbsp	87	—	1
Thousand Island	1 tbsp	65	—	7

SALADS AND SALAD BARS

FOOD	PORTION	CALS.	FIB.	CHOL.
Bread Bowl	1 serv	290	—	0
Roasted Chicken Breast Fillet	1 serv	143	—	49
Subway Club	1 serv	123	—	37
Subway Seafood & Crab	1 serv	238	—	34
Subway Seafood & Crab w/ Light Mayonnaise	1 serv	155	—	32
Tuna	1 serv	345	—	35
Tuna w/ Light Mayonnaise	1 serv	194	—	31
Turkey Breast	1 serv	99	—	20
Veggie Delight	1 serv	45	—	0

SUBS AND SANDWICHES

FOOD	PORTION	CALS.	FIB.	CHOL.
6-Inch Cold Classic Italian B.M.T.	1	434	—	54
6-Inch Cold Cold Cut Trio	1	347	—	56
6-Inch Cold Ham	1	273	—	24
6-Inch Cold Roast Beef	1	299	—	42
6-Inch Cold Subway Club	1	300	—	37
6-Inch Cold Subway Seafood & Crab	1	415	—	34
6-Inch Cold Subway Seafood & Crab w/ Light Mayonnaise	1	333	—	32

FOOD	PORTION	CALS.	FIB.	CHOL.
6-Inch Cold Tuna	1	522	—	35
6-Inch Cold Tuna w/ Light Mayonnaise	1	372	—	31
6-Inch Cold Turkey Breast	1	276	—	20
6-Inch Cold Turkey Breast & Ham	1	275	—	22
6-Inch Cold Veggie Delight	1	223	—	0
6-Inch Hot Meatball	1	411	—	34
6-Inch Hot Roasted Chicken Breast Fillet	1	321	—	49
6-Inch Hot Steak & Cheese	1	363	—	22
6-Inch Hot Subway Melt	1	361	—	40
Bacon	2 strips	45	—	8
Cheese	2 triangles	41	—	10
Jumbo Deli Bologna	1	446	—	57
Jumbo Deli Ham	1	259	—	36
Jumbo Deli Roast Beef	1	335	—	84
Jumbo Deli Subway Seafood & Crab	1	472	—	52
Jumbo Deli Subway Seafood & Crab w/ Light Mayonnaise	1	348	—	48
Jumbo Deli Tuna w/ Light Mayonnaise	1	406	—	47
Jumbo Deli Tuna w/ Light Mayonnaise	1	632	—	52
Jumbo Deli Turkey Breast	1	290	—	40
Junior Deli Bologna	1	270	—	19
Junior Deli Ham	1	218	—	13
Junior Deli Roast Beef	1	232	—	12
Junior Deli Subway Seafood & Crab	1	279	—	17
Junior Deli Subway Seafood & Crab w/ Light Mayonnaise	1	238	—	16
Junior Deli Tuna	1	332	—	17
Junior Deli Tuna w/ Light Mayonnaise	1	257	—	16
Junior Deli Turkey Breast	1	218	—	13
Light Mayonnaise	1 tsp	18	—	2
Mayonnaise	1 tsp	37	—	3
Mustard	2 tsp	8	—	0
Olive Oil Blend	1 tsp	45	—	0
Vinegar	1 tsp	1	—	0

TACO BELL

Bean Burrito	1 (6.9 oz)	390	8	5

FOOD	PORTION	CALS.	FIB.	CHOL.
Burrito Supreme	1 (8.7 oz)	440	5	45
Burrito Beef	1	431	2	57
Burrito Combo	1	407	3	33
Chilito	1	383	2	47
Cinnamon Twists	1 serv	171	1	0
Green Sauce	1 oz	4	tr	0
Guacamole	0.6 oz	34	5	0
Jalapeno Peppers	3.5 oz	20	tr	0
Light 7-Layer Burrito	1 (9.7 oz)	440	10	5
Light Bean Burrito	1 (6.9 oz)	330	8	5
Light Burrito Supreme	1 (8.7 oz)	350	4	25
Light Chicken Burrito	1 (6 oz)	290	2	30
Light Chicken Burrito Supreme	1 (8.7 oz)	410	2	65
Light Soft Taco	1 (3.5 oz)	180	2	25
Light Soft Taco Chicken	1 (4.2 oz)	180	1	30
Light Soft Taco Supreme	1 (4.5 oz)	200	2	25
Light Taco	1 (2.7 oz)	140	2	20
Light Taco Salad w/ Chips	1 (18.8 oz)	680	10	50
Light Taco Salad w/o Chips	1 (16.2 oz)	330	10	50
Light Taco Supreme	1 (5.6 oz)	160	2	20
MexiMelt Beef	1	266	2	38
MexiMelt Chicken	1	257	2	48
Mexican Pizza	1	575	3	52
Nacho Cheese Sauce	2 oz	103	tr	9
Nachos	1 serv	346	1	9
Nachos Bellgrande	1	649	4	36
Nachos Supreme	1	367	2	18
Pico De Gallo	1 oz	6	tr	1
Pintos 'N Cheese	1	190	2	16
Ranch Dressing	2.5 oz	236	tr	35
Red Sauce	1 oz	10	tr	0
Salsa	0.3 oz	18	4	0
Soft Taco	1 (3.5 oz)	220	2	30
Soft Taco Supreme	1 (4.5 oz)	270	2	45
Sour Cream	0.66 oz	46	tr	0
Taco	1 (2.7 oz)	180	1	30
Taco Salad	1 (18.8 oz)	860	10	80
Taco Salad w/o Shell	1	484	3	80
Taco Sauce	1 pkg	2	tr	0
Taco Sauce Hot	1 pkg	3	tr	0
Taco Supreme	1	230	1	32
Taco Supreme	1 (5.6 oz)	230	1	45
Tostada	1	243	2	16

FOOD	PORTION	CALS.	FIB.	CHOL.

TACO JOHN'S
CHILDREN'S MENU SELECTIONS

FOOD	PORTION	CALS.	FIB.	CHOL.
Kid's Meal Softshell Taco	1 serv (8.5 oz)	623	—	32
Kid's Meal Taco Burger	1 serv (8.75 oz)	668	—	35
Kid's Meal Crispy Taco	1 serv (8 oz)	575	—	31
DESSERTS				
Choco Taco	1 serv (3.5 oz)	320	—	20
Churro	1 serv (1.5 oz)	147	—	4
Flauta Apple	1 serv (2 oz)	84	—	0
Flauta Cherry	1 serv (2 oz)	143	—	0
Flauta Cream Cheese	1 serv (2 oz)	181	—	10
MAIN MENU SELECTIONS				
Bean Burrito	1 (6 oz)	294	7	10
Beans Refried	1 serv (9.25 oz)	301	—	8
Beef Burrito	1 (5.25 oz)	309	3	23
Chicken Fajita Burrito	1 (6.25 oz)	294	2	36
Chicken Fajita Salad w/o Bowl	1 serv (11 oz)	254	4	38
Chicken Fajita Salad w/o Dressing	1 serv (12.25 oz)	561	—	55
Chicken Fajita Softshell	1 (4 oz)	149	1	26
Chili Texas Style w/ 2 Saltines	1 serv (9.25 oz)	297	—	47
Chimichanga Platter	1 serv (18.5 oz)	922	—	50
Combination Burrito	1 (6 oz)	378	—	30
Crispy Tacos	1 serv (3 oz)	178	—	22
Double Enchilada Platter	1 serv (18.5 oz)	901	—	73
Mexi Rolls w/ Guacamole	1 serv (9.75 oz)	839	—	46
Mexi Rolls w/ Nacho Cheese	1 serv (9.75 oz)	813	—	46
Mexi Rolls w/ Salsa	1 serv (9.75 oz)	754	—	46
Mexi Rolls w/ Sour Cream	1 serv (9.75 oz)	854	—	46
Mexican Pizza	1 (9.75 oz)	636	—	55
Mexican Rice	1 serv (8 oz)	567	—	0
Nachos	1 serv (3.5 oz)	294	—	6
Potato Oles w/ Nacho Cheese	1 serv (7.55 oz)	523	—	6
Salad Dressing House	1 serv (2 oz)	114	—	tr
Sampler Platter	1 serv (25 oz)	1276	—	97
Sierra Chicken Fillet Sandwich	1 (8.5 oz)	500	—	41
Smothered Burrito Platter	1 serv (19 oz)	972	—	61
Softshell Taco	1 (4 oz)	165	2	16
Super Burrito	1 (8.5 oz)	424	—	45
Super Nachos	1 serv (13 oz)	848	—	50
Taco Bravo	1 (6 oz)	332	—	23
Taco Burger	1 (5 oz)	275	—	26
Taco Salad w/o Bowl	1 (11 oz)	276	4	24
Taco Salad w/o Dressing	1 (10.5 oz)	469	—	22

FOOD	PORTION	CALS.	FIB.	CHOL.
TACOTIME				
Beef	1 serv (2.5 oz)	115	—	31
Burrito Casita	1 (12 oz)	602	—	67
Burrito Casita w/o Sour Cream Dressing	1 (11 oz)	537	—	54
Burrito Crisp Bean	1 (5.25 oz)	391	—	11
Burrito Crisp Meat	1 (5.25 oz)	393	—	45
Burrito Soft Bean	1 (9 oz)	547	—	20
Burrito Soft Bean w/o Cheese	1 (8.25 oz)	462	—	0
Burrito Soft Combo	1 (9 oz)	550	—	48
Burrito Soft Combo w/o Cheese	1 (8.25 oz)	465	—	26
Burrito Soft Meat	1 (9 oz)	552	—	75
Burrito Soft Meat w/o Cheese	1 (8.25 oz)	467	—	53
Burrito Veggie	1 (11.25 oz)	535	—	20
Burrito Veggie w/o Sour Cream	1 (10.75 oz)	502	—	14
Burrito Veggie w/o Sour Cream & Cheese	1 (10.25 oz)	477	—	0
Casa Sauce	1 serv (1 oz)	40	—	0
Cheese	1 serv (0.75 oz)	85	—	22
Chicken	1 serv (3 oz)	135	—	57
Crustos	1 serv (3.5 oz)	373	—	0
Empanada Cherry	1 (4 oz)	250	—	0
Hot Sauce	1 serv (1 oz)	10	—	0
Lettuce	1 serv (0.5 oz)	2	—	0
Mexi-Fries	1 reg (4 oz)	266	—	0
Mexi-Fries	1 lg (8 oz)	532	—	0
Mexican Brown Rice	1 serv (4 oz)	160	—	0
Mexican Dressing No Fat	1 serv (2 oz)	20	—	0
Olives	1 serv (0.50 oz)	16	—	0
Ranchero Salsa	1 serv (2 oz)	18	—	0
Refritos	1 serv (7 oz)	378	—	20
Refritos w/o Cheese	1 serv (6.25 oz)	293	—	0
Sauce	1 serv (1 oz)	14	—	0
Side Salad w/o Dressing	1 serv (3.75 oz)	106	—	13
Side Salad w/o Dressing & Cheese	1 serv (3.25 oz)	51	—	0
Soft Flour Taco	1 (6.5 oz)	416	—	48
Soft Flour Taco w/o Cheese	1 (5.75 oz)	331	—	26
Soft Taco Chicken	1 (6.5 oz)	390	—	70
Soft Taco Chicken w/o Cheese	1 (6 oz)	335	—	56
Sour Cream	1 serv (1 oz)	65	—	13
Taco	1 (4 oz)	218	—	34
Taco Cheese Burger	1 (8.25 oz)	589	—	48
Taco Cheese Burger w/o Thousand Island Dresssing	1 (7.25 oz)	482	—	39

FOOD	PORTION	CALS.	FIB.	CHOL.
Taco Cheese Burger w/o Thousand Island Dresssing & Cheese	1 (6.5 oz)	397	—	17
Taco Salad	1 serv (9.25 oz)	447	—	41
Taco Salad Chicken	1 serv (11 oz)	571	—	70
Taco Salad Chicken w/o Sour Cream Dressing	1 serv (9.5 oz)	436	—	70
Taco Salad Chicken w/o Sour Cream Dressing & Cheese	1 serv (9 oz)	381	—	56
Taco Salad w/o Sour Cream Dressing	1 serv (7.75 oz)	347	—	35
Taco Salad w/o Sour Cream Dressing & Cheese	1 serv (7 oz)	262	—	13
Thousand Island Dressing	1 serv (1 oz)	107	—	9
Tomato	1 serv (0.50 oz)	3	—	0
Tostada Meat	1 serv (7.5 oz)	409	—	31
Tostada Meat w/o Cheese	1 serv (6.75 oz)	324	—	9
Tostada Delight Meat	1 (9.75 oz)	560	—	60
Tostada Delight Meat w/o Sour Cream	1 (8.75 oz)	495	—	47
Tostada Delight Meat w/o Sour Cream & Cheese	1 (8 oz)	410	—	25
Veggie Salad w/o Dressing	1 serv (8.5 oz)	357	—	14
Veggie Salad w/o Dressing & Cheese	1 serv (8 oz)	302	—	0

TCBY

FOOD	PORTION	CALS.	FIB.	CHOL.
Nonfat All Flavors	1 reg (8.2 fl oz)	226	—	<5
Nonfat All Flavors	1 kiddie (3.2 fl oz)	88	—	<5
Nonfat All Flavors	1 lg (10.5 fl oz)	289	—	<5
Nonfat All Flavors	1 giant (31.6 fl oz)	869	—	<5
Nonfat All Flavors	1 sm (5.9 fl oz)	162	—	<5
Nonfat All Flavors	1 super (15.2 fl oz)	418	—	<5
Regular All Flavors	1 lg (10.5 fl oz)	341	—	26
Regular All Flavors	1 giant (31.6 fl oz)	1027	—	79
Regular All Flavors	1 sm (5.9 fl oz)	192	—	15
Regular All Flavors	1 kiddie (3.2 fl oz)	104	—	8
Regular All Flavors	1 super (15.2 fl oz)	494	—	38
Sugar Free All Flavors	1 sm (5.9 fl oz)	118	—	<5
Sugar Free All Flavors	1 lg (10.5 fl oz)	210	—	<5
Sugar Free All Flavors	1 reg (8.2 fl oz)	164	—	<5
Sugar Free All Flavors	1 super (15.2 fl oz)	304	—	<5
Sugar Free All Flavors	1 kiddie (3.2 fl oz)	64	—	<5
Sugar Free All Flavors	1 giant (31.6 fl oz)	632	—	<5

FOOD	PORTION	CALS.	FIB.	CHOL.

TGI FRIDAY'S

FOOD	PORTION	CALS.	FIB.	CHOL.
Fresh Vegetable Medley w/ Potato	1 serv	470	—	25
Fresh Vegetable Medley w/ Rice	1 serv	407	—	<2
Friday's Gardenburger	1	445	—	13
Garden Dagwood Sandwich	1 serv	375	—	<2
Pacific Coast Chicken	1 serv	415	—	70
Pacific Coast Tuna	1 serv	410	—	70
Pea Salsa	1 serv (6.4 oz)	175	—	0
Salad & Baked Potato	1 serv	250	—	<2
Turkey Burger	1 (9.8 oz)	410	—	95

T.J. CINNAMONS

FOOD	PORTION	CALS.	FIB.	CHOL.
Doughnuts Cake	2	454	tr	98
Doughnuts Raised	2	352	tr	98
Mini-Cinn Plain	1	75	tr	3
Mini-Cinn With Icing	1	80	tr	3
Original Gourmet Cinnamon Roll Plain	1	630	1	38
Original Gourmet Cinnamon Roll With Icing	1	686	1	38
Petite Cinnamon Roll Plain	1	185	tr	11
Petite Cinnamon Roll With Icing	1	202	tr	11
Sticky Bun Cinnamon Pecan	1	607	tr	29
Sticky Bun Petite Cinnamon Pecan	1	255	tr	11
Triple Chocolate Classic Roll Plain	1	412	tr	28
Triple Chocolate Classic Roll With Icing	1	462	tr	28

TROPIGRILL

(Restaurants in this chain may also be called Pollo Tropical. Menu items are the same for both.)

FOOD	PORTION	CALS.	FIB.	CHOL.
Banana Tropical	1 serv (7.55 oz)	498	9	0
Black Beans (combo meal portion)	1 serv (4.78 oz)	153	10	0
Black Beans (side)	1 serv (8.39 oz)	269	18	0
Boiled Yuca	1 serv (12 oz)	334	5	0
Boneless Breast	1 serv (3.14 oz)	140	tr	83
Cheese Potatoes	1 serv (7.42 oz)	177	2	10
Chicken ¼ Dark Meat	1 serv (4.52 oz)	298	tr	187
Chicken ¼ Dark Meat w/o Skin	1 serv (3.42 oz)	170	tr	144
Chicken ¼ White Meat	1 serv (5.09 oz)	295	tr	170
Chicken ¼ White Meat w/o Skin	1 serv (3.82 oz)	167	tr	117
Chicken Caesar Sandwich	1 (6.4 oz)	457	tr	97
Chicken Sandwich	1 (7.92 oz)	442	tr	89
Congri	1 serv (7.08 oz)	439	7	0

FOOD	PORTION	CALS.	FIB.	CHOL.
Vegetable Kabob	1 (3.07 oz)	106	5	0
White Rice	1 serv (6.82 oz)	341	2	0
Yellow Rice	1 serv (7 oz)	294	3	0
Yucatan Fries	1 serv (5.3 oz)	440	3	0

UNO RESTAURANT

FOOD	PORTION	CALS.	FIB.	CHOL.
DeepDish Pizza	1 serv	770	6	45

VILLAGE INN

FOOD	PORTION	CALS.	FIB.	CHOL.
French Toast Cinnamon Raisin	1 serv	809	—	9
Fruit & Nut Pancakes Low Cholesterol	1 serv	936	—	2
Omelette Chicken & Cheese	1 serv	721	—	120
Omelette Fresh Veggie	1 serv	704	—	102
Omelette Mushroom & Cheese	1 serv	680	—	102
Turkey & Vegetable Scrambled Sensation	1 serv	726	—	124

WENDY'S
BEVERAGES

FOOD	PORTION	CALS.	FIB.	CHOL.
Coffee Decaffeinated Black	1 cup (6 fl oz)	0	0	0
Coffee Black	1 cup (6 fl oz)	0	0	0
Cola	1 sm (8 fl oz)	90	0	0
Diet Cola	1 sm (8 fl oz)	0	0	0
Hot Chocolate	1 cup (6 fl oz)	80	0	0
Lemon-Lime	1 sm (8 fl oz)	90	0	0
Lemonade	1 sm (8 fl oz)	90	0	0
Milk 2%	1 (8 fl oz)	110	0	15
Tea Hot	1 cup (6 fl oz)	0	0	0
Tea Iced	1 cup (6 fl oz)	0	0	0

CHILDREN'S MENU SELECTIONS

FOOD	PORTION	CALS.	FIB.	CHOL.
Kid's Meal Cheeseburger	1 (4.3 oz)	320	2	45
Kid's Meal Hamburger	1 (3.9 oz)	270	2	30

DESSERTS

FOOD	PORTION	CALS.	FIB.	CHOL.
Chocolate Chip Cookie	1 (2 oz)	270	3	15
Frosty Dairy Dessert	1 sm (12 oz)	340	3	40
Frosty Dairy Dessert	1 lg (20 fl oz)	570	5	70
Frosty Dairy Dessert	1 med (16 fl oz)	460	4	55

MAIN MENU SELECTIONS

FOOD	PORTION	CALS.	FIB.	CHOL.
¼ lb Hamburger Patty	1 (2.6 oz)	200	0	65
2 oz Hamburger Patty	1 (1.3 oz)	100	0	30
American Cheese	1 slice (0.6 oz)	70	0	15
American Cheese Jr.	1 slice (0.4 oz)	45	0	10
Bacon	1 strip (0.2 oz)	30	0	5
Baked Potato Bacon & Cheese	1 (13.3 oz)	540	7	20

FOOD	PORTION	CALS.	FIB.	CHOL.
Baked Potato Broccoli & Cheese	1 (14.4 oz)	470	9	5
Baked Potato Cheese	1 (13.4 oz)	570	7	30
Baked Potato Chili & Cheese	1 (15.4 oz)	620	9	40
Baked Potato Plain	1 (10 oz)	310	7	0
Baked Potato Sour Cream & Chives	1 (11 oz)	380	8	15
Big Bacon Classic	1 (10.1 oz)	610	3	105
Breaded Chicken Fillet	1 (3.5 oz)	230	0	55
Breaded Chicken Sandwich	1 (7.3 oz)	440	2	60
Cheddar Cheese Shredded	2 tbsp (0.6 oz)	70	0	15
Chicken Club Sandwich	1 (7.7 oz)	500	2	70
Chicken Nuggets	6 pieces (3.3 oz)	280	0	50
Chili	1 sm (8 oz)	210	5	30
Chili	1 lg (12 oz)	310	7	45
French Fries	1 med (4.6 oz)	380	5	0
French Fries	1 Biggie (5.6 oz)	460	6	0
French Fries	1 sm (3.2 oz)	260	3	0
Grilled Chicken Fillet	1 (2.5 oz)	100	0	50
Grilled Chicken Sandwich	1 (6.2 oz)	290	2	55
Honey Mustard Reduced Calorie	1 tsp (0.2 oz)	25	0	0
Jr. Bacon Cheeseburger	1 (6 oz)	410	2	60
Jr. Cheeseburger	1 (4.5 oz)	320	2	45
Jr. Cheeseburger Deluxe	1 (6.3 oz)	360	3	45
Jr. Hamburger	1 (4.1 oz)	270	2	30
Kaiser Bun	1 (2.4 oz)	190	2	0
Ketchup	1 tsp (0.2 oz)	10	0	0
Lettuce	1 leaf (0.5 oz)	0	0	0
Mayonnaise	1½ tsp (0.3 oz)	30	0	5
Mustard	½ tsp (0.2 oz)	5	0	0
Nuggets Sauce Barbeque	1 pkg (1 oz)	50	—	0
Nuggets Sauce Honey	1 pkg (0.5 oz)	45	0	0
Nuggets Sauce Sweet & Sour	1 pkg (1 oz)	45	—	0
Nuggets Sauce Sweet Mustard	1 pkg (1 oz)	50	—	0
Onion	4 rings (0.5 oz)	0	0	0
Pickles	4 slices (0.4 oz)	0	0	0
Plain Single	1 (4.7 oz)	360	2	65
Saltines	2 (0.2 oz)	25	0	0
Sandwich Bun	1 (2 oz)	160	2	0
Single With Everything	1 (7.7 oz)	420	3	70
Sour Cream	1 pkt (1 oz)	60	0	10
Whipped Margarine	1 pkg (0.5 oz)	60	0	0
SALAD DRESSINGS				
Blue Cheese	2 tbsp (1 oz)	170	0	15
French	2 tbsp (1 oz)	120	0	0

FOOD	PORTION	CALS.	FIB.	CHOL.
French Fat Free	2 tbsp (1 fl oz)	30	0	0
French Sweet Red	2 tbsp (1 oz)	130	0	0
Hidden Valley Ranch	2 tbsp (1 oz)	90	0	10
Hidden Valley Ranch Reduced Fat Reduced Calorie	2 tbsp (1 oz)	60	0	10
Italian Caesar	2 tbsp (1 fl oz)	150	0	15
Italian Caesar	2 tbsp (1 oz)	150	0	20
Italian Reduced Fat Reduced Calorie	2 tbsp (1 oz)	40	0	0
Salad Oil	1 tbsp (0.5 fl oz)	130	0	0
Thousand Island	2 tbsp (1 oz)	130	0	10
Wine Vinegar	1 tbsp (0.5 fl oz)	0	0	0
SALADS AND SALAD BARS				
Applesauce	2 tbsp (1.4 oz)	30	0	0
Bacon Bits	2 tbsp (0.5 oz)	45	0	10
Bananas & Strawberry Glaze	¼ cup (1.6 oz)	30	1	0
Broccoli	¼ cup (0.5 oz)	0	0	0
Cantaloupe	1 piece (1.6 oz)	15	0	0
Carrots	¼ cup (0.6 oz)	5	0	0
Cauliflower	¼ cup (0.6 g)	0	0	0
Caesar Side Salad	1 (3.1 oz)	110	2	10
Cheese Shredded Imitation	2 tbsp (0.6 oz)	50	0	0
Chicken Salad	2 tbsp (1.2 oz)	70	0	0
Chow Mein Noodles	¼ cup (0.2 oz)	35	0	0
Cole Slaw	2 tbsp (1.3 oz)	45	1	5
Cottage Cheese	2 tbsp (1.1 oz)	30	0	5
Croutons	2 tbsp (0.2 oz)	30	0	0
Cucumbers	2 slices (0.5 oz)	0	0	0
Deluxe Garden Salad	1 (9.5 oz)	110	4	0
Eggs Hard Cooked	2 tbsp (0.9 oz)	40	0	110
Green Peas	2 tbsp (0.7 oz)	15	1	0
Green Peppers	2 pieces (0.3 oz)	0	0	0
Grilled Chicken Salad	1 (11.9 oz)	200	4	50
Honeydew Melon Sliced	1 piece (1.8 oz)	20	0	0
Lettuce Iceberg/Romaine	1 cup (2.6 oz)	10	1	0
Mushrooms	¼ cup (0.5 oz)	0	0	0
Orange Sliced	2 slices (1.1 oz)	15	1	0
Parmesan Cheese Grated	2 tbsp (0.5 oz)	70	0	10
Pasta Salad	2 tbsp (1.2 oz)	35	1	0
Peaches Sliced	1 piece (1 oz)	15	0	0
Pepperoni Sliced	6 slices (0.2 oz)	30	0	5
Pineapple Chunks	4 pieces (1.1 oz)	20	0	0
Potato Salad	2 tbsp (1.3 oz)	80	0	5
Pudding Chocolate	¼ cup (1.8 oz)	70	0	0

FOOD	PORTION	CALS.	FIB.	CHOL.
Pudding Vanilla	¼ cup (1.8 oz)	70	0	0
Red Onions	3 rings (0.5 oz)	0	0	0
Seafood Salad	¼ cup (1.3 oz)	70	0	0
Sesame Breadstick	1 (0.1 oz)	15	0	0
Side Salad	1 (5.4 oz)	60	2	0
Soft Breadstick	1 (1.5 oz)	130	1	5
Strawberries	1 (0.9 oz)	10	1	0
Sunflower Seeds & Raisins	2 tbsp (0.5 oz)	80	1	0
Taco Salad	1 (17.9 oz)	590	10	65
Tomatoes Wedged	1 piece (0.9 oz)	5	0	0
Turkey Ham Diced	2 tbsp (0.8 oz)	50	0	25
Watermelon Wedged	1 piece (2.2 oz)	20	0	0

WHATABURGER
BAKED SELECTIONS

FOOD	PORTION	CALS.	FIB.	CHOL.
Apple Turnover	1	215	—	0
Blueberry Muffin	1	239	—	0
Buttermilk Biscuit	1	280	—	3
Cookie Chocolate Chunk	1	247	—	28
Cookie Macadamia Nut	1	269	—	34
Cookie Oatmeal Raisin	1	222	—	28
Cookie Peanut Butter	1	262	—	39
Pecan Danish	1	270	—	11

BEVERAGES

FOOD	PORTION	CALS.	FIB.	CHOL.
Coffee	1 sm	5	—	0
Coke Cherry	16 fl oz	151	—	0
Coke Classic	16 fl oz	141	—	0
Creamer	1 pkg	10	—	0
Diet Coke	16 fl oz	1	—	0
Dr Pepper	16 fl oz	138	—	0
Iced Tea	16 fl oz	3	—	0
Lemon Juice	1 pkg	1	—	0
Milk 2%	1 serv	113	—	18
Orange Juice	1 serv	77	—	0
Root Beer	16 fl oz	158	—	0
Shake Chocolate	1 (12 fl oz)	364	—	36
Shake Strawberry	1 (12 fl oz)	352	—	35
Shake Vanilla	1 (12 fl oz)	325	—	37
Sprite	16 fl oz	141	—	0
Sugar	1 pkg	15	—	0
Sweet And Low	1 pkg	4	—	0

BREAKFAST SELECTIONS

FOOD	PORTION	CALS.	FIB.	CHOL.
Biscuit With Bacon	1	359	—	15
Biscuit With Egg And Cheese	1	434	—	202

FOOD	PORTION	CALS.	FIB.	CHOL.
Biscuit With Egg, Cheese And Bacon	1	511	—	213
Biscuit With Egg, Cheese And Sausage	1	601	—	236
Biscuit With Gravy	1	479	—	20
Biscuit With Sausage	1	446	—	37
Breakfast Platter With Bacon	1 serv	695	—	389
Breakfast Platter With Sausage	1 serv	785	—	412
Breakfast On A Bun	1	455	—	232
Breakfast On A Bun Bacon	1	365	—	210
Butter	1 pkg	36	—	11
Egg Omelette Sandwich	1	288	—	198
Grape Jelly	1 pkg	38	—	0
Hash Brown	1	150	—	0
Honey	1 pkg	27	—	0
Margarine	1 pkg	25	—	0
Pancake Syrup	1 pkg	169	—	0
Pancakes	3	259	—	0
Pancakes w/ Sausage	1 serv	426	—	34
Scrambled Eggs	2 eggs	189	—	374
Strawberry Jam	1 pkg	37	—	0
MAIN MENU SELECTIONS				
Bacon	1 slice	38	—	6
Baked Potato	1	310	—	0
Baked Potato w/ Broccoli Cheese Topping	1	453	—	17
Baked Potato w/ Cheese Topping	1	510	—	22
Baked Potato w/ Mushroom Topping	1	360	—	0
Cheese Large	1 serv	89	—	22
Cheese Small	1 serv	46	—	12
Chicken Sandwich Grilled	1	442	—	66
Chicken Sandwich Grilled w/o Dressing	1	385	—	66
Club Crackers	1 pkg	31	—	0
Croutons	1 serv	29	—	0
Fajita Taco Beef	1	326	—	28
Fajita Taco Chicken	1	272	—	33
French Fries	1 junior	221	—	0
French Fries	1 reg	332	—	0
French Fries	1 lg	442	—	0
Garden Salad w/o dressing	1	56	—	0
Grilled Chicken Salad	1 serv	150	—	49
Jalapeno Pepper	1	3	—	0

FOOD	PORTION	CALS.	FIB.	CHOL.
Justaburger	1	276	—	34
Onion Rings	1 reg	329	—	0
Onion Rings	1 lg	493	—	0
Picante Sauce	1 pkg	5	—	0
Sour Cream	1 serv (2 oz)	121	—	25
Steak Sandwich	1	387	—	61
Taquito Bacon	1 serv	335	—	286
Taquito Potato	1 serv	446	—	281
Taquito Sausage	1 serv	443	—	315
Turkey Sandwich Grilled	1	439	—	46
Whataburger	1	598	—	84
Whataburger Double Meat	1	823	—	168
Whataburger Jr.	1	300	—	34
Whatacatch	1	475	—	32
Whatachick'n Deluxe	1	573	—	56
Whatachick'n Sandwich	1	501	—	40
SALAD DRESSINGS				
French	1 pkg	249	—	5
Ranch	1 pkg	364	—	5
Thousand Island	1 pkg	280	—	0
Vinaigrette Lite	1 pkg	36	—	0

WHITE CASTLE

FOOD	PORTION	CALS.	FIB.	CHOL.
Cheeseburger	2 (3.6 oz)	310	8	30
Grilled Chicken Sandwich	2 (4 oz)	250	5	20
Grilled Chicken Sandwich w/ Sauce	2 (4.8 oz)	290	5	20
Hamburger	2 (3.2 oz)	270	5	20

ZUZU

FOOD	PORTION	CALS.	FIB.	CHOL.
Bean & Cheese Burrito Platter	1 serv	475	—	15
Beans	1 cup	210	—	0
Cheese Enchilada Platter	1 serv	395	—	15
Chicken Burrito Platter	1 serv	580	—	60
Chicken Taco Platter	1 serv	440	—	70
Chicken Taco w/o Mexican Cream	1	125	—	35
Frozen Yogurt	1 serv	200	—	0
Green Salad w/o Dressing or Avocado	1	20	—	0
Grilled Chicken Salad w/o Dressing	1 serv	305	—	70
Rice	1 cup	150	—	0
Salsa Roja Epazote	¼ cup	8	—	0
Tortilla Corn	1	35	—	0
Tortilla Flour	1	60	—	0

ABOUT THE AUTHORS

ANNETTE B. NATOW, Ph.D., R.D., and JO-ANN HESLIN, M.A., R.D., are the authors of twenty-two books on nutrition. Both are former faculty members of Adelphi University and the State University of New York, Downstate Medical Center. They are editors of the *Journal of Nutrition for the Elderly*, serve as editorial board members for the *Environmental Nutrition Newsletter*, and are contributors to magazines and journals.